# Gynecological Cancers: Recent Progress in Diagnosis and Treatment

# Gynecological Cancers: Recent Progress in Diagnosis and Treatment

Edited by Isabella Dawson

hayle
medical

New York

Hayle Medical,
750 Third Avenue, 9th Floor,
New York, NY 10017, USA


Visit us on the World Wide Web at:
www.haylemedical.com

ISBN: 978-1-63241-698-8

**Cataloging-in-Publication Data**

Gynecological cancers : recent progress in diagnosis and treatment / edited by Isabella Dawson.
     p. cm.
Includes bibliographical references and index.
ISBN 978-1-63241-698-8
1. Generative organs, Female--Cancer. 2. Generative organs, Female--Cancer--Diagnosis.
3. Generative organs, Female--Cancer--Treatment. 4. Cancer in women. 5. Generative organs, Female--Tumors.
6. Gynecology. 7. Oncology. I. Dawson, Isabella.
RC280.G5 G96 2019
616.994 65--dc23

# Table of Contents

# Preface

Gynecology is the field of medicine that deals with female reproductive health pertaining to the uterus, vagina and ovaries. Gynecological cancers can occur in the ovaries, uterus, vagina, fallopian tubes, cervix and vulva. Pap test, biopsy, CT and MRI scans, etc. assist the diagnosis of such cancers. Gynecologic ultrasonography for the imaging of the pelvic organs particularly the ovaries, the uterus and the fallopian tubes is used extensively to diagnose gynecological cancers. Radical hysterectomy involving a complete removal of the cervix, upper vagina, uterus and parametrium is a common treatment strategy. Ovaries, lymph nodes and fallopian tubes are often removed in such cases. Another gynecological procedure is the vulvectomy. It involves the partial or complete removal of the vulva to manage certain cancers. An inguinofemoral lymphadenectomy may be performed in addition to a radical vulvectomy procedure if metastasis of a cancer is suspected. This book is compiled in such a manner, that it will provide in-depth knowledge about gynecological cancers. The topics covered in this extensive book deal with the core clinical aspects of such conditions. It will help the readers in keeping pace with the rapid changes in this field.

This book is a comprehensive compilation of works of different researchers from varied parts of the world. It includes valuable experiences of the researchers with the sole objective of providing the readers (learners) with a proper knowledge of the concerned field. This book will be beneficial in evoking inspiration and enhancing the knowledge of the interested readers.

In the end, I would like to extend my heartiest thanks to the authors who worked with great determination on their chapters. I also appreciate the publisher's support in the course of the book. I would also like to deeply acknowledge my family who stood by me as a source of inspiration during the project.

**Editor**

# Differentiating pelvic actinomycosis from advanced ovarian cancer: a report of two cases, management reflections

Alex Laios[1*], Iryna Terekh[1], Hooman Soleymani Majd[1], Pubudu Pathiraja[1], Sanjiv Manek[2] and Krishnayan Haldar[1]

## Abstract

Pelvic actinomycosis comprises a rare, subacute to chronic bacterial infection characterised by suppurative and granulomatous inflammation. Diagnosis is difficult as it may simulate pelvic malignancies. Laboratory and radiological findings are non-specific. We reported on 2 cases of pelvic actinomycosis mimicking ovarian malignancy with different management approaches that lead to opposite outcomes. We reviewed the literature on pelvic actinomycosis imitating ovarian cancer with a focus on its surgical management. Despite agreement on the duration of antibiotic therapy following surgical management, consensus regarding surgical approach was rather equivocal. We concluded that pelvic actinomycosis should be strongly suspected in women with presumed ovarian cancer of atypical presentation and a history of intrauterine devices (IUD).

## Background

Actinomycosis comprises a subacute to chronic bacterial infection caused by filamentous, gram-positive, nonacid-fast, anaerobic bacteria. It is characterised by contiguous, suppurative and granulomatous inflammation. Pelvic actinomycosis although rare, occurs almost only in women. It may simulate pelvic malignancies or retroperitoneal tumours [1], which often makes it difficult to diagnose. Pelvic organs can be affected leading to different clinical presentations. A high index of disease suspicion in patients with a history of intrauterine devices (IUD) can prevent unnecessary extensive surgical procedures [2]. Radiological findings are non-specific, however computed tomography (CT) appears to be the most useful imaging modality. We presented 2 case reports of pelvic actinomycosis with different management approaches that lead to opposite outcomes. We also conducted a literature review to add on the understanding of this rare disease.

## Case presentation

### Case report 1

A 57-year old, mother of two, postmenopausal caucasian woman was referred to our centre following MDT discussion for a 4-month long, persistent, progressively worsening lower abdominal pain. This was associated with mild, offensive vaginal discharge but no vaginal bleeding. She had a significant weight loss (19 kg over 1 month), loss of appetite, dysuria and constipation. Her past medical history included bipolar disorder, hypothyroidism and hypertension. She had a recent psychotic episode following discontinuation of her medication due to lithium toxicity. She had no previous abdominal or pelvic surgeries, abdominal wall trauma or immunosuppression. The patient was previously on HRT for 8 years and had a copper IUD *in situ* for the last 9 years. Her family history was unremarkable.

Physical examination demonstrated a large abdominal mass protruding through the anterior abdominal wall between the umbilicus and symphysis pubis. She was afebrile and had mild generalised abdominal tenderness but no rigidity or guarding. Pelvic examination revealed a 20-week sized gravid uterus and a fixed solid abdomino-pelvic mass with no cervical motion tenderness. Laboratory investigations demonstrated mild anaemia (Hb: 9 g/dL), raised CRP at 118 mg/l and leucocytosis (WCC 27 × 10$^3$/μl).

* Correspondence: alex.laios@obs-gyn.ox.ac.uk
[1]Gynaecologic Oncology Unit, Churchill Hospital, Oxford University Hospitals, NHS Trust, Oxford, UK
Full list of author information is available at the end of the article

A pelvic US showed bilateral complex, predominantly cystic pelvic masses, inseparable from each other. This was confirmed by CT, which additionally reported a soft anterior abdominal wall mass 60 × 25 × 60 mm situated below the umbilicus involving the right rectus abdominis muscle. A small amount of fluid in the right paracolic gutter was seen in addition to generalised peritoneal disease and sigmoid involvement. The overall picture was suggestive of malignant ovarian disease (Figure 1a-b).

CA125 was 39 U/ml, CEA and CA199 were normal. The patient was transfused preoperatively due to low haemoglobin and scheduled for an exploratory laparotomy preceded by laparoscopy. Unfortunately, due to deterioration of her symptoms, she underwent an emergency procedure. Following initial laparoscopic assessment to assess the disease operability, she underwent an en bloc pelvic resection with total abdominal hysterectomy and bilateral salpingo-ophorectomy, omentectomy, bladder peritonectomy, rectosigmoid resection with re-anastomosis and excision of an anterior abdominal wall tumour. Subsequently, she required a defunctioning stoma due to pelvic sepsis and partial closure of the abdominal defect with a prolene mesh. Further debridement was required, which was followed by a split skin graft from her right thigh. Histology revealed widespread abdominal and pelvic actinomycosis with a florid inflammatory and fibrotic response comprising of microabscesses (Figures 1c and 2). A tumour mass effect was seen (Figure 3). Active chronic inflammation in the endometrial cavity, most likely associated with the IUD was reported. She remained on IV benzylpenicillin 1.8 mg/4 h for a total of 6 weeks. She was discharged at 2 months with a low grade wound infection

secondary to foreign mesh material reaction and a rather erratic colostomy performance required supportive management. She became systemically well. Oral amoxicillin 500 mg 3 times daily was initially considered until reversal of the colostomy. At 9 months follow-up, endoscopy showed mild active proctitis and as it deemed unsafe to restore GI continuity, a revision of her end colostomy with reconstruction of abdominal wall was undertaken. The total duration of oral antibiotics was 12 months.

## Case report 2

A 37-year old, mother of two, caucasian woman was initially presented to the gastroenterology team for investigation of a 3-month long persistent, progressively worsening lower abdominal pain. This was severe in nature, predominant in the left flank, lasting for a few seconds and spontaneously resolving. It was associated with significant weight loss (15 kg over 2 months), pyrexia, night sweats, anorexia and altered bowel habits. Her medical history included asthma. She had no previous abdominal surgery, trauma or immunosuppression. She had a copper IUD *in situ* for 4 years. There was a family history of colon cancer and Crohn's disease.

On physical examination, there was no pyrexia. There was left flank and iliac fossa tenderness with no rigidity or guarding and mild left lower limb oedema. Pelvic examination revealed a tender, solid, fixed pelvic mass extending to the left pelvic side wall and the posterior sacral region. Doppler ultrasonography (US) of the left lower limb ruled out deep vein thrombosis and superficial thrombophlebitis. Laboratory investigations demonstrated

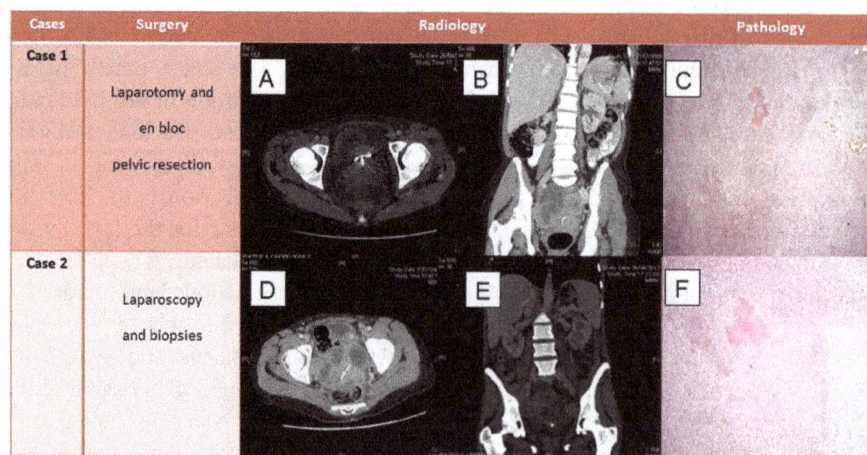

**Figure 1 Surgical procedures, imaging and pathological findings.** Case 1 - **a)** Axial preoperative abdominopelvic CT scan showing inseparable bilateral ovarian masses with coil in situ **b)** coronal view **c)** colony of Actinomyces organisms surrounded by inflammatory cells with adjacent fibrosis which had disrupted the smooth muscle of bowel wall rendering a 'mass' (H&E stain, 10×). Case 2 - **d)** preoperative abdominopelvic computed tomography (CT) scan showing right complex adnexal mass (axial) **e)** preoperative abdominopelvic CT showing presacral mass with IUD in situ (coronal) **f)** colony of Actinomyces surrounded by acute and chronic inflammatory cells. To the right of the image, there is fibrosis (H&E stain, 10×).

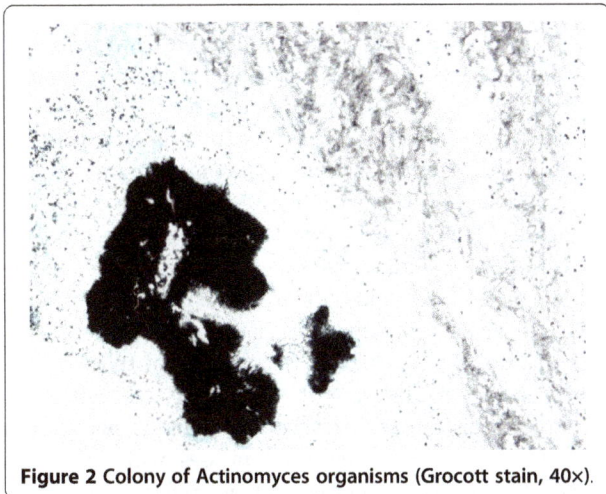

**Figure 2** Colony of Actinomyces organisms (Grocott stain, 40×).

anaemia (Hb: 7.9 g/dL), raised CRP at 133 mg/l and leucocytosis (WCC $14.3 \times 10^3/\mu l$).

Gastro-duodenoscopy revealed mild chronic gastritis and reactive gastropathy whilst colonoscopy ruled out the possibility of inflammatory bowel disease. CT thorax-abdomen-pelvis scan revealed a $75 \times 61$ mm complex right adnexal mass and a $52 \times 41$ mm heterogeneous pre-sacral mass. Multiple smaller masses were seen in the left flank, left iliac fossa and anterior pelvis, consistent with metastatic disease (Figure 1d-e). Several loops of small bowel appeared to be tethered in the pelvis and were partially obstructed. The rectum was thought to be infiltrated by the pre-sacral mass. There were bilateral hydronephroses. There was small volume of ascites with some associated peritoneal enhancement and mild left pleural effusion with no evidence of lung parenchymal metastases.

The case was discussed at the gynaecologic oncology multidisciplinary team (MDT) due to high suspicion of

advanced ovarian cancer. Tumour markers included elevated CA125 at 83 U/ml, CA199 at 51 U/ml; AFP and CEA were normal. A US-guided percutaneous biopsy of the left adnexal mass was performed as per MDT decision, which was abandoned as there was no safe path to the lesion and hence diagnostic laparoscopy and biopsies were planned instead.

At laparoscopy, there were multiple omental and large bowel adhesions to the anterior and lateral abdominal wall. The right adnexal mass was not visualised as the adjacent small bowel was obscuring the right ovary. A left pelvic side wall biopsy was taken and ascitic fluid was drained. Histology confirmed a benign peritoneal nodule showing fibrosing inflammation in association with actinomyces colonies. The latter were surrounded by acute suppurative exudate within chronic inflammation and prominent foamy macrophages (Figure 1f). The fibrous band rendered a mass effect. No dysplasia or malignancy was present. Cytology was negative for malignancy too. This was therefore a case of severe pelvic inflammatory disease secondary to actinomyces infection. The patient made an uneventful recovery. She had a negative STD work-up and the IUD was removed. However, IUD culture failed to isolate actinomyces. Blood cultures were negative for bacteraemia. She was advised against reinsertion of the IUD.

The patient was commenced on intravenous (IV) benzylpenicilline 1.8 mg 4-hourly followed by IV ceftriaxone 2 g daily for 6 weeks. She was then switched to oral amoxicillin 500 mg 3 times daily totalling 6 months. As a result, her weight increased steadily whilst her night sweats and abdominal discomfort subsided. All haematological parameters returned to normal. Abdominopelvic examination prior to discharge was unremarkable. She returned to follow-up appointments at 6 weeks and 6 months and was completely asymptomatic.

### Literature review

We searched the MEDLINE and EMBASE databases for articles published between 1988 and 2013 using medical subject heading (MeSH) terms. Key terms included "pelvic actinomycosis" and "ovar* cancer or tumour or carcinoma or neoplasm". The search was limited to the words "humans and adult female". Additional publications were identified via cross-referencing from reference lists within the retrieved publications. Only case series published in English language but with no geographical restrictions were included in the literature review.

### Results

The electronic search initially yielded 36 citations. Eleven reports were published in language other than english. There were two duplicate studies. Five studies were unrelated after screening titles; one study was a review, 3

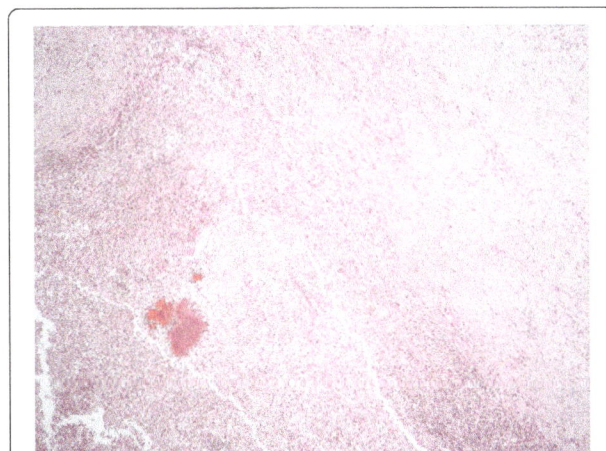

**Figure 3 Mass effect.** Another area in the exenteration sample in case 1 showing the inflammation and fibrosis which has caused a mass effect (H&E stain, 10×).

studies referred to bladder cancer, intrauterine myomas and tubo-ovarian abscesses respectively and one study was on a pediatric patient. In 2 studies, abstracts were not available and they were further excluded. A total of 16 publications were finally included in the literature review (Figure 4). The main characteristics of those case report studies with an emphasis to their management are shown in Table 1.

## Discussion

Our institution is a tertiary referral cancer centre; as large numbers of patients are referred with presumed metastatic ovarian or primary peritoneal cancer, it is important to determine the frequency and nature of diseases that mimic malignancy. In this context, pelvic actinomycosis, although difficult to diagnose by virtue of its rarity [18], should be included in the differential diagnosis of ovarian cancer, especially if atypical presentation occurs.

We reported 2 cases of women who were diagnosed with extensive pelvic actinomycosis following surgical intervention. All management decisions were MDT approved and documented in MDT proformas. Their different management demonstrates the importance of making the diagnosis in an evocative clinical context, performing the necessary investigations to confirm suspicions, favouring medical treatment and possibly reserving surgical treatment for specific situations (Figure 5).

Both patients had a long standing history of copper IUD use. Pelvic actinomycosis accompanied by IUD accounts for about 3% of all actinomycosis [19]. Although

uncommon, a long duration of IUD appears to confer the greatest risk [1]. Signs of infection such as fever, night sweats and leucocytosis also add suspicion towards an infective cause or accurately predict the severity of the condition [20]. In our cases, abdominopelvic pain associated with significant weight loss constituted the prominent symptoms. As ovarian malignancy was presumed in both cases, staging CT scans were included in the diagnostic work-up. CT findings although useful in the preoperative diagnosis were non-specific to differentiate between malignancy and actinomycocis. They are quite often, similar to those in Crohn's disease or intestinal tuberculosis. However, they might show the aggressive, infiltrative nature of the disease with disruption of tissue planes and demonstrate one or more solid masses with thickened walls [21]. The first patient was initially referred from a regional hospital for MDT discussion. In the light of suspected advanced ovarian cancer and while waiting for an elective procedure with the intention-to-treat, she deteriorated and transferred to our centre. She underwent an emergency laparoscopy proceeding to exploratory laparotomy with en bloc resection. In the absence of emergency, a more conservative surgical approach should have been pursued. Performing such an extensive operation in such an infected surgical field added to the complications encountered in the postoperative period. The learning experience from that first case was reflected on the MDT discussion of the second case, yet ovarian malignant disease was the working diagnosis. A biopsy taken at the time of a diagnostic laparoscopy confirmed actinomycosis infection [22]. Frozen section should be considered in cases

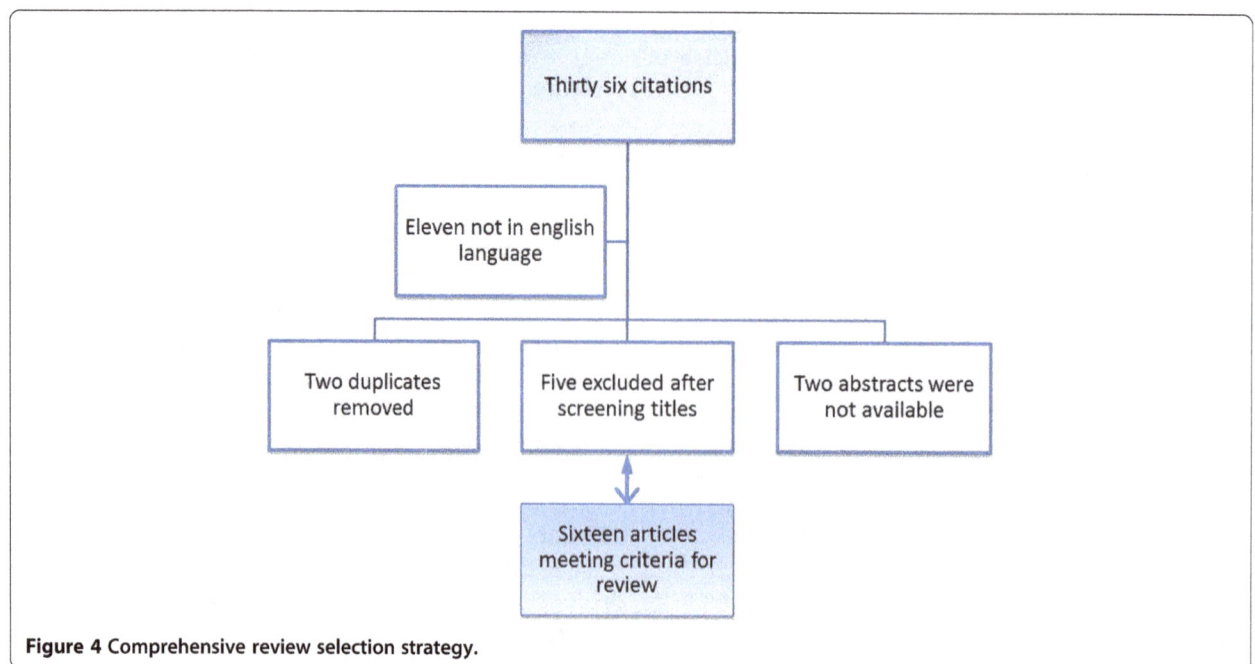

**Figure 4** Comprehensive review selection strategy.

**Table 1 Case report studies on pelvic actinomycosis mimicking advanced ovarian cancer**

| | | Case report studies on pelvic actinomycosis mimicking advanced ovarian cancer | | |
|---|---|---|---|---|
| Reference | Age (years) | Title | Duration of copper IUD (years) | Diagnosis/Management algorithm/ complications |
| Gungor T et al. [3], 2013 (n = 1) | 43 | Pelvic actinomycosis: a disease that should not be overlooked in cases with suspected ovarian cancer | 7 | Explorative laparotomy and debulking surgery |
| Kim YS et al. [4], 2012 (n = 1) | 41 | Metastatic hepatic actinomycosis masquerading as distant metastases of ovarian cancer | 15 | Hepatic actinomycosis misdiagnosed as distant metastases of ovarian cancer, exploratory laparotomy with frozen section of pelvic mass, penicillin totalling 5 months |
| Ong C et al. [5], 2012 (n = 1) | 73 | Actinomyces turicensis infection mimicking ovarian tumour | No IUD | Pelvic mass and enlarged supraclavicular LN, non-diagnostic FNA, blood cultures positive for actinomyces, penicillin totalling 7 months |
| Pusiol T et al. [2], 2011 (n = 1) | 46 | Abdomino-pelvic actinomycosis mimicking malignant neoplasm | 3 | Uncomplicated explorative laparotomy and debulking surgery but incomplete staging, penicillin totalling 6 months |
| Hwang JH et al. [6], 2010 (n = 1) | 59 | Primary serous papillary carcinoma of the peritoneum mimicking pelvic actinomycosis: a case report and brief literature review | No IUD | Pelvic CT and MRI suggestive of pelvic actinomycosis. Full staging debulking surgery confirmed primary peritoneal carcinoma followed by adjuvant chemotherapy |
| Kumar N et al. [7], 2010 (n = 1) | 32 | Pelvic actinomycosis mimicking an advanced ovarian cancer | 2 | IUD removed 4 months prior to admission, uncomplicated explorative laparotomy and debulking surgery, incomplete staging |
| Lee YK et al. [8], 2008 (n = 1) | 42 | Pelvic actinomycosis with hydronephrosis and colon stricture simulating an advanced ovarian cancer | 8 | Imaging guided needle biopsy made correct nonsurgical diagnosis, antibiotic treatment, no surgery required |
| Akhan SE et al. [9], 2008 (n = 3) | 38, 37, 51 | Pelvic actinomycosis mimicking ovarian malignancy: three cases | >7 | Debulking surgeries in all cases, complete/ incomplete staging, second case was complicated by need for colostomy and fascial necrosis |
| Kim HS et al. [10], 2007 (n = 1) | 47 | A case of pelvic actinomycosis with hepatic actinomycotic pseudotumor | 18 | FNA of hepatic tumour and explorative laparotomy of pelvis masses followed by penicillin totalling 4 months |
| Sehouli J et al. [11], 2006 (n = 1) | 35 | Actinomycotic inflammatory disease and misdiagnosis of ovarian cancer | 10 | Ureteric stenting followed by uncomplicated explorative laparotomy, patient received ampicillin and sulbactam totalling 6 weeks |
| Atay Y et al. [12], 2005 (n = 3) | 37, 45, 47 | Ovarian actinomycosis mimicking malignancy | No IUD | Explorative laparotomy and intraoperative frozen section diagnosis of actinomycosis, long-term penicillin totalling 3 months |
| Oztekin K et al. [13], 2004 (n = 1) | 49 | Pelvic actinomycosis in a postmenopausal patient with systemic lupus erythematosus mimicking ovarian malignancy; case report and review of literature | No IUD | Rare occurrence of actinomycosis with an autoimmune disease that predisposed to infections, patient had laparotomy |
| Koshiyama M et al. [14], 1999 (n = 1) | 52 | Ovarian actinomycosis complicated by diabetes mellitus simulating an advanced ovarian carcinoma | No IUD | MRI detected solid pelvic tumour mimicking advanced ovarian carcinoma invasive to bladder, rectum and uterus, patient denied initial explorative laparotomy, had neodjuvant chemotherapy followed by incomplete staging laparotomy and long-term penicillin, colostomy secondary to rec-tovaginal fistula |
| Hawnaur JM et al. [15], 1999 (n = 1) | 43 | Magnetic resonance imaging of actinomycosis presenting as pelvic malignancy | 10 | MRI confirmed regression of pelvic disease in response to antibiotic therapy |
| Kirova YM et al. [16], 1997 (n = 1) | 37 | IUD-associated pelvic actinomycosis: a rare disease mimicking advanced ovarian cancer; a case report | 4 | CT detected pelvic mass with liver metastases mimicking advanced ovarian carcinoma, exploratory laparotomy and debulking surgery, incomplete staging |
| Hoffman MS et al., [17], 1991 (n = 2) | N/A | Advanced actinomycotic pelvic inflammatory disease simulating gynecologic malignancy. A report of two cases. | Plastic IUCD, 7, 17 | Laparotomy and long-term penicillin, some resolution of the pelvic fibrosis |

| | Case 1 | | Case 2 |
|---|---|---|---|
| | 57 | Age (years) | 37 |
| | 9 | Duration of IUD use (years) | 4 |
| | Moderate | Abdominal pain | Moderate |
| | Severe | Weight loss | Severe |
| | Mild | Abnormal vaginal bleeding/discharge | None |
| | 9 | Hb (g/dl) | 7.9 |
| | No | Pyrexia | No |
| | Mild | Ascites | Mild |
| | 39 | Ca125 (U/ml) | 83 |
| | 118 | CRP (mg/l) | 133 |
| | 27 | WCC (x$10^3$/µl) | 14.3 |
| | Pelvic ultrasound, CT scan | Investigations | CT scan, endoscopy, colonoscopy |
| | 60 | Max size of pelvic mass (mm) | 75 |
| | Laparotomy and en block pelvic resection | Operative procedure | Laparoscopy and biopsies |
| | Bilateral ovarian cysts, rectosigmoid involvement, abdominal wall lesion | Surgical findings | Multiple adhesions, pelvic side wall lesion |
| | Yes | Complications | No |

**Figure 5** Differentiation between the two reported cases with pelvic actinomycosis.

of atypical adnexal masses before undertaking extensive surgery [23]. Recently, a high detection rate of actinomyces by cytology has been suggested adding on the diagnosis [24].

Several case reports of pelvic actinomycosis mimicking ovarian malignancies have been published [3,25-27] and (Table 1). Pelvic actinomycosis has been known to present as a rectal mass with hydronephrosis [28], following hysteroscopic removal of IUD [29] or incarcerated inguinal hernia [30]. In the presence of an abdominopelvic mass with suspected deposits, laparoscopy was a less invasive approach of establishing a definitive diagnosis, thereby minimising the risk for mutilating surgery. In most reports pelvic actinomycosis was diagnosed in women younger than 50 years old, who would not benefit from extensive surgery, especially as medical treatment was likely to be successful. Adjuvant debulking surgery could have taken place later if medical treatment was unsuccessful or if the patient developed complications [31]. Nonetheless, Nagler suggested that patients may not respond well to antibiotics before lesion resection, possibly due to compartmentalisation of organisms within granulation tissue [32]. Aggressive surgical management including extensive surgery –full debulking- is overwhelmingly supported in the literature [3,9,11,14,33,34] taking into consideration the extent of the disease and patient's condition (Table 1). Alternatively, incomplete staging may be offered [2,7,16,17] as an intermediate approach with lower morbidity risk while histology is pending.

According to this review, there was no consensus with respect to surgical management of actinomycosis. Agreement came only with the approximate duration of antibiotic treatment. Once diagnosis was made, high-dose and long-term use of penicillin was recommended to eradicate actinomycosis. IV benzylpenicillin was administered daily for up to 6 weeks following surgery. Oral treatment should be continued for a period of at least 6 months due to low penetration in the fibrosis and the tendency to recur [4].

## Conclusion

Despite advanced imaging and diagnostics, it is important to suspect actinomycosis in women who present with a presumed ovarian cancer and a history of IUD. This will spare patients from unnecessary, potentially extensive surgery.

**Competing interests**

The authors declare that they have no competing interests.

**Authors' contributions**

AL conceived the subject of this manuscript, performed the literature review and drafted the manuscript. IT contributed to the written material and authored the manuscript. HSM selected the CT images and contributed to the written material. SM selected and described the histological images and revised the manuscript. PP and KH critically appraised and revised the manuscript. All authors read and approved the final manuscript.

**Acknowledgements**

We are grateful to our patients who agreed on the publication of their case reports and to all participating site staff. We would like to thank Professor Ahmed Ahmed and Miss Nicola Jones for helpful discussions. We also thank Zoe Risk for administrative support and proof editing.

## Author details

[1]Gynaecologic Oncology Unit, Churchill Hospital, Oxford University Hospitals, NHS Trust, Oxford, UK. [2]Department of Cellular Pathology, Oxford University Hospitals, Oxford, UK.

## References

1. Westhoff C: IUDs and colonization or infection with Actinomyces. *Contraception* 2007, **75**:S48–S50.
2. Pusiol T, Morichetti D, Pedrazzani C, Ricci F: Abdominal-Pelvic actinomycosis mimicking malignant neoplasm. *Infect Dis Obstet Gynecol* 2011, **2011**:747059.
3. Gungor TC, Baser E, Sirvan L, Erdogan K: Pelvic actinomycosis: a disease that should not be overlooked in cases with suspected advanced ovarian cancer. *J Obstet Gynaecol* 2013, **33**:212–213.
4. Kim YS, Lee BY, Jung MH: Metastatic hepatic actinomycosis masquerading as distant metastases of ovarian cancer. *J Obstet Gynaecol Res* 2012, **38**:601–604.
5. Ong C, Barnes S, Senanayake S: Actinomyces turicensis infection mimicking ovarian tumour. *Singapore Med J* 2012, **53**(1):e9–e11.
6. Hwang JH, Song SH, Kim KA, Shin BK, Lee JK, Lee NW, Lee KW: Primary serous papillary carcinoma of the peritoneum mimicking pelvic actinomycosis: a case report and brief literature review. *Eur J Gynaecol Oncol* 2010, **31**:214–216.
7. Kumar N, Das P, Kumar D, Kriplani A, Ray R: Pelvic actinomycosis mimicking an advanced ovarian cancer. *Indian J Pathol Microbiol* 2010, **53**:164–165.
8. Lee YK, Bae JM, Park YJ, Park SY, Jung SY: Pelvic actinomycosis with hydronephrosis and colon stricture simulating an advanced ovarian cancer. *J Gynecol Oncol* 2008, **19**:154–156.
9. Akhan SE, Dogan Y, Akhan S, Iyibozkurt AC, Topuz S, Yalcin O: Pelvic actinomycosis mimicking ovarian malignancy: three cases. *Eur J Gynaecol Oncol* 2008, **29**:294–297.
10. Kim HS, Park NH, Park KA, Kang SB: A case of pelvic actinomycosis with hepatic actinomycotic pseudotumor. *Gynecol Obstet Invest* 2007, **64**(2):95–99.
11. Sehouli JSJ, Schlieper U, Kuemmel S, Henrich W, Denkert C, Dietel M, Lichtenegger W: Actinomycotic inflammatory disease and misdiagnosis of ovarian cancer. a case report. *Anticancer Res* 2006, **26**:1727–1731.
12. Atay Y, Altintas A, Tuncer I, Cennet A: Ovarian actinomycosis mimicking malignancy. *Eur J Gynaecol Oncol* 2005, **26**:663–664.
13. Oztekin K, Akerkan F, Yucebilgin MS, Kazandi M, Terek MC, Sendag F, Zekioglu O: Pelvic actinomycosis in a postmenopausal patient with systemic lupus erythematosus mimicking ovarian malignancy: case report and review of the literature. *Clin Exp Obstet Gynecol* 2004, **31**:154–157.
14. Koshiyama M, Yoshida M, Fujii H, Nanno H, Hayashi M, Tauchi K, Kaji Y: Ovarian actinomycosis complicated by diabetes mellitus simulating an advanced ovarian carcinoma. *Eur J Obstet Gynecol Reprod Biol* 1999, **87**:95–99.
15. Hawnaur JM, Reynolds K, McGettigan C: Magnetic resonance imaging of actinomycosis presenting as pelvic malignancy. *Br J Radiol* 1999, **72**:1006–1011.
16. Kirova YM, Belda-Lefrère MA, Le Bourgeois JP: Intrauterine device–associated pelvic actinomycosis: a rare disease mimicking advanced ovarian cancer. a case report. *Eur J Gynaecol Oncol* 1997, **18**:502–503.
17. Hoffman MS, Roberts WS, Solomon P, Gunasekarin S, Cavanagh D: Advanced actinomycotic pelvic inflammatory disease simulating gynecologic malignancy. a report of two cases. *J Reprod Med* 1991, **36**:543–545.
18. Bernet C, De Brabant F, Gonzalez M, Jung B, Millet O: Pelvic actinomycosis: a misleading picture. *Ann Fr Anesth Reanim* 2010, **29**(1):50–52.
19. Merki-Feld GS, Lebeda E, Hogg B, Keller PJ: The incidence of actinomyces-like organisms in Papanicolaou-stained smears of copper- and levonorgestrel-releasing intrauterine devices. *Contraception* 2000, **61**:365–368.
20. Koo YJ, Kwon YS, Shim JU, Mok JE: Predictors associated with severity of pelvic actinomycosis. *J Obstet Gynaecol Res* 2011, **37**:1792–1796.
21. Bae JH, Song R, Lee A, Park JS, Kim MR: Computed tomography for the preoperative diagnosis of pelvic actinomycosis. *J Obstet Gynaecol Res* 2011, **37**:300–304.
22. Lee YC, Min D, Holcomb K, Buhl A, DiMaio T, Abulafia O: Computed tomography guided core needle biopsy diagnosis of pelvic actinomycosis. *Gynecol Oncol* 2000, **79**:318–323.
23. Marret H, Wagner N, Ouldamer L, Jacquet A, Body G: Actinomycose pelvienne: est-ce prévisible? *Gynecol Obstet Fertil* 2010, **38**:307–312.
24. Matsuda K, Nakajima H, Khan KN, Tanigawa T, Hamaguchi D, Kitajima M, Hiraki K, Moriyama S, Masuzaki H: Preoperative diagnosis of pelvic actinomycosis by clinical cytology. *Int J Womens Health* 2012, **4**:527–533.
25. Acevedo F, Baudrand R, Letelier LM, Gaete P: Actinomycosis: a great pretender. case reports of unusual presentations and a review of the literature. *Int J Infect Dis* 2008, **12**:358–362.
26. Baltoyiannis G, Skopelitou AS, Gloustianou G, Batsis C, Kappas AM: Pelvic actinomycosis mimicking frozen pelvis: report of an unusual case. *J Obstet Gynaecol* 2000, **20**:548–549. 12.
27. Wadhwa N, Jain G, Panikar N: Actinomycotic oophoritis misdiagnosed as an ovarian tumor. *J Obstet Gynaecol Res* 2011, **37**:969–970.
28. Yilmaz M, Akbulut S, Samdanci ET, Yilmaz S: Abdominopelvic actinomycosis associated with an intrauterine device and presenting with a rectal mass and hydronephrosis: a troublesome condition for the clinician. *Int Surg* 2012, **97**:254–259.
29. Wunderink HF, Lashley EELO, van Poelgeest MIE, Gaarenstroom KN, Claas ECJ, Kuijper EJ: Pelvic actinomycosis-like disease due to propionibacterium propionicum after hysteroscopic removal of an intrauterine device. *J Clin Microbiol* 2011, **49**:466–468.
30. Dharmadhikari D, Dharmadhikari R, Macdonald J, Beukenholdt R: Intrauterine contraceptive device-related actinomycosis infection presenting as an incarcerated inguinal hernia. *J Obstet Gynaecol Res* 2007, **33**:595–597.
31. Lely RJ, van Es HW: Case 85: pelvic actinomycosis in association with an intrauterine device. *Radiology* 2005, **236**:492–494.
32. Nagler R, Peled M, Laufer D: Cervicofacial actinomycosis: a diagnostic challenge. *Oral Surg Oral Med Oral Pathol Oral Radiol Endod* 1997, **83**:652–656.
33. Simsek A, Perek A, Cakcak IE, Durgun AV: Pelvic actinomycosis presenting as a malignant pelvic mass: a case report. *J Med Case Reports* 2011, **5**:40.
34. de Feiter PW: Gastrointestinal actinomycosis: an unusual presentation with obstructive uropathy: report of a case and review of the literature. *Dis Colon Rectum* 2001, **44**:1521–1525.

# 2

# Genetic testing in a gynaecological oncology care in developing countries—knowledge, attitudes and perception of Nepalese clinicians

Hanoon P Pokharel[1*], Neville F Hacker[2,3] and Lesley Andrews[3,4]

## Abstract

**Background:** Genetic testing for an inherited susceptibility to cancer is an emerging technology in medical practice. Little information is currently available about physicians' attitudes towards these tests in developing countries.

**Methods:** We conducted an email survey of Nepalese physicians practicing in academic and non-academic settings in Nepal, regarding knowledge, attitudes and perception towards genetic testing for gynaecologic cancer.

**Results:** Responses were received from 251 of 387 practitioners (65%). Only 46% of all respondents felt prepared to answer patients' questions about genetic testing for gynaecologic cancer, despite 80% reporting that patients had asked questions about genetic testing, and 55% being asked more than 5 times in the past year. 42% reported more than 10 of their patients having had genetic testing for cancer, the majority for *BRCA1/2*. Access (40%), cost (37%) and lack of physicians' information (24%) were cited as the main barriers to testing. The most commonly identified concerns regarding genetic testing were the potential for increased patient anxiety, misinterpretation of results by patients, and maintaining confidentiality of results (64%, 47% and 38% of respondents respectively).

**Conclusion:** This study shows the gap among the health care providers in developing countries and the available modern scientific tools and skills in regard to the benefits of genetic testing for gynaecological cancers in a developing nation. These findings indicate the need for the introduction of further genetic counselling education and support into gynaecological care in Nepal.

**Keywords:** Physician survey, Genetic testing, Physician attitudes, Nepal, Hereditary gynaecological cancer

## Background

It is known that a diagnosis of ovarian, fallopian tube, peritoneal or endometrial cancer may be the first indicator of a *BRCA1* or *BRCA2* mutation or Lynch Syndrome due to germline mutations in one of the mismatch repair genes: *MLH1, MSH2, MSH6 or PMS2* [1, 2]. These syndromes account for the majority of inherited gynaecological cancers. *BRCA1/2* mutations account for 14% of all non-mucinous ovarian cancer and 22% of the high grade serous subtype [3]. Evidence of Lynch Syndrome is found in 2% of ovarian cancer cases unselected for age

[4, 5] and 9% of endometrial cancer cases under the age of 50 years [2, 6].

Identifying mutation carriers now has important implications for the management of these gynaecological cancers, as well as long term surveillance and risk reduction of other cancers. Additionally, at-risk relatives can be offered testing, and appropriate risk management if found to be mutation carriers, or reassured if not. Gynaecologists and gynaecological oncologists have a major role to play in not only identifying women at risk of inherited cancer syndromes and referring appropriate patients to genetic services, but also in managing them appropriately [7].

The issue is much more complex than just referring women for genetic testing and offering them prophylactic

---

* Correspondence: hanoon.pokharel@bpkihs.edu
[1]Department of Obstetrics & Gynaecology, B P Koirala Institute of Health Sciences, Dharan, Nepal
Full list of author information is available at the end of the article

treatment. The genetics of hereditary gynaecological cancer is continually evolving and our understanding of the molecular basis of inherited susceptibility to gynaecological cancer has improved considerably [8]. Thus, it is the responsibility of clinicians to keep up to date with advances in this area, so as to support patients to make informed decisions (Tables 1 and 2). A study from Australia revealed that doctors feel it is their duty to inform individuals at risk for hereditary cancer about the availability of genetic counselling [9]. The doctors' knowledge on the subject, however, seemed to be suboptimal. Indeed, studies have shown that a high proportion of patients do not receive adequate familial cancer risk assessment [10–12]. There has been a steady increase in the availability and application of genetic tests during the past decade [13]. In the USA genetic testing for hereditary cancer is offered by multiple private laboratories. The cost of testing is generally covered by the patient's health insurer, while in United Kingdom, hereditary cancer genetic testing is covered by the National Health Service. Cancer predisposition genetic testing is not covered by Australia's national healthcare provider, Medicare, but through the public genetic service ordering the test. Each nation has national guidelines for eligibility for funded testing, with many offering mutation searching where there is an estimated likelihood of finding a mutation of at least 10%.

Genetic testing for susceptibility for gynaecological cancers is widely available in western countries, whereas in developing countries it is still in a rudimentary level.

In Nepal National Academy of Medical Sciences, Bir Hospital is in the process of establishing a genetic laboratory. Currently, Nepalese patients are referred to India for genetic testing, where the current cost of BRCA1/2 testing is approximately US$1400.

The hereditary cancer burden in Nepal is unknown, however a recent study of 50 women with breast cancer diagnosed in Kathmandu found the prevalence of a single mutation (BRCA1 185delAG) to be 8%, which is considerably higher than in unselected breast cancer cases in a western population [14], suggesting that hereditary cancer may be just as common, if not more so, than in other populations. Compared with the western developed countries, genetic testing and risk assessment for familial cancer in Asia has been shown to be less available, thus prohibiting the appropriate surveillance, clinical strategies and cancer management of patients and their relatives [15].

Nepal has a population of 27.8 million, and a land area of 147,181 km$^2$. The size of the country, relative inaccessibility of mountainous regions and the demographic factors all contribute to difficulties in providing accurate cancer statistics. No population based cancer registry program exists to assess the incidence, prevalence, morbidity and mortality of cancer. The importance of cancer registry data for development of national cancer control programs has been stressed in the context of South Asia [16]. Pooling the cases presented in the main urban centres has been used as a surrogate for

**Table 1** Risk management for an Unaffected Female BRCA1/2 Mutation Carrier

| Cancer type | Recommendation | |
| --- | --- | --- |
| Breast | Surgical | • offer bilateral risk-reducing mastectomy followed by self-surveillance of breast area. The greatest benefit is predicted when surgery occurs at age ≤40 years |
| | | • alternatively in the absence of bilateral risk-reducing mastectomy, recommend RRSO preferably around age 40 years |
| | Surveillance | • in families with breast cancer diagnosed under age 35 years, individualised screening recommendations may apply |
| | | • otherwise screening should start at age 30 years |
| | | • 30–50 years – annual MRI + MMG (+/– US) |
| | | • >50 years – annual MMG +/– US |
| | | • pregnant - no MRI or MMG, consider US |
| | Risk-reducing medication | • careful assessment of risks and benefits in the individual case by an experienced medical professional is required when considering the use of medication, such as tamoxifen or raloxifene to reduce risk of developing breast cancer in unaffected women. See Cancer Australia Risk-reducing medication resource |
| Ovarian/fallopian tube | Surgical | • recommend RRBSO after family completion or around age 40 years[3] with peritoneal lavage and close histological examination to exclude occult malignancy |
| | Surveillance | • do not offer serum CA125 and/or transvaginal ultrasound (TVU) |
| Pancreatic | | • no evidence of benefit from surveillance |

https://www.eviq.org.au Risk Management for an unaffected Female BRCA1 Mutation Carrier
https://www.eviq.org.au Risk Management for an unaffected Female BRCA2 Mutation Carrier
Abbreviations: RRSO: Risk-reducing salpingo-oophorectomy, RRBSO: Risk-reducing bilateral salpingo-oophorectomy, US: ultrasound, MMG: mammogram (digital if available), MRI: magnetic resonance imaging

**Table 2** Lynch Syndrome risk management guidelines. All patients should be entered on a local hereditary cancer registry for information and surveillance reminders

| Cancer type | Recommendations | |
|---|---|---|
| Colorectal | Surgical | • consider subtotal colectomy in selected individuals |
| | Surveillance MSH6/PMS2 | • annual colonoscopy from age 30 years or 5 years younger than youngest affected if <35 years |
| | | • review frequency of colonoscopy at age 60 years with a view to reduced frequency |
| | Surveillance MLH1/MSH2 | • annual colonoscopy from age 25 years or 5 years younger than youngest affected if <30 years |
| | | • review frequency of colonoscopy at age 60 years with a view to 2nd yearly frequency |
| | Risk-reducing medication | • there may be a reduction of risk in taking aspirin however the appropriate dose is not yet defined (preliminary data) |
| Endometrial | Surgical | • recommend hysterectomy after childbearing complete or from age 40 years, or 5 years younger than the youngest affected, whichever comes first |
| | Surveillance | • there is no evidence for transvaginal ultrasound (TVU) and/or aspiration biopsy |
| Ovarian | Surgical | • recommend risk reducing salpingo-oophorectomy (RRSO) at time of hysterectomy |
| | | • recommend HRT at the time of RRSO and continue until the usual time of menopause |
| | Surveillance | • do not offer serum CA125 and/or transvaginal ultrasound (TVU). See Cancer Australia for further information |
| Gastric | Surveillance | • consider second yearly gastroscopy from age 30 years in families with gastric cancer or those at high ethnic risk - e.g. Chinese, Korean, Chilean and Japanese |
| Urothelial | Surveillance | • no evidence of benefit but patients encouraged to report symptoms e.g. haematuria |

https://www.eviq.org.au Risk Management for Lynch Syndrome

a central cancer registry; however these figures are likely to be an underestimate of incidence, as many of the patients go to India or abroad for their further treatment.

A hospital based cancer registry (HBCR) program was started from 1997 in 3 cancer diagnosing and treating hospitals in Kathmandu. Since 2003, with the support of WHO-Nepal, the HBCR program has expanded to cover seven major cancer diagnosis and treatment hospitals in Nepal, which are cooperating to provide relevant data coordinated by the BP Koirala Memorial Cancer Hospital. An initial assessment of incidence at 4 major hospitals found that of 2340 cancers in females overall in 2004, the most common site was cervix uteri (21%), followed by breast (16%), lung (11%) and ovary (6%). However breast and ovarian were the most common cancers amongst women aged 15–34 [17]. This high incidence at young ages raises the possibility of an inherited basis for some of these cancers. In 2012, almost 4000 female cancer cases were registered amongst 7 hospitals, with the most prevalent age group being 50–54 years (12.8%). There was a decrease in cervical and lung cancers, but an increase in breast cancers [18].

There is currently no specialised hereditary cancer service. The level of knowledge of hereditary cancer amongst practitioners seeing women with gynaecological cancer in Nepal is unknown. It is also unknown if these practitioners are currently referring women for genetic testing, and if so, to where. The present study is the first of its kind to be conducted among the Nepalese

practitioners regarding the awareness and knowledge about genetic testing of patients with gynaecological malignancy diagnosis.

**Method**

A self-administered 15 min survey consisting of 23 questions was designed after a focus group discussion among doctors working at the B.P. Koirala Institute of Health Sciences (BPKIHS) and a literature search of similar topics (Additional file 1). The questionnaire included demographic characteristics, physician practice parameters of speciality, patients seen per week, years of practice and practice setting.

Questionnaires were emailed to 387 general practitioners and specialists of government and private hospitals in Nepal. Their fields included Gynaecologic Oncology, General Gynaecology, Internal Medicine, Family Medicine, Community Medicine/Public health and Primary Care. Practitioners were identified through the Nepal Society of Obstetricians and Gynaecologists and the faculties of the B.P. Koirala Institute of Health Sciences (BPKIHS).

The questionnaire was sent with a cover letter explaining the aims of the study and reassuring the respondents that their responses would be de-identified. Two reminder emails were sent to non-responders at two-week intervals. The email also gave the option of requesting another questionnaire if the original one had been misplaced/discarded.

Doctors' consent to participate was inferred by completion and return of the questionnaire.

The study was approved by the UNSW Human Research Ethics Advisory (HREA) Panel, University of New South Wales, Sydney, Project number-HC16248.

## Results

Responses were received from 251 of 387 practitioners (65%) – 118 gynaecologists (47%), 36 gynaecological oncologists (14%) and 97 clinicians from other fields (39%). There was a trend for gynaecologists to be older (36% aged over 50, vs 17% both of gynaecological oncologists and other clinicians) and more likely to be female (72% vs 33% of gynaecological oncologists and 47% of other clinicians), but differences did not reach significance.

Overall, half of the respondents saw less than 3 patients per week regarding gynaecological cancer (which included 30% of non-gynaecologists who reported seeing none). No respondent reported seeing more than 10 gynaecological cancer patients per week, with 64% of gynaecological oncologists, 90% of gynaecologists and all clinicians from other fields seeing less than 6 patients per week regarding gynaecological cancer (Fig. 1).

Approximately half of all respondents felt prepared to answer patient's questions about genetic testing for gynaecologic cancer (46%). However, while 94% of gynaecologic oncologists felt prepared, only 47% of gynaecologists and 26% of other clinicians did so, despite 86% of gynaecologists and 71% of other clinicians reporting that patients had asked questions about genetic testing. Non-gynaecologic clinicians had lower requests for information with a third reporting never being asked, and half being asked on less than 5 occasions in the past year. Gynaecologists and gynaecological-oncologists had similar requests with around 58% of each group reporting less than 5 requests in the past year and 39% and 36% respectively being asked on 6–10 occasions.

All groups demonstrated a bimodal distribution of the number of patients having had genetic testing for cancer

predisposition, with overall 40% reporting less than 6 patients having had testing and 42% reporting more than 10 of their patients having had genetic testing for cancer. The majority of tests were for *BRCA1/2* (70%), with 10% for mismatch repair *genes* (Lynch Syndrome) and 22% reporting other genetic tests. 27% of respondents reported that the results never influenced management, 45% said that they did sometimes and 27% said most of the time.

Access (40%), cost (37%) and lack of physicians' information (24%) were cited as the main barriers to testing. When asked about how genetic test results influenced their patients' care, preventive surgery was the most cited option (47%) followed by screening (33%), lifestyle changes (31%) and medication (14%). The vast majority of respondents thought that genetic testing was clinically useful. Of the 23 respondents who did not think genetic testing was clinically useful, the majority ($n = 17$) were non gynaecological clinicians. They cited difficulties in interpreting results, failure to affect patient care and patient anxiety as the main reasons. Amongst all respondents, the most commonly identified concerns regarding genetic testing were the potential for increased patient anxiety, misinterpretation of results by patients, and maintaining confidentiality of results (64%, 47% and 38% of respondents respectively). Approximately one quarter of all respondents noted concerns regarding the provision of post-test counselling, the potential for discrimination, the clinical utility of results, and the accuracy of results. However, 91% of all respondents said that if a patient brought genetic test results, it would be likely or very likely to influence their care.

## Discussion

This is the first analysis of Nepalese clinicians regarding genetic testing for gynaecological cancer. Similar to Baars MJ et al. [19] who surveyed Dutch medical practitioners regarding genetic testing in 2005, we had a pleasing response rate of 65%. Our findings should however be viewed in light of several limitations. We have no criteria to estimate if decliners would answer differently to our respondents. The replies are self-reported with no objective measures, and sub group analysis was limited by the sample size.

Our cohort reported low preparedness to answer patients' questions about genetic testing for gynaecological cancer, particularly from non-gynaecologists. Remaining respondents were primary care physicians (39%), which is consistent with a study conducted by Keating NL et al., [20] where it was emphasized that wider participation by community-based physicians successfully incorporated genetic testing into practice. The trend is seen that with their involvement, chances of early detection care and referral will increase. This will ultimately

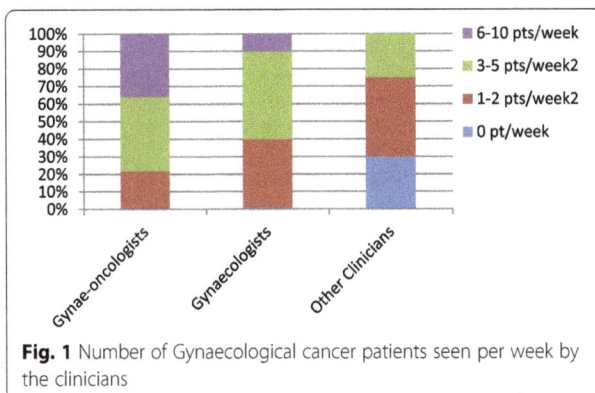

**Fig. 1** Number of Gynaecological cancer patients seen per week by the clinicians

facilitate and increase the promotion of genetic testing facilities, and expand Gynaecologists' role in counselling and testing.

Self-reported utilisation of genetic information was high. This cohort has experienced the need for better clinicians' education and confidence to discuss results. A number of the issues concerning patient anxiety and confidentiality may be improved by more extensive use of genetic counsellors in the testing process. Western models of care include genetic counsellors as a source of assessment and care of patients suitable for genetic assessment, and our findings that less than half of gynaecologists and a quarter of other clinicians feel prepared to answer questions about genetic testing for hereditary cancer, indicate that there is a need for genetic professionals to assist clinicians in Nepal. The limited access to genetic counsellors is unlikely to change with no tertiary institution in Nepal currently offering this course.

Access and cost of genetic testing may not be such significant barriers with the establishment of the planned genetic service in Nepal. Additionally, the ongoing reduction in the cost of testing panels of multiple genes through next generation sequencing, combined with the ease of saliva and cheek swab testing, is anticipated to facilitate Nepalese doctors ordering testing for hereditary cancers in the future.

Our survey of the Royal Hospital for Women in Sydney [21], found that 23% of all gynaecological cancer patients warranted a genetic assessment. At this hospital, a Hereditary Cancer expert attends all Tumour Board meetings and this allows optimal identification of patients requiring genetic assessment.

Almost half of the respondents cited possible misinterpretation of results by patients as a concern, further highlighting a need for genetic counselling expertise.

Until there are data on the prevalence of hereditary gynaecological cancer in Nepal, estimates of the need for improved genetic care need to be based on outside data. A comparison of the BPKMCH 2010–2012 annual report compared with a recent audit of cases from Sydney [21], indicates there are approximately twice as many gynaecological cancer patients seen at BPKMCH compared with the Royal Hospital for Women. If the mutation prevalence is similar to that of Australia, 20 women diagnosed with gynaecological cancer in BPKMCH each year would be found to carry either a *BRCA1/2* or MMR mutation, providing the opportunity for improved care for themselves and their relatives.

We did not enquire about frequency of patients reporting a family history of relevant cancers, as participant recall may not have been robust. A future prospective audit of consultations from a similar cohort would provide further data to assess the need for hereditary cancer services in Nepal.

In Nepal women diagnosed with gynaecological cancer are treated by general gynaecologists and the women who are referred to Nepal Cancer Hospital and Research centre, Bhaktapur Cancer Hospital and B.P. Koirala Memorial Cancer Hospital are treated by Gynaecologists with additional expertise in Gynaeoncology. There are very few specialist gynaecological Oncologists in Nepal.

## Conclusion

This survey highlights clinicians' concerns about genetic testing for hereditary gynaecological cancer in Nepal, and provides a basis for consideration of measures to improve knowledge and consideration of testing for affected Nepalese women and their families.

### Acknowledgements

We are grateful to all the Nepalese Practitioners and Specialists who participated in the study by giving their valuable time. Special gratitude goes to Dr Shyam Sundar Budhathoki, Assistant Professor, School of Public Health and Community Medicine, BPKIHS, Nepal, for his generous contribution in doing statistical analysis.

### Funding

No funding was received.

### Authors' contributions

Conception and design: HPP, NFH, LA. Collection and assembly of data: HPP, LA. Data analysis and interpretation: HPP, LA. Manuscript writing: HPP, NFH, LA. Final approval of manuscript: HPP, NFH, LA. All authors agree to be accountable for all aspects of the work related to the integrity of the work.

### Competing interests

The authors declare that they have no competing interests.

### Author details

[1]Department of Obstetrics & Gynaecology, B P Koirala Institute of Health Sciences, Dharan, Nepal. [2]Royal Hospital for Women, Randwick, Australia. [3]School of Women's and Children's Health, University of New South Wales, Sydney, Australia. [4]Prince of Wales Hospital, Randwick, Australia.

### References

1. Lu KH, Schorge JO, Rodabaugh KJ, Daniels MS, Sun CC, Soliman PT, et al. Prospective determination of prevalence of Lynch syndrome in young women with endometrial cancer. J Clin Oncol. 2007;25:5158–64.
2. Kulkarni A, Brady AF. Management of Women with a Gentic Predisposition to Gynaecological Cancers. Royal College of Obstetrics & Gynaecologists. Scientific Impact paper. 2015;48:2–9.
3. Alsop K, Fereday S, Meldrum C, DeFazio A, Emmanuel C, George J, et al. BRCA mutation frequency and patterns of treatment response in BRCA mutation-positive Women with ovarian cancer. A report from the Australian ovarian cancer study group. J Clin Oncol. 2012;30(21):2654–63.
4. Rubin SC, Blackwood MA, Bandera C, Behbakht K, Benjamin I, Rebbeck TR. BRCA1, BRCA2, and hereditary nonpolyposis colorectal cancer gene mutations is an unselected ovarian cancer population: Relationship to family history and implications for genetic testing. Am J Obstet Gynecol. 1998;178:670–7.
5. Malander S, Rambech E, Kristoffersson U, Halvarsson B, Ridderheim M, Borg

A, et al. The contribution of the hereditary nonpolyposis colorectal cancer syndrome to the development of ovarian cancer. Gynecol Oncol. 2006;101: 238–43.

6. Berends MJ, Wu Y, Sijmons RH, Van der Sluis T, EK WB, Ligtenberg MJ. Towards new strategies to select young endometrial cancer patients for mismatch repair gene mutation analysis. J Clin Oncol. 2003;21:4364–70.

7. Brown K, Bunting M. Genetics and gynaecological cancer. Genetics. 2016; 18(2):43–5.

8. Beirne J, Irwin G, McIntosh SA, Harley IJG, Harkin DP. The molecular and genetic basis of inherited cancer risk in gynaecology. Obstet Gynaecol. 2015;17:233–41.

9. Teng I, Spigelman A. Attitudes and knowledge of medical practitioners to hereditary cancer clinics and cancer genetic testing. Familial Cancer. 2014; 13(2):311–24.

10. Murff HJ, Byrne D, Syngal S. Cancer risk assessment: quality and impact of the family history interview. Am J Prev Med. 2004;27(3):239–45.

11. Meyer LA, Anderson ME, Lacour RA, Suri A, Daniels MS, Urbauer DL, et al. Evaluating women with ovarian cancer for BRCA1 and BRCA2 mutations: missed opportunities. Obstet Gynecol. 2010;115(5):945–52.

12. Lanceley A, Eagle Z, Ogden G, Gessler S, Razvi K, Ledermann JA, et al. Family history and women with ovarian cancer: is it asked and does it matter? An observational study. Int J Gynecol Cancer. 2012;22(2):254–9.

13. Bellcross CA, Kolor K, Goddard KA, Coates RJ, Reyes M, Muin J, et al. Awareness and utilization of BRCA1/2 testing among U.S. primary care physicians. Am J Prev Med. 2011;40(1):61–6.

14. Bhatta B, Thapa R, Shahi S, Bhatta Y, Pandeya DR, Paudel BH. A Pilot Study on Screening of BRCA1 Mutations (185delAG, 1294del40) in Nepalese Breast Cancer Patients. Asian Pac J Cancer Prev. 2016;17(4):1829–32.

15. Nakamura S, Kwong A, Kim SW, Patmasiriwat PLP, Dofitas R, Aryandono T, et al. Current Status of the management of Hereditary Breast and Ovarian Cancer in Asia: First Report by the Asian BRCA Consortium. Public health genomics. 2016;19(1):53–60.

16. Bhurgri Y. Karachi cancer registry data - implications for the national cancer control program of Pakistan. Asian Pac J Cancer Prev. 2004;5(1):77–82.

17. Pradhananga KK, Baral M, Shrestha BM. Multi-institution hospital-based cancer incidence data for Nepal: an initial report. Asian Pac J Cancer Prev. 2009;10(2):259–62.

18. Pun CB, Pradhananga KK, Siwakoti B, Subedi K, Moore AM. Malignant Neoplasm Burden in Nepal - Data from the Seven Major Cancer Service Hospitals for 2012. Asian Pac J Cancer Prev. 2015;16(18):8659–63.

19. Baars MJ, Henneman L, Ten Kate LP. Deficiency of knowledge of genetics and genetic tests among general practitioners, gynecologists, and pediatricians: a global problem. Genet Med. 2005;7(9):605–10.

20. Keating NL, Stoeckert KA, Regan MM, DiGianni L, Garber JE. Physicians' Experience with BRCA1/2 Testing in Community Settings. J Clin Oncol. 2008; 26(35):5789–95.

21. Pokharel HP, Hacker NF, Andrews L, et al. Changing patterns of referrals and outcomes of genetic participation in gynaecological-oncology multidisciplinary care. Aust N Z J Obstet Gynaecol. 2016. Accepted 17 Aug 2016. doi:10.1111/ajo.12504.

# 3

# Immunotherapy in endometrial cancer - an evolving therapeutic paradigm

Teresa C. Longoria and Ramez N. Eskander[*]

## Abstract

Endometrial cancer is the only gynecologic malignancy with a rising incidence and mortality. While cure is routinely achieved with surgery alone or in combination with adjuvant pelvic radiotherapy when disease is confined to the uterus, patients with metastatic or recurrent disease exhibit limited response rates to cytotoxic chemotherapy, targeted agents, or hormonal therapy. Given the unmet clinical need in this patient population, exploration of novel therapeutic approaches is warranted, and attention is turning to immunomodulation of the tumor microenvironment. Existing evidence suggests that endometrial cancer is sufficiently immunogenic to be a reasonable candidate for active and/or passive immunotherapy. In this review, we critically examine what is known about the microenvironment in endometrial cancer and what has been learned from preliminary immunotherapy trials that enrolled endometrial cancer patients, encouraging further attempts at immunomodulation in the treatment of aggressive forms of this disease.

**Keywords:** Adoptive cellular therapy, Bispecific T-cell engager antibodies, Endometrial cancer, Immune checkpoint inhibitors, Therapeutic vaccination, Tumor microenvironment

## Background

As the most common cancer of the female genital tract, it is estimated that in 2015 endometrial cancer will be diagnosed in over 54,000 women and will be responsible for over 10,000 deaths in the United States [1]. At the time of diagnosis, 67 % of women have disease confined to the uterus and an associated 5-year survival rate of 95 % [1]. In contrast, the 8 % of patients with distant metastases at the time of diagnosis have a 5-year survival rate of 17 % [1] and face the prospect of cytotoxic chemotherapy (primarily with taxanes, anthracyclines, and platinum drugs) with limited response.

Since the completion of Gynecologic Oncology Group (GOG) protocol 177, which explored the triplet regimen of paclitaxel, doxorubicin and cisplatin (TAP) in patients with advanced stage and recurrent endometrial cancer, demonstrating an overall response rate of 57 % and median overall survival of 15.3 months, results have been clinically disappointing. Furthermore, the toxicity associated with the 3-drug regimen has limited its clinical utility [2]. The GOG, in the 229 queue, has evaluated a

series of targeted agents [3–9] including bevacizumab (229E), aflibercept (229 F), bevacizumab/temsirolimus (229G), AZD6244 (229H), brivanib (229I), cediranib (229 J), AMG386 (229 L) and BIBF 1120 (229 K) with modest overall response rates, ranging from 0 % - 24.5 % (Table 1). Hormonal therapy is better tolerated but results in response rates between 18 % and 34 % [10]. With taxanes alone showing response rates of greater than 20 % in select patients (taxane-naïve) with recurrent disease [11, 12], effective second-line chemotherapeutic options are limited. Given the above unmet clinical need, exploration of novel therapeutic approaches is warranted in this patient population.

Within cancer drug development, a shift in focus from the tumor cell itself to the tumor microenvironment (TME) has been gradually gaining momentum. This shift has come with the recognition of the limitations of targeted therapy, which act by blocking essential biochemical pathways or mutant proteins that are required for tumor cell growth and survival. The ideal use of targeted therapies is in cancers with a single dominant driver mutation and a small mutational load, the classic example being chronic myeloid leukemia (CML) bearing the Philadelphia chromosome (bcr-abl gene translation)

---
* Correspondence: eskander@uci.edu
University of California, Irvine Medical Center, 101 The City Drive South, Bldg 56, Ste 800, Orange, CA 92868, USA

**Table 1** Clinical end points in the GOG 229 queue

| GOG Trial | N | ORR | PFS > 6mo | Median PFS (mo.) | Median OS (mo.) |
| --- | --- | --- | --- | --- | --- |
| 229 N [7] | 28 | 0 % | 11 % | 2.1 | 9.4 |
| 229 K [6] | 37 | 9.4 % | 22 % | 3.3 | 10.1 |
| 229 I [8] | 45 | 18.6 % | 30 % | 3.3 | 10.7 |
| 229 G* [5] | 53 | 24.5 % | 47 % | 5.6 | 16.9 |
| 229 F* [4] | 49 | 8.9 % | 40 % | 2.9 | 14.6 |
| 229 E [3] | 56 | 13.5 % | 40.4 % | 4.2 | 10.5 |
| 229 J [9] | 53 | 12.5 % | 29 % | 3.5 | 12.5 |

*Significant Grade 3/4 adverse events were encountered on these studies preventing subsequent development of a phase 3 trial; GOG = gynecologic oncology group; ORR = overall response rate; PFS = progression free survival; OS = overall survival

[13]. Most cancers, however, exhibit genetic heterogeneity. Fortunately, this same genetic heterogeneity that translates into limited therapeutic responses with targeted agents, may result in enhanced tumor immunogenicity, provoking an adaptive immune response. This concept of tumor immunogenicity is well appreciated for its role in determining the efficacy of immunotherapy [14]. Currently, our understanding of the somatic mutational load in endometrial cancer is evolving, and work is being done to identify the correlation between mutations and immunogenicity [15].

In this review, we critically examine what is known about the microenvironment in endometrial cancer and what has been learned from preliminary immunotherapy trials that enrolled endometrial cancer patients, encouraging further attempts at immunomodulation in the treatment of aggressive forms of this disease.

## Characterizing the Tumor Microenvironment

Exploiting the immune system in cancer therapeutics relies on characterizing its components within the TME. This has proven to be a major endeavor, given the differences in the immune cell composition between different types of cancer, as well as between cancers of the same type. This diversity results from the phenotypic and functional plasticity of immune cells, which are responsible for a diverse set of tasks within the immune system's overarching objective of host protection and tissue homeostasis. In both innate and adaptive immunity, immune cells are simultaneously responsible for promoting host defense while limiting collateral tissue damage. It is well established that the microenvironment has the capacity to regulate the phenotype and function of differentiated myeloid or lymphoid cells at the level of their progenitors, during their lineage-specific differentiation, and after they have matured into the fully differentiated cell types [16]. This plasticity lends support to the idea that differentiated hematopoietic cells should be viewed on a dynamic continuum rather than in distinct subcategories.

The lack of success in developing a cohesive picture of endometrial cancer on the molecular level may be explained, in part, by the fluctuations in immune cell composition of the endometrium that result from hormonal influences. As described in two recent reviews [17, 18], the immune system within the endometrium faces a unique challenge; it must be competent enough to provide protection against sexually transmitted pathogens while being permissive enough to allow the development of an allogeneic fetus. As such, this site within the female reproductive tract has evolved in such a way that sex hormones precisely regulate immune function to accomplish both tasks. The number of macrophages, neutrophils, and natural killer (NK) cells steadily increase throughout the menstrual cycle and are most abundant before menstruation, perhaps reflecting their role in the breakdown of the endometrium and in host defense during disruption of the mucosal barrier. Similarly, adaptive immune cells, which are present in the endometrium as unique aggregates consisting of a B-cell core surrounded by T cells and an outer halo of macrophages, increase in number throughout the proliferative phase and temporarily lose cytotoxic capabilities during the secretory phase, when conception may occur. These findings highlight the exceptional responsiveness of the immune system to hormonal fluctuations in this particular microenvironment.

In regards to the composition of the TME and corresponding associations with prognosis, endometrial cancer has been relatively understudied in comparison to other malignancies. In ovarian cancer, for example, it is well established that the presence of intraepithelial tumor infiltrating lymphocytes (TILs) is a robust predictor of a more favorable outcome, as demonstrated in a recent meta-analysis including 10 studies [19]. Early clinicopathologic studies were conflicting in regards to whether TILs were more common in low-grade [20] vs. high-grade endometrial cancers [21] and whether the location of TILs has prognostic implications. A perivascular lymphocytic infiltrate has been shown to correlate with poor overall survival (OS) on univariate analysis

[22] while an intraepithelial lymphocytic infiltrate at the invasive border [23] has been shown to correlate with improved OS on multivariate analysis. On the whole, given the limited data set, and study heterogeneity, comparing studies to draw meaningful conclusions has been problematic.

Contemporary studies have not only examined the presence of intra-tumoral, cytotoxic T cells but also the ratio of CD8+ TILs to regulatory T cells (Tregs: CD4+ CD25+ FOXP3+), which are well known for their physiologic role in peripheral tolerance and their pathological role in antitumor immunity. After adjusting for well known prognostic factors in multivariate analysis, de Jong and colleagues [24] found that the presence of high numbers of CD8+ TILs was an independent predictor of increased OS (whole cohort and type II) and that the presence of a high CD8+/FoxP3+ ratio was an independent predictor of increased disease-free survival (DFS) in type I, though not type II, endometrial cancer patients. The importance of the ratio of CD8+ to FoxP3 + T cells to DFS was confirmed in an additional study that did not stratify by tumor type [25]. The amount of intra-tumoral Tregs alone has not been shown to impact recurrence and survival curves [26, 27], though a statistically significant correlation has been shown between the presence of Tregs and tumor stage, grade, and presence of myometrial invasion [28].

There appears to be a better understanding of the role of myeloid cells, in comparison to lymphoid cells, in endometrial pathology. While myeloid-derived suppressor cells (MDSCs) have been detected in tumor specimens [29], tumor associated macrophages (TAMs) have been consistently identified as the dominant contributor to a pro-tumorigenic environment [30]. TAM density, particularly within the stromal compartment, has been shown to steadily increase with disease progression from precancerous endometrial lesions (various forms of hyperplasia) to endometrial cancer [31, 32]. The presence of TAMs has been repeatedly correlated to aggressive features within the primary tumor, specifically higher stage and grade and the presence of lymphovascular and myometrial invasion [27, 33–36]. The results of only one study, containing a small and heterogeneous cohort of type I and II carcinomas, has differed from these consistent findings [31]. Additionally, the presence of TAMs has been strongly associated with pelvic lymph node metastases [27, 32, 35, 37] and an angiogenic profile [34–36, 38, 39].

Recently, Kubler and colleagues [27] were the first to demonstrate that TAM density is an independent prognostic factor for recurrence-free survival, finding that a high density compared to a low density of TAMs increased the risk of recurrence by a factor of 8.3. In their study, a significant relationship between the presence of

TAMs and overall survival was found on univariate analysis but not on multivariate analysis. They hypothesize that detecting significance may not have been possible in this cohort of patients of mostly early stage disease due to the length of follow-up and the treatment of relapsed cases with curative intent. These same factors may explain why previous studies were only able to document a trend towards significance [32, 33, 35].

## Immunotherapy in Endometrial Cancer
### Therapeutic Vaccination

Therapeutic cancer vaccination is a form of active immunotherapy (Table 2). Active immunotherapies stimulate the host's own immune system to mount an antitumor immune response and induce immunological memory, theoretically producing a durable effect after treatment is stopped. Cancer vaccines exploit the cellular arm of the immune system, inciting a cytotoxic T-lymphocyte response against tumor-associated antigens (TAAs). In concept, cancer vaccines offer the prospect of high specificity, low toxicity, and prolonged activity, though these properties have yet to be reliably translated in clinical practice [40].

The product of Wilms tumor gene 1 (WT1) has been identified as a TAA with therapeutic potential in endometrial cancer. WT1 is located on chromosome 11p13 and encodes a transcription factor that plays an essential role in the normal development of the urogenital system. It has been detected in 0 % to 79 % of endometrial cancer, depending on the immunohistochemical staining technique [41]. The safety and tolerability of a weekly WT1 peptide vaccine (HLA-A2402-restricted, modified 9-mer WT1 peptide emulsified with Montanide ISA51 adjuvant) in 12 patients with recurrent or progressive gynecologic malignancies was demonstrated in a recent phase I trial [42]. Adverse events were limited to erythema at the injection site, and the disease control rate in the initial 3 months was 25 % (stable disease [SD] in 3 patients, progressive disease [PD] in 9 patients). Unfortunately, the only subject with recurrent uterine carcinosarcoma failed to respond to treatment, with disease progression after 11 vaccine injections (3 months on therapy). Utilizing an alternative approach, Cooseman and colleagues have reported the vaccination of 4 patients with advanced serous endometrial cancer with autologous dendritic cells loaded with WT1 mRNA [43, 44]. After 4 weekly injections, 3 of 4 patients demonstrated an immunological response (defined as an increase in the percentage of WT1-specific T-cells or NK cells among peripheral blood mononuclear cells), 2 of 4 patients demonstrated a molecular response (defined as a decrease in CA-125), but no patients were found to have a decrease in tumor size on repeat CT scan. Similar to the experience in the WT1 peptide trial, adverse events were limited to

**Table 2** Immunotherapeutic approaches and their application to endometrial cancer[a]

| Cancer Immunotherapy: The treatment of cancer by inducing, enhancing, or suppressing an immune response. | Active Therapy: Stimulation of the host's own immune system to mount an anti-tumor immune response • Delayed response • Durable effect • Induces immunological memory • Decreased efficacy in the immunosuppressed | Vaccination | Peptides & Proteins • Ohno et al. [44] • Kaumaya et al. [57] |
|---|---|---|---|
| | | | Whole tumor cell |
| | | | Dendritic cell • Coosemans et al. [45] • Coosemans et al. [46] • Santin et al. [62] |
| | | | Nucleic-acid based |
| | | | Viral or Bacterial Vectors • Jager et al. [51] |
| | Passive Therapy: Administration of immune system components that are exogenously produced or manipulated to promote an anti-tumor immune response • Immediate response • Short-term effect • Does not induce immunological memory • Beneficial in the immunosuppressed | Adoptive Cellular Therapy • Inoue et al. [58] • Shimizu et al. [59] • Steis et al. [60] • Santin et al. [61] | |
| | | Antibodies | Bispecific T-cell Engager Antibodies • Bellone et al. [65] |
| | | | Immune Checkpoint Inhibitors • Le et al. [69] |
| | | Cytokines | |
| | Immunomodulation: Nonspecific approaches that enhance general immune responsiveness, such as Indoleamine-2,3-dioxygenase (IDO) inhibitors and cyclooxygenase-2 (COX-2) inhibitors | | |

[a]It is important to note that there is significant overlap between categories. For example, immune checkpoint inhibitors have many of the features of active immunotherapy. Antibodies that are often referred to as 'targeted therapies' are also not included in this table.

erythema at the injection site and 1 local allergic reaction. The investigators hypothesized that the limited clinical response may be partially attributable to the advanced stage of the patients and the early termination of therapy once radiological progression was demonstrated.

Cancer testis (CT) antigens, expressed exclusively in male germ cells and placental tissue in healthy adults but ectopically in tumor cells of multiple types of human cancer, have emerged as excellent candidates for therapeutic manipulation. The restricted nature of their expression lends to high tumor-specificity and immunogenicity [45]. To date, several CT antigens have been identified in endometrial cancer. NY-ESO-1 and MAGE-A4 have been reported in 19 % and 12 % of endometrioid adenocarcinomas, respectively [46]. These numbers increase to 32 % and 63 % of USC, respectively. Additionally, KU-CT-1 has been identified in 64 % of cases of endometrial cancer [47] and SSX-4 in 24 % of cases [48]. In a two-part, open-label cohort study designed to test the safety and immunogenicity of recombinant vaccinia-NY-ESO-1 and recombinant fowlpox-NY-ESO-1, 36 patients with a wide range of tumor types experienced a similar, minor reaction to the vaccine (erythema and pruritis at the injection site) but differed significantly in their immunologic response [49]. The sole patient with endometrial cancer was one of three patients to demonstrate NY-ESO-1 sero-conversion and both a CD8+ and CD4+ T-cell response.

Additionally, human epidermal growth factor receptor 2 (HER-2/neu), the transmembrane receptor encoded by the *ERBB2* gene, has exciting potential in the treatment of endometrial cancer. In USC, specifically, overexpression of HER-2/neu ranges from 16 % to 80 % and is associated with worse overall survival [50–52]. The success of targeted therapy with trastuzumab, a recombinant humanized monoclonal antibody against HER2, in producing impressive response rates and prolonged disease-free survival in patients with metastatic breast cancer [53, 54] has encouraged the development of active immunotherapies that may produce a more durable anti-tumor immune response. In a phase I, dose-escalating, safety trial in patients with various metastatic, heavily pretreated cancers, Kaumaya and colleagues [55] tested a novel peptide combination vaccine consisting of 2 B-cell epitopes derived from the HER2 extracellular domain. In utilizing B-cell epitopes rather than T-cell epitopes, they were able to overcome the requirement for specific HLA restrictions in their patient population and engage the humoral arm of the immune system. Between the 2 endometrial cancer patients enrolled in the study, 1 patient has a partial response, experiencing extended clinical benefit at 4 years after the initial vaccination. In functional studies, the vaccine elicited antibodies in this patient that disrupted 2 different HER2 signaling methods, ultimately suppressing HER2 phosphorylation and inhibiting cell proliferation. Vaccines such as this one offer hope that we may overcome the limitations of antibody therapy, namely the short half-life of IgG, requiring frequent treatments and accruing high costs.

### Adoptive Cellular Therapy

Adoptive cellular therapy is a form of passive immunotherapy (Table 2). Passive immunotherapies involve the administration of immune system components (i.e. antibodies, cytokines, lymphocytes) that are exogenously produced or manipulated to promote an anti-tumor immune response. Unable to induce immunological memory, they offer immediate but short-term protection. In adoptive cellular therapy, cells from the blood or bone marrow are isolated, activated and expanded in vitro, and re-infused into the same patient (autologous) or a different patient (allogeneic). The technology has evolved substantially and now includes the generation of tumor-reactive T cells that are genetically engineered to express recombinant or chimeric T-cell receptors directed against common TAAs (CAR T cells).

Adoptive cellular therapy in the treatment of endometrial cancer has not yet exploited these most recent technological advances. The earliest animal studies involved the infusion of lymphokine-activated killer (LAK) cells with and without additional immuno-stimulatory components (Il-2, lentinan) [56, 57]. This therapy produced growth retardation of tumor

in nude mice. Intraperitoneal adoptive transfer of LAK cells with IL-2 has also been tested in a phase I trial that enrolled 12 colorectal cancer patients, 10 ovarian cancer patients, and 1 endometrial cancer patient with abdominal metastases [58]. Thirty percent of patients had a laparoscopy- or laparotomy-documented PR, though this did not include the patient with endometrial cancer. While the majority of adverse events (minor to moderate hypotension, fever, chills, rash, nausea, vomiting, abdominal pain and distension, diarrhea, oliguria, fluid retention, thrombocytopenia, and minor elevations of liver function tests) were attributable to Il-2, intraperitoneal fibrosis (14 patients) was a notable toxic side effect of the therapy that led to treatment discontinuation in 5 patients. Adding to the question of safety, one patient had a grand mal seizure and another had colonic perforation.

The infusion of peripheral blood T cells stimulated with tumor lysate-pulsed autologous dendritic cells has been reported by Santin and colleagues [59] in a 65-year-old patient with advanced, chemoresistant endometrial cancer. Prior to the treatment, which consisted of 3 infusions administered every 3 to 4 weeks, the patient's liver metastasis had substantially increased in size (9.5 X 8 cm to 14 X 10 cm in 3 weeks). During treatment, stabilization of the liver metastasis was achieved as a result of a tumor-specific, cytotoxic T-cell response. A more dramatic response was likely limited by the inability of the activated T cells to deeply infiltrate the large tumor mass, as evaluated in 3 dimensions by single photon emission computerized tomography (SPECT) imaging. Since publication of this report, these investigators have also demonstrated the ability to induce a tumor-specific, cytotoxic T-cell response in vitro through vaccination with tumor lysate-pulsed autologous dendritic cells in 3 patients with USC [60].

### Bispecific T-cell Engager (BiTE) Antibodies

The diverse array of molecules employed within passive immunotherapeutic approaches now includes bispecific T-cell engager (BiTE) antibodies [61]. These novel molecules induce a transient cytolytic synapse between a cytotoxic T cell and the cancer target cell. This interaction results in discharge of cytotoxic T-cell contents following perforin fusion with the T-cell membrane resulting in direct tumor cell lysis. Currently, the only drug within this class with United States FDA approval is blinatumomab (BiTE for CD 19 and CD3) for patients with acute lymphoblastic leukemia (ALL), based on an impressive complete remission rate in a phase 2 clinical trial [62].

Solitomab, which targets epithelial-cell-adhesion-molecule (EpCAM) on tumor cells while also containing a CD3 binding region, is being pursued as treatment for metastatic, recurrent, or persistent USC overexpressing EpCAM (86 % of USC cell lines tested by flow cytometry) [63]. After exposure to peripheral blood lymphocytes in vitro, EpCAM positive

USC cells were found to be resistant to NK or T-cell-mediated killing. This resistance was overcome by incubating the cell lines with solitomab. Additionally, ex vivo incubation of autologous tumor associated lymphocytes (TAL) with EpCAM expressing malignant cells in ascites with solitomab resulted in a significant increase in both CD4+ and CD8+ T-cell proliferation, an increase in T-cell activation markers, and a reduction in number of viable USC cells in ascites.

### Immune Checkpoint Inhibitors

The therapies discussed thus far involve activating the immune system to achieve tumor cell death. However, recognition that the effectiveness of both active and passive immunotherapies are reduced by tumor immune evasion [40] has led to a recent paradigm shift within immunotherapeutics away from a focus on stimulating the immune system to a focus on inhibiting the inhibitors of an adequate immune response. Among the emerging strategies of tackling immune tolerance, immune checkpoint inhibitors are the most promising.

Immune checkpoints refer to a variety of inhibitory pathways employed by the immune system to maintain self-tolerance and minimize collateral damage during physiologic responses to pathogens. Many of these pathways are initiated by ligand-receptor interactions on the surface of immune cells and, thus, are logical targets for monoclonal antibodies. Cytotoxic T-lymphocyte-associated protein-4 (CTLA-4) and programmed cell death protein-1 (PD-1) were the first, and remain the most relevant, immune-checkpoint receptors to be clinically targeted [64]. Although PD-1 and CTLA-4 belong to the same CD28 family of T-cell receptors, they assume very different roles in the down regulation of an inflammatory response. While CTLA-4 predominately regulates T cell activation within secondary lymphoid organs, PD-1 predominately regulates T cell effector function within peripheral tissues.

Importantly, immunohistochemical studies on endometrial cancer specimens have detailed PD-1 and PD-L1 expression levels surpassing those seen in ovarian and cervical carcinoma. Specifically, Vanderstraeten et al. described PD-L1 expression levels of 67-100 % in primary, recurrent and metastatic endometrial cancer specimens [29]. At the 2015 annual meeting of the Society of Gynecologic Oncology, Herzog et al. reported PD-1 expression levels of 75 %, and PD-L1 expression levels ranging from 25-47 %, once again surpassing all examined cervical and ovarian cancer specimens [65] (Table 3). Given the above, investigation of immune checkpoint inhibitors in patients with metastatic and recurrent endometrial cancer may represent a promising alternative to traditional cytotoxic therapies.

While preliminary evidence exists that tumor cell surface PD-L1 expression correlates with the likelihood of response

**Table 3** PD-1 and PD-L1 expression levels in uterine cancer (450 specimens) [67]

| Histology | PD-1 | PD-L1 |
|---|---|---|
| | % Expression based on IHC staining* | |
| Endometrioid | 77.9 | 39.7 |
| Serous Carcinoma | 68.2 | 10.2 |
| Carcinosarcoma | 80.0 | 22.2 |
| Leiomyosarcoma | 46.9 | 36.0 |
| Stromal Sarcoma | 64.3 | 64.3 |
| Clear Cell Carcinoma | 69.2 | 23.1 |

* IHC antibody = Spring Bioscience (Rabbit anti-Human IgG)

to PD-1 pathway inhibition [66], the best argument for the use of checkpoint inhibitors in select endometrial cancer cases was recently put forth by a phase 2 trial of pembrolizumab, a humanized monoclonal antibody to the PD-1 receptor, in patients with mismatch repair- (MMR-) deficient tumors [67]. This trial was designed to test the hypothesis that MMR-deficient tumors are more responsive to PD-1 blockade than MMR-proficient tumors, due to the high somatic mutational load, resulting in neoantigen formation and a more prominent lymphocytic infiltrate. As predicted, the two cohorts with MMR-deficient cancers (one with colorectal cancer patients and the other with non-colorectal cancer patients, including 2 patients with endometrial cancer) had significantly higher objective response rates by immune-related response criteria and by Response Evaluation Criteria in Solid Tumors (RECIST). They also had a significantly better immune-related PFS at 20 weeks and disease control rate by RECIST. Interestingly, patients with sporadic MMR-deficient tumors responded more frequently to treatment than those with Lynch syndrome (100 % vs 27 %). This study provides preliminary clinical evidence that immune checkpoint inhibitors may be used effectively in the treatment of MMR-deficient endometrial cancers, and trials exploring this hypothesis are currently in development.

More recently, Howitt et al. specifically examined the hypothesis that microsatellite unstable endometrial cancers would exhibit more tumor specific neoantigens, resulting in increased tumor infiltrating lymphocytes and a compensatory up-regulation of immune checkpoints (9). Microsatellite unstable tumors exhibited higher numbers of CD3+ and CD8+ tumor infiltrating lymphocytes. Furthermore, PD-1 was overexpressed in tumor infiltrating lymphocytes, and peri-tumoral lymphocytes of microsatellite unstable tumors.

### Conclusion

Despite existing evidence that endometrial cancer, particularly the most aggressive forms of the disease, is sufficiently immunogenic to be a reasonable candidate for immunomodulation, attempts to expand the role of active and/or passive immunotherapy in the treatment of this condition have been limited. At a time when the U.S. FDA-approved indications for immune checkpoint inhibitors is steadily amassing, progress in the endometrial cancer arena has been slow. Uniquely, endometrial cancer is the only gynecologic cancer with a rising incidence and mortality, and identifying effective therapies for patient with metastatic or recurrent disease is critical.

As reviewed here, these patients have been enrolled in small preclinical and phase I trials assessing the utility of immunotherapy. These studies have demonstrated encouraging immunologic responses but few clinical responses, provoking questions regarding the ability to establish therapeutic efficacy in a small number of heavily pretreated patients with advanced disease and short follow-up. The most urgent questions in identifying the utility of immunotherapy for the treatment of endometrial cancer are: how do we identify the subset of individuals most likely to respond to immunotherapy, the biomarkers most likely to predict successful treatment, and the therapy combinations most likely to enhance drug performance while limiting toxicity.

## Abbreviations

ALL: Acute lymphoblastic leukemia; BiTE antibody: Bispecific T-cell engager antibody; CML: Chronic myeloid leukemia; CR: Complete responses; CT antigen: Cancer testis antigen; CTLA-4: Cytotoxic T-lymphocyte-associated protein-4; DFS: Disease-free survival; EpCAM: Epithelial-cell-adhesion-molecule; GOG: Gynecologic Oncology Group; HER-2/neu: Human epidermal growth factor receptor 2; LAK cells: Lymphokine-activated killer cells; MDSCs: Myeloid-derived suppressor cells; MMR: Mismatch repair; NK cells: Natural killer cells; OS: Overall survival; PD: Progressive disease; PD-1: Programmed cell death protein-1; RECIST: Response Evaluation Criteria in Solid Tumors; PR: Partial responses; SD: Stable disease; SPECT: Single photon emission computerized tomography; TAAs: Tumor-associated antigens; TALs: Tumor associated lymphocytes; TAMs: Tumor associated macrophages; TAP: Paclitaxel, doxorubicin and cisplatin; TILs: Tumor infiltrating lymphocytes; TME: Tumor microenvironment; Tregs: Regulatory T cells; WT1: Wilms tumor gene 1.

## Competing interests

The authors declare that they have no competing interest.

## Authors' contributions

All authors contributed substantially to the concept of this review article, evaluation of the existing literature, preparation and editing of the manuscript. All authors have given final approval for publication, and agree to be accountable for all aspects of the work.

## Acknowledgments

Financial Support: This research was supported by an institutional NIH-T32 training grant (Ruth L. Kirschenstein NRSA Institutional Research Grant, 2 T32 CA06039611).

## References

1. National Cancer Institute: SEER Stat Fact Sheets: Endometrial Cancer. http://seer.cancer.gov/statfacts/html/corp.html. Accessed August 23 2015.
2. Fleming GF, Brunetto VL, Cella D, Look KY, Reid GC, Munkarah AR, et al. Phase III trial of doxorubicin plus cisplatin with or without paclitaxel plus filgrastim in advanced endometrial carcinoma: a Gynecologic Oncology Group Study. J Clin Oncol. 2004;22(11):2159–66. doi:10.1200/JCO.2004.07.184.
3. Aghajanian C, Sill MW, Darcy KM, Greer B, McMeekin DS, Rose PG, et al. Phase II trial of bevacizumab in recurrent or persistent endometrial cancer:
   a Gynecologic Oncology Group study. J Clin Oncol. 2011;29(16):2259–65. doi:10.1200/JCO.2010.32.6397.
4. Coleman RL, Sill MW, Lankes HA, Fader AN, Finkler NJ, Hoffman JS, et al. A phase II evaluation of aflibercept in the treatment of recurrent or persistent endometrial cancer: a Gynecologic Oncology Group study. Gynecol Oncol. 2012;127(3):538–43. doi:10.1016/j.ygyno.2012.08.020.
5. Alvarez EA, Brady WE, Walker JL, Rotmensch J, Zhou XC, Kendrick JE, et al. Phase II trial of combination bevacizumab and temsirolimus in the treatment of recurrent or persistent endometrial carcinoma: a Gynecologic Oncology Group study. Gynecol Oncol. 2013;129(1):22–7. doi:10.1016/j.ygyno.2012.12.022.
6. Dizon DS, Sill MW, Schilder JM, McGonigle KF, Rahman Z, Miller DS, et al. A phase II evaluation of nintedanib (BIBF-1120) in the treatment of recurrent or persistent endometrial cancer: an NRG Oncology/Gynecologic Oncology Group Study. Gynecol Oncol. 2014;135(3):441–5. doi:10.1016/j.ygyno.2014.10.001.
7. Makker V FV, Chen L, Darus C, Kendrick JE, Sutton G, Moxley K, Aghajanian C. Phase II evaluation of dalantercept, a soluble recombinant activin receptor-like kinase 1 (ALK1) receptor-fusion protein, for treatment of recurrent/persistent endometrial cancer: GOG 0229 N. J Clin Oncol. 2014;32(5 s):Abst#5594.
8. Powell MA, Sill MW, Goodfellow PJ, Benbrook DM, Lankes HA, Leslie KK, et al. A phase II trial of brivanib in recurrent or persistent endometrial cancer: an NRG Oncology/Gynecologic Oncology Group Study. Gynecol Oncol. 2014;135(1):38–43. doi:10.1016/j.ygyno.2014.07.083.
9. Bender DP SM, Lankes H, Darus CJ, Delmore J, Rotmensch J, Gray HJ, Mannel RS, Schilder JM, Leslie KK. A phase II evaluation of cediranib in the treatment of recurrent or persistent endometrial cancer: An NRG Oncology/Gynecologic Oncology Group (GOG) study. Gynecol Oncol. 2015;SGO Annula Meeting 2015:Late Breaking Abstract 3.
10. Pectasides D, Pectasides E, Economopoulos T. Systemic therapy in metastatic or recurrent endometrial cancer. Cancer Treat Rev. 2007;33(2):177–90. doi:10.1016/j.ctrv.2006.10.007.
11. Dellinger TH, Monk BJ. Systemic therapy for recurrent endometrial cancer: a review of North American trials. Expert Rev Anticancer Ther. 2009;9(7):905–16. doi:10.1586/era.09.54.
12. Dizon DS. Treatment options for advanced endometrial carcinoma. Gynecol Oncol. 2010;117(2):373–81. doi:10.1016/j.ygyno.2010.02.007.
13. Shekarian T, Valsesia-Wittmann S, Caux C, Marabelle A. Paradigm shift in oncology: targeting the immune system rather than cancer cells. Mutagenesis. 2015;30(2):205–11. doi:10.1093/mutage/geu073.
14. Longoria TC, Eskander RN. Immune checkpoint inhibition: therapeutic implications in epithelial ovarian cancer. Recent Pat Anticancer Drug Discov. 2015;10(2):133–44.
15. Alexandrov LB, Nik-Zainal S, Wedge DC, Aparicio SA, Behjati S, Biankin AV, et al. Signatures of mutational processes in human cancer. Nature. 2013;500(7463):415–21. doi:10.1038/nature12477.
16. Galli SJ, Borregaard N, Wynn TA. Phenotypic and functional plasticity of cells of innate immunity: macrophages, mast cells and neutrophils. Nat Immunol. 2011;12(11):1035–44. doi:10.1038/ni.2109.
17. Wira CR, Fahey JV, Ghosh M, Patel MV, Hickey DK, Ochiel DO. Sex hormone regulation of innate immunity in the female reproductive tract: the role of epithelial cells in balancing reproductive potential with protection against sexually transmitted pathogens. American journal of reproductive immunology (New York, NY : 1989). 2010;63(6):544–65. doi:10.1111/j.1600-0897.2010.00842.x.
18. Vanderstraeten A, Tuyaerts S, Amant F. The immune system in the normal endometrium and implications for endometrial cancer development. J Reprod Immunol. 2015;109:7–16. doi:10.1016/j.jri.2014.12.006.
19. Hwang WT, Adams SF, Tahirovic E, Hagemann IS, Coukos G. Prognostic significance of tumor-infiltrating T cells in ovarian cancer: a meta-analysis. Gynecol Oncol. 2012;124(2):192–8. doi:10.1016/j.ygyno.2011.09.039.
20. Deligdisch L. Morphologic correlates of host response in endometrial carcinoma. Am J Reproduc Immunol (New York, NY: 1989). 1982;2(1):54–7.
21. Silverberg SG, Sasano N, Yajima A. Endometrial carcinoma in Miyagi Prefecture, Japan: histopathologic analysis of a cancer registry-based series and comparison with cases in American women. Cancer. 1982;49(7):1504–10.
22. Ambros RA, Kurman RJ. Combined assessment of vascular and myometrial invasion as a model to predict prognosis in stage I endometrioid adenocarcinoma of the uterine corpus. Cancer. 1992;69(6):1424–31.

23. Kondratiev S, Sabo E, Yakirevich E, Lavie O, Resnick MB. Intratumoral CD8+ T lymphocytes as a prognostic factor of survival in endometrial carcinoma. Clin Cancer Res. 2004;10(13):4450–6. doi:10.1158/1078-0432.ccr-0732-3.

24. de Jong RA, Leffers N, Boezen HM, ten Hoor KA, van der Zee AG, Hollema H, et al. Presence of tumor-infiltrating lymphocytes is an independent prognostic factor in type I and II endometrial cancer. Gynecol Oncol. 2009;114(1):105–10. doi:10.1016/j.ygyno.2009.03.022.

25. Yamagami W, Susumu N, Tanaka H, Hirasawa A, Banno K, Suzuki N, et al. Immunofluorescence-detected infiltration of CD4 + FOXP3+ regulatory T cells is relevant to the prognosis of patients with endometrial cancer. Int J Gynecol Cancer. 2011;21(9):1628–34. doi:10.1097/IGC.0b013e31822c271f.

26. Giatromanolaki A, Bates GJ, Koukourakis MI, Sivridis E, Gatter KC, Harris AL, et al. The presence of tumor-infiltrating FOXP3+ lymphocytes correlates with intratumoral angiogenesis in endometrial cancer. Gynecol Oncol. 2008;110(2):216–21. doi:10.1016/j.ygyno.2008.04.021.

27. Kubler K, Ayub TH, Weber SK, Zivanovic O, Abramian A, Keyver-Paik MD, et al. Prognostic significance of tumor-associated macrophages in endometrial adenocarcinoma. Gynecol Oncol. 2014;135(2):176–83. doi:10.1016/j.ygyno.2014.08.028.

28. Chang WC, Li CH, Huang SC, Chang DY, Chou LY, Sheu BC. Clinical significance of regulatory T cells and CD8+ effector populations in patients with human endometrial carcinoma. Cancer. 2010;116(24):5777–88. doi:10.1002/cncr.25371.

29. Vanderstraeten A, Luyten C, Verbist G, Tuyaerts S, Amant F. Mapping the immunosuppressive environment in uterine tumors: implications for immunotherapy. Cancer Immunol Immunother. 2014;63(6):545–57. doi: 10.1007/s00262-014-1537-8.

30. Zsiros E, Odunsi K. Tumor-associated macrophages: co-conspirators and orchestrators of immune suppression in endometrial adenocarcinoma. Gynecol Oncol. 2014;135(2):173–5. doi:10.1016/j.ygyno.2014.10.012.

31. Dun EC, Hanley K, Wieser F, Bohman S, Yu J, Taylor RN. Infiltration of tumor-associated macrophages is increased in the epithelial and stromal compartments of endometrial carcinomas. Int J Gynecol Pathol. 2013;32(6):576–84. doi:10.1097/PGP.0b013e318284e198.

32. Jiang XF, Tang QL, Li HG, Shen XM, Luo X, Wang XY, et al. Tumor-associated macrophages correlate with progesterone receptor loss in endometrioid endometrial adenocarcinoma. J Obstet Gynaecol Res. 2013;39(4):855–63. doi:10.1111/j.1447-0756.2012.02036.x.

33. Salvesen HB, Akslen LA. Significance of tumour-associated macrophages, vascular endothelial growth factor and thrombospondin-1 expression for tumour angiogenesis and prognosis in endometrial carcinomas. Int J Cancer. 1999;84(5):538–43.

34. Hashimoto I, Kodama J, Seki N, Hongo A, Miyagi Y, Yoshinouchi M, et al. Macrophage infiltration and angiogenesis in endometrial cancer. Anticancer Res. 2000;20(6c):4853–6.

35. Soeda S, Nakamura N, Ozeki T, Nishiyama H, Hojo H, Yamada H, et al. Tumor-associated macrophages correlate with vascular space invasion and myometrial invasion in endometrial carcinoma. Gynecol Oncol. 2008;109(1):122–8. doi:10.1016/j.ygyno.2007.12.033.

36. Espinosa I, Jose Carnicer M, Catasus L, Canet B, D'Angelo E, Zannoni GF, et al. Myometrial invasion and lymph node metastasis in endometrioid carcinomas: tumor-associated macrophages, microvessel density, and HIF1A have a crucial role. Am J Surg Pathol. 2010;34(11):1708–14. doi:10.1097/PAS.0b013e3181f32168.

37. Ohno S, Ohno Y, Suzuki N, Kamei T, Koike K, Inagawa H, et al. Correlation of histological localization of tumor-associated macrophages with clinicopathological features in endometrial cancer. Anticancer Res. 2004; 24(5c):3335–42.

38. Fujimoto J, Aoki I, Khatun S, Toyoki H, Tamaya T. Clinical implications of expression of interleukin-8 related to myometrial invasion with angiogenesis in uterine endometrial cancers. Ann Oncol. 2002;13(3):430–4.

39. Tanaka Y, Kobayashi H, Suzuki M, Kanayama N, Suzuki M, Terao T. Thymidine phosphorylase expression in tumor-infiltrating macrophages may be correlated with poor prognosis in uterine endometrial cancer. Hum Pathol. 2002;33(11):1105–13. doi:10.1053/hupa.2002.129203.

40. Melero I, Gaudernack G, Gerritsen W, Huber C, Parmiani G, Scholl S, et al. Therapeutic vaccines for cancer: an overview of clinical trials. Nat Rev Clin Oncol. 2014;11(9):509–24. doi:10.1038/nrclinonc.2014.111.

41. Coosemans A, Moerman P, Verbist G, Maes W, Neven P, Vergote I, et al. Wilms' tumor gene 1 (WT1) in endometrial carcinoma. Gynecol Oncol. 2008; 111(3):502–8. doi:10.1016/j.ygyno.2008.08.032.

42. Ohno S, Kyo S, Myojo S, Dohi S, Ishizaki J, Miyamoto K, et al. Wilms' tumor 1 (WT1) peptide immunotherapy for gynecological malignancy. Anticancer Res. 2009;29(11):4779–84.

43. Coosemans A, Vanderstraeten A, Tuyaerts S, Verschuere T, Moerman P, Berneman ZN, et al. Wilms' Tumor Gene 1 (WT1)–loaded dendritic cell immunotherapy in patients with uterine tumors: a phase I/II clinical trial. Anticancer Res. 2013;33(12):5495–500.

44. Coosemans A, Wolfl M, Berneman ZN, Van Tendeloo V, Vergote I, Amant F, et al. Immunological response after therapeutic vaccination with WT1 mRNA-loaded dendritic cells in end-stage endometrial carcinoma. Anticancer Res. 2010;30(9):3709–14.

45. Gjerstorff MF, Andersen MH, Ditzel HJ. Oncogenic cancer/testis antigens: prime candidates for immunotherapy. Oncotarget. 2015;6(18):15772–87.

46. Resnick MB, Sabo E, Kondratev S, Kerner H, Spagnoli GC, Yakirevich E. Cancer-testis antigen expression in uterine malignancies with an emphasis on carcinosarcomas and papillary serous carcinomas. Int J Cancer. 2002; 101(2):190–5. doi:10.1002/ijc.10585.

47. Okada T, Akada M, Fujita T, Iwata T, Goto Y, Kido K, et al. A novel cancer testis antigen that is frequently expressed in pancreatic, lung, and endometrial cancers. Clin Cancer Res. 2006;12(1):191–7. doi:10.1158/1078-0432.ccr-05-1206.

48. Hasegawa K, Koizumi F, Noguchi Y, Hongo A, Mizutani Y, Kodama J, et al. SSX expression in gynecological cancers and antibody response in patients. Cancer Immun. 2004;4:16.

49. Jager E, Karbach J, Gnjatic S, Neumann A, Bender A, Valmori D, et al. Recombinant vaccinia/fowlpox NY-ESO-1 vaccines induce both humoral and cellular NY-ESO-1-specific immune responses in cancer patients. Proc Natl Acad Sci U S A. 2006;103(39):14453–8. doi:10.1073/pnas.0606512103.

50. Santin AD, Bellone S, Gokden M, Palmieri M, Dunn D, Agha J, et al. Overexpression of HER-2/neu in uterine serous papillary cancer. Clin Cancer Res. 2002;8(5):1271–9.

51. Slomovitz BM, Broaddus RR, Burke TW, Sneige N, Soliman PT, Wu W, et al. Her-2/neu overexpression and amplification in uterine papillary serous carcinoma. J Clin Oncol. 2004;22(15):3126–32. doi:10.1200/jco.2004.11.154.

52. Odicino FE, Bignotti E, Rossi E, Pasinetti B, Tassi RA, Donzelli C, et al. HER-2/neu overexpression and amplification in uterine serous papillary carcinoma: comparative analysis of immunohistochemistry, real-time reverse transcription-polymerase chain reaction, and fluorescence in situ hybridization. Int J Gynecol Cancer. 2008;18(1):14–21. doi:10.1111/j.1525-1438.2007.00946.x.

53. Piccart-Gebhart MJ, Procter M, Leyland-Jones B, Goldhirsch A, Untch M, Smith I, et al. Trastuzumab after adjuvant chemotherapy in HER2-positive breast cancer. N Engl J Med. 2005;353(16):1659–72. doi:10.1056/NEJMoa052306.

54. Romond EH, Perez EA, Bryant J, Suman VJ, Geyer Jr CE, Davidson NE, et al. Trastuzumab plus adjuvant chemotherapy for operable HER2-positive breast cancer. N Engl J Med. 2005;353(16):1673–84. doi:10.1056/NEJMoa052122.

55. Kaumaya PT, Foy KC, Garrett J, Rawale SV, Vicari D, Thurmond JM, et al. Phase I active immunotherapy with combination of two chimeric, human epidermal growth factor receptor 2, B-cell epitopes fused to a promiscuous T-cell epitope in patients with metastatic and/or recurrent solid tumors. J Clin Oncol. 2009;27(31):5270–7. doi:10.1200/jco.2009.22.3883.

56. Inoue M, Shimizu H, Shimizu C, Sasagawa T, Ueda G, Tanizawa O, et al. Antitumor efficacy of recombinant interleukin 2-activated killer cells against endometrial cancers. Nihon Sanka Fujinka Gakkai zasshi. 1987;39(1):143–4.

57. Shimizu H, Inoue M, Tanizawa O. Adoptive cellular immunotherapy to the endometrial carcinoma cell line xenografts in nude mice. Gynecol Oncol. 1989;34(2):195–9.

58. Steis RG, Urba WJ, VanderMolen LA, Bookman MA, Smith 2nd JW, Clark JW, et al. Intraperitoneal lymphokine-activated killer-cell and interleukin-2 therapy for malignancies limited to the peritoneal cavity. J Clin Oncol. 1990; 8(10):1618–29.

59. Santin AD, Hermonat PL, Ravaggi A, Bellone S, Cowan C, Coke C, et al. Development and therapeutic effect of adoptively transferred T cells primed by tumor lysate-pulsed autologous dendritic cells in a patient with metastatic endometrial cancer. Gynecol Obstet Invest. 2000;49(3):194–203. doi:10.1246.

60. Santin AD, Bellone S, Ravaggi A, Roman JJ, Pecorelli S, Parham GP, et al. Induction of tumour-specific CD8(+) cytotoxic T lymphocytes by tumour lysate-pulsed autologous dendritic cells in patients with uterine serous papillary cancer. Br J Cancer. 2002;86(1):151–7. doi:10.1038/sj.bjc.6600026.

61. Wickramasinghe D. Tumor and T cell engagement by BiTE. Discov Med. 2013;16(88):149–52.

62. Topp MS, Gokbuget N, Zugmaier G, Klappers P, Stelljes M, Neumann S, et al. Phase II trial of the anti-CD19 bispecific T cell-engager blinatumomab shows hematologic and molecular remissions in patients with relapsed or refractory B-precursor acute lymphoblastic leukemia. J Clin Oncol. 2014; 32(36):4134–40. doi:10.1200/jco.2014.56.3247.

63. Bellone S, Black J, English DP, Schwab CL, Lopez S, Cocco E et al. Solitomab, an EpCAM/CD3 bispecific antibody construct (BiTE(R)), is highly active against primary uterine serous papillary carcinoma cell lines in vitro. American journal of obstetrics and gynecology. 2015. doi:10.1016/j.ajog. 2015.08.011.

64. Pardoll DM. The blockade of immune checkpoints in cancer immunotherapy. Nat Rev Cancer. 2012;12(4):252–64. doi:10.1038/nrc3239.

65. Herzog T, Arguello D, Reddy S, Gatalica Z. PD-1 and PD-L1 expression in 1599 gynecological malignancies - implications for immunotherapy. Gynecol Oncol. 2015;137:Suppl. 1.

66. Brahmer JR, Tykodi SS, Chow LQ, Hwu WJ, Topalian SL, Hwu P, et al. Safety and activity of anti-PD-L1 antibody in patients with advanced cancer. N Engl J Med. 2012;366(26):2455–65. doi:10.1056/NEJMoa1200694.

67. Le DT, Uram JN, Wang H, Bartlett BR, Kemberling H, Eyring AD, et al. PD-1 Blockade in Tumors with Mismatch-Repair Deficiency. N Engl J Med. 2015; 372(26):2509–20. doi:10.1056/NEJMoa1500596.

# 4

# Long term follow-up of a phase II trial of multimodal therapy given in a "sandwich" method for stage III, IV, and recurrent endometrial cancer

Michelle Glasgow[1], Rachel Isaksson Vogel[1,2], Jennifer Burgart[3], Peter Argenta[1], Kathryn Dusenbery[4] and Melissa A. Geller[1,5*]

## Abstract

**Background:** Our objective was to determine if previously reported overall survival (OS) and progression-free survival (PFS) rates are maintained long term following multimodal therapy for advanced and recurrent endometrial cancer and to assess the lymphedema rates associated with this therapy.

**Methods:** Women with advanced-stage or recurrent endometrial cancer were recruited between 9/2004 and 6/2009 to our previously published Phase II trial. Patients received intravenous docetaxel (75 mg/m2) and carboplatin (AUC = 6) every 3 weeks for 3 cycles before and after radiation therapy. Patient outcomes were updated in July 2014. Data abstracted included presence of lymphedema, disease progression, and death. OS and PFS estimates at 5 years were calculated using Kaplan-Meier methods.

**Results:** Of the 41 patients enrolled, 10 (24 %) had stage IIIA and 21 (51 %) had stage IIIC disease; 32 (78 %) had endometrioid histology; and 35 (85 %) completed the protocol. With a median follow-up of 5 years, 15 of 41 patients have died. The Kaplan–Meier estimate and 95 % CI for OS at 5 years was 70 % (53–82 %). Excluding the two patients with recurrent disease at enrollment, 15 of 39 patients progressed or died during follow-up. The Kaplan–Meier estimate and 95 % CI for PFS at 5 years was 66 % (48–78 %). Fifteen patients (37 %) had medical record documentation of lymphedema following treatment.

**Conclusions:** After additional follow-up, OS and PFS estimates remain high and in-field recurrences low following "sandwich" therapy. The "sandwich" method remains efficacious for women with stage III-IV or recurrent endometrial cancer.

**Keywords:** Endometrial cancer, Sandwich therapy, Lymphedema

* Correspondence: gelle005@umn.edu
Preliminary data from this study were presented at the Annual Meeting of the Society of Gynecologic Oncologists in March 2015.
[1]Department of Obstetrics, Gynecology and Women's Health, Division of Gynecologic Oncology, University of Minnesota, Minneapolis, MN, USA
[5]University of Minnesota, MMC 395, 420 Delaware St. SE, Minneapolis, MN 55445, USA
Full list of author information is available at the end of the article

## Background

Endometrial cancer is the most common gynecologic malignancy in the United States with an estimated 52,630 new cases occurring in 2014 [1]. While most patients present with early stage disease and can be cured with surgery alone, survival is poor for those with advanced disease [2]. Adjuvant chemotherapy has been shown to control distant recurrence while adjuvant radiation has demonstrated control of local disease [3]. Several studies in recent years have shown that the combination of these two treatment modalities may be the most promising option for patients with advanced disease.

In 2011, we presented the results of a Phase II trial examining the use of carboplatin and docetaxel followed by radiation treatment and additional chemotherapy, according to the "sandwich" method in women with advanced stage or recurrent endometrial cancer [4]. With a median follow up of 28 months of 41 evaluable patients, the Kaplan-Meier (KM) estimates for overall survival (OS) at 1 year were 95 %, at 3 years 90 %, and at 5 years 71 %; the KM estimates for progression-free survival (PFS) at 1 year were 87 %, at 3 years 71 %, and at 5 years 64 %.

Several others have published retrospective and prospective studies supporting our conclusions that the "sandwich" method for the treatment of advanced stage endometrial cancer is effective and well tolerated (Table 1). Abaid et al. [5] reported that among 32 patients with advanced stage endometrial cancer (or early stage with high risk features, such as high grade and presence of lymphovascular space invasion) treated with the "sandwich" approach, PFS was

84 %, with a mean duration of follow-up of 18.9 months. Einstein et al. [6] examined the use of the "sandwich" method in 72 patients with both early and advanced stage uterine papillary serous carcinoma in a prospective Phase II trial; they estimated 3-year OS at 84 % for patients with early stage disease and 50 % for patients with advanced stage disease. In both of these studies, the rates of treatment completion were high (>90 %) and reported toxicity profiles acceptable. The hematologic and non-hematologic toxicities were mostly self-limited. However, the retrospective nature of these studies and their limited follow up prohibited a comprehensive assessment of long term treatment toxicities.

While these studies support the effectiveness of the "sandwich" method, toxicities do exist. Dogan et al. [7] examined acute toxicity following the "sandwich" approach in 25 women with stage IIIC endometrial cancer and compared their toxicities with those of women of the same stage who received chemotherapy followed by radiation alone. These authors found higher toxicity rates with more required dose reductions and treatment breaks, especially when pelvic and para-aortic lymph nodes were included in the radiation field. Published studies to date have not examined the long-term toxicities associated with the "sandwich" method. One of the most concerning toxicities is that of lymphedema, given the physical discomfort, pain, reduction in mobility, and negative impact on body image. [8–11]. Beesley et al. [9] recently reported the cumulative incidence of lymphedema after treatment for endometrial cancer in the Australian National

**Table 1** Reported progression-free and overall survival for endometrial cancer patients treated with "sandwich" chemotherapy and radiation therapy

| Lead Author, Year | Overall survival | | | | | Progression-free survival | | |
|---|---|---|---|---|---|---|---|---|
| | N | UPSC/clear cell/ mixed | Deaths | 3-years OS | Median follow-up (months) | N | Recur, progression or death (N) | 3-years PFS |
| Gehrig, 2004 [25] | 9 | 100 %/0 %/0 % | 0 | 100 % | 38 | N/A | 1 | N/A |
| [a]Lupe, 2007 [26] | 33 | 33 %/9 %/15 % | 13 | 55 % (2-years) | 21 | 33 | 14 | 55 % (2-years) |
| Secord, 2007 [27] | 51 | N/A | 5 | 91 % | 36 | 51 | 13 | 69 % |
| [a]Fields, 2008 [28] | 30 | 100 %/0 %/0 % | 10 | 52 % | N/A | 29 | 12 | 54 % |
| [a]Lupe, 2009 [16] | 43 | 35 %/7 %/14 % | 14 | 68 % | 30 | 41 | 35 | 53 % |
| Secord, 2009 [29] | 45 | 13 %/4 %/29 % | 7 | 88 % | 36 | 45 | 11 | 69 % |
| Geller, 2010 [17] | 23 | 52 %/4 %/0 % | 3 | 88 % | 44 | 23 | 5 | 80 % |
| [a]Geller, 2011 [4] | 41 | 9 %/NA/2 % | 7 | 90 % | 28 | 39 | 11 | 71 % |
| Abaid, 2012 [5] | 32 | 13 %/9 %/9 % | 3 | N/A | 19 | 8 | 8 | 84 % |
| [a]Einstein, 2012 [6] | | 100 %/0 %0 % | | 84 % (early stage); 50 % (advanced stage) | 9 | 20 | 20 | N/A |
| Dogan, 2013 [7] | 11 | 18 %/18 %/0 % | 0 | N/A | 18 | 1 | 5 | N/A |
| Lan, 2013 [30] | 35 | N/A | 4 | 82 % | 36 | 35 | 9 | 62 % |
| [a]Geller, 2011 - updated | 41 | 9 %/NA/2 % | 15 | 75 % | 60 | 39 | 15 | 71 % |

*UPSC* uterine papillary serous carcinoma, *PFS* progression-free survival

[a]Prospective study

Endometrial Cancer Study to be 13 %, consistent with previous reports which documented incidence rates between 1 and 18 %.

The primary aim of our current study is to present updated estimates of OS and PFS among women with advanced stage endometrial cancer who participated in our previously published Phase II trial [4]. Although important to review long term toxicity data such as gastrointestinal or genitourinary side effects, the symptoms associated with these side effects are often difficult to ascertain from a retrospective chart review. In this review, we focused on development of lymphedema instead of other long-term toxicities given few studies have reported lymphedema rates following multi-modality therapy.

## Methods

### Patient selection

Detailed methods for this Phase II trial are provided elsewhere [4]. Briefly, women with newly diagnosed advanced stage endometrial cancer (e.g. Stage IIIA-IVB according to the International Federation of Gynecology (FIGO) 1988 staging classification) or recurrent disease were recruited from the University of Minnesota Gynecologic Cancer Clinic and Methodist Hospital between 9/2004 and 6/2009. Patients were ineligible if they had received previous pelvic radiation or chemotherapy. Informed consent was obtained for all study participants for the original Phase II trial and University of Minnesota IRB approval (IRB#1406M51501) was granted for the follow-up medical chart review.

### Treatment regimen

Patients received 3 cycles (once weekly for 3 weeks) of IV docetaxel at 75 mg/m$^2$ administered over 60 min followed by carboplatin area under the curve (AUC) of 6 administered over 30 min, prior to radiation therapy. Radiotherapy was initiated within 4 weeks of the third cycle of chemotherapy and was delivered using a 4-field technique to the pelvis. All patients received pelvic irradiation; the fields were expanded to encompass the para-aortic nodal chains for those with positive para-aortic nodes. The total dose to the pelvic isocenter was 45.5 Gy and to the center of the paraaortic nodal tissue between 43 and 45 Gy. HDR brachytherapy vaginal cuff boost was delivered for vaginal extension, cervical involvement, lower uterine segment involvement, parametrial extension or at the discretion of the treating radiation oncologist. Following radiation, three identical cycles of chemotherapy were initiated within 6 weeks of completing radiotherapy.

### Patient follow-up

Patients were evaluated before every chemotherapy cycle and weekly during radiation therapy. Adverse events were assessed and reported. After completion of treatment, participants underwent disease assessment with imaging 4–6 weeks following their final chemotherapy. Patients were evaluated for disease progression and recurrence every 3 months for 2 years and then every 6 months thereafter for an additional 3 years. Symptoms or exam findings concerning for disease progression and/or recurrence were confirmed with imaging and biopsy. Recurrences were defined as local if they occurred within the radiation field. Initial results were reported in 2011. Following approval from the University of Minnesota's Institutional Review Board, a retrospective medical chart review was conducted May-July 2014 to obtain updated follow-up on all participants in this trial. Clinical data abstracted included: reported lymphedema (defined as any documentation of patient-reported lymphedema confirmed by physical exam following treatment), date of disease progression, site of recurrence and additional treatment, and date of death or date of last follow-up for those last known to be alive.

### Statistical methods

Patient demographic and clinical data were summarized and presented as frequencies (number, percent) or means ± standard deviations as appropriate unless otherwise noted. OS was calculated from date of study enrollment to death or was censored at date of last contact for patients still alive. PFS was calculated from study enrollment date to the date of first known progression or death or was censored at date of last contact for patients still alive; two patients with recurrent disease at the time of study entry were excluded from the analysis of this outcome. Kaplan-Meier estimates and 95 % confidence intervals (CI) at 3 and 5 years are reported [12]. Median OS and PFS are provided as well, however there were an insufficient number of deaths to accurately estimate the 95 % CIs. The rate of lymphedema was calculated as the proportion of participants in the study with documented lymphedema.

### Results

Forty-two patients enrolled in this trial between July 2004 and July 2009, however, ultimately 41 patients were evaluable as one patient withdrew prior to receiving any treatment. Table 2 describes the demographic and clinical characteristics of the study population. Of this group, ten patients had Stage IIIA disease, 21 had Stage IIIC disease, 1 had Stage IVA disease and 7 had Stage IV disease. The mean age at study entry was 59.0 ± 11.5 years, the majority had Stage IIIC endometrioid adenocarcinoma (51.2 %), and grades 2 and 3 histology were most common (41.5 % each). Other histologies included serous (9.8 %), mucinous (2.4 %), adenosquamous (7.3 %), and mixed serous and endometrioid (2.4 %). Two patients were treated at disease recurrence; the initial stages for these patients were Stage IC and IIA. Thirty-five patients completed the protocol as

**Table 2** Demographic and Clinical Data for all Participants (*N* = 41)

|  | Number | Percent (%) |
|---|---|---|
| Age, years, mean (SD) | 41 | 59.0 (11.5) |
| Race |  |  |
| White | 35 | 85.4 |
| Other | 5 | 12.2 |
| Missing | 1 | 2.4 |
| Disease Status |  |  |
| Primary | 39 | 95.1 |
| Recurrence | 2 | 4.9 |
| Stage |  |  |
| IC (recurrence) | 1 | 2.4 |
| IIA (recurrence) | 1 | 2.4 |
| IIIA | 10 | 24.4 |
| IIIC | 21 | 51.2 |
| IVA | 1 | 2.4 |
| IVB | 7 | 17 |
| Grade |  |  |
| 1 | 7 | 17.1 |
| 2 | 17 | 41.5 |
| 3 | 17 | 41.5 |
| Histology |  |  |
| Endometrioid | 32 | 78.1 |
| Serous | 4 | 9.8 |
| Mucinous | 1 | 2.4 |
| Adeno Squamous | 3 | 7.3 |
| Endometrioid + Serous | 1 | 2.4 |
| Surgery Type |  |  |
| Open | 32 | 84.2 |
| Minimally Invasive | 6 | 15.8 |
| *Missing* | *3* |  |
| Extent of lymphadenectomy |  |  |
| Any lymphadenectomy | 36 | 92.3 |
| Pelvic lymphadenectomy | 5 | 13.9 |
| Para-aortic lymphadenectomy | 1 | 2.8 |
| Both | 30 | 83.3 |

prescribed. Two participants were taken off protocol due to disease progression, one due to liver toxicity and three withdrew at their request.

Of the 39 patients with newly diagnosed disease, 36 patients had lymph nodes removed; five patients underwent pelvic lymphadenectomy alone, one patient underwent a para-aortic lymphadenectomy alone and 30 patients underwent both pelvic and para-aortic lymphadenectomy. The median number of pelvic lymph nodes removed was 17 (range: 0–32); the median number of para-aortic lymph nodes removed was 6 (range: 0–22). Twenty-six patients received pelvic radiation only, while eight patients received extended-field radiation. Two received incomplete radiation; one due to disease progression and one at patient request. The median dose of external beam pelvic radiation was 45.5 Gy (range = 21–60 Gy) in 25 fractions. The median length of time for completion of radiation was 38 days (15–55 days). Twenty-five patients were administered brachytherapy at a dose of 7 Gy in a single fraction to the proximal 4 cm of vagina at a depth of 0.5 cm and four patients received brachytherapy at a dose of 18 Gy in 3 fractions of 6 Gy, each prescribed to the proximal 4 cm of the vaginal surface.

Updated data resulted in patients being followed for a median of 5 years (range: 0.5–9.6 years). One patient was lost to follow-up after treatment completion due to moving out of the country. There have been eight additional deaths since the initial report. Of the 41 patients enrolled, 15 patients died since the start of treatment (Fig. 1). The Kaplan–Meier estimate and 95 % CI for OS at 3 years was 75 % (59–86 %) and 5 years was 70 % (53–82 %); estimated median OS was 8.2 years.

After excluding the two patients who enrolled at recurrence, 15 of the 39 patients progressed or died during follow-up (Fig. 2). The Kaplan–Meier estimate and 95 % CI for PFS at 3 years was 71 % (54–83 %) and 5 years was 66 % (48–78 %); estimated median PFS was 8.5 years in this subgroup. As reported in the initial manuscript, the majority of relapses occurred distantly. There was one additional recurrence to the liver since the original manuscript, occurring 56 months after study entry. In total there were two local relapses (one of which was both a local and distant failure) that occurred within the radiated field and nine distant recurrences (Fig. 3).

A total of 15 patients (36.6 %) had documented lymphedema in their medical record following treatment. Lymphedema was unilateral in nine patients and bilateral in six patients. The median time from completion of study treatment to patient report of lymphedema was 18.6 months (range 1–60 months). Stage and treatments were not consistently reported. The median time from completion of radiation treatment to patient report of lymphedema was 15 months (range 2.5–62.5 months). The extent of surgery (e.g. performance of both pelvic and para-aortic lymphadenectomy) and the radiation doses were similar between patients who developed lymphedema and those who did not. Five (33.3 %) of the patients with subsequent lymphedema were treated with extended radiation to the para-aortic chains. No relationship was observed between recurrence, location of recurrence, or surgical approach (laparotomy versus minimally invasive) and risk of subsequent lymphedema.

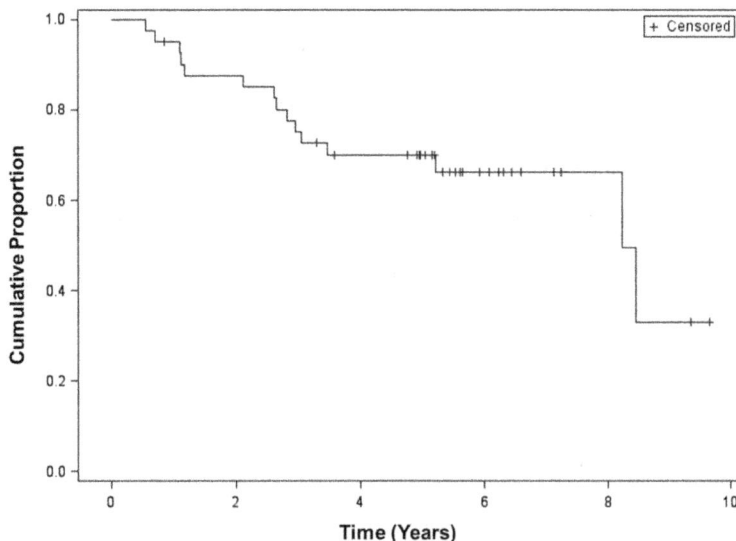

**Fig. 1** Overall survival for study participants

## Discussion

This follow-up study of women with advanced stage and recurrent endometrial cancer receiving adjuvant chemotherapy and radiation using the "sandwich" method indicates the treatment demonstrates high long-term efficacy. With a median follow-up of 5 years, estimates of OS and PFS at 5 years remain high at 70 and 66 %, respectively. Importantly, there have been no additional pelvic recurrences since the original publication, supporting the use of radiation treatment to prevent local recurrence. There has only been one additional distant recurrence during the follow-up period. This is the longest follow-up data available for this treatment modality to our knowledge.

In this prospective trial we chose to use docetaxel based on the increased neurotoxicity associated with paclitaxel in an endometrial cancer population that often has baseline neuropathy. The activity of docetaxel in endometrial cancer has been previously reported by Katsumata et al. who used docetaxel at 70 mg/m$^2$ every 3 weeks in stage III, IV or recurrent endometrial cancer with an overall response rate of 31 % [13]. Günthert et al. reported response rates of 21 % in a similar previously untreated population [14]. The GOG has conducted a phase II study in previously treated recurrent endometrial cancer patients studying docetaxel 36 mg/m$^2$ administered weekly every 28 days. They reported modest activity with two (7.7 %)

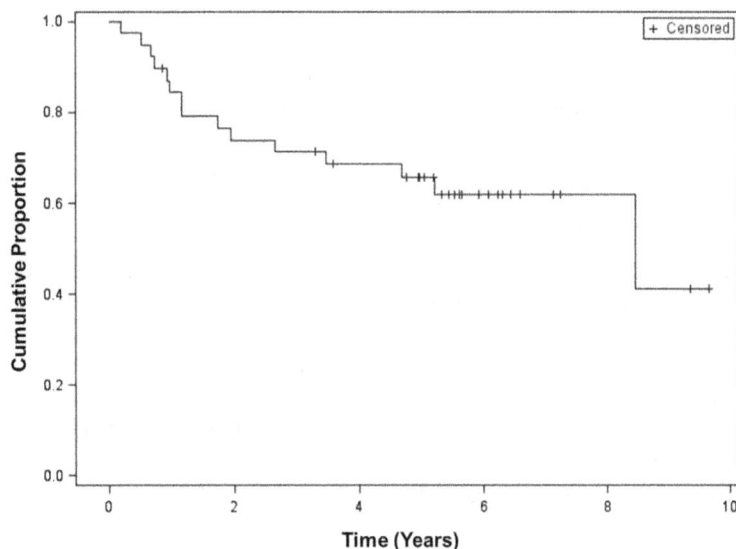

**Fig. 2** Progression-free survival for study participants. Excludes two patients who were recurrent at time of study entry

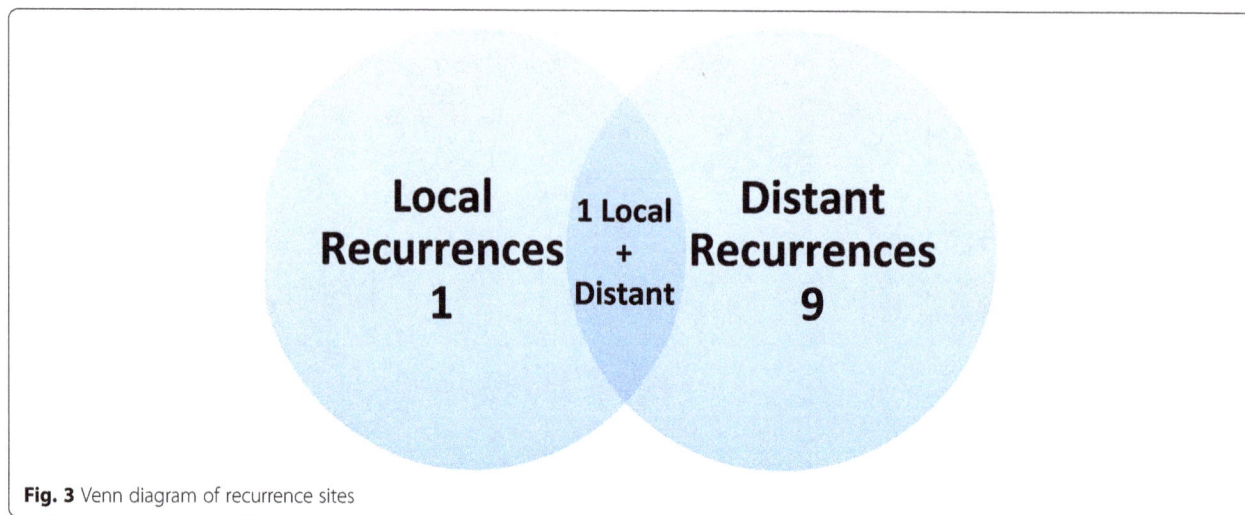

**Fig. 3** Venn diagram of recurrence sites

partial responses and eight (30.8 %) with stable disease [15]. In our study, during treatment only two patients reported grade 2 neuropathy; none experienced grade 3 or 4 neuropathy. Lupe et al. reported that 31 % of their patients receiving paclitaxel and carboplatin interposed by radiation experienced grade 3 or 4 toxicity with peripheral neuropathy and neutropenia being the most commonly cited [16]. The decision to use docetaxel as opposed to paclitaxel and carboplatin over cisplatin is largely due to the grades 3 and 4 neuropathy observed in approximately 40 % of patients receiving cisplatin and paclitaxel. Endometrial cancer patients often are older and many have previously-diagnosed diabetes, therefore neuropathy tends to be a significant issue in this population. We believed that administration of docetaxel instead of paclitaxel decreased neurotoxicity allowing for completion of six total prescribed courses of chemotherapy.

In GOG 258, the primary objective was to determine if treatment with cisplatin and volume-directed radiation followed by carboplatin and paclitaxel for 4 cycles (experimental arm) reduced the rate of recurrence or death when compared to chemotherapy consisting of carboplatin and paclitaxel for 6 cycles (control arm) in patients with Stages III-IVA endometrial carcinoma. Historically for Stage III endometrial carcinoma, patients underwent surgery followed by radiation therapy. Often, systemic failure beyond treatment fields is an issue in advanced stage endometrial cancer. Alternatively, chemotherapy for this population allows for good systemic control, but poor local control. We choose to study the "sandwich" approach because in theory, sequential rather than concurrent delivery of the two treatment modalities should limit the overall toxicity and allow for maximum therapeutic dosing of both radiation and chemotherapy. Despite thorough surgical staging and cytoreduction, remaining microscopic disease can be present outside the pelvis at the time of adjuvant therapy initiation. Typically following surgery, initiation of therapy

can be delayed for 2–3 weeks. If radiation therapy is given initially, as was seen in our patient population we have previously reported, it took a median of 42.5 days (range 34–62) to complete radiation therapy [17].

A multimodality regimen similar to GOG 258 was used in RTOG 9708 [18]. In RTOG 9708, pathologic requirements included grade 2 or 3 endometrial adenocarcinoma with either >50 % myometrial invasion, cervical stromal invasion, or pelvic-confined extrauterine disease. Patients received 45 Gy in 25 fractions to the pelvis along with cisplatin (50 mg/m2) on days 1 and 28. Vaginal brachytherapy was performed after the external beam radiation. Patients then went on to receive four courses of cisplatin (50 mg/m2) and paclitaxel (175 mg/m2) at 4-week intervals following completion of radiotherapy. Unlike our population that consisted only of advanced stage disease (Stages III and IV) and included serous histology, the patient population in RTOG 9708 represented an earlier stage group (stages I to IIIC); with 39 % having Stage I or II disease. The inclusion of earlier stage disease may account for the slightly higher 4-year overall survival (OS) and disease-free survival (DFS) of 85 and 81 %, respectively. In their stage III patients, the 4-year rates for OS and DFS were 77 and 72 %, respectively. In our more advanced stage population, our 4-year rates were OS and DFS was 0.70 (0.53–0.82) and 0.69 (0.51–0.81), respectively.

As we await the results from GOG 258, the protocol we follow is based on the observation that following radiation therapy there often is a treatment break before beginning chemotherapy. Theoretically, this delay could lead to disease progression prior to beginning systemic therapy in areas outside of the radiation field. Often times, if all six courses of chemotherapy are given followed by tumor directed radiotherapy, patients may have difficulty in finishing the radiation therapy due to toxicity related to the chemotherapy. Administering three cycles of chemotherapy followed by radiation allows for both modalities, with the ability to give at least some systemic therapy prior to initiating the radiation phase of the protocol.

In addition to long-term survival, we also examined the rates of lymphedema associated with the "sandwich" method. We found that 15 patients (36.6 %) were diagnosed with clinically observable lymphedema after treatment. No consistent relationship was observed between the presence of subsequent lymphedema and the extent of surgery, radiation dose, or radiation fields. Many factors may contribute to lymphedema among patients with endometrial cancer, including patient habitus, disease, and treatment-related factors. There is no consensus on the individual weight of these factors in contributing to this treatment toxicity. Several studies have demonstrated that the risk of lymphedema increases with removal of a greater number of lymph nodes. For instance, Abu-Rustum et al. [10] reported that patients who had ten or more regional lymph nodes removed were at higher risk for developing lymphedema. This association has not been found in all studies [10, 19–21]. Additionally, other studies have proposed the risk of lymphedema varies according to which lymph nodes are removed. In opposition, Yost et al. [20] found no difference in lymphedema rates in women with endometrial cancer according to the extent of lymphadenectomy (e.g. pelvic compared with pelvic and para-aortic node dissection) and Todo et al. [19] did not find para-aortic lymphadenectomy to be a risk factor for lymphedema in their review of 286 women with endometrial cancer. Hareyama et al. [22] examined the effect of preserving the circumflex iliac lymph nodes in 329 women with various gynecologic malignancies who underwent both pelvic and para-aortic lymphadenectomies. They found a lower incidence of lymphedema in the patients whose circumflex iliac lymph nodes were not removed. In our study, no significant differences were seen regarding the location of lymphadenectomy (e.g. pelvic versus pelvic and para-aortic) or in the number of lymph nodes removed in women who developed lymphedema.

The literature also suggests that radiation impacts the risk of lymphedema. Todo et al. [19] reported that whole pelvic radiation therapy was an independent risk factor for developing lower-extremity lymphedema, and this risk was reiterated by Yost et al. [20]. This association however, has not been identified in all studies. In a study of 150 women with vulvar cancer there was no increase in the risk of lymphedema in women who had previously received radiation [23]. Ryan et al. reports that in a sample population of women with lower limb lymphedema after gynecologic cancer treatment, more than half of the women with lymphedema reported having to change their daily activities as a result of lymphedema [8]. More attention is now being given to defining the effect lymphadenectomy has on the risk of lymphedema. We await the findings of GOG 244, the LEG study, a prospective longitudinal trial

examining the incidence and risk factors for lymphedema and its impact on quality of life in women who have undergone radical gynecologic surgery [24].

The strengths of this study include its ability to report long-term outcomes in patients treated with the "sandwich" method. Additionally, it is the first study to describe the risk of lymphedema with this multimodal treatment. However, given the retrospective approach to identifying post-treatment lymphedema and the loss of follow-up in some patients, it is likely that the reported incidence of lymphedema is underestimated in our study. Additionally, the severity of lymphedema was not always reported, therefore limiting the utility of these data for fully counseling patients on the risk associated with this treatment modality.

## Conclusions

Our study confirms that the "sandwich" approach is a promising treatment for women with advanced and recurrent endometrial cancer, but its subsequent risk of lymphedema is not negligible. It is important to recognize this risk and to counsel patients appropriately, especially as studies have shown that lymphedema can have a significant negative impact on a patient's quality of life after cancer treatment [20]. As the medical community develops better treatment protocols for patients with gynecologic cancers, which will hopefully lead to improved prognoses, it is also important to treat and care for conditions that may result from these cancer treatments. Studies that focus on lymphedema and other long term sequela of treatments in gynecologic cancer patients are necessary to estimate the true prevalence of these unwanted side-effects. We are currently prospectively collecting lymphedema risks and incidence in our endometrial cancer patients being treated in the "sandwich" method. This information will improve our ability to counsel patients on long-term risks of therapy and hopefully, in the future, will inform us on methods of prevention.

**Funding source**

The original study was supported financially by Sanofi-Aventis. Statistical data analysis was supported in part by NIH grant P30 CA77598 utilizing the Biostatistics and Bioinformatics Core shared resource of the Masonic Cancer Center, University of Minnesota and by the National Center for Advancing Translational Sciences of the National Institutes of Health Award Number UL1TR000114.

**Authors' contributions**

MG wrote the introduction and discussion sections and finalized manuscript. RV wrote the initial draft of methods, performed the statistical data analysis and wrote the results sections of the manuscript. JB performed the collection of follow-up data and also conducted a literature review. Both PA and KD were Co-Investigators on the original trial and provided significant input on this manuscript. MA was the Principle Investigator on the original trial, conceived the idea for the follow-up study, and provided significant input on the manuscript. All authors read and approved the final manuscript.

**Competing interests**

The authors declare that they have no competing interests.

## Consent section

Written informed consent was obtained from the patients enrolled in this trial for the publication of the original trial results as well as accompanying images. A copy of the written consent is available for review by the Editor-in-Chief of this journal.

## Author details

[1]Department of Obstetrics, Gynecology and Women's Health, Division of Gynecologic Oncology, University of Minnesota, Minneapolis, MN, USA. [2]Biostatistics and Bioinformatics Core, Masonic Cancer Center, University of Minnesota, Minneapolis, MN, USA. [3]Eastern Virginia Medical School, Norfolk, VA, USA. [4]Radiation Oncology, University of Minnesota, Minneapolis, MN, USA. [5]University of Minnesota, MMC 395, 420 Delaware St. SE, Minneapolis, MN 55445, USA.

## References

1. Siegel R, Ma J, Zou Z, Jemal A. Cancer statistics, 2014. CA Cancer J Clin. 2014;64:9–29.
2. Amant F, Moerman P, Neven P, Timmerman D, Van Limbergen E, Vergote I. Endometrial cancer. Lancet. 2005;366:491–505.
3. Deleon MC, Ammakkanavar NR, Matei D. Adjuvant therapy for endometrial cancer. J Gynecol Oncol. 2014;25:136–47.
4. Geller MA, Ivy JJ, Ghebre R, Downs Jr LS, Judson PL, Carson LF, et al. A phase II trial of carboplatin and docetaxel followed by radiotherapy given in a "Sandwich" method for stage III, IV, and recurrent endometrial cancer. Gynecol Oncol. 2011;121:112–7.
5. Abaid LN, Rettenmaier MA, Brown 3rd JV, Micha JP, Mendivil AA, Wabe MA, et al. Sequential chemotherapy and radiotherapy as sandwich therapy for the treatment of high risk endometrial cancer. J Gynecol Oncol. 2012;23:22–7.
6. Einstein MH, Frimer M, Kuo DY, Reimers LL, Mehta K, Mutyala S, et al. Phase II trial of adjuvant pelvic radiation "sandwiched" between combination paclitaxel and carboplatin in women with uterine papillary serous carcinoma. Gynecol Oncol. 2012;124:21–5.
7. Dogan NU, Yavas G, Yavas C, Ata O, Yilmaz SA, Celik C. Comparison of "sandwich chemo-radiotherapy" and six cycles of chemotherapy followed by adjuvant radiotherapy in patients with stage IIIC endometrial cancer: a single center experience. Arch Gynecol Obstet. 2013;288:845–50.
8. Ryan M, Stainton MC, Jaconelli C, Watts S, MacKenzie P, Mansberg T. The experience of lower limb lymphedema for women after treatment for gynecologic cancer. Oncol Nurs Forum. 2003;30:417–23.
9. Beesley VL, Rowlands IJ, Hayes SC, Janda M, O'Rourke P, Marquart L, et al. Incidence, risk factors and estimates of a woman's risk of developing secondary lower limb lymphedema and lymphedema-specific supportive care needs in women treated for endometrial cancer. Gynecol Oncol. 2015;136:87–93.
10. Abu-Rustum NR, Alektiar K, Iasonos A, Lev G, Sonoda Y, Aghajanian C, et al. The incidence of symptomatic lower-extremity lymphedema following treatment of uterine corpus malignancies: a 12-year experience at Memorial Sloan-Kettering Cancer Center. Gynecol Oncol. 2006;103:714–8.
11. Ghezzi F, Uccella S, Cromi A, Bogani G, Robba C, Serati M, et al. Lymphoceles, lymphorrhea, and lymphedema after laparoscopic and open endometrial cancer staging. Ann Surg Oncol. 2012;19:259–67.
12. Kaplan E, Meier P. Nonparametric estimation from incomplete observations. J Am Stat Assoc. 1958;53:457–81.
13. Katsumata N, Noda K, Nozawa S, Kitagawa R, Nishimura R, Yamaguchi S, et al. Phase II trial of docetaxel in advanced or metastatic endometrial cancer: a Japanese Cooperative Study. Br J Cancer. 2005;93:999–1004.
14. Gunthert AR, Ackermann S, Beckmann MW, Camara O, Kiesel L, Rensing K, et al. Phase II study of weekly docetaxel in patients with recurrent or metastatic endometrial cancer: AGO Uterus-4. Gynecol Oncol. 2007;104:86–90.
15. Garcia AA, Blessing JA, Nolte S, Mannel RS. A phase Ii evaluation of weekly docetaxel in the treatment of recurrent or persistent endometrial carcinoma: a study by the Gynecologic Oncology Group. Gynecol Oncol. 2008;111:22–6.
16. Lupe K, D'Souza DP, Kwon JS, Radwan JS, Harle IA, Hammond JA, et al. Adjuvant carboplatin and paclitaxel chemotherapy interposed with involved field radiation for advanced endometrial cancer. Gynecol Oncol. 2009;114:94–8.
17. Geller MA, Ivy J, Dusenbery KE, Ghebre R, Isaksson Vogel R, Argenta PA. A single institution experience using sequential multi-modality adjuvant chemotherapy and radiation in the "sandwich" method for high risk endoemtrial carcinoma. Gynecol Oncol. 2010;118:19–23.
18. Greven K, Winter K, Underhill K, Fontenesci J, Cooper, Burke T. Final analysis of RTOG 9708: adjuvant postoperative irradiation combined with cisplatin/paclitaxel chemotherapu following surgery for patients with high-risk endometrial cancer. Gynecol Oncol. 2006;103:155–9.
19. Todo Y, Yamamoto R, Minobe S, Suzuki Y, Takeshi U, Nakatani M, et al. Risk factors for postoperative lower-extremity lymphedema in endometrial cancer survivors who had treatment including lymphadenectomy. Gynecol Oncol. 2010;119:60–4.
20. Yost KJ, Cheville AL, Al-Hilli MM, Mariani A, Barrette BA, McGree ME, et al. Lymphedema after surgery for endometrial cancer: prevalence, risk factors, and quality of life. Obstet Gynecol. 2014;124:307–15.
21. Tada H, Teramukai S, Fukushima M, Sasaki H. Risk factors for lower limb lymphedema after lymph node dissection in patients with ovarian and uterine carcinoma. BMC Cancer. 2009;9:47.
22. Hareyama H, Ito K, Hada K, Uchida A, Hayakashi Y, Hirayama E, et al. Reduction/prevention of lower extremity lymphedema after pelvic and para-aortic lymphadenectomy for patients with gynecologic malignancies. Ann Surg Oncol. 2012;19:268–73.
23. Carlson JW, Kauderer J, Walker JL, Gold MA, O'Malley D, Tuller E, et al. A randomized phase III trial of VH fibrin sealant to reduce lymphedema after inguinal lymph node dissection: a Gynecologic Oncology Group study. Gynecol Oncol. 2008;110:76–82.
24. Gynecologic Oncology Group. The Lymphedema and Gynecologic Cancer (LEG) Study: Incidence, Risk Factors, and Impact in Newly Diagnosed Patients. Bethesda: ClinicalTrials.gov; 2014.
25. Gehrig PA, Boggess JF, Moller KA, Boruta DM, Dunlap AP, Fowler WC, et al. Paclitaxel and carboplatin sequenced with radiotherapy in women with advanced uterine serous carcinoma: is this optimal therapy? J Clin Oncol. 2004;22:5084.
26. Lupe K, Kwon J, D'Souza D, Gawlik C, Stitt L, Whiston F, et al. Adjuvant paclitaxel and carboplatin chemotherapy with involved field radiation in advanced endometrial cancer: a sequential approach. Int. J Radiat Oncol Biol Phys. 2007;67:110–116.
27. Alvarez Secord A, Havrilesky LJ, Bae-Jump V, Chin J, Calingaert B, Bland A, et al. The role of multi-multimodality adjuvant chemotherapy and radiation in women with advanced stage endometrial cancer. Gynecol Oncol. 2007;107: 285–291.
28. Fields AL, Einstein MH, Novetsky AP, Gebb J, Goldberg GL. Pilot phase II trial of radiation "sandwiched" between combination paclitaxel/platinum chemotherapy in patients with uterine papillary serous carcinoma (UPSC). Gynecol Oncol. 2008;108:201–206.
29. Secord AA, Havrilesky LJ, O'Malley DM, Bae-Jump V, Fleming ND, Broadwater G, et al. A multicenter evaluation of sequential multimodality therapy and clinical outcome for the treatment of advanced endometrial cancer. Gynecol Oncol. 2009;114:442–447.
30. Lan C, Huang X, Cao X, Huang H, Feng Y, Huang Y, et al. Adjuvant docetaxel and carboplatin chemotherapy administered alone or with radiotherapy in a "sandwich" protocol in patients with advanced endometrial cancer: a single-institution experience. Expert Opin Pharmacother. 2013;14:535–42.

# 5

# Analysis of in vitro chemoresponse assays in endometrioid endometrial adenocarcinoma: an observational ancillary analysis

Brittany A. Davidson[1*], Jonathan Foote[1], Stacey L. Brower[2], Chunqiao Tian[2], Laura J. Havrilesky[1] and Angeles Alvarez Secord[1]

## Abstract

**Background:** Chemotherapy plays a role in the treatment of endometrioid endometrial cancer (EEC); however, tumor grade may affect response. Our objective was to evaluate associations between tumor grade and in vitro chemoresponse.

**Methods:** We conducted an analysis of primary tumor samples from women with EEC undergoing in vitro chemoresponse testing. Results were classified as sensitive (S), intermediate (I), or resistant (R) to each drug tested. Correlations between tumor grade and response were examined.

**Results:** Data was collected from 159 patients: 28 with grade 1 (18%), 52 with grade 2 (32%), and 79 (50%) with grade 3 tumors. Median age of patients was 62 (range 31–92). Most patients were Caucasian (83%) with advanced disease (Stage III: 50.9%; Stage IV: 13.2%). Overall chemoresponse was similar across all grades. Fifty percent, 56 and 51% for grade 1, 2, and 3 tumors, respectively, demonstrated S results to at least 1 agent. There was no association between grade and in vitro response to chemotherapy agents ($p > 0.05$) except a marginal association between grade and doxorubicin response ($p = 0.08$). Grade 1 and 2 cancers were more likely to demonstrate R results for doxorubicin compared to grade 3 cancers (G1: 19% vs G2: 25% vs G3: 8%; $p = 0.08$). In a subset tested for all 7 agents, only one patient tumor was pan-R and 4 were pan-S.

**Conclusions:** Based on our data, grades 1–3 EEC have similar in vitro chemoresponse. These findings suggest that chemotherapy may be useful in advanced low grade EECs, but further clinical correlation is needed.

**Keywords:** Endometrial cancer, Chemosensitivity, Tumor grade, Endometrioid

## Background

Endometrial cancer (EC) is the most common gynecologic malignancy, with nearly 55,000 new cases and more than 10,000 deaths predicted for 2015 [1]. While 5 year survival trends have improved for other gynecologic malignancies, the survival rate for patients diagnosed with EC between 2004 and 2010 is lower than that of patients diagnosed between 1975 and 1977 (83 vs. 87% $p = <0.05$) [1]. Undoubtedly, many factors account for this trend; however it is yet unknown if chemoresistance plays an important role.

The mechanism underlying chemoresistance in EC is uncertain, however current dogma suggests that low grade Type I endometrioid endometrial cancers (EEC) are less likely to respond to chemotherapy. Type I tumors represent the majority of sporadic EC, characterized predominantly by endometrioid histology and expression of estrogen and/or progesterone receptors [2]. In contrast, Type II EC is less common and often of serous or clear cell histology, arising in atrophic endometrium, rather than estrogen excess [3]. There is

* Correspondence: Brittany.davidson@duke.edu
[1]Division of Gynecologic Oncology, Duke University Medical Center, Duke University, DUMC Box 3079, Durham, NC 27710, USA
Full list of author information is available at the end of the article

conflicting data regarding chemotherapy response and tumor grade and histology in endometrial cancers.

Response rate (RR) to chemotherapy was not significantly different between endometrioid (44%), clear cell (32%) and serous tumors (44%) in a pooled analysis of patients with advanced or recurrent EC treated on 1 of 4 GOG trials (GOG 107, GOG 139, GOG 163, GOG 177) (clear cell $p = 0.13$; serous $p = 0.99$) [4]. In a subgroup analysis of over 600 patients with endometrioid histology alone enrolled in these same 4 GOG trials, grade 3 tumors had an estimated odds of response of approximately 1.5 times that of grade 1 tumors, although these results were not statistically significant ($p = 0.09$) [4]. However, these two analyses were based on a retrospective assessment of investigator-determined response which may be prone to subjective assessment and error.

We previously explored the association between tumor grade and cytotoxic treatment response in patients with advanced or recurrent EEC ($N = 91$). Contrary to expectations, grade 2 cancers were more likely to respond to all types of chemotherapy (72 vs 43% $p = 0.02$) and to carboplatin/paclitaxel doublets (72 vs 41% $p = 0.02$) compared to grade 3 cancers [5]. However, this study was limited by lack of central pathology review, small sample size, and paucity of patients with grade 1 EEC.

Given the contradictory data and limitations of prior studies, we explored in vitro chemoresponse profiles to obtain insight into the relationship between chemotherapeutic anti-tumor activity and grade in EEC specimens from women enrolled in observational studies.

## Methods

The study population included women with endometrioid endometrial cancer whose primary cancer specimens were submitted for in vitro chemoresponse assay testing on prospectively-accrued observational studies between 2006 and 2010. These were longitudinal, observational multi-center studies examining the outcomes associated with chemosensitivity assays in women with gynecologic malignancies. Participants had not received chemotherapy prior to specimen collection. Tumor grades were assigned by the institutions submitting the specimens for testing. Assays were conducted for up to 7 cytotoxic agents including carboplatin, cisplatin, doxorubicin, paclitaxel, docetaxel, gemcitabine, and topotecan.

Details regarding the particular chemoresponse assay used in this study (ChemoFx®, Helomics Corporation, Pittsburgh, PA) have been described elsewhere [6, 7]. Assay preparation included an immunocytochemistry step to aid in the confirmation that cells were of epithelial, rather than stromal, origin. All cultures required a majority of epithelial cells to proceed to chemoresponse testing. A board-certified pathologist assessed cell morphology.

Inhibition of tumor growth was measured at several serially-diluted concentrations of each cytotoxic agent tested. For each drug, the area under the dose–response curve (AUC) was calculated. Greater sensitivity to the therapy tested was indicated by a smaller AUC. Using established criteria, tumor chemoresponse was classified using the in vitro AUC score into one of three categories: sensitive (S), intermediate sensitive (I), or resistant (R). The in vitro tumor response rate (RR) for each agent was then defined as the proportion of patients with tumors testing either S or I for that agent.

The primary endpoint of this ancillary study was to assess the association between tumor grade and in vitro chemoresponse assay results in EEC. Patient demographics were also collected, including age and stage at diagnosis. Correlations of tumor grade with assay results were examined using Cochran-Armitage test for trend using SAS version 9.4 (SAS Institute, Cary, NC).

## Results

A total of 159 patients were included for this analysis. Twenty-eight patients had grade 1 (18%), 52 had grade 2 (32%), and 79 (50%) had grade 3 tumors. The median age of patients was 62 (range 31–92). Most patients were Caucasian (83%) and had advanced stage disease (Stage III: 50.9%; Stage IV: 13.2%) at diagnosis [Table 1].

As mentioned previously, the chemotherapeutic agents tested in this assay included carboplatin, cisplatin, doxorubicin, and paclitaxel, which are commonly used in EC. In addition, other cytotoxics incorporated in the panel

**Table 1** Patient Characteristics by Tumor Grade

|  | Grade 1 ($n = 28$) | Grade 2 ($n = 52$) | Grade 3 ($n = 79$) | Total ($n = 159$) |
|---|---|---|---|---|
|  | No. (%) | No. (%) | No. (%) | No. (%) |
| Age (years) |  |  |  |  |
| Median (Range) | 63.5 (42–92) | 62 (32–87) | 62 (31–89) | 62 (31–92) |
| < 50 | 2 (7.1) | 8 (15.4) | 9 (11.4) | 19 (11.9) |
| 50–64 | 13 (46.4) | 22 (42.3) | 36 (45.6) | 71 (44.7) |
| 65–74 | 8 (28.6) | 14 (26.9) | 24 (30.4) | 46 (28.9) |
| ≥ 75 | 5 (17.9) | 8 (15.4) | 10 (12.7) | 23 (14.5) |
| Race |  |  |  |  |
| White | 24 (85.7) | 45 (86.5) | 63 (79.7) | 132 (83) |
| Black | 1 (3.6) | 4 (7.7) | 12 (15.2) | 17 (10.7) |
| Other | 3 (10.7) | 3 (5.8) | 4 (5.1) | 10 (6.3) |
| FIGO Stage |  |  |  |  |
| I | 11 (39.3) | 8 (15.4) | 21 (26.6) | 40 (25.2) |
| II | 0 (0.0) | 8 (15.4) | 7 (8.9) | 15 (9.4) |
| III | 15 (53.6) | 28 (53.8) | 38 (48.1) | 81 (50.9) |
| IV | 2 (7.1) | 6 (11.5) | 13 (16.5) | 21 (13.2) |
| Unknown | 0 (0.0) | 2 (3.8) | 0 (0.0) | 2 (1.3) |

were evaluated including docetaxel, gemcitabine, and topotecan. Not all patients had their tumors tested for all 7 cytotoxic agents. Assay results were available for the following cytotoxic agents stratified by grade 1, 2, and 3: carboplatin (25/28[89%], 41/52[79%], 66/79[84%]), paclitaxel (24/28[86%], 40/52[77%], 65/79[82%]), doxorubicin (27/28[96%], 48/52[92%], 77/79[97%]), cisplatin (24/28[86%], 43/52[83%], 67/79[85%]), docetaxel (19/28[68%], 35/52[67%], 61/79[77%]), gemcitabine (14/28[50%], 26/52[50%], 45/79[56%]), and topotecan (22/28[71%], 41/52[79%], 61/79[77%]) [Table 2].

The number of R results, defined as responses that were neither S nor I, was similar across grades. Twenty seven percent, 21, and 17% for grade 1, 2, and 3 tumors, respectively, demonstrated resistant chemoresponse results for

**Table 2** In Vitro Tumor Responses to Seven Drugs

| Drug | Tumor Grade | No. patients | R (%) | I (%) | S (%) | P value[a] |
|------|-------------|--------------|-------|-------|-------|---------|
| Assay Result[b] | | | | | | |
| Carboplatin | | | | | | .928 |
| | 1 | 25 | 28.0 | 40.0 | 32.0 | |
| | 2 | 41 | 24.4 | 39.0 | 36.6 | |
| | 3 | 66 | 19.7 | 53.0 | 27.3 | |
| Cisplatin | | | | | | .322 |
| | 1 | 24 | 29.2 | 41.7 | 29.2 | |
| | 2 | 43 | 18.6 | 55.8 | 25.6 | |
| | 3 | 67 | 13.4 | 58.2 | 28.4 | |
| Docetaxel | | | | | | .812 |
| | 1 | 19 | 26.3 | 42.1 | 31.6 | |
| | 2 | 35 | 8.6 | 54.3 | 37.1 | |
| | 3 | 61 | 18.0 | 47.5 | 34.4 | |
| Doxorubicin | | | | | | .080 |
| | 1 | 27 | 18.5 | 55.6 | 25.9 | |
| | 2 | 48 | 25.0 | 56.3 | 18.8 | |
| | 3 | 77 | 7.8 | 61.0 | 32.2 | |
| Gemcitabine | | | | | | .238 |
| | 1 | 14 | 28.6 | 28.6 | 42.9 | |
| | 2 | 26 | 30.8 | 23.1 | 46.2 | |
| | 3 | 45 | 22.2 | 62.2 | 15.6 | |
| Paclitaxel | | | | | | .670 |
| | 1 | 24 | 33.3 | 33.3 | 33.3 | |
| | 2 | 40 | 15.0 | 37.5 | 47.5 | |
| | 3 | 65 | 15.4 | 53.9 | 30.8 | |
| Topotecan | | | | | | .861 |
| | 1 | 22 | 27.3 | 45.5 | 27.3 | |
| | 2 | 41 | 24.4 | 48.8 | 26.8 | |
| | 3 | 61 | 23.0 | 50.8 | 26.2 | |

[a]Correlation of tumor grade with assay result examined by Cochran-Armitage test
[b]R resistant, I intermediately sensitive, S sensitive

any of the agents tested. There was no association between tumor grade and in vitro response to various chemotherapy agents ($p > 0.05$) other than a marginal association between grade and response to doxorubicin ($p = 0.08$) (Table 2). Specifically, grade 1 and 2 cancers were more likely to demonstrate R assay results for doxorubicin compared to grade 3 cancers (G1: 18% vs G2: 25% vs G3: 8%; $p = 0.08$).

Ten of 28 (36%) grade 1, 21/52 (38%) grade 2, and 33/79 (42%) grade 3 tumors were tested for all 7 cytotoxic agents (Fig. 1). Of those grade 1 tumors tested for all 7 cytotoxic agents, 6/10 (60%) were pan-sensitive (defined as S + I), and none were pan-resistant. Of the 21 grade 2 tumors tested for all 7 agents, 10 (47.6%) were pan-sensitive and 1 (5%) pan-resistant. Similarly, 19 of 33 (57.6%) grade 3 tumors were pan-sensitive while none were pan-resistant. When examining the entire cohort of tumors, 14/ 28 (50%) grade 1 tumors exhibited a sensitive (S only) chemoresponse assay to at least 1 agent. Similarly, 29/52 (56%) of grade 2 tumors and 40/79 (51%) grade 3 tumors also showed in vitro sensitivity to at least one cytotoxic agent. If S + I responses are considered, these RRs increase to 73, 79 and 83% for grades 1, 2 and 3 tumors, respectively.

## Discussion

Our data suggests there is no difference in in vitro chemoresponse among EECs of various grades. When stratified by tumor grade, RRs were similar for 7 chemotherapeutic agents with the exception of doxorubicin, where grade 3 tumors exhibited a non-significant increased RR (92% (S + I)) compared to grade 1 (81%) and grade 2 (75%) tumors. Overall our results are similar to the clinical findings reported by McMeekin and colleagues examining the relationship between tumor histology and chemotherapeutic response in 4 GOG endometrial cancer trials (GOG#107, GOG#139, GOG#163, GOG#177). To date, this GOG ancillary analysis is the largest study to examine the association between tumor grade and chemotherapy response in EEC [4]. These trials encompassed both advanced and recurrent EC treated with a variety of cytotoxic agents, including doxorubicin, a doxorubicin/cisplatin doublet, a doxorubicin/paclitaxel doublet, and a doxorubicin/cisplatin/paclitaxel triplet administered in various intervals and doses [8–11]. The majority of patients included in these studies had also received prior radiation therapy. In a subgroup analysis of over 600 patients with endometrioid histology only, there was no difference in response of grade 3 versus grade 1 tumors ($p = 0.09$). Furthermore, tumor grade was not associated with progression free survival (PFS) or overall survival [4]. This may be due, in part, to the fact that patients had advanced or recurrent disease associated with a

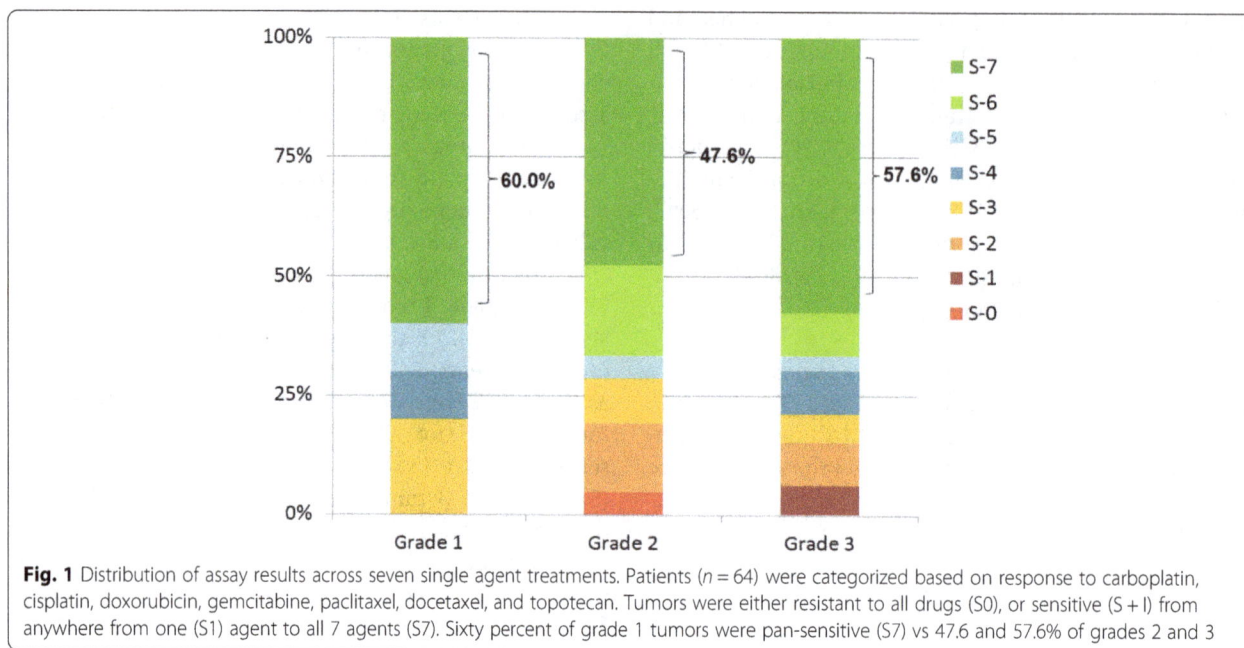

**Fig. 1** Distribution of assay results across seven single agent treatments. Patients ($n = 64$) were categorized based on response to carboplatin, cisplatin, doxorubicin, gemcitabine, paclitaxel, docetaxel, and topotecan. Tumors were either resistant to all drugs (S0), or sensitive (S + I) from anywhere from one (S1) agent to all 7 agents (S7). Sixty percent of grade 1 tumors were pan-sensitive (S7) vs 47.6 and 57.6% of grades 2 and 3

poor prognosis, limiting the ability to detect differences in subgroups. While there was heterogeneity among these various studies, the strength of the ancillary analysis of the GOG trials is the uniform delivery of therapy in a prospective clinical trial setting, and pathologic confirmation of tumor grade and histology required for enrollment.

The correlation between in vitro chemoresponse & tumor grade, as well as the correct definition of this response (S + I vs S) in women with EC is unknown. We compared our in vitro chemotherapy response to the RR reported in the literature for combination carboplatin/paclitaxel (CT) or cisplatin/doxorubicin/paclitaxel (TAP), the current standard of care therapy for advanced or recurrent EC. In our study, RRs based on in vitro chemotherapy response defined as S + I, were noted for the following agents: carboplatin, 77%; paclitaxel, 81%; cisplatin, 82%; and doxorubicin, 85%. These in vitro chemotherapy RRs are nearly twice the RRs reported in the 4 GOG trials studied by McMeekin et al. [4] However, when only S results are considered (carboplatin, 31%; paclitaxel, 36%; cisplatin, 28%; doxorubicin: 26%), our in vitro results are similar to those reported in several small phase II trials evaluating the use of single agents in chemo naïve patients with EC. For example, 20% of women with chemo naïve advanced or recurrent EC receiving single agent cisplatin achieved a response [12], compared to a 28% in vitro response in our analysis. Furthermore, our in vitro results were nearly identical to those seen with paclitaxel (14.3% CR, 21.4% PR) in GOG-860 and doxorubicin (RR 25%) in GOG-107 [10, 13]. No in vitro doublet assays were

performed for comparison with in vivo studies. Comparisons between the populations in these prior studies and our results are limited due to different dosing schedules as well as the in vitro vs. in vivo differences. However, the results suggest that in vitro studies may be applicable in predicting tumor response in vivo.

Data from epithelial ovarian cancer (EOC) specimens have compared in vitro assay response to clinical outcomes. Krivak and colleagues reported that in vitro assay resistance to carboplatin is associated with decreased PFS in women with advanced-stage EOC treated with platinum based therapy. Specifically, women whose tumor specimens demonstrated in vitro platinum resistance were at higher risk for disease progression compared to those with sensitive or intermediate sensitive assay results (median PFS: 11.8 vs 16.6 months, respectively, $P < .001$) [6]. In addition, our group compared in vitro assay response between Type I and Type II EOC and found that, despite the dogmatic belief that Type I EOC are chemoresistant, the majority (86%) of Type I tumors were chemosensitive to at least one cytotoxic agent and 35.7% were pan-S to all 7 agents tested [14]. Multi-drug resistance was twice as likely in women with Type I EOC compared to Type II EOC (pan-R, 14.3 vs. 6.8% ($p = 0.268$); pan-S, 35.7 vs. 51.2% ($p = 0.183$)), but did not reach statistical significance. Similarly, in our analysis in EC, 20% of grade 1 tumors were pan-sensitive. None of the grade 1 ECs were resistant to the 7 agents included in the cytotoxic panel, indicating that chemotherapy may be useful in the treatment of grade 1 advanced or recurrent disease. These recent studies demonstrate the clinical validity and utility of in vitro chemotherapy assays to direct therapy. Continued evaluation could further support the role of this test in clinical practice, especially given the interest in precision and personalized medicine.

Understanding the intricacies of molecular differences in EC histologies may be fundamental in directing targeted therapies. Data from The Cancer Genome Atlas (TCGA) have identified molecular signatures that may account for heterogeneity in treatment response for endometrioid endometrial tumors. While only a small percentage of grade 1 and 2 EECs have genetic fingerprints similar to serous endometrial cancers, almost 25% of grade 3 EECs possess signatures closely related to these more aggressive tumors [15]. This data supports the possibility of including grade 3 EECs with other Type II EECs. However, it is uncertain if these molecular signatures are associated with or can differentially predict response to chemotherapy in endometrioid cancers and Type II cancers. Additional analyses into molecular fingerprints of these malignancies have also helped to characterize pathways that may be involved in low grade, yet aggressive EEC in young women. While the PI3K pathway is a source of frequent mutations in EEC, differential expression of hotspot mutations have been noted in microsatellite stable vs. instable endometrial tumors [16]. As we learn more about the intricacies of the cancer genome, it is apparent that histology and tumor grade may not be the only factors that determine the behavior of these endometrial malignancies.

Limitations of this study include the lack of size equivalence between the tumor grade cohorts (namely, fewer tumors in the grade 1 cohort). In addition, not all tumors underwent chemosensitivity testing to all 7 agents as physicians could choose which drugs to submit, thus introducing a selection bias. Strengths of this study include the prospective collection of data that was routinely and comprehensively monitored, as well as the uniform preparation and performance of the chemosensitivity assay. Less than 20% of submitted samples fail the assay due to insufficient cell growth in culture or contamination. We were unable to assess the association between in vitro response results and clinical RR and survival outcomes due to limited clinical data.

## Conclusion

Based on our results, there does not appear to be an association between tumor grade and in vitro chemoresponse assay results. Specifically low grade EECs are not more likely to have resistant assay results compared to higher grade EECs. In addition, 50% of grade 1 EECs demonstrated in vitro sensitivity to at least one cytotoxic therapy, suggesting that chemotherapy may be useful in advanced low grade EECs. However, further clinical correlation is needed to assess assay sensitivity/resistance to

in vivo response and clinical outcomes to determine if chemoresponse assays may be useful to direct therapy in women with endometrioid endometrial cancer.

**Abbreviations**
AUC: Area under the dose response curve; C/T: Carboplatin/paclitaxel; EC: Endometrial cancer; EEC: Endometrioid endometrial cancer; EOC: Epithelial ovarian cancer; I: Intermediate; R: Resistant; RR: Response Rate; S: Sensitive; TAP: Cisplatin/doxorubicin/paclitaxel

**Acknowledgements**
Not applicable

**Authors' contributions**
BD designed and interpreted the statistical analyses and is the lead author of the manuscript. JF was a major contributor in the writing of the manuscript. SB provided the raw data & contributed to the statistical analysis. CT performed the majority of the statistical analyses. A.S. served as the primary mentor to BD on this research project and was a major contributor in writing the manuscript. L.H. served as the secondary mentor to BD and was a major contributor in writing the manuscript. All authors read and approved the final manuscript.

**Competing interests**
A.S. has served on Advisory Boards for Precision Therapeutics (now known has Helomics). The authors declare that they have no competing interests.

**Author details**
[1]Division of Gynecologic Oncology, Duke University Medical Center, Duke University, DUMC Box 3079, Durham, NC 27710, USA. [2]Product Development, Helomics Corporation, Pittsburgh, PA, USA.

**References**
1. Siegel RL, Miller KD, Jemal A. Cancer statistics, 2015. CA Cancer J Clin. 2015; 65(1):5–29.
2. Dottino JA, Cliby WA, Myers ER, Bristow RE, Havrilesky LJ. Improving NCCN guideline-adherent care for ovarian cancer: value of an intervention. Gynecol Oncol. 2015.
3. Doll A, Abal M, Rigau M, Monge M, Gonzalez M, Demajo S, et al. Novel molecular profiles of endometrial cancer-new light through old windows. J Steroid Biochem Mol Biol. 2008;108(3–5):221–9.
4. McMeekin DS, Filiaci VL, Thigpen JT, Gallion HH, Fleming GF, Rodgers WH, et al. The relationship between histology and outcome in advanced and recurrent endometrial cancer patients participating in first-line chemotherapy trials: a gynecologic oncology group study. Gynecol Oncol. 2007;106(1):16–22.
5. Davidson BFJ, Clarke LH, et al. Tumor grade and chemotherapy response in endometrioid endometrial cancer. 2015.
6. Krivak TC, Lele S, Richard S, Secord AA, Leath 3rd CA, Brower SL, et al. A chemoresponse assay for prediction of platinum resistance in primary ovarian cancer. Am J Obstet Gynecol. 2014;211(1):68. e1-8.
7. Rutherford T, Orr Jr J, Grendys Jr E, Edwards R, Krivak TC, Holloway R, et al. A prospective study evaluating the clinical relevance of a chemoresponse assay for treatment of patients with persistent or recurrent ovarian cancer. Gynecol Oncol. 2013;131(2):362–7.
8. Fleming GF, Brunetto VL, Cella D, Look KY, Reid GC, Munkarah AR, et al. Phase III trial of doxorubicin plus cisplatin with or without paclitaxel plus filgrastim in advanced endometrial carcinoma: a gynecologic oncology group study. J Clin Oncol. 2004;22(11):2159–66.
9. Fleming GF, Filiaci VL, Bentley RC, Herzog T, Sorosky J, Vaccarello L, et al. Phase III randomized trial of doxorubicin + cisplatin versus doxorubicin +

24-h paclitaxel + filgrastim in endometrial carcinoma: a gynecologic oncology group study. Ann Oncol. 2004;15(8):1173–8.

10. Thigpen JT, Brady MF, Homesley HD, Malfetano J, DuBeshter B, Burger RA, et al. Phase III trial of doxorubicin with or without cisplatin in advanced endometrial carcinoma: a gynecologic oncology group study. J Clin Oncol. 2004;22(19):3902–8.

11. Gallion HH, Brunetto VL, Cibull M, Lentz SS, Reid G, Soper JT, et al. Randomized phase III trial of standard timed doxorubicin plus cisplatin versus circadian timed doxorubicin plus cisplatin in stage III and IV or recurrent endometrial carcinoma: a gynecologic oncology group study. J Clin Oncol. 2003;21(20):3808–13.

12. Thigpen JT, Blessing JA, Homesley H, Creasman WT, Sutton G. Phase II trial of cisplatin as first-line chemotherapy in patients with advanced or recurrent endometrial carcinoma: a gynecologic oncology group study. Gynecol Oncol. 1989;33(1):68–70.

13. Ball HG, Blessing JA, Lentz SS, Mutch DG. A phase II trial of paclitaxel in patients with advanced or recurrent adenocarcinoma of the endometrium: a gynecologic oncology group study. Gynecol Oncol. 1996;62(2):278–81.

14. Previs R, Leath 3rd CA, Coleman RL, Herzog TJ, Krivak TC, Brower SL, et al. Evaluation of in vitro chemoresponse profiles in women with type I and type II epithelial ovarian cancers: an observational study ancillary analysis. Gynecol Oncol. 2015;138(2):267–71.

15. Cancer Genome Atlas Research N, Kandoth C, Schultz N, Cherniack AD, Akbani R, Liu Y, et al. Integrated genomic characterization of endometrial carcinoma. Nature. 2013;497(7447):67–73.

16 Marchio C, De Filippo MR, Ng CK, Piscuoglio S, Soslow RA, Reis-Filho JS, et al. PIKing the type and pattern of PI3K pathway mutations in endometrioid endometrial carcinomas. Gynecol Oncol. 2015;137(2):321–8.

# 6

# Diagnostic, therapeutic and evolutionary characteristics of cervical cancer in Department of Radiotherapy, Mohamed V Military Hospital – Rabat in Morocco

Mohammed Elmarjany[1], Abdelhak Maghous[2*], Rachid Razine[3], Elamin Marnouche[2], Khalid Andaloussi[1], Amine Bazine[1], Issam Lalya[1], Noha Zaghba[1], Khalid Hadadi[1], Hassan Sifat[1], Baba Habib[4], Jaouad Kouach[4] and Hamid Mansouri[1]

## Abstract

**Background:** Cancer of uterine cervix is the second most common cause of cancer related deaths among women. The aim of this study is to report the experience of Military Hospital Mohamed V in the management of cervical cancer and their results.

**Methods:** All cervical cancer managed at the radiotherapy department of Military Hospital Mohamed V between January 2005 and February 2010, were included for investigation of their demographic, histological, therapeutic and follow-up characteristics. Of the 162 cases managed, 151 (93.2 %) cases were treated in our department.

**Results:** In our study the median age was 51.5 years (33–82). The median duration of symptoms before diagnosis was four [3, 7] months. The major presenting complaints were abnormal vaginal bleeding (89.8 %). Squamous cell carcinoma cervix was seen in 86.2 % ($n = 137$), adenocarcinoma in 11.3 % ($n = 18$) and adenosquamous carcinoma in 2.4 % ($n = 4$). One hundred seventeen (84.8 %) cases were seen at late stage. An abdominal and pelvic computed tomography (CT) scan was performed in 34.6 % ($n = 56$) of cases, magnetic resonance imaging (MRI) in 62.9 % ($n = 102$). The pelvic lymph nodes were achieved in 16.6 % of cases.

Over half of patients 58.3 % ($n = 88$) were treated with a combination of external beam radiation therapy (EBRT) and a concurrent cisplatin based chemotherapy (40 mg /m2 weekly).

With a mean of 51.6 months (2 to 109), we recorded 19 (12.6 %) pelvic relapse and 15 (9.9 %) metastases. The median time to onset was 19.4 months (2–84 months). The local control rate was 63.6 % ($n = 96$) and 21 (13.9 %) patients were lost to follow-up. The overall survival (OS) at 3 years and 5 years was respectively 78.3 % and 73.6 % and the relapse-free survival (RFS) was respectively 80 % and 77.2 %.

**Conclusion:** Most of cervical cancer patients in Morocco are seen at late stage necessitating referral for radiotherapy, chemotherapy or palliative care. This may reflect lack of cervical screening in order to early detect and treat pre-malignant disease stage.

**Keywords:** Cancer of uterine cervix, Radiotherapy, Concomitant radio-chemotherapy

* Correspondence: magabdelhak@gmail.com
[2]National Institute of Oncology, Rabat, Morocco
Full list of author information is available at the end of the article

## Background

Cervical cancer is the second most common cancer in women worldwide [1]. It is estimated that there are more than 529 000 new cases diagnosed annually and more than 274,000 deaths in the world in 2008, of which more than 87 % occur in developing countries [2, 3]. Cervical cancer continues to be related to socio-economic and demographic (SEDS) disparities in both developing and developed countries. In the U.S., although the overall downward trend in cervical cancer there still exists a disproportion in mortality rates for cervical cancer related deaths among ages, racial, geographic and socio-economic groups [4, 5]. Analyses of the USA cancer data have shown that mortality due to cervical cancer increases with poverty and decreasing education [6]. Studies have publicized that late stage at diagnosis is correlated with lower survival rates [7]. It has also been reported that longer durations of symptoms as well as of treatment prolongation negatively affect survival [8, 9]. These two factors can therefore be useful predictors for the severity of illness and likelihood of survival.

In Morocco, cervical cancer is the second most common cancer of women after breast cancer [10]. According to GLOBOCAN 2008 [2], the world age-standardized incidence of cervical cancer among women in Morocco was 14.1 new cases/100 000 inhabitants/year (1979 new cases/year). The mortality rate from this cancer was 8.4 per 100 000. The stage of diagnosis is the most important independent factor of prognosis [11, 12]. In Morocco, a recent study [13] showed a late diagnosis of cervical cancer. Indeed, 43.7 % were presented with stage II at diagnosis (FIGO) and 38.1 % were presented in advanced stages (stages III and IV).

The aim of this study is to report the experience of Military Hospital Mohamed V in the management of cervical cancer, the various treatment modalities used and their results.

## Methods

This is a retrospective analytic study of 162 cervical cancer patients managed at the radiotherapy department of Military Hospital Mohamed V of Rabat in Morocco, between January 2005 and February 2010.

Data was collected using a well structured checklist containing important study parameters. The record collection includes patient demographic data (age of diagnosis, of marriage and age of first pregnancy (years)), menopausal status (premenopausal or postmenopausal) and parity was separated on three groups (0, 1–4 and ≥ 5). Data includes also clinical presenting symptoms (abnormal vaginal bleeding, offensive vaginal discharge, pelvis pain...), duration of symptoms (months), vaginal invading (free, upper, medium or lower vaginal wall) and other

clinical data such as classification FIGO of disease (IA, IB, IIA, IIB, IIIB, IVA, IVB), histological type (squamous, adenocarcinoma or adenosquamous), pelvic and/or lateral aortic adenopathy, parametrial invasion, date of primary diagnosis. The type and modalities of primary treatment (radiotherapy, chemotherapy, both or/and surgery), date and sites of relapse (pelvic and/or metastases), the follow up data, death date and date of last follow-up visit were also recorded.

Statistical analysis of the data was carried out by the SPSS for Windows (SPSS, Inc., Chicago, IL, USA). Qualitative variables were presented as number and percentages. Quantitative variables were presented as mean ± standard deviation for variables with normal distribution, and as median and interquartile range (IQR) for variables with skewed distributions. The survival rate was analyzed with the Kaplan-Meier method.

## Results

Of the 162 cases of cervical cancer managed, 151 (93.2 %) cases were treated in our department. Table 1 shows their epidemiological characteristics. Their ages ranged from 33 to 82 years old with a mean of 51.5 (±11.5) years. More than half of patients were post menopausal 85 (52.5 %) and married early 58 (63.7 %) Age of first pregnancy ranged from 14 to 36 with a mean of 20.3 (±4.2). Also, their parity ranged from 0 to 12 with a mean of 4.9 (±2.6).

Abnormal vaginal bleeding was the most common symptom reported by 143 (89.9 %) patients. Other symptoms were offensive vaginal discharge 91 (57.2) and pelvic pain 44 (27.7). The median duration of symptoms before diagnosis was four months [3, 7]. Tumor size was 4.8 cm (±1.6) clinically and in 64 (57.7 %) patient's upper vaginal wall was invaded. Squamous cell carcinoma 137 (86.2 %) was the leading histological type, whereas adenocarcinoma contributed 18 (11.3 %) and 4 (2.5 %) were adenosquamous carcinoma.

An abdominal and pelvic CT was performed in 34.6 % ($n = 56$) of cases, MRI in 62.9 % ($n = 102$). The pelvic lymph nodes were achieved in 16.6 % of cases. In MRI Tumor size was 41.6 (±16.8) mm and parametrial was invaded in 57 (55.9 %) of cases.

Based on International Federation of Gynaecology and Obstetrics classification for staging cervical cancer (ACS, 2008), 2 (1.4 %), 17 (12.3 %), 18 (13 %), 5 (3.6 %), 31 (22.5 %), 27 (19.6 %), 3 (2.2 %), 29 (21 %), 4 (2.9 %) and 2 (1.4 %) of cases, cancer stages were respectively IA, IB1, IB2, IIA, IIB proximal, distal IIB, IIIA, IIIB, VIA and VIB (Fig. 1).

One hundred fifty one (93.2 %) cases were treated in our department. Table 2 shows their modalities. Over half of patients 58.3 % ($n = 88$) were treated with a combination of external beam radiation therapy (EBRT) and

**Table 1** Clinical and para-clinical epidemiological characteristics (n = 162)

| Item | Frequency (%) | Range | Mean (±standard deviation) |
|---|---|---|---|
| Age of diagnosis (years) | | 33-82 | 51.5 (±11.5) |
| ≤39 | 21 (12.9) | | |
| 40–49 | 61 (37.6) | | |
| 50–59 | 45 (27.7) | | |
| 60–69 | 18 (11.1) | | |
| ≥70 | 17 (10.5) | | |
| Menopausal status | | | |
| Premenopausal | 77 (47.5) | | |
| Postmenopausal | 85 (52.5) | | |
| Age of marriage (years) | | 12-30 | 17.9 (±3.6) |
| ≤18 | 58 (63.7) | | |
| >18 | 33 (36.3) | | |
| Age of first pregnancy (years) | | 14-36 | 20.3 (±4.2) |
| Parity | | 0-12 | 4.9 (±2.6) |
| 0 | 5 (3.7) | | |
| 1-4 | 65 (47.8) | | |
| ≥5 | 66 (48.5) | | |
| Duration of symptoms (months) | | | 4 [3, 7] |
| Presenting complaints | | | |
| Abnormal vaginal bleeding | 143 (89.9) | | |
| Offensive vaginal discharge | 91 (57.2) | | |
| Pelvic pain | 44 (27.7) | | |
| Haematuria | 2 (1.3) | | |
| Clinically review | | | 4.8 (±1.6) |
| Tumor size (cm) | | | |
| Vaginal invading | | | |
| Upper | 64 (57.7) | | |
| Medium | 15 (13.5) | | |
| Lower | 4 (3.6) | | |
| Free | 28 (25.2) | | |
| Parametrial invasion | 95 (67.4) | | |
| Histological type | | | |
| Squamous cell carcinoma | 137 (86.2) | | |
| Adenocarcinoma | 18 (11.3) | | |
| Adenosquamous carcinoma | 4 (2.5) | | |
| Para clinical review | | | |
| Abdominal and pelvic CT | 56 (34.6) | | |
| Pelvic adenopathy | 12 (21.4) | | |

**Table 1** Clinical and para-clinical epidemiological characteristics (n = 162) *(Continued)*

| | | | |
|---|---|---|---|
| Lateral aortic adenopathy | 1 (1.8) | | |
| Pelvic MRI | | | 41.6 (±16.8) |
| Tumor size (mm) | 102 (93) | | |
| Pelvic adenopathy | 16 (15.7) | | |
| Parametrial invasion | 57 (55.9) | | |
| Hemoglobin (g/dl) | | | 11.8 (±1.8) |

a concurrent cisplatin based chemotherapy (40 mg /m2 weekly). Fifty (34 %) patients underwent surgery as their initial treatment. Forty six (31.4 %) of these received post operative radiotherapy or concomitant radio-chemotherapy following surgery due to positive pelvic lymphnodes, narrow or positive surgical margins or other poor risk factors. The surgical procedure was Piver II; a modified radical hysterectomy with annexectomy, which includes removal of the uterus, cervix, upper one-fourth of the vagina, and parametria. The surgeon also performs a bilateral pelvic lymphadenectomy via laparotomy in 57 (85.1 %) cases, who brought $4.7 \pm 3.9$ nodes on the right and $4.1 \pm 3.7$ nodes on the left, of which was only invaded in 18/471 (3.82 %). Conventional laparoscopy or robot-assisted laparoscopy was not available in our hospital.

Table 3, summarizes the various therapeutic modalities of different stages. Essentially our series contains 87 (63.1 %) patients with stage IIB and IIIB. These two stages are essentially treated with concomitant radio-chemotherapy.

With a mean follow-up of 51.6 months (2 to 109), we recorded 19 (12.6 %) pelvic relapse and 15 (9.9 %) metastases. The median time to onset was 19.4 months [2–33] and [34-84]. The local control rate was 63.6 % (n = 96) and 21 (13.9 %) patients were lost to follow-up. The overall survival (OS) at 3 years and 5 years was respectively 78.3 % and 73.6 % and the relapse-free survival (RFS) was

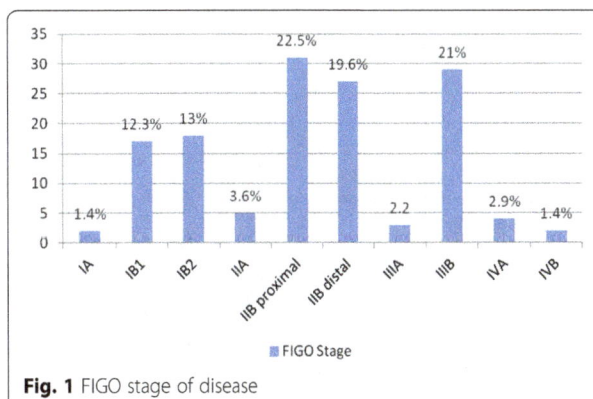

**Fig. 1** FIGO stage of disease

**Table 2** Therapeutic modalities ($n = 151$)

| Therapeutic modalities | Frequency (%) |
|---|---|
| Concomitant radio-chemotherapy | 66 (43.7) |
| Concomitant radio chemotherapy followed by surgery | 22 (14.9) |
| Exclusive radiotherapy | 12 (7.9) |
| Surgery followed by exclusive radiotherapy | 25 (16.6) |
| Surgery followed by concomitant radio chemotherapy | 21 (13.9) |
| Surgery alone | 4 (2.6) |
| Palliative chemotherapy | 1 (0.7) |

respectively 80 % and 77.2 % (Fig. 2). We tried to contact all patients who were lost to follow-up by phone and by sending correspondence letter without resulting from response.

As shown in Table 4, univariate analysis for clinical parameters as risk factors for relapse, the only independently significant variables were the Menopausal status ($p = 0.043$) and parity ($p = 0.010$). Women with advanced cervical cancer (distal IIB, III and IV) have a higher rate of relapse 16 (25.8 %) than those with early stage disease (I, IIA and proximal IIB) but there's statistically no significant.

Multivariate analysis was not performed for our patient because of the small number of events.

## Discussion

Cervical cancer has continued to have a devastating impact on women's health globally, and particularly in developing countries like Morocco where it has remained the second most common cancer of women after breast cancer [10].

The demographic characteristics of the patients in this study share similarities with results from several other centers in Morocco and North Africa. For instance, the mean age of patients in this study was 51.5 ($\pm11.5$) years and the high mean parity 4.9 ($\pm2.6$) agrees with the results from other studies [14, 15]. Elsewhere in Africa, the mean age was lower: 35 years in Dakar and 48 years in Burkina Faso [16] and Madagascar [17]. The older mean age in our study probably indicates a later exposure to risk factors or reflects the belated consultation and the lack of screening. These findings affirm that menopausal status and grand multiparity were significant causal risk factor for relapse.

The presenting complaints were essentially similar to the reports in the literatures reviewed. The higher incidence of abnormal vaginal bleeding reported in literature, affirm that is an important sign in cervical cancer. Abnormal vaginal bleeding normally occurs as post-coital, inter-menstrual, or postmenopausal bleeding. Should every case of abnormal vaginal bleeding be promptly investigated, cervical cancers would be diagnosed in early stages, at a time when there could be hopes of cure. However, due to the illiteracy, poverty, ignorance, non-utilization of screening services, the majority of the women present in late stage disease [13]. Initial evaluation of lymph nodes is commonly performed with CT or RMI to minimize expense, biopsy of suspected lymph nodes was not performed because it is not a standard in cervical cancer but PET and PET/CT are the imaging modalities used to provide information for treatment decisions [18–21]. In our study, no patients have PET because we do not have a pet scan this period. Actually, since 2012, we perform a PET/CT prior

**Table 3** Therapeutic modalities based on clinical stage

| Modalities | FIGO stage | | | | | | | | | |
|---|---|---|---|---|---|---|---|---|---|---|
| | IIIA | IA | IB1 | IB2 | IIA | IIB proximal | IIB distal | IIIB | IVA | IVB |
| Exclusive radiotherapy | 0 | 0 | 2 | 0 | 0 | 0 | 3 | 5 | 2 | 0 |
| | 0,0 % | 0,0 % | 16,7 % | 0,0 % | 0,0 % | 0,0 % | 25,0 % | 41,7 % | 16,7 % | 0,0 % |
| Concomitant radio-chemotherapy | 2 | 0 | 1 | 7 | 1 | 18 | 18 | 16 | 1 | 1 |
| | 3,1 % | 0,0 % | 1,5 % | 10,8 % | 1,5 % | 27,7 % | 27,7 % | 24,6 % | 1,5 % | 1,5 % |
| Surgery followed by exclusive radiotherapy | 0 | 1 | 10 | 3 | 0 | 3 | 0 | 0 | 0 | 0 |
| | 0,0 % | 5,9 % | 58,8 % | 17,6 % | 0,0 % | 17,6 % | 0,0 % | 0,0 % | 0,0 % | 0,0 % |
| Surgery followed by concomitant radio chemotherapy | 0 | 0 | 3 | 4 | 1 | 0 | 0 | 0 | 0 | 0 |
| | 0,0 % | 0,0 % | 37,5 % | 50,0 % | 12,5 % | 0,0 % | 0,0 % | 0,0 % | 0,0 % | 0,0 % |
| Concomitant radio chemotherapy followed by surgery | 1 | 0 | 0 | 2 | 2 | 9 | 5 | 3 | 0 | 0 |
| | 4,5 % | 0,0 % | 0,0 % | 9,1 % | 9,1 % | 40,9 % | 22,7 % | 13,6 % | 0,0 % | 0,0 % |
| Surgery alone | 0 | 1 | 0 | 1 | 0 | 0 | 0 | 0 | 0 | 0 |
| | 0,0 % | 50,0 % | 0,0 % | 50,0 % | 0,0 % | 0,0 % | 0,0 % | 0,0 % | 0,0 % | 0,0 % |
| Palliative chemotherapy | 0 | 0 | 0 | 0 | 0 | 0 | 0 | 0 | 0 | 1 |
| | 0,0 % | 0,0 % | 0,0 % | 0,0 % | 0,0 % | 0,0 % | 0,0 % | 0,0 % | 0,0 % | 100,0 % |

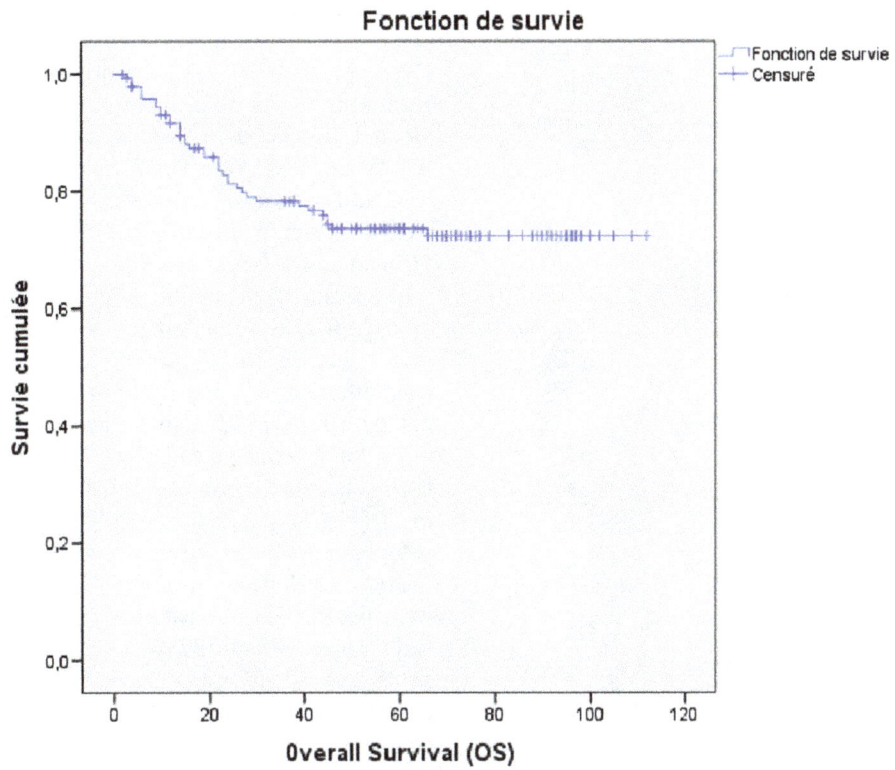

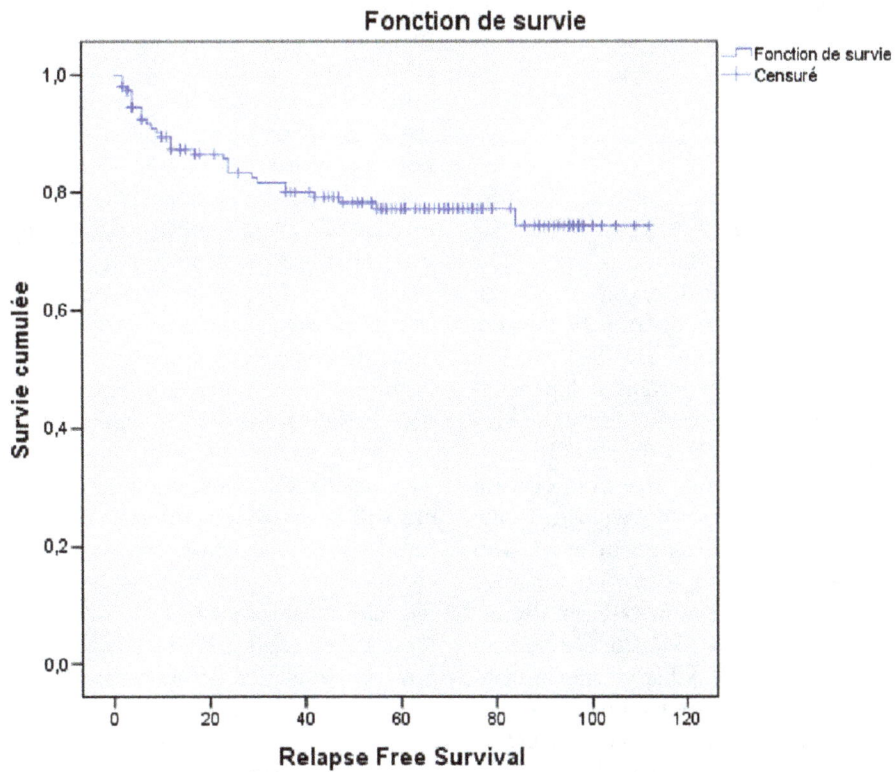

**Fig. 2** Global survival (GS) and relapse free survival (RFS)

**Table 4** Univariate analysis for clinical parameters associated with the occurrence of relapse and/or metastasis

| Characteristic | Pelvic relapse and/or metastases | | P value |
|---|---|---|---|
| | Yes (n = 31) | No (n = 120) | |
| Age | 47.97 ± 10.317 | 52.11 ± 11.54 | 0.071 |
| Menopausal status | | | 0.043 |
| Premenopausal | 20 (27.4 %) | 53 (72.6 %) | |
| Postmenopausal | 11 (14.1 %) | 67 (85.9 %) | |
| Age of marriage (years) | 18.57 ± 2.84 | 17.79 ± 3.86 | 0.393 |
| Age of first pregnancy (years) | 21.86 ± 4.26 | 19.97 ± 4.97 | 0.124 |
| Parity | 3.79 ± 2.04 | 5.19 ± 2.65 | 0.010 |
| Tumor size (cm) | 5.19 ± 2.01 | 4.62 ± 1.50 | 0.168 |
| Parametrial invasion | 21 (22.1 %) | 74 (77.9 %) | 0.596 |
| Histological type | | | 0.281 |
| Squamous cell carcinoma | 24 (18.8 %) | 104 (81.2 %) | |
| Adenocarcinoma | 6 (35.3 %) | 11 (64.7 %) | |
| Pelvic adenopathy | 4 (23.5 %) | 13 (76.5 %) | 0.658 |
| Hemoglobin (g/dl) | 11.62 ± 1.61 | 11.97 ± 1.88 | 0.448 |
| FIGO stage | | | 0.052 |
| I, IIA and proximal IIB | 8 (12.3 %) | 57 (87.7 %) | |
| Distal IIB, III and IV | 16 (25.8 %) | 46 (74.2 %) | |
| Therapeutic Modalities | | | 0.151 |
| Concomitant radio-chemotherapy | 18 (27.3 %) | 48 (72.7 %) | |
| Radio-surgery | 10 (14.7 %) | 58 (85.3 %) | |

to treatment to evaluate the extent of disease with particular attention to lymph node metastases to provide information to design radiation fields.

This study confirmed a delayed diagnosis of cervical cancer in Morocco. In fact, the majority of patients were presented in advanced stage (IB2-IVA) 117 (84.8 %). The stage of diagnosis is the most important independent prognostic factor [11, 12] and the survival rate at 5 years decreases with stage of diagnosis: 85 % for stage IB to 0-20 % for stage IV [22]. The mortality rate from cervical cancer is greatly dependent on stage of diagnosis. In the same way, the risk of pelvic recurrence increases with the stage, 10 % for stage IB to more than 75 % for stage IV [22, 23]. Finally, the risk of distant metastases also increases with the stage, respectively 16 %, 26 %, 39 % and 75 % for stages I, II, III and IV [24]. Early Clinical diagnosis has been responsible for the reduction of cervical cancer mortality achieved in developed countries before cervical screening programs were adopted [25–27].

Our pathological data joined those already described with the large predominance of squamous cell carcinoma [28, 29]; the most represented histological type in our study was squamous cell carcinoma 137 (86.2 %);

adenocarcinomas in 18 (11.3 %) and adenosquamous cell carcinomas represented only 4 (2.5 %) of cervical cancer. Over the past 40 years, multiple reports have documented the increase in relative distribution of adenocarcinoma compared to SCC in developed countries [30, 31]. In the USA, from 1973 to 1977, the proportions of SCC and adenocarcinoma were 88 % and 12 %, respectively; however, from 1993 to 1996, the proportions were 76 % and 24 % respectively [30].

In our study, treatment varied depending on the stage of diagnosis. Radiotherapy was indicated for the different stages. For advanced tumors (≥ stage II) concomitant chemotherapy was associated with radiotherapy and /or brachytherapy which join, in general, the recommendations for the management of invasive cervical cancer [32]. Whereas surgery was a part of treatment modalities in 71 (47.7 %) patients, which 50 (33.6 %) were operated before admission to our department without multidisciplinary consultation meetings. The reasons of surgery were intricate in our patients. It was indicated for very early stages (IA and IB2) in 15 (21.1 %) cases and for patients with adenocarcinoma in 14 (19.7 %) cases. It was also performed in 21 (29.5 %) case of poor response to concomitant chemoradiotherapy. Some locally advanced cervical cancer did not receive concomitant chemotherapy because of 6 (25 %) kidney failure and 11 (45.8 %) medical comorbidities or poor performance status associated.

In our population, the rate of relapse increased with the stage of diagnosis. This association shows the importance of early diagnosis. Morocco is endowed, since March 2010, of a National Plan for the Prevention and Control of Cancer (PNPCC). Screening and treatment of cervical cancer in Morocco represent the most crucial priorities for PNPCC. A screening program for cervical cancer is being introduced as well as other measures in order to improve the opportunities of access to early diagnosis by reducing geographical obstacles, multiply the number of centers of diagnosis confirmation, reduce economic barriers and provision facilities and resources. The installation of a screening program for cervical cancer will be based on infrastructure and personnel, primarily general practitioners, of primary level of health care delivery. A pilot mass screening performed in Lyon has clearly shown that intensive action, involving all local stakeholders including general practitioners, could reach a population of women who do not benefit from an adequate gynecological following-up [33].

We conducted our study in radiotherapy department of Military Hospital Mohamed V between January 2005 and February 2010. Despite recruits a small proportion of cancer cases, our center is accounted the one of public centers of cancer management in Morocco and we believe that our population can be considered as a representative sample of cases of cervical cancer who access to health system in Morocco.

## Conclusion

Cervical cancer most often afflicts women in developing countries. Our study confirmed a delayed diagnosis of cervical cancer in Morocco and affirmed that menopausal status and grand multiparity were significant causal risk factor for relapse. As in the literature, advanced stages are essentially treated with concomitant radio-chemotherapy.

Despite the limitation of our study, the results may represent an important tool in guiding the actions and measures of early diagnosis of cervical cancer in Morocco.

### Competing interests
The authors declare that they have no competing interests.

### Authors' contributions
AM and ME, performed research and share the first position on article; AM, RR and ME, analyzed data statistically; EM and AM, collected the clinical data; KA, AB, IL, KH, HS, BH, JK, NZ and HM, designed and coordinated research and drafted the manuscript. All authors read and approved the final manuscript.

### Acknowledgement
All the authors are thankful for providing the necessary facilities for the preparation the manuscript.
Special thanks are due to the Faculty of Medicine and Pharmacy of Rabat; the source(s) of funding for all authors.

### Author details
[1]Department of Radiotherapy, Mohamed V Military Hospital, Rabat, Morocco. [2]National Institute of Oncology, Rabat, Morocco. [3]Department of Public Health, Laboratory of Biostatics, Clinical Research and Epidemiology, School of Medicine and Pharmacy of Rabat, Rabat, Morocco. [4]Department of Gynecology, Mohamed V Military Hospital, Rabat, Morocco.

### References
1. Arbyn M, Castellsagué X, de Sanjosé S, Bruni L, Saraiya M, Bray F, et al. Worldwide burden of cervical cancer in 2008. Ann Oncol. 2011;22(12):2675–86.
2. Ferlay J, Shin HR, Bray F, Forman D, Mathers C, Parkin DM. Estimates of worldwide burden of cancer in 2008: GLOBOCAN 2008. Int J Cancer. 2010;127(12):2893–917.
3. Jemal A, Bray F, Center MM, Ferlay J, Ward E, Forman D. Global cancer statistics. CA Cancer J Clin. 2011;61(2):69–90.
4. Nelson DE, Bohen J, Marcus S, Wells HE, Meissner H. Cancer screening estimates for US metropolitan areas. Am J Prev Med. 2003;24(4):301–9.
5. Coughlin SS, King J, Richards TB, Ekwueme DU. Cervical cancer screening among women in metropolitan areas of the United States by individual-level and area-based measures of socioeconomic status, 2000 to 2002. Cancer Epidemiol Biomarkers Prev. 2006;15:2154–60.
6. Singh G, Miller B, Hankey B, Edwards B. Persistent socioeconomic disparities in US incidence of cervical cancer, mortality, stage and survival, 1975, 2000. Cancer. 2004;101:1051–7.
7. Vinh-Hung V, Bourgain C, Vlastos G, Cserni G, De Ridder M, Storme G, et al. Prognostic value of histopathology and trends in cervical cancer: a SEER population study. BMC Cancer. 2007;7:164.
8. Chen SW, Liang JA, Yang SN, Ko HL, Lin FJ. The adverse effect of treatment prolongation in cervical cancer by high-dose-rate intracavitary brachytherapy. Radiother Oncol. 2003;67(1):69–76.
9. Choan E, Dahrouge S, Samant R, Mirzaei A, Price J. Radical radiotherapy for cervix cancer: the effect of waiting time on outcome. Int J Radiat Oncol Biol Phys. 2005;61(4):1071–7.
10. Bouchbika Z, Haddad H, Benchakroun N, Eddakaoui H, Kotbi S, Megrini A, et al. Cancer incidence in Morocco: report from Casablanca registry 2005–2007. Pan Afr Med J. 2013;16:31.
11. Barillot I, Horiot JC, Pigneux J, Schraub S, Pourquier H, Daly N, et al. Carcinoma of the intact uterine cervix treated with radiotherapy alone: a French cooperative study: update and multivariate analysis of prognostics factors. Int J Radiat Oncol Biol Phys. 1997;38(5):969–78.
12. Fyles AW, Pintilie M, Kirkbride P, Levin W, Manchul LA, Rawlings GA. Prognostic factors in patients with cervix cancer treated by radiation therapy: results of a multiple regression analysis. Radiother Oncol. 1995;35(2):107–17.
13. Berraho M, Obtel M, Bendahhou K, Zidouh A, Errihani H, Benider A, et al. Sociodemographic factors and delay in the diagnosis of cervical cancer in Morocco. Pan Afr Med J. 2012;12:14. Epub 2012 May 25.
14. Berraho M, Bendahhou K, Obtel M, Zidouh A, Benider A, Errihani H, et al. Cervical cancer in Morocco: epidemiological profile from two main oncological centers. Asian Pac J Cancer Prev. 2012;13(7):3153–7.
15. Missaoui N, Hmissa S, Trabelsi A, Frappart L, Mokni M, Korbi S. Cervix cancer in Tunisia: clinical and pathological study. Asian Pac J Cancer Prev. 2010;11(1):235–8.
16. Lankoande J, Sakande B, Ouedraogo A, Ouedraogo C, Ouatara T, Bonane B, et al. Le cancer du col utérin: aspects épidémiocliniques et anatomopathologiques. Med Afr Noire. 1998;45(7):442–5.
17. Pignon T, Ratovonarivo H, Rafaramino F, Ruggieri S. La curiethérapie dans le traitement des cancers du col utérin à Madagascar. Bull Cancer Radiother. 1993;80:118–24.
18. Kumar R, Chauhan A, Jana S, Dadparvar S. Positron emission tomography in gynecological malignancies. Expert Rev Anticancer Ther. 2006;6:1033.
19. Rajendran JG, Greer BE. Expanding role of positron emission tomography in cancer of the uterine cervix. J Natl Compr Canc Netw. 2006;4:463.
20. Wolfson AH. Magnetic resonance imaging and positron-emission tomography imaging in the 21st century as tools for the evaluation and management of patients with invasive cervical carcinoma. Semin Radiat Oncol. 2006;16:186.
21. Sironi S, Buda A, Picchio M, Perego P, Moreni R, Pellegrino A, et al. Lymph node metastasis in patients with clinical early-stage cervical cancer: detection with integrated FDG PET/CT. Radiology. 2006;238:272–9.
22. Perez CA, Grigsby PW, Nene SM, Camel HM, Galakatos A, Kao MS, et al. Effect of tumor size on the prognosis of carcinoma of the uterine cervix treated with irradiation alone. Cancer. 1992;69(11):2796–806.
23. Rose PG, Java J, Whitney CW, Stehman FB, Lanciano R, Thomas GM, et al. Nomograms predicting progression-free survival, overall survival, and pelvic recurrence in locally advanced cervical cancer developed from an analysis of identifiable prognostic factors in patients from NRG ncology/Gynecologic Oncology Group randomized trials of chemoradiotherapy. J Clin Oncol. JCO.2014.57.7122. [Epub ahead of print].
24. Fagundes H, Perez CA, Grigsby PW, Lockett MA. Distant metastases after irradiation alone in carcinoma of the uterine cervix. Int J Radiat Oncol Biol Phys. 1992;24(2):197–204.
25. Ponten J, Adami HO, Bergstrom R, Dillner J, Friberg LG, Gustafsson L, et al. Strategies for global control of cervical cancer. Int J Cancer. 1995;60(1):1–26.
26. Sparen P, Gustafsson L, Friberg LG, Pontén J, Bergström R, Adami HO. Improved control of invasive cervical cancer in Sweden over six decades by earlier clinical detection and better treatment. J Clin Oncol. 1995;13(3):715–25.
27. Jacqueme B, Coudert C, Mabriez JC, Bonnier P, Piana L. Antécédents de dépistage cytologique chez les patientes traitées pour cancer infiltrant du col de l'utérus. Bull Cancer. 2002;89(2):234–40.
28. Gien LT, Beauchemin MC, Thomas G. Adenocarcinoma: a unique cervical cancer. Gynecol Oncol. 2010;116(1):140–6.
29. Karimi Zarchi M, Akhavan A, Fallahzadeh H, Gholami H, Dehghani A, Teimoori S. Outcome of cervical cancer in Iranian patients according to tumor histology, stage of disease and therapy. Asian Pac J Cancer Prev. 2010;11(5):1289–91.
30. Smith HO, Tiffany MF, Qualls CR, Key CR. The rising incidence of adenocarcinoma relative to squamous cell carcinoma of the uterine cervix in the United States: a 24-year population-based study. Gynecol Oncol. 2000;78(2):97–105.
31. Wang SS, Sherman ME, Hildesheim A, Lacey Jr JV, Devesa S. Cervical adenocarcinoma and squamous cell carcinoma incidence trends among white women and black women in the United States for 1976–2000. Cancer. 2004;100(5):1035–44.

# 7

# New classification of endometrial cancers: the development and potential applications of genomic-based classification in research and clinical care

A. Talhouk[1] and J. N. McAlpine[2*]

## Abstract

Endometrial carcinoma (EC) is the fourth most common cancer in women in the developed world. Classification of ECs by histomorphologic criteria has limited reproducibility and better tools are needed to distinguish these tumors and enable a subtype-specific approach to research and clinical care. Based on the Cancer Genome Atlas, two research teams have developed pragmatic molecular classifiers that identify four prognostically distinct molecular subgroups. These methods can be applied to diagnostic specimens (e.g., endometrial biopsy) with the potential to completely change the current risk stratification systems and enable earlier informed decision making. The evolution of genomic classification in ECs is shared herein, as well as potential applications and discussion of the essential research still needed in order to optimally integrate molecular classification in to current standard of care.

**Keywords:** Endometrial carcinoma, Histotype, The Cancer Genome Atlas (TCGA), Risk stratification, Prognosis, *POLE* mutations, Mismatch repair deficiencies, p53, Molecular classification

## Background

Cancer care in the last decade has featured a concerted move towards the personalization of patient care, often called precision medicine. In the field of cancer, this has meant a progression from broad categorization of tumors by anatomic site, to distinguishing subgroups by histomorphology, and more recently defining tumors by molecular features. This evolution has not happened over night and pace of change has varied by tumor site. Paradoxically, despite endometrial cancer being the most common gynecologic malignancy in women in Canada and the United States [1, 2] and the 6th most common cancer in women globally [3], research and clinical advancement have arguably lagged as compared to other cancers. This may be because over 75% of women diagnosed with endometrial cancer have early stage disease (stage I or II) and favorable outcomes (5-year overall survival 75–90%)

[4–6]. However, for those women who recur or for those who present with more advanced disease, response rates to conventional chemotherapy are low and clinical outcomes are extremely poor [7–10].

Renewed research focus on this disease site has been prompted by a dramatic increase in incidence observed in the developed world [2, 11–13]. In addition, there has been frustration with contemporary practice, in part due to inconsistent EC histomorphologic categorization, imprecise risk stratification, and diverse treatment strategies. Multidisciplinary panel recommendations on management of ECs [14] have emerged in an effort to make treatment (surgery, chemotherapy, radiotherapy, surveillance) more consistent. Multiple reviews on state of the art care of EC's have been published, and increasingly the repercussions of treatment on patient quality of life are being assessed in addition to survival parameters [6, 15–20]. Attention to this balance of treatment and sequelae may be even more essential in this disease site as there is concern that many women are likely over-treated or under-treated.

* Correspondence: jessica.mcalpine@vch.ca
[2]Department of Gynecology and Obstetrics, Division of Gynecologic Oncology, University of British Columbia, 2775 Laurel St. 6th Floor, Vancouver, BC, CanadaV5Z 1M9
Full list of author information is available at the end of the article

There has been a call for the incorporation of molecular features in to both classification and risk determination of ECs in order to better assess the biological behavior of an individual's disease and ultimately to improve treatment decisions and outcomes [21, 22]. The objective of this review is to focus on the new genomic framework used to categorize endometrial carcinomas. Herein we describe the evolution of molecular classification systems and how genomic characterization will impact both research approach and clinical management for this disease.

## Historical/Pathogenetic Classification of Endometrial Cancer

Thirty years ago, Bokhman hypothesized there were two pathogenetic types of endometrial carcinomas driven by very different metabolic and endocrine signals [23]. Type 1 is more common (~70–80%), consisting of endometrioid, low grade, diploid, hormone-receptor positive tumors that are moderately- or well-differentiated and more common in obese women. Patients presenting with Type 1 tumors tend to have localized disease confined to the uterus and a favourable prognosis. In contrast, Type 2 tumors (20–30%) are more common in non-obese women, of non-endometrioid histology, high-grade, aneuploid, poorly differentiated, hormone receptor negative and associated with higher risk of metastasis and poor prognosis. While this historical system of taxonomy has been useful, substantial heterogeneity within and overlap between Type I and II cancers is now recognized. Type I and Type II designation has never been part of the formal staging nor risk stratification, and thus has no clinical utility beyond providing a conceptual framework for understanding endometrial cancer pathogenesis.

## Endometrial classification by histomorphology and current systems of risk stratification

Tumor grade and histologic subtype assessment are subjectively assigned according to appearance under the microscope and predefined pathologic criteria. Nuclear features and the proportion of solid tumor vs. identifiable glands defines grade 1–3. Histologic subtype is assigned by morphologic criteria and often aided by immunostains. Pathologic accuracy is hampered by poor diagnostic reproducibility, especially in the case of high-grade subtypes (e.g. grade 3 endometrioid, serous). Studies describe inter-observer disagreement or lack of consensus on histologic subtype diagnosis in one-third or higher of ECs [24–27]. The overall kappa statistics for FIGO grade assignment between pathologists is 0.41–0.68, indicative of only moderate levels of inter-observer agreement [24, 28]. Agreement between diagnostic specimens and final hysterectomy is also limited [29–32]. In short, histologic classification is not accurate or precise

enough to effectively triage patients into optimal treatment groups.

Endometrial carcinoma has been a surgically staged disease since 1988. Surgery traditionally involves hysterectomy with bilateral salpingo-oophorectomy +/- lymph node dissection or sampling and omentectomy with several safe options in surgical approach [14, 33–35]. Extent of staging may vary according to patient age, comorbidities, cancer histology, grade, disease distribution, surgeon preference and institutional practice. Surgery alone is typically sufficient to cure early-stage EC [14, 36, 37], however, it is recognized that tumors with 'high-risk' features have a high likelihood of recurrence and adjuvant treatment (radiation and/or chemotherapy) is recommended [8, 16, 38, 39]. The major challenge is in distinguishing the features that comprise 'low-', 'intermediate-', and 'high-risk' disease in ECs. Multiple different risk predictive clinical models have been developed to guide treatment [14, 37, 40–48]. These have evolved with new FIGO staging and through interpretation of large clinical trials, however all incorporate the key pathological parameters of histotype, grade, and stage. As mentioned previously, the reproducibility of both histotype and grade have been demonstrated to be poor in EC's [24, 26, 27], thus two of three major criteria for risk group assignment which directly impacts recommendations for adjuvant treatment have limited reproducibility. Understandably, this makes it challenging to confidently make treatment decisions. We know that some women are undertreated who could have benefited from aggressive surgery, chemotherapy and/or radiation, and many may be overtreated having been cured by surgery alone.

The adequacy of risk stratification systems in EC have recently been compared and challenged [22, 49]. There are five major risk stratification systems in EC, of which the modified European Society of Medical Oncologists (ESMO) classification was demonstrated to best discriminate for recurrence and nodal metastases in apparent early stage disease [49]. However, none of the existing schemes were deemed highly accurate. In addition, all current systems stratify women based on pathologic data obtained *after* surgical staging (stage is a component of risk assignment). There is great need to obtain *earlier* and more *biologically informative* data from EC tumors that could assist in planning the optimal course of treatment for the individual. In addition, diagnostic tools that could objectively and consistently categorize ECs into distinct subgroups would enable stratification of clinical trials and study of treatment efficacy within biologically 'like' subgroups. Stemming from clinical need and a recognized inadequate/unsustainable system a call was made for the integration of molecular features.

## A new genomic era: molecular classification of endometrial carcinomas

Several research teams have defined immunohistochemical and/or mutation profiles to aid in distinguishing EC subtypes [50–58]. In one series, a set of seven immunohistochemical markers was able to improve the distinction between high-grade EC histotypes [28] and more recently, another team demonstrated a nine protein panel improved identification of both low and high-grade EC subtypes [57]. Sequencing has enabled further improvement, with a nine-gene panel, demonstrating distinct mutational profiles for the major EC histotypes [52]. Molecular data has also been used to further stratify risk categories; using gene expression profiling and copy number analysis to determine risk of recurrence [59, 60], even in apparent low stage disease [61]. Molecular characterization has also been pursued for potential therapeutic targets in EC, focusing on frequently mutated pathways such as PI3K/PTEN/AKT/mTOR. Further work is needed to define molecular biomarkers that more accurately reflect tumor susceptibility [62–66].

The most comprehensive molecular study of ECs to date has been The Cancer Genome Atlas (TCGA) project, which included a combination of whole genome sequencing, exome sequencing, microsatellite instability (MSI) assays, and copy number analysis [67]. Molecular information was used to classify 232 endometrioid and serous endometrial cancers into four groups - POLE ultramutated, MSI hypermutated, copy-number (CN) low, and CN high - that correlate with progression-free survival.

The ultramutated POLE subgroup was a novel finding from the TCGA, and generated interest due to its very favorable outcomes even within high-grade tumors. In TCGA, ultramutated cases were characterized by POLE exonuclease domain mutations (EDM), a high percent of C > A transversions, a low percent of C > G transversions, as well as more than 500 SNVs. POLE encodes the major catalytic and proofreading subunits of the Polε (Polymerase Epsilon) DNA polymerase enzyme complex responsible for leading strand DNA replication. The exonuclease proofreading function and the high fidelity incorporation of bases by POLE ensures a low mutation rate in the daughter strand. In ECs, POLE EDMs are mostly found in hotspot regions with V411L and P286R being the most common mutations. Substitutions in DNA polymerases were shown to inactivate or suppress proofreading abilities, thus causing increased replicative error rates and resulting in the ultra-mutated phenotype. In the TCGA, whole genome or exome sequencing was used to assess POLE status. Other series have subsequently assessed POLE status using more focused methods including Sanger sequencing [68, 69], gene panels [69–71], digital PCR [72–74] or functional assays [75] and confirmed very favourable outcomes for women with POLE aberrant ECs.

TCGA also described a molecular subgroup that exhibited microsatellite instability (MSI). MSI arises from defects in post-replicative DNA mismatch repair system. In the TCGA, MSI was determined by a panel of four mononucleotide repeat loci (polyadenine tracts BAT25, BAT26, BAT40, and transforming growth factor receptor type II) and three dinucleotide repeat loci (CA repeats in D2S123, D5S346, & D17S250) in addition to the recommended markers from the National Cancer Institute [76], tumor DNA was classified as microsatellite- stable (MSS) if zero markers were altered, low level MSI (MSI-L) if one to two markers (less than 40%) were altered and high level MSI (MSI-H) if three or more markers (greater than 40%) were altered. Mismatch repair deficiencies can result from i) an inherited cancer syndrome (e.g., Lynch), ii) acquired/somatic mutations or iii) epigenetic events e.g. methylation of one of the genes involved in mismatch DNA repair, most commonly MLH1.

Finally TCGA distinguished a distinct molecular subgroup by copy number analysis. Copy number was determined using Affymetrix SNP 6.0 microarrays using DNA originating from frozen tissue. Hierarchical clustering identified significantly reoccurring amplifications or deletions regions and a 'copy number (CN) high' subgroup. All remaining samples that did not belong to the POLE ultramutated group, the MSI group, or the CN high group, were termed CN low. The appeal of objective molecular categorization of new EC cases into one of four prognostic subgroups was immediately apparent. However, methodologies used for the TCGA study were costly, complex and unsuitable for wider clinical application.

Two research teams, including our own, have subsequently developed more pragmatic methodologies to evaluate molecular features of ECs, working in standard formalin-fixed paraffin-embedded tissue. These methods do not identify molecular subgroups that are identical to TCGA but do recapitulate the four survival curves observed in TCGA [69, 71, 73, 77] (Fig. 1). Stelloo et al. [69, 71] used a combination of TP53 mutational testing and p53 IHC to determine p53 status obtained from sequencing as a surrogate for CN high TCGA subgroup. The promega MSI analysis system was used to determine MSI status. For tumors exhibiting low levels of instability or from which extracted DNA quality was poor, immunohistochemistry for mismatch repair (MMR) proteins (MLH1, MSH2, MSH6, and PMS2) was performed. POLE EDM hotspot mutations were identified by Sanger sequencing. This team also tested for hotspot mutations (159) across 13 genes (BRAF, CDKNA2, CTNNB1, FBXW7, FGFR2, FGFR3, FOXL2, HRAS, KRAS, NRAS, PIK3CA, PPP2R1A, and PTEN). Testing ultimately yielded four molecular subgroups: group 1 - p53 (mutation identified), group 2- MSI, group 3 –POLE (POLE EDM identified), and

**a**  Leiden/TransPORTEC molecular classification

New sample

- Failed molecular classification
- Multiple classifying alterations

······▶ unclassifiable

| Group 1 p53 | Group 2 MSI | Group 3 POLE | Group 4 NSMP |
|---|---|---|---|
| p53 mutation (assessed by IHC validated by sequencing) | MSI assay validated by IHC (MLH1, MSH2, MSH6, PMS2) | POLE EDM by sequencing exon 9 and 13 | |

**b**  ProMisE /Vancouver group molecular classification

New sample

MMR-Deficient / MMR intact

MMR IHC missing ······▶ unclassifiable

MMR-D

POLE mutated / POLE wild type

POLE missing ······▶ unclassifiable

POLE EDM

p53 IHC missing ······▶ unclassifiable

p53 IHC(1+) / p53 IHC (0 or 2+)

p53 wt    p53 abn

Fig. 1 Schematic of the **a** Leiden/TransPORTEC and **b** ProMisE/Vancouver molecular classification systems including testing performed, molecular subgroups identified, and by what criteria cases would be considered unclassifiable

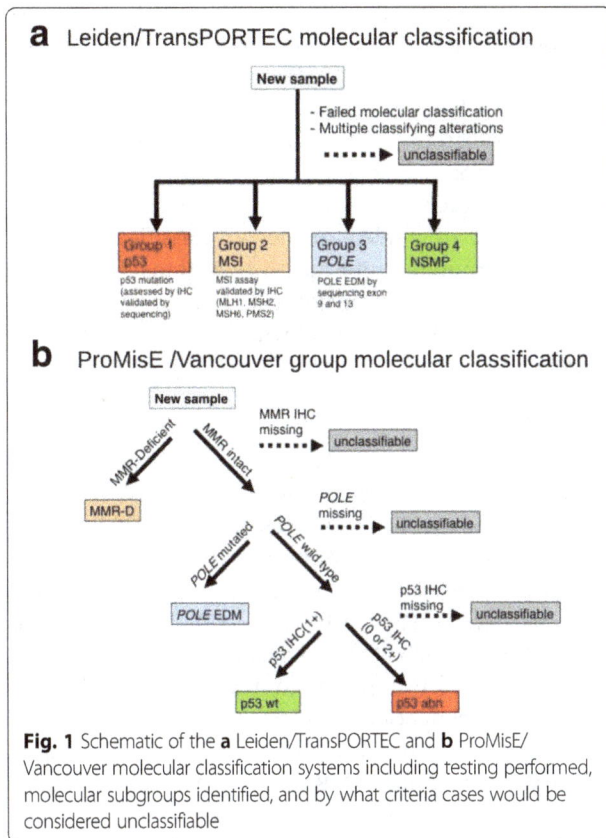

finally group 4 –NSMP, a group with 'no specific molecular profile' (Fig. 1a). Tumors with insufficient tissue to perform all molecular testing were not classified and tumors with more than one molecular feature, constituting 2–3% of the cohort, were also not classified. Due to this exclusion, the order of mutational testing was irrelevant. This research team initially assessed ECs from the PORTEC3 trial (n = 116), with known high risk features. Recurrence-free survival and time to distance metastasis were assessed within the four molecular subgroups. They observed that patients belonging to the POLE and the MSI subgroups showed similar and much better survival outcomes in comparison to the p53 mutant group and the NSMP group which exhibited worse recurrence and distance metastasis outcomes even within the endometrioid histology cases. Differences in survival patterns relative to the TCGA results were attributed to a greater proportion of high-risk features in the PORTEC 3 cohort.

The Leiden/TransPORTEC group has since applied the same series of molecular tests to a larger, more diverse cohort [71]. However, survival analysis and assessment of prognostic ability was restricted to endometrioid subtype and stage 1 tumors of patients with intermediate clinical risk. Within this very specific group, the observed outcomes associated with each molecular subgroup more closely mirrored TCGA.

Our research team has also developed a molecular classification system that uses practical methodologies to assign ECs to one of four molecular subgroups with distinct survival outcomes. We have followed the Institute of Medicine (IOM) guidelines for the development of 'omics based tests [78], initially exploring 16 models in a 'discovery' cohort (n = 141) [73], next locking down sequence of testing and methods to a single model termed ProMisE (Proactive Molecular Risk Classifier for Endometrial Cancer) on a new 'confirmation' cohort (n = 319) [77, 79] to prove feasibility and confirm the association with outcomes/prognosis, and finally testing in a large 'validation' cohort (n = ~500) of ECs from collaborators at the University of Tübingen (Germany). Molecular decision tree analysis for ProMisE is outlined in Fig. 1b. Specific methodologies include immunohistochemistry (IHC) for the detection of the presence/absence of two mismatch repair (MMR) proteins: MSH6 and PMS2. This identifies 'MMR-D' (deficient) subgroup. Cases are then sequenced using digital PCR to identify POLE exonuclease domain mutations ('POLE EDM'). Finally, cases are assessed using IHC for p53 (wild type vs. null or missense mutations; 'p53wt' and 'p53abn', respectively). We have demonstrated that women within each molecular subgroup have clinicopathological characteristic that have consistently been shown to be typical of that group. For example, the p53 abn subgroup usually encompasses the highest proportion of high grade, advanced stage, non-endometrioid histotypes and arises in older, thinner women. Similarly, the emerging phenotype of women whose EC harbor POLE EDMs is of particular interest since it generally includes younger, thinner and with surprisingly aggressive pathologic features (large proportion of grade 3 tumors, many with deep myometrial invasion and LVSI) yet consistently exhibit favorable outcomes. The MMR-D subgroup have very similar 'uterine factors' (clinicopathologic features in the uterus itself) [48] to the POLE subgroup, i.e. a comparable proportion of high grade tumors and deep myometrial invasion and LVSI, yet they have worst observed outcomes of any group next to p53abn [77, 79]. On multivariable analysis, ProMisE molecular subgroup assignment maintained its association with overall survival (OS), progression free survival (PFS) and recurrence free survival (RFS) even after correction of other clinicopathologic parameters of known prognostic significance available at time of diagnosis/collection of diagnostic specimen for molecular analysis (e.g., age, BMI, grade, histotype but not stage).

Both ProMisE (across all tumors tested), and the Leiden classifier (within the intermediate-risk group examined) demonstrate comparable risk discriminatory ability to the ESMO risk stratification system. Furthermore when clinical and pathological features were integrated with molecular features they resulted in improved risk stratification. Through evaluation of the collective cohort (discovery +

confirmation + validation cohorts = ~ 1000 ECs) we plan to evaluate which key clinicopathological parameters can add value to molecular classification giving high priority to those features available at time of diagnosis (e.g., age, BMI).

Our goal has consistently been to develop a molecular classification tool that could be applied to diagnostic specimens (endometrial biopsy or curettage) and therefore inform treatment at the earliest time point. Biologically relevant information about an individual's tumor could guide surgical urgency and aggressiveness, fertility or hormonal function sparing management options, adjuvant therapy, and/or surveillance schedules. We have demonstrated high concordance between ProMisE molecular classification in diagnostic vs. final hysterectomy samples, far superseding concordance of grade, or histotype as assigned on original pathology reports or within or between reviews by expert gynecologic cancer pathologists [80]. The Leiden team has also shown high concordance of molecular tumor alterations between pre-operative curettage specimens and final hysterectomy specimens (13 gene panel and MSI assay) [81] and a multicenter, prospective trial in Holland is in process to see if surgical management can be improved [82]. As diagnostic specimens are fixed immediately (in contrast to a hysterectomy specimen that may sit for hours in an operating room before processing in pathology), the quality of DNA extracted and fixation for IHC is high. We believe one of the most exciting aspects of molecular classification and what will be most impactful in directing care for women with EC will be this capability of determining earlier prognostic (and possibly predictive) information.

Ultimately, integration of molecular classification by either method into current practice, as performed on diagnostic specimens or final hysterectomy, will need to be studied in the context of a prospective clinical trial; comparing survival outcomes, quality of life and health economic implications to conventional/historical standard of care.

## Challenges with molecular classification: key components

The Leiden/TransPORTEC and Vancouver/ProMisE pragmatic molecular classification systems incorporate the same integral components: identification of ECs with mismatch repair deficiency/microsatellite instability, POLE exonuclease domain mutations and aberrant p53. Similarities and differences are shown in Fig. 1. Prognostic strength of molecular classification is at least equivalent to other clinicopathological features or risk stratification systems but offers the advantage of objective results (e.g., presence or absence of a protein or mutation). We believe these key molecular components are unlikely to be outperformed by any single clinicopathological parameter or biomarker. Notably, as yet none of the additional immunohistochemical

markers we have tested across our endometrial cancer cases have outperformed ProMisE. Although we and others are investigating the immune landscape and specific immunohistochemical biomarkers within the context of these major molecular subgroups these studies will not be covered in this manuscript. Should any parameter improve the ability to discern outcomes and guide management beyond the ProMisE or Leiden molecular classification, they can be incorporated into future algorithms. Herein, we focus on some of the major challenges and considerations for future implementation of molecular classification.

### MMR/MSI

There are different techniques for the identification of mismatch repair deficiency [76, 83–87]. Both TCGA and the Leiden series use microsatellite instability (MSI) assays. These have primarily been utilized in research, not clinical practice settings (there are no FDA-approved MSI tests) and require DNA extraction from tumor as well as normal tissue or blood for comparison. ProMisE tests for the presence of two mismatch repair proteins (MSH6, PMS2) by immunohistochemistry and we have shown high concordance between MMR IHC and MSI assay methods [83]. IHC staining for MMR and interpretation is routine for most pathology laboratories. Unfortunately, although histomorphologic surrogates for MMR deficiency or Lynch syndrome have been explored (e.g., tumor infiltrating and/or peritumoral lymphocytes, dedifferentiated histology, lower uterine segment origin) [88, 89], as yet they have not proven to be equivalent to molecular confirmation.

Although all MMR deficiencies are often grouped together, for inherited mutations (Lynch syndrome), the lifetime risk and age of penetration of Lynch-associated cancers can vary substantially according which gene is aberrant [90]. This may impact recommendations regarding the timing of screening or intervention e.g., lower lifetime risk and later average age of penetration for individuals with aberrant MSH6 [90–93] might enable delay of recommended risk reducing surgery as compared to other Lynch mutations.

Prognostic and predictive implications of mismatch repair may also vary according to specific MMR gene mutation or protein loss identified. It has been hypothesized that epigenetic/methylation events in mismatch repair likely have different implications on tumor characteristics and clinical outcomes than germline defects e.g. an age-related somatic event would not be expected to promote the development of tumor that is equivalent to one arising in a young individual harboring a germline mutation. Immune environment, intrinsic biologic behavior, toleration of adjuvant therapy/response to cell injury may vary significantly in these individuals. This may partially explain the relatively wide range of response to immunotherapy within

MMR-D cases. At present, all mismatch repair deficiencies are lumped together but further interrogation of these differences (e.g. subgroups of subgroups) is warranted. Recently, over 1000 women with EC had their tumors evaluated for microsatellite instability, *MLH1* methylation, and MMR protein expression as part of a combined NRG Oncology/Gynecologic Oncology Group Study (GOG210) [94]. Categories of normal mismatch repair, epigenetic defect and probable mutation (somatic or germline) were compared to clinicopathologic variables and clinical outcomes in the trial cohort. Even with this large number of cases, these three broad categories of MMR status were not shown to be associated with PFS or DSS. Univariate analysis did suggest potentially worse PFS for women whose tumors had epigenetic defects (trend, *p* = 0.1) but this association was not maintained after adjusting for other factors, including the highly relevant parameter of age in this cohort. In addition, the authors observed a trend to improved PFS in tumors with MMR mutations and a suggestion that these patients received greater benefit from adjuvant chemotherapy compared to women with normal mismatch repair. Similar results for probable germline/Lynch syndrome mismatch repair deficient tumors were observed in a smaller series of 221 ECs, with no prognostic nor predictive associations noted in the tumors with methylation events [95].

## POLE

Several research teams have characterized *POLE* mutated tumors by histomorphology and immune environment [96–101]. Obvious clinical implications for tumors with substantial immune infiltrates include selection for anti-PD-1 therapy. However, the highly favorable outcomes observed in women with *POLE* mutated tumors would suggest that costly targeted therapy might better be reserved for the very rare cases of recurrent or advanced disease [102, 103]. *POLE* somatic mutations are found in less than 10% of endometrial carcinomas and recurrence is seldom observed; thus, it has been difficult for a single study to be adequately powered to determine optimal management of women whose tumors harbour this molecular feature. Adjuvant treatment is commonly administered due to the frequency of 'high-risk' features in ECs with *POLE* EDMs (e.g., relatively high frequency of grade 3, deep myometrial invasion, LVSI) but whether this is over treatment of women who would do well based on their *POLE* genotype alone or whether treatment is needed and favorable outcomes are secondary to exquisite sensitivity to DNA damaging agents in these tumors is as yet unclear.

The paradox of observed aggressive histopathologic features but excellent survival outcomes may in part be explained by the high neoantigen load and immune rich microenvironment in tumors with *POLE* EDMS (and to a lesser degree, also described in MMR-D tumors).

Both sequencing and functional assays currently employed for *POLE* mutation testing are more costly than IHC and utilize methods that require a skilled team to perform and interpret. We, and others, continue to search for surrogates for *POLE* sequencing. Although the clinical and pathological phenotype of women with *POLE* mutated tumors is beginning to be characterized; on average younger, lower BMI, high proportion of grade 3, LVSI+, predominantly endometrioid, and low stage, these parameters overlap with other molecular subgroups. At present there is no single pathognomonic surrogate for this feature.

## p53

The mutational spectrum of *TP53* mutations within ECs was recently described in Schultheis et al. [104], both in the context of histotype and across TCGA molecular subgroups. This study confirmed the very high proportion (91%) of *TP53* mutations in the 'CN high' TCGA category but also seen in 35% of the *POLE* genomic subgroup. No clinical correlative data was provided with their paper but our series and others confirm the highly favorable outcome of POLE mutation carriers even with the identification of other mutations traditionally associated with high risk disease. The order of our categorization: identification and removal of *POLE* subgroup prior to p53 stratification thus seems to be of great importance (see tumors with >1 molecular feature below). Also described in this series was the presence of frameshift or nonsense TP53 mutations (22% of *TP53* mutant subset) of which they acknowledge would yield different IHC results (loss or IHC score 0) than missense variants (IHC score 2). Identification of both aberrant states is essential. Our team, in collaboration with others is in the process of further characterizing both *TP53* mutational and IHC status in ECs in order to better guide interpretation in this disease site.

## Tumors with more than one molecular feature

Both Talhouk et al. [77, 79] and Stelloo [71] et al. describe approximately 2-3% of endometrial tumors having more than one of the key molecular features described. Reported frequency of post-replication *POLE* proofreading defect *and* a DNA mismatch repair defects varies in the literature, but in series where co-occurrence is higher, this has been attributed to somatic MMR mutations which may be secondary to the ultra-mutated *POLE* phenotype. [67, 70, 98]. Similarly, it is perhaps not surprising that in both the *POLE* and MMR-D subgroups of ECs with high mutational loads, tumors may also harbour *TP53* mutations (as evidenced by either sequencing, or complete loss or overexpression of p53 protein on

IHC) [71, 77, 79, 104]. The order of testing for molecular classification is therefore critically important. Determination of *POLE* status prior to p53 testing will categorize a given EC as *POLE* EDM. Favorable outcomes are therefore anticipated for that individual, and indeed for cases reported thus far with dual features, that has been observed [77]. We believe testing for MMR-D first is still valid, as that information is arguably more actionable than *POLE* status (referral for hereditary testing, consideration of immunotherapy) which is not currently integrated into treatment algorithms. Ultimately, distinguishing between what are likely passenger mutations or late events without functional consequence as compared to mutations that define biologic behavior is essential. Molecular classification tools that utilize large gene panels may detect a plethora of coexisting mutations in *POLE* EDM ECs and need to be interpreted with caution e.g., discovery of *BRCA1* or *BRCA2* mutation in a *POLE* mutated EC may not indicate homologous recombination deficiency / PARPi efficacy [105].

Clinical outcomes may be harder to discern between ECs demonstrating both MMR deficiency and p53 mutations and the 'best' categorization of these tumors remains to be determined. At present, molecular classification will first identify the MMR deficiency at least enabling patients to be referred for hereditary counselling and providing opportunities in genotype specific clinical trials.

### Genotype-phenotype interplay

Genotype-phenotype interactions have been appreciated and characterized in recent years. Although not the focus of this review, we will take this opportunity to describe one highly relevant example.

It is now appreciated that PTEN loss has different prognostic implications in lean vs obese individuals. Mutations in the central relay pathways of insulin signals (phosphatidylinositol 3-kinase (PI3K) pathway including mutations specifically in PIK3CA, PIK3R1 and PTEN) are extremely common in ECs yet prior studies on the prognostic significance of PTEN mutations had markedly discordant results. Westin et al. stratified cases by body mass index (BMI) revealed improved progression free survival in obese (BMI >30) women with endometrioid endometrial carcinoma suggesting an interaction between metabolic state and genetics [106]. Subsequently, a constellation of 'obesity related' genes are observed to be upregulated with increasing BMI among endometrioid carcinomas in the TCGA cohort [107], and different targets for treatment were suggested in obese vs non-obese individuals [108]. Given the global epidemic of obesity and associated 'metabolic syndrome', this clinical context is essential to know in guiding clinical management and in research/ interpretation of data. In our own series, for example, we anticipate, that further stratification of cases within

the p53 wt subgroup (and possibly within MMR-D) by BMI status may refine prognosis further. We are in the process of examining the interaction of PTEN and BMI within the ProMisE molecular subgroups across all of our evaluable cohorts.

### Rare histotypes and diversity within tumors

The role of molecular classification in rare histotypes of endometrial carcinoma has not been determined. The TCGA was restricted to cases of endometrioid and serous histology, however, the TransPORTEC cohorts and our own series included other histologies; 15% clear cell, and a combination of 6% clear cell, carcinosarcoma, undifferentiated, and mixed, in the cohorts respectively [69, 77, 79]. Fundamental features of the immunophenotype for dedifferentiated, clear cell, and mixed carcinomas have been reported [50, 54, 109–111]. Assessment of mixed tumors show that despite morphologic differences/mimicry, the majority of molecular aberrations are shared across the tumor [112]. Thus the application of ProMisE or Leiden classification systems to these cancers may be of value. Indeed in the small number of non-serous, non-endometrioid cases studied thus far, histotypes were distributed across the molecular subgroups (not confined to p53 abn subgroup). We anticipate there will be deeper characterization of unique genomic categories; e.g., dedifferentiated carcinomas within p53 wt subgroup with mutations in the SWI/ SNF pathway.

Intratumoral heterogeneity in EC has been described [113, 114], and might be predicted to weaken the utility of ProMisE. However, in the cases examined, although single nucleotide variations and copy number analysis revealed some diversity between anatomic sites within an individual (at time of diagnosis) the ProMisE molecular subgroup categorization was concordant across all tumor sites (6–14 anatomic sites examined per individual) [114]. We have reported on a case of discordant ProMisE categorization between a diagnostic endometrial biopsy and final hysterectomy specimen in an individual with a dedifferentiated endometrial carcinoma [80]. This was secondary to concurrent low grade and high grade areas within the endometrium and myometrium where mismatch repair profiles differed. In rare cases, in which diverse tumor morphology is observed it may be that more than one area needs to undergo molecular testing. Certainly, gross and microscopic assessment of endometrial cancers by pathologists will need to continue just as relevant post staging data on metastases may be weighed in management. Successful integration of molecular classification will require addressing all of these issues over time, but in the interim, we anticipate a mix of current practice (histomorphologic categorization) and molecular tools for assessment of newly diagnosed ECs.

## Conclusions

We have harboured too long in a system of irreproducible categorization of endometrial carcinomas, inconsistent management within and across cancer centers, and inappropriate research investigations that grouped diverse tumors for study, making advances in research and clinical management slow or impossible in this disease site. It is essential that biologically relevant molecular features are assessed and considered for categorization of tumors, and in deciding surgical management and adjuvant therapy. This does not require abandonment of clinicopathologic parameters, many of which have been demonstrated to maintain prognostic relevance even in the post-TCGA era, but rather not to rely on them as the only or most important feature to guide management.

We have shown that in the hands of two independent research teams molecular classification of endometrial carcinomas is feasible, and identifies four prognostically distinct subgroups. Historical segregation of Type I (mostly CN low, p53 wt cases) and Type II ECs (mostly CN high, p53 abn subgroups) is inadequate and do not account for the approximately 30% of cases that are MMR-D or *POLE* EDM. All components of the molecular classifier together can be achieved at a cost* comparable to other commonly utilized clinical assays in cancer care. At minimum, this system provides objective reproducible categorization of EC's. Familiarity with MMR and p53 IHC testing and interpretation lends to rapid adoption in any pathology department. The reproducibility of ProMisE across Canadian cancer centers is currently being evaluated.

Additional benefits of molecular classification include early identification of women who may have an inherited genetic syndrome (Lynch) who would benefit from additional screening or interventions for other Lynch-associated cancers or in whom specific therapies for their

**Table 1** Potential changes in practice through molecular categorization

| | Immediate? | Future Studies |
|---|---|---|
| **Overall** | • Reproducible categorization<br>• Stratification of trials: past and future, e.g. GOG 210, PORTEC4a | • Characterization of tumours with two or more molecular features<br>• Modeling: which features (clinical, pathological, IHC)* can be added to molecular classification to improve the ability to discern outcomes<br>• Health economic implications<br>• QoL and patient reported outcomes |
| **MMR-D** | • Referred for hereditary cancer counselling and testing<br>• Options in immunotherapy | • Further characterization of predictive and prognostic differences within MMR-D: specific mutations, germline vs. somatic, and epigenetic |
| **POLE EDM** | • Options in immunotherapy (for rare recurrence or advanced disease unresponsive to conventional Rx) | • Can adjuvant therapy be withheld? Determination of role of treatment in tumors with POLE EDMs: are favorable outcomes independent of therapy?<br>• Possible hormonal management/fertility sparing Rx in young women desiring childbearing |
| **p53 wt** | • Lower likelihood metastatic disease: hysterectomy/BSO, managed in community (?) | • Possible hormonal management/fertility sparing Rx in young women desiring childbearing<br>• What additional parameters* can further direct management within this subgroup? |
| **p53 abn** | • Fertility sparing Rx not recommended<br>• Complete/aggressive surgical staging<br>• High likelihood will require adjuvant chemotherapy +/- radiation | • Stratification of clinical trials within molecular subgroup |

*Features that have been historically used in risk classification or are considered prognostic markers in other series

endometrial carcinomas may be more effective. For young women with EC considering delay of hysterectomy for fertility reasons (e.g., progesterone therapy), molecular classification of her diagnostic endometrial specimen could help guide management as either MMR-D (depending on germline results post hereditary cancer referral) or p53 abn categorization would discourage a conservative approach. It is still unclear how knowing the *POLE* mutation status within an individual's EC will impact her clinical management, as favorable outcomes observed in these individuals may be either independent or secondary to increased sensitivity to DNA damaging agents (chemotherapy, radiation), and withholding treatment cannot yet be advised. Plausibly, women with p53 abn tumors with higher association of metastatic disease and aggressive clinical course would be recommended to undergo more comprehensive surgical staging and closer surveillance.    Conversely, biologically indolent tumors may be cured by simplified surgery alone and perhaps spared toxic treatment and managed by community gynecologists.

We are at an exciting juncture, but aware of the many questions still remaining (Table 1). Through clinical trials, we need to determine how molecular classification can be best integrated in to current clinical care and how will it impact outcomes. What, if any, additional parameters can better inform management? Interrogation of genotypic and phenotypic features may provide additional prognostic and predictive information. These can now be explored within the context of the four major molecular categories of tumors, and even within molecular subgroups. How reliable are IHC surrogates for mutational data in endometrial cancer? Characterization of p53 and other markers, as has been achieved in ovarian cancer [115] is needed for this disease site. Can molecular classification help interpret the natural history and direct management of cases that have historically been a great challenge to manage e.g., grade 3 endometrioid carcinoma? What is the natural history of ECs with two molecular features e.g. MMR-deficient and aberrant p53? How often are these tumors encountered and how should they be categorized? Is there a surrogate that could replace sequencing for *POLE*? Are favorable outcomes in *POLE* patients independent of treatment (e.g., can these women be spared adjuvant therapy?) Although there may be many questions to address we anticipate that molecular classification will facilitate rapid progress in research and clinical care as has been achieved through a subtype specific approach in other tumor sites.

In summary, whilst the combination of histomorphology and clinical factors has proven to be insufficiently reproducible, prognostic and predictive, two molecular classifiers based on the TCGA study show great potential as pragmatic and effective tools to stratify patient risk and subsequent care decisions. Given the high and increasing incidence of endometrial cancer and the societal cost of over- and under-treatment there is urgent need for prospective clinical studies to determine how best to utilize these tools.

*For ProMisE; the materials, assay and interpretation costs total < $300 USD

**Abbreviations**

EC: Endometrial cancer; TCGA: The cancer genome atlas; ESMO: European Society for Medical Oncology; LVSI: Lymph-vascular space invasion; *POLE* EDM: Polymerase epsilon exonuclease domain mutation; MMR: Mismatch repair; MMR-D: Mismatch repair deficiency

**Acknowledgements**

The authors are part of OVCARE, British Columbia's gynecologic cancer research team and are grateful for the intellectual contributions and encompassing work towards the development and implementation of the molecular classifier. In particular, our lab team of Samuel Leung, Melissa McConechy, Winnie Yang, Amy Lum, and Janine Senz, mentors and collaborators Blake Gilks and David Huntsman, and local and international collaborators Janice Kwon, Rob Soslow, Lien Hoang, Martin Kobel, and Cheng Han Lee. We are also grateful for supportive funding through the Canadian Institute of Health Research (CIHR New investigator award, McAlpine and CIHR Proof of Principal Phase I grant (201509-PPP-355221-PPP-CAAA-168787)) and the BC Cancer Foundation (Clinical Investigator Award (McAlpine) and the Sarabjit Gill Fund).

**Funding**

No specific funding is associated with this review article. The research from our center described herein has in part been funded by the sources acknowledged above.

**Authors' contributions**

AT and JM authored this manuscript and continue to work in translational research on endometrial carcinomas. Both authors read and approved the final manuscript.

**Competing interests**

US patent 62192230 for the ProMisE molecular classifier has been filed (pending) by the BC cancer agency.

**Author details**

[1]Department of Pathology and Laboratory Medicine, University of British Columbia and BC Cancer Agency, Vancouver, BC, Canada. [2]Department of Gynecology and Obstetrics, Division of Gynecologic Oncology, University of British Columbia, 2775 Laurel St. 6th Floor, Vancouver, BC, CanadaV5Z 1M9.

**References**

1. Siegel RL, Miller KD, Jemal A. Cancer statistics, 2015. CA Cancer J Clin. 2015; 65(1):5–29.

2. Society CC. Canadian Cancer. Statistics. 2016;2016(2016):1–142.

3. Ferlay J, Soerjomataram I, Dikshit R, Eser S, Mathers C, Rebelo M, et al. Cancer incidence and mortality worldwide: sources, methods and major patterns in GLOBOCAN 2012. Int J Cancer. 2015;136(5):E359–86.

4. Rose PG. Endometrial carcinoma. N Engl J Med. 1996;335(9):640–9.

5. Creasman WT, Odicino F, Maisonneuve P, Beller U, Benedet JL, Heintz AP, et al. Carcinoma of the corpus uteri. J Epidemiol Biostat. 2001;6(1):47–86.

6. Morice P, Leary A, Creutzberg C, Abu-Rustum N, Darai E. Endometrial cancer. Lancet. 2016;387(10023):1094–108.

7. Ueda SM, Kapp DS, Cheung MK, Shin JY, Osann K, Husain A, et al. Trends in demographic and clinical characteristics in women diagnosed with corpus cancer and their potential impact on the increasing number of deaths. Am J Obstet Gynecol. 2008;198(2):218 e1–6.

8. Hamilton CA, Cheung MK, Osann K, Chen L, Teng NN, Longacre TA, et al. Uterine papillary serous and clear cell carcinomas predict for poorer survival compared to grade 3 endometrioid uterus cancers. Br J Cancer. 2006;94(5):642–6. Pubmed Central PMCID: 2361201.

9. del Carmen MG, Birrer M, Schorge JO. Uterine papillary serous cancer: a review of the literature. Gynecol Oncol. 2012;127(3):651–61.

10. Del Carmen MG, Boruta 2nd DM, Schorge JO. Recurrent endometrial cancer. Clin Obstet Gynecol. 2011;54(2):266–77.

11. Jung KW, Won YJ, Kong HJ, Oh CM, Lee DH, Lee JS. Prediction of cancer incidence and mortality in Korea, 2014. Cancer Res Treat. 2014;46(2):124–30. Pubmed Central PMCID: 4022820.

12. Lim MC, Moon EK, Shin A, Jung KW, Won YJ, Seo SS, et al. Incidence of cervical, endometrial, and ovarian cancer in Korea, 1999–2010. J Gynecol Oncol. 2013;24(4):298–302. Pubmed Central PMCID: 3805909.

13. Rahib L, Smith BD, Aizenberg R, Rosenzweig AB, Fleshman JM, Matrisian LM. Projecting cancer incidence and deaths to 2030: the unexpected burden of thyroid, liver, and pancreas cancers in the United States. Cancer Res. 2014;74(11):2913–21.

14. Colombo N, Creutzberg C, Amant F, Bosse T, Gonzalez-Martin A, Ledermann J, et al. ESMO-ESGO-ESTRO consensus conference on endometrial cancer: diagnosis, treatment and follow-up. Int J Gynecol Cancer. 2016;26(1):2–30. Pubmed Central PMCID: 4679344.

15. Bestvina CM, Fleming GF. Chemotherapy for endometrial cancer in adjuvant and advanced disease settings. Oncologist. 2016;21(10):1250–9. Pubmed Central PMCID: 5061541.

16. Galaal K, Al Moundhri M, Bryant A, Lopes AD, Lawrie TA. Adjuvant chemotherapy for advanced endometrial cancer. Cochrane Database Syst Rev. 2014;5:CD010681.

17. Galaal K, Bryant A, Fisher AD, Al-Khaduri M, Kew F, Lopes AD. Laparoscopy versus laparotomy for the management of early stage endometrial cancer. Cochrane Database Syst Rev. 2012;12(9):CD006655.

18. de Boer SM, Powell ME, Mileshkin L, Katsaros D, Bessette P, Haie-Meder C, et al. Toxicity and quality of life after adjuvant chemoradiotherapy versus radiotherapy alone for women with high-risk endometrial cancer (PORTEC-3): an open-label, multicentre, randomised, phase 3 trial. Lancet Oncol. 2016;17(8):1114–26.

19. Joly F, McAlpine J, Nout R, Avall-Lundqvist E, Shash E, Friedlander M, et al. Quality of life and patient-reported outcomes in endometrial cancer clinical trials: a call for action! Int J Gynecol Cancer. 2014;24(9):1693–9.

20. McAlpine JN, Greimel E, Brotto LA, Nout RA, Shash E, Avall-Lundqvist E, et al. Quality of life research in endometrial cancer: what is needed to advance progress in this disease site? Methodological considerations from the Gynecologic Cancer InterGroup Symptom Benefit Working Group brainstorming session, Leiden 2012. Int J Gynecol Cancer. 2014;24(9):1686–92.

21. Murali R, Soslow RA, Weigelt B. Classification of endometrial carcinoma: more than two types. Lancet Oncol. 2014;15(7):e268–78.

22. Bendifallah S, Darai E, Ballester M. Predictive modeling: a new paradigm for managing endometrial cancer. Ann Surg Oncol. 2016;23(3):975–88.

23. Bokhman JV. Two pathogenetic types of endometrial carcinoma. Gynecol Oncol. 1983;15(1):10–7.

24. Gilks CB, Oliva E, Soslow RA. Poor interobserver reproducibility in the diagnosis of high-grade endometrial carcinoma. Am J Surg Pathol. 2013;37(6):874–81.

25. Clarke BA, Gilks CB. Endometrial carcinoma: controversies in histopathological assessment of grade and tumour cell type. J Clin Pathol. 2010;63(5):410–5.

26. Hussein YR, Broaddus R, Weigelt B, Levine DA, Soslow RA. The genomic heterogeneity of FIGO grade 3 endometrioid carcinoma impacts diagnostic accuracy and reproducibility. Int J Gynecol Pathol. 2016;35(1):16–24. Pubmed Central PMCID: 4934379.

27. Han G, Sidhu D, Duggan MA, Arseneau J, Cesari M, Clement PB, et al. Reproducibility of histological cell type in high-grade endometrial carcinoma. Mod Pathol. 2013;26(12):1594–604.

28. Alkushi A, Kobel M, Kalloger SE, Gilks CB. High-grade endometrial carcinoma: serous and grade 3 endometrioid carcinomas have different immunophenotypes and outcomes. Int J Gynecol Pathol. 2010;29(4):343–50.

29. Karateke A, Tug N, Cam C, Selcuk S, Asoglu MR, Cakir S. Discrepancy of pre- and postoperative grades of patients with endometrial carcinoma. Eur J Gynaecol Oncol. 2011;32(3):283–5.

30. Sany O, Singh K, Jha S. Correlation between preoperative endometrial sampling and final endometrial cancer histology. Eur J Gynaecol Oncol. 2012;33(2):142–4.

31. Wang XY, Pan ZM, Chen XD, Lu WG, Xie X. Accuracy of tumor grade by preoperative curettage and associated clinicopathologic factors in clinical stage I endometrioid adenocarcinoma. Chin Med J. 2009;122(16):1843–6.

32. Batista TP, Cavalcanti CL, Tejo AA, Bezerra AL. Accuracy of preoperative endometrial sampling diagnosis for predicting the final pathology grading in uterine endometrioid carcinoma. Eur J Surg Oncol. 2016;26.

33. Guy MS, Sheeder J, Behbakht K, Wright JD, Guntupalli SR. Comparative outcomes in older and younger women undergoing laparotomy or robotic surgical staging for endometrial cancer. Am J Obstet Gynecol. 2016;214(3):350 e1–e10.

34. Walker JL, Piedmonte MR, Spirtos NM, Eisenkop SM, Schlaerth JB, Mannel RS, et al. Laparoscopy compared with laparotomy for comprehensive surgical staging of uterine cancer: Gynecologic Oncology Group Study LAP2. J Clin Oncol. 2009;27(32):5331–6. Pubmed Central PMCID: 2773219.

35. Peters 3rd WA, Andersen WA, Thornton Jr WN, Morley GW. The selective use of vaginal hysterectomy in the management of adenocarcinoma of the endometrium. Am J Obstet Gynecol. 1983;146(3):285–9.

36. Cornelison TL, Trimble EL, Kosary CL. SEER data, corpus uteri cancer: treatment trends versus survival for FIGO stage II, 1988–1994. Gynecol Oncol. 1999;74(3):350–5.

37. Creutzberg CL, van Putten WL, Koper PC, Lybeert ML, Jobsen JJ, Warlam-Rodenhuis CC, et al. Surgery and postoperative radiotherapy versus surgery alone for patients with stage-1 endometrial carcinoma: multicentre randomised trial. PORTEC Study Group. Post Operative Radiation Therapy in Endometrial Carcinoma. Lancet. 2000;355(9213):1404–11.

38. Di Cello A, Rania E, Zuccala V, Venturella R, Mocciaro R, Zullo F, et al. Failure to recognize preoperatively high-risk endometrial carcinoma is associated with a poor outcome. Eur J Obstet Gynecol Reprod Biol. 2015;194:153–60.

39. Zhang C, Hu W, Jia N, Li Q, Hua K, Tao X, et al. Uterine carcinosarcoma and high-risk endometrial carcinomas: a clinicopathological comparison. Int J Gynecol Cancer. 2015;25(4):629–36.

40. Imai K, Kato H, Katayama K, Nakanishi K, Kawano A, Iura A, et al. A preoperative risk-scoring system to predict lymph node metastasis in endometrial cancer and stratify patients for lymphadenectomy. Gynecol Oncol. 2016;142(2):273–7.

41. Colombo N, Preti E, Landoni F, Carinelli S, Colombo A, Marini C, et al. Endometrial cancer: ESMO clinical practice guidelines for diagnosis, treatment and follow-up. Ann Oncol. 2013;24 Suppl 6:vi33–8.

42. Mariani A, Dowdy SC, Cliby WA, Gostout BS, Jones MB, Wilson TO, et al. Prospective assessment of lymphatic dissemination in endometrial cancer: a paradigm shift in surgical staging. Gynecol Oncol. 2008;109(1):11–8. Pubmed Central PMCID: 3667391.

43. AlHilli MM, Mariani A, Bakkum-Gamez JN, Dowdy SC, Weaver AL, Peethambaram PP, et al. Risk-scoring models for individualized prediction of overall survival in low-grade and high-grade endometrial cancer. Gynecol Oncol. 2014;133(3):485–93.

44. Kang S, Lee JM, Lee JK, Kim JW, Cho CH, Kim SM, et al. A Web-based nomogram predicting para-aortic nodal metastasis in incompletely staged patients with endometrial cancer: a Korean multicenter study. Int J Gynecol Cancer. 2014;24(3):513–7.

45. Keys HM, Roberts JA, Brunetto VL, Zaino RJ, Spirtos NM, Bloss JD, et al. A phase III trial of surgery with or without adjunctive external pelvic radiation therapy in intermediate risk endometrial adenocarcinoma: a gynecologic oncology group study. Gynecol Oncol. 2004;92(3):744–51.

46. Barlin JN, Soslow RA, Lutz M, Zhou QC, St Clair CM, Leitao Jr MM, et al. Redefining stage I endometrial cancer: incorporating histology, a binary grading system, myometrial invasion, and lymph node assessment. Int J Gynecol Cancer. 2013;23(9):1620–8. Pubmed Central PMCID: 4405774.

47. Kong TW, Chang SJ, Paek J, Lee Y, Chun M, Ryu HS. Risk group criteria for tailoring adjuvant treatment in patients with endometrial cancer:

a validation study of the gynecologic oncology group criteria. J Gynecol Oncol. 2015;26(1):32–9. Pubmed Central PMCID: 4302283.

48. Kwon JS, Qiu F, Saskin R, Carey MS. Are uterine risk factors more important than nodal status in predicting survival in endometrial cancer? Obstet Gynecol. 2009;114(4):736–43.

49. Bendifallah S, Canlorbe G, Collinet P, Arsene E, Huguet F, Coutant C, et al. Just how accurate are the major risk stratification systems for early-stage endometrial cancer?. Brit J cancer. 2015;12.

50. Hoang LN, McConechy MK, Kobel M, Han G, Rouzbahman M, Davidson B, et al. Histotype-genotype correlation in 36 high-grade endometrial carcinomas. Am J Surg Pathol. 2013;37(9):1421–32.

51. Lax SF, Kurman RJ. A dualistic model for endometrial carcinogenesis based on immunohistochemical and molecular genetic analyses. Verh Dtsch Ges Pathol. 1997;81:228–32.

52. McConechy MK, Ding J, Cheang MC, Wiegand KC, Senz J, Tone AA, et al. Use of mutation profiles to refine the classification of endometrial carcinomas. J Pathol. 2012;228(1):20–30. Pubmed Central PMCID: 3939694.

53. Mcconechy MK, Ding J, Senz J, Yang W, Melnyk N, Tone AA, et al. Ovarian and endometrial endometrioid carcinomas have distinct CTNNB1 and PTEN mutation profiles. Mod Pathol. 2014;27(1):128–34. Pubmed Central PMCID: 3915240.

54. Hoang LN, Lee YS, Karnezis AN, Tessier-Cloutier B, Almandani N, Coatham M, et al. Immunophenotypic features of dedifferentiated endometrial carcinoma Insights from BRG1/INI1-deficient tumors. Histopathology. 2016.

55. Hoang LN, McConechy MK, Meng B, McIntyre JB, Ewanowich C, Gilks CB, et al. Targeted mutation analysis of endometrial clear cell carcinoma. Histopathology. 2014.

56. Alvarez T, Miller E, Duska L, Oliva E. Molecular profile of grade 3 endometrioid endometrial carcinoma: is it a type I or type II endometrial carcinoma? Am J Surg Pathol. 2012;36(5):753–61.

57. Santacana M, Maiques O, Valls J, Gatius S, Abo AI, Lopez-Garcia MA, et al. A 9-protein biomarker molecular signature for predicting histologic type in endometrial carcinoma by immunohistochemistry. Hum Pathol. 2014;45(12):2394–403.

58. Coenegrachts L, Garcia-Dios DA, Depreeuw J, Santacana M, Gatius S, Zikan M, et al. Mutation profile and clinical outcome of mixed endometrioid-serous endometrial carcinomas are different from that of pure endometrioid or serous carcinomas. Virchows Archiv. 2015;466(4):415–22.

59. Ferguson SE, Olshen AB, Viale A, Barakat RR, Boyd J. Stratification of intermediate-risk endometrial cancer patients into groups at high risk or low risk for recurrence based on tumor gene expression profiles. Clin Cancer Res. 2005;11(6):2252–7.

60. Salvesen HB, Carter SL, Mannelqvist M, Dutt A, Getz G, Stefansson IM, et al. Integrated genomic profiling of endometrial carcinoma associates aggressive tumors with indicators of PI3 kinase activation. Proc Natl Acad Sci U S A. 2009;106(12):4834–9. Pubmed Central PMCID: 2660768.

61. Wik E, Trovik J, Kusonmano K, Birkeland E, Raeder MB, Pashtan I, et al. Endometrial Carcinoma Recurrence Score (ECARS) validates to identify aggressive disease and associates with markers of epithelial-mesenchymal transition and PI3K alterations. Gynecol Oncol. 2014;134(3):599–606.

62. Wik E, Birkeland E, Trovik J, Werner HM, Hoivik EA, Mjos S, et al. High phospho-Stathmin(Serine38) expression identifies aggressive endometrial cancer and suggests an association with PI3K inhibition. Clin Cancer Res. 2013;19(9):2331–41.

63. Myers AP. New strategies in endometrial cancer: targeting the PI3K/mTOR pathway-the devil is in the details. Clin Cancer Res. 2013;19(19):5264–74.

64. Krakstad C, Birkeland E, Seidel D, Kusonmano K, Petersen K, Mjos S, et al. High-throughput mutation profiling of primary and metastatic endometrial cancers identifies KRAS, FGFR2 and PIK3CA to be frequently mutated. PloS one. 2012;7(12):e52795. Pubmed Central PMCID: 3531332.

65. Salvesen HB, Haldorsen IS, Trovik J. Markers for individualised therapy in endometrial carcinoma. Lancet Oncol. 2012;13(8):e353–61.

66. Iglesias DA, Yates MS, van der Hoeven D, Rodkey TL, Zhang Q, Co NN, et al. Another surprise from Metformin: novel mechanism of action via K-Ras influences endometrial cancer response to therapy. Mol Cancer Ther. 2013; 12(12):2847–56. Pubmed Central PMCID: 3883498.

67. Cancer Genome Atlas Research N, Kandoth C, Schultz N, Cherniack AD, Akbani R, Liu Y, et al. Integrated genomic characterization of endometrial carcinoma. Nature. 2013;497(7447):67–73. Pubmed Central PMCID: 3704730.

68. Meng B, Hoang LN, McIntyre JB, Duggan MA, Nelson GS, Lee CH, et al. POLE exonuclease domain mutation predicts long progression-free survival in grade 3 endometrioid carcinoma of the endometrium. Gynecol Oncol. 2014;134(1):15–9.

69. Stelloo E, Bosse T, Nout RA, MacKay HJ, Church DN, Nijman HW, et al. Refining prognosis and identifying targetable pathways for high-risk endometrial cancer; a TransPORTEC initiative. Mod Pathol. 2015.

70. Billingsley CC, Cohn DE, Mutch DG, Stephens JA, Suarez AA, Goodfellow PJ. Polymerase varepsilon (POLE) mutations in endometrial cancer: Clinical outcomes and implications for Lynch syndrome testing. Cancer. 2015;121(3): 386–94. Pubmed Central PMCID: 4304930.

71. Stelloo E, Nout RA, Osse EM, Jurgenliemk-Schulz IJ, Jobsen JJ, Lutgens LC, et al. Improved risk assessment by integrating molecular and clinicopathological factors in early-stage endometrial cancer - combined analysis of PORTEC cohorts. Clin Cancer Res. 2016;22.

72. Church DN, Stelloo E, Nout RA, Valtcheva N, Depreeuw J, ter Haar N, et al. Prognostic significance of POLE proofreading mutations in endometrial cancer. J Natl Cancer Inst. 2015;107(1):402.

73. Talhouk A, McConechy MK, Leung S, Li-Chang HH, Kwon JS, Melnyk N, et al. A clinically applicable molecular-based classification for endometrial cancers. Br J Cancer. 2015;113(2):299–310. Pubmed Central PMCID: 4506381.

74. McConechy MK, Talhouk A, Leung S, Chiu DS, Yang W, Senz J, et al. Endometrial carcinomas with POLE exonuclease domain mutations have a favorable prognosis. Clin Cancer Res. 2016;13.

75. Cancer Genome Atlas Research N, Weinstein JN, Collisson EA, Mills GB, Shaw KR, Ozenberger BA, et al. The cancer genome atlas pan-cancer analysis project. Nat Genet. 2013;45(10):1113–20. Pubmed Central PMCID: 3919969.

76. Umar A, Boland CR, Terdiman JP, Syngal S, de la Chapelle A, Ruschoff J, et al. Revised Bethesda guidelines for hereditary nonpolyposis colorectal cancer (Lynch syndrome) and microsatellite instability. J Natl Cancer Inst. 2004;96(4):261–8. Pubmed Central PMCID: 2933058.

77. Talhouk A, McConechy M, Leung S, Yang W, Lum A, Senz J, et al. Confirmation of ProMisE: a simple genomics-based clinical classifier for endometrial cancer. Cancer. 2016; Accepted, In Press.

78. In: Micheel CM, Nass SJ, Omenn GS, editors. Evolution of translational omics: Lessons learned and the path forward. Washington (DC): National Academies Press; 2012.

79. Talhouk A, McConechy MK, Leung S, Yang W, Senz J, et al. A clinically applicable molecular-based classification system for endometrial cancers. J Clin Oncol. 2016; ASCO poster presentation: Abstract No: 5518.

80. Talhouk A, Hoang LN, McConechy MK, Nakonechny Q, Leo J, Cheng A, et al. Molecular classification of endometrial carcinoma on diagnostic specimens is highly concordant with final hysterectomy: earlier prognostic information to guide treatment. Gynecol Oncol. 2016;143(1):46–53.

81. Stelloo E, Nout RA, Naves LC, Ter Haar NT, Creutzberg CL, Smit VT, et al. High concordance of molecular tumor alterations between pre-operative curettage and hysterectomy specimens in patients with endometrial carcinoma. Gynecol Oncol. 2014;133(2):197–204.

82. Visser NC, Bulten J, van der Wurff AA, Boss EA, Bronkhorst CM, Feijen HW, et al. PIpelle Prospective ENDOmetrial carcinoma (PIPENDO) study, pre-operative recognition of high risk endometrial carcinoma: a multicentre prospective cohort study. BMC Cancer. 2015;15:487. Pubmed Central PMCID: 4485884.

83. McConechy MK, Talhouk A, Li-Chang HH, Leung S, Huntsman DG, Gilks CB, et al. Detection of DNA mismatch repair (MMR) deficiencies by immunohistochemistry can effectively diagnose the microsatellite instability (MSI) phenotype in endometrial carcinomas. Gynecol Oncol. 2015;28.

84. Goodfellow PJ, Billingsley CC, Lankes HA, Ali S, Cohn DE, Broaddus RJ, et al. Combined microsatellite instability, MLH1 methylation analysis, and immunohistochemistry for lynch syndrome screening in endometrial cancers from GOG210: An NRG oncology and gynecologic oncology group study. J Clin Oncol Off J Am Soc Clin Oncol. 2015;33(36):4301–8. Pubmed Central PMCID: 4678181.

85. Hall G, Clarkson A, Shi A, Langford E, Leung H, Eckstein RP, et al. Immunohistochemistry for PMS2 and MSH6 alone can replace a four antibody panel for mismatch repair deficiency screening in colorectal adenocarcinoma. Pathology. 2010;42(5):409–13.

86. Burgart LJ. Testing for defective DNA mismatch repair in colorectal carcinoma: a practical guide. Arch Pathol Lab Med. 2005;129(11):1385–9.

87. Yamamoto H, Imai K. Microsatellite instability: an update. Arch Toxicol. 2015; 89(6):899–921.

88. Rabban JT, Calkins SM, Karnezis AN, Grenert JP, Blanco A, Crawford B, et al. Association of tumor morphology with mismatch-repair protein status in older endometrial cancer patients: implications for universal versus

selective screening strategies for Lynch syndrome. Am J Surg Pathol. 2014;38(6):793–800.

89. Garg K, Soslow RA. Lynch syndrome (hereditary non-polyposis colorectal cancer) and endometrial carcinoma. J Clin Pathol. 2009; 62(8):679–84.

90. Bonadona V, Bonaiti B, Olschwang S, Grandjouan S, Huiart L, Longy M, et al. Cancer risks associated with germline mutations in MLH1, MSH2, and MSH6 genes in Lynch syndrome. Jama. 2011;305(22):2304–10.

91. Hendriks YM, Wagner A, Morreau H, Menko F, Stormorken A, Quehenberger F, et al. Cancer risk in hereditary nonpolyposis colorectal cancer due to MSH6 mutations: impact on counseling and surveillance. Gastroenterology. 2004;127(1):17–25.

92. Carayol J, Bonaiti-Pellie C. Estimating penetrance from family data using a retrospective likelihood when ascertainment depends on genotype and age of onset. Genet Epidemiol. 2004;27(2):109–17.

93. Bonaiti B, Bonadona V, Perdry H, Andrieu N, Bonaiti-Pellie C. Estimating penetrance from multiple case families with predisposing mutations: extension of the 'genotype-restricted likelihood' (GRL) method. Eur J Hum Genet. 2011;19(2):173–9. Pubmed Central PMCID: 3025788.

94. McMeekin DS, Tritchler DL, Cohn DE, Mutch DG, Lankes HA, Geller MA, et al. Clinicopathologic significance of mismatch repair defects in endometrial cancer: an NRG oncology/gynecologic oncology group study. J Clin Oncol. 2016;34(25):3062–8. Pubmed Central PMCID: 5012715.

95. Shikama A, Minaguchi T, Matsumoto K, Akiyama-Abe A, Nakamura Y, Michikami H, et al. Clinicopathologic implications of DNA mismatch repair status in endometrial carcinomas. Gynecol Oncol. 2016;140(2):226–33.

96. Bakhsh S, Kinloch M, Hoang LN, Soslow R, Kobel M, Lee CH, et al. Histopathological features of endometrial carcinomas associated with POLE mutations: implications for decisions about adjuvant therapy. Histopathology. 2015.

97. Bellone S, Centritto F, Black J, Schwab C, English D, Cocco E, et al. Polymerase epsilon (POLE) ultra-mutated tumors induce robust tumor-specific CD4+ T cell responses in endometrial cancer patients. Gynecol Oncol. 2015;138(1):11–7. Pubmed Central PMCID: 4469551.

98. Hussein YR, Weigelt B, Levine DA, Schoolmeester JK, Dao LN, Balzer BL, et al. Clinicopathological analysis of endometrial carcinomas harboring somatic POLE exonuclease domain mutations. Mod Pathol. 2015;28(4):505–14.

99. Howitt BE, Shukla SA, Sholl LM, Ritterhouse LL, Watkins JC, Rodig S, et al. Association of polymerase e-mutated and microsatellite-instable endometrial cancers with neoantigen load, number of tumor-infiltrating lymphocytes, and expression of PD-1 and PD-L1. JAMA Oncol. 2015;1(9):1319–23.

100. Gargiulo P, Della Pepa C, Berardi S, Califano D, Scala S, Buonaguro L, et al. Tumor genotype and immune microenvironment in POLE-ultramutated and MSI-hypermutated endometrial cancers: new candidates for checkpoint blockade immunotherapy? Cancer Treat Rev. 2016;48:61–8.

101. van Gool IC, Bosse T, Church DN. POLE proofreading mutation, immune response and prognosis in endometrial cancer. Oncoimmunology. 2016;5(3): e1072675. Pubmed Central PMCID: 4839358.

102. Santin AD, Bellone S, Buza N, Choi J, Schwartz PE, Schlessinger J, et al. Regression of chemotherapy-resistant Polymerase epsilon (POLE) ultra-mutated and MSH6 hyper-mutated endometrial tumors with nivolumab. Clin Cancer Res. 2016.

103. Mehnert JM, Panda A, Zhong H, Hirshfield K, Damare S, Lane K, et al. Immune activation and response to pembrolizumab in POLE-mutant endometrial cancer. J Clin Invest. 2016;126(6):2334–40. Pubmed Central PMCID: 4887167.

104. Schultheis AM, Martelotto LG, De Filippo MR, Piscuglio S, Ng CK, Hussein YR, et al. TP53 mutational spectrum in endometrioid and serous endometrial cancers. Int J Gynecol Pathol. 2016;35(4):289–300.

105. Hansen JM, Baggerly KA, Wang Y, Wu S, Previs RA, Zand B, et al. Homologous recombination deficiency in endometrioid uterine cancer: an unrecognized phenomenon. Gynecol Oncol. 2015;137(1):21.

106. Westin SN, Ju Z, Broaddus RR, Krakstad C, Li J, Pal N, et al. PTEN loss is a context-dependent outcome determinant in obese and non-obese endometrioid endometrial cancer patients. Mol Oncol. 2015;9(8):1694–703. Pubmed Central PMCID: 4584169.

107. Roque DR, Makowski L, Chen TH, Rashid N, Hayes DN, Bae-Jump V. Association between differential gene expression and body mass index among endometrial cancers from the cancer genome atlas project. Gynecol Oncol. 2016;142(2):317–22. Pubmed Central PMCID: 4961559.

108. Berg A, Hoivik EA, Mjos S, Holst F, Werner HM, Tangen IL, et al. Molecular profiling of endometrial carcinoma precursor, primary and metastatic lesions suggests different targets for treatment in obese compared to non-obese patients. Oncotarget. 2014.

109. Hoang LN, Han G, McConechy M, Lau S, Chow C, Gilks CB, et al. Immunohistochemical characterization of prototypical endometrial clear cell carcinoma–diagnostic utility of HNF-1beta and oestrogen receptor. Histopathology. 2014;64(4):585–96.

110. Coatham M, Li X, Karnezis AN, Hoang LN, Tessier-Cloutier B, Meng B, et al. Concurrent ARID1A and ARID1B inactivation in endometrial and ovarian dedifferentiated carcinomas. Mod Pathol. 2016.

111. Karnezis AN, Hoang LN, Coatham M, Ravn S, Almadani N, Tessier-Cloutier B, et al. Loss of switch/sucrose non-fermenting complex protein expression is associated with dedifferentiation in endometrial carcinomas. Mod Pathol. 2016;29(3):302–14. Pubmed Central PMCID: 4980656.

112. Kobel M, Meng B, Hoang LN, Almadani N, Li X, Soslow RA, et al. Molecular analysis of mixed endometrial carcinomas shows clonality in most cases. Am J Surg Pathol. 2016;40(2):166–80.

113. Gibson WJ, Hoivik EA, Halle MK, Taylor-Weiner A, Cherniack AD, Berg A, et al. The genomic landscape and evolution of endometrial carcinoma progression and abdominopelvic metastasis. Nat Genet. 2016;48(8):848–55. Pubmed Central PMCID: 4963271.

114. Wang Y, McConechy M, Gilks B, Huntsman D, Shah SP, McAlpine J. Genome-wide copy number analysis and mutational profiling provides evidence of intratumoral heterogeneity in endometrial cancers. Int J Gyne Cancer. 2014;24(Suppl 49).

115. Kobel M, Reuss A, du Bois A, Kommoss S, Kommoss F, Gao D, et al. The biological and clinical value of p53 expression in pelvic high-grade serous carcinomas. J Pathol. 2010;222(2):191–8.

# 8

# Fertility preservation in women with cervical, endometrial or ovarian cancers

Michael Feichtinger[1,2,4] and Kenny A. Rodriguez-Wallberg[3,4*]

## Abstract

**Background:** Although cancer in general affects an aged population, a significant number of women develop cancer at childbearing age. Long-term survival rates after gynecological cancer, especially in young patients are increasing and all quality-of-life aspects, including preservation of fertility have become of major relevance.

**Outcomes:** Surgical techniques aimed at sparing reproductive organs and preserving fertility have been developed for women presenting with gynecological cancer found at early stages. Indications for fertility-sparing surgery are in general restricted to women presenting with a well-differentiated low-grade tumor in its early stages or with low malignant potential. Up to now, use of fertility-sparing techniques in well-selected patients has not been shown to affect overall survival negatively and fertility outcomes reported have been favorable. Still larger amounts of data and longer follow-up periods are needed. Several current fertility-sparing cancer treatments may result in sub-fertility and in those cases assisted reproductive techniques are indicated. Overall quality of life has been satisfactory in cancer patients after fertility-sparing surgery.

**Conclusions:** Fertility-sparing surgery is a viable tool to enable gynecological cancer patients of young age to fulfill their family building without impairment of oncological outcome. Cancer patients of reproductive age should undergo fertility counseling to analyze this sensitive subject. Further studies are needed to investigate the role of fertility-sparing treatment and combined adjuvant therapy in higher-grade cancers.

**Keywords:** Fertility preservation, Gynecological cancer, QoL, IVF, Cervical cancer, Ovarian cancer, Endometrial cancer, Pregnancy

## Background

The overall cancer risk in women below the age of 39 years is estimated to be one in 39 [1]. Of all gynecological cancer cases, young women comprise 2 % of cervix cancer cases, 5 % of endometrial cancers and up to approximately 12 % of ovarian cancers [1]. Five-year survival rates range from 46 % in ovarian cancer to more than 80 % in endometrial cancer and over 90 % in cases of borderline ovarian tumors [2, 3]. Infertility following cancer treatment has been recognized as a main concern as regards quality of life (QoL) in cancer patients [4, 5]. As a result of improved long-term survival rates in young people, all QoL aspects are of major importance. Additionally, due to current social trends, childbearing nowadays is delayed, hence an increasing number of women that present with cancer at a young age might have not yet fulfilled their family building plans and will be interested in undergoing treatments that would preserve their chances to have children in the future [6]. Most oncologic treatments have detrimental effects on female reproductive potential, in particular those including chemotherapy with agents of high gonadotoxicity, or radiation therapy in a field involving the ovaries, the uterus and the vagina, which may be compromised and damaged by direct irradiation [7]. The resumption of menstrual cycles indicates that some ovarian function is maintained, but it does not guarantee fertility, and early onset of menopause in women previously treated for cancer is a common finding [7–9].

Surgery is currently the most effective treatment for cancer and eventually up to 100 % of patients may be cured when complete removal of a tumor is achieved. Surgery may also be indicated for treatment of

* Correspondence: kenny.rodriguez-wallberg@karolinska.se
[3]Department of Oncology – Pathology, Karolinska Institutet, Stockholm, Sweden
[4]Department of Obstetrics and Gynecology, Section of Reproductive Medicine, Karolinska University Hospital, Novumhuset Plan 4, SE-141 86 Stockholm, Sweden
Full list of author information is available at the end of the article

premalignant disease of the cervix or the endometrium in female patients, as cancer prophylaxis. Conization, for example, may lead to completely disease-free follow-up, but it may induce sub-fertility by affecting the normal function of the cervix and its glandular secretion. Infertility induced by such forms of intervention may be overcome by treatments involving assisted reproductive technologies, such as intrauterine insemination or in vitro fertilization, IVF.

In gynecologic oncologic surgery, there has been gradual development of fertility-sparing surgery with the aim of preserving the reproductive organs. Survival should not be compromised and thus indications are restricted to patients of a young age with a desire to preserve fertility and presenting with a well-differentiated cervical, ovarian or endometrial low-grade tumor in its early stages or with low malignant potential.

In this article we will discuss indications for fertility-sparing methods available to women with gynecological cancer, and up-to-date data on safety and efficacy as regards oncologic outcomes and reproductive outcomes including obstetric outcomes and quality of life.

## Cervical cancer

Cervical cancer makes up 1.5 % of all new cancer cases in females. In 2015, 12 900 patients with a median age of 49 years had newly diagnosed cervical cancer in the US. Of these, 38.5 % were under the age of 45 years [1, 2]. The different approaches regarding fertility-sparing surgery in cases of cervical cancer are summarized in Table 1.

In cases of micro-invasion (< 3 mm), FIGO stage IA1, cervical carcinoma can be treated with simple large loop excision of the transformation zone (LLETZ), without further affecting fertility potential. Compared with this approach, hysterectomy has not been associated with improved survival rates if no lymph vascular space invasion and negative cancer margins are confirmed [10]. This approach can be applied in micro-invasive squamous cell carcinoma as well as adenocarcinoma, with similar outcomes [11].

In patients affected by cervical cancer at FIGO stages IA2–IB1 who wish to preserve fertility, radical trachelectomy with pelvic lymphadenectomy (confirming negative lymph node status) is the treatment of choice [12, 13]. Radical trachelectomy was first described by Dargent in 1994 [14] and it represents the most established surgical procedure for fertility preservation in women. The procedure has been reported for the treatment of squamous cell carcinomas and adenocarcinomas, with similar outcomes [15]. As operative techniques, vaginal, laparascopic, abdominal and robot-assisted trachelectomy have been described [13]. Long-term oncologic outcomes of trachelectomy seem not to differ compared with radical hysterectomy, and a long-term survival rate of 98.4 % and a relapse rate of only 4.5 % have been reported [16, 17].

Perioperative complications have also been similar when compared with radical hysterectomy [13]. Further development of non-invasive nuclear methods to identify lymph nodes in patients with early-stage cervical cancer might improve future patient selection for this type of fertility-sparing surgery [18].

After trachelectomy, over 60 % of tissue samples have demonstrated absence of residual tumor [19]. Therefore, conization in combination with laparoscopic lymphadenectomy has also been described as an appropriate procedure in selected patients presenting with early-stage cervical cancer (FIGO IA2 and IB1) and tumors < 20 mm. Women thus treated have succeeded in conceiving in 47 % of cases and the 5-year disease free survival reported of 97 % [20, 21]. However, although data are promising, the number of cases published is still small and further research is needed to implement this technique as a clinical routine.

In cases of more advanced disease with a tumor size >2 cm, initial neoadjuvant chemotherapy followed by radical trachelectomy and lymphadenectomy has been suggested by some authors [22, 23]. This approach has been shown to correlate with high fertility rates and no differences in oncologic outcome compared with immediate trachelectomy without chemotherapy [24]. Because of few reported cases and no long-term follow-up outcomes, this procedure should still be regarded as experimental.

In selected cases where radiotherapy or chemoradiation are necessary, the ovaries can be protected by ovarian transposition to remove them from the radiation field [25–27]. However, depending on the radiation dose and radiation scatter, the efficacy of this procedure has been reported to be about 50 % [28, 29]. If assisted reproductive treatments involving IVF are needed thereafter, the ovaries are often difficult to access for ovum pickup. Ovarian stimulation in connection with subsequent cryopreservation of oocytes or embryos before cancer treatment is thus indicated in such cases [6, 30–34]. However, even if ovarian function is preserved, or oocytes or embryos have been cryopreserved, irradiation of the uterus may cause irreversible damage. Although cases of good obstetric outcome have been reported after fertility preservation among women with a heavily irradiated uterus [35], unsuccessful results should be expected and in many cases surrogacy will be necessary [36].

If oocyte or embryo cryopreservation are not feasible, the emerging technique of cryopreserving ovarian tissue for later retransplantation might serve as a viable tool to preserve fertility in some cancer patients. Heterotopic and orthotopic transplantation sites have been described, with resumption of ovarian function [35, 37–39]. Up to now more than 60 children have been born worldwide after ovarian tissue transplantation [39, 40].

In cases of ovarian tissue cryopreservation, concerns have been raised as regards the risk of reseeding cancer

**Table 1** Fertility-sparing interventions in women with cervical or endometrial cancer

| Diagnosis | Type of Surgery | Description | Reproductive and Obstetric Outcomes | Oncologic Outcome | Quality of Life |
|---|---|---|---|---|---|
| Cervical Cancer FIGO Stage IA1 (microinvasion <3 mm) | Large loop excision of the transformation zone (LLETZ) or conization if absence of lymph vascular space invasion and negative margins are confirmed | Complete resection of the transformation zone | No fertility impairment reported. OR 1.7 for preterm delivery and 2.69 for premature rupture of membranes; associated with resection size. No difference in neonatal outcome [130] | Similar oncologic outcomes reported in comparison with hysterectomy [10] | Conization has not been associated with reduced quality of life or sexual satisfaction [49] |
| FIGO Stages IA2, IB1 < 2 cm | Cervical conization and laparoscopic lymphadenectomy | Conization of the cervix and laparoscopic pelvic lymphadenectomy | Spontaneous conceptions of about 47 %. Prematurity rates reported with 14.3 % of infants born <32 weeks of gestation [21] | Excellent rates of 5-year disease-free survival (97 %) [21] | Conization with laparoscopic lymphadenectomy has not been associated with reduced quality of life or sexual satisfaction [49] |
| FIGO Stages IA2, IB1 | Radical trachelectomy. Techniques described for vaginal, abdominal, laparoscopic or robotic trachelectomy | Resection of the cervix and surrounding parametria with conservation of the uterus and the ovaries, pelvic lymphadenectomy | Spontaneous pregnancy rates in >60 % of patients Preterm deliveries with 28 % of infants born <32 weeks of gestation [17, 132] | Rates of recurrence and mortality are comparable with those described for similar cases treated with radical hysterectomy; long-term survival 98.4 %. Low relapse rates (4.5 %) [16, 17] | Lower quality of life than healthy controls but similar to radical hysterectomy No significant impairment in sexual satisfaction Long-term bladder complications (40 %) and lymphedema (10 %) [46–48] |
| FIGO Stage IB1, >2 cm | Neoadjuvant chemotherapy followed by radical trachelectomy | Three cycles of paclitaxel, cisplatin and ifosfamide followed by radical trachelectomy | After neoadjuvant chemotherapy and trachelectomy up to 86 % live-birth rates with 86 % spontaneous conception rate [134] | Reported relapse rate of 7.6 % with 90 % survival [23, 24] | Lack of data |
| Endometrial Cancer FIGO stage IA | Medical conservative treatment with hormone therapy using progestational agents either orally or by IUD for >6 months  Myometrial evaluation by MRI should be performed to confirm absence of myometrial infiltration and no extrauterine involvement [52]. | Follow-up by hysteroscopic exams with endometrial biopsies every 3 months | Pregnancy rates of >60 % Uneventful pregnancies reported [63, 72] | Positive response rate to progesterone treatment of 72 %. Either oral or local IUD treatments proposed, as well as a combination of both. Relapse rate of 50 %. A second round of progesterone therapy in cases of relapse has been associated with a response rate of up 89 % [55, 57, 60, 62]. A levonorgestrel IUD has shown greater regression on histology, lower relapse rates and lower rates of hysterectomy for treatment of complex endometrial hyperplasia vs. oral progesterone [57–59]. | Levonorgestrel IUD treatment has been associated with fewer systemic side effects compared with oral progesterone administration [79, 80] |

Modified from: Rodriguez-Wallberg KA, Oktay K. Fertility preservation during cancer treatment: clinical guidelines. Cancer management and research. 2014;6:105-17
Abbreviations: *FIGO* International Federation of Gynecology and Obstetrics, *LLETZ* large loop excision of the transformation zone; *IUD* intrauterine device, *OR* odds ratio

cells at time of retransplantation, if they are present in the tissue preserved. Ovarian metastasis has been reported in 6 % of patients with adenocarcinoma of the cervix and 1 % of patients with squamous cell carcinoma [41]. Nevertheless, of five published cases of retransplantation of ovarian tissue in women with previous cervical carcinoma, none have resulted in relapse [32, 37].

For women undergoing radical surgery with hysterectomy, the chance of childbearing is only possible by means of a womb transplant. Successful results have been obtained by a Swedish team that has led this project over many years [42] and these procedures are expected to extend to several US centers in the future [43].

Data on assisted reproductive treatments after cervical cancer are scarce. In one study a prevalence of infertility of 13.5 % among patients with previous vaginal trachelectomy was reported [44]. Of these, cervical factor infertility was found in about 40 % of cases, indicating a need for intrauterine insemination as the first-line treatment approach. In other series of cases reported, 80 % of women conceived after subsequent fertility treatments [44, 45].

Regarding quality of life, compared with women with radical hysterectomy who had at least one ovary, patients who had undergone trachelectomy had similar sexual satisfaction and quality of life after surgery [46]. However, another study group reported low sexual satisfaction in the first year after surgery compared with healthy subjects and patients after abdominal hysterectomy. However, this effect decreased over time and after one year these patients had similar sexual satisfaction (but with a persistently reduced QoL) when compared with healthy controls [47]. These results are consistent with those of another study reporting bladder-emptying problems in more than 40 % and lymphedema in more than 10 % of cases, reflecting a lower QoL in patients after vaginal or abdominal trachelectomy compared with healthy controls [48].

Cold-knife conization and laparoscopic lymphadenectomy, on the other hand, are not associated with reduced sexual satisfaction and quality of life [49].

### Endometrial cancer

Endometrial cancer comprises 7.1 % of all new cancer cases in females. In the US, 55,000 new cases of endometrial cancer cases were expected in 2015, with a median patient age of 62 years. Seven percent of endometrial cancer patients are under the age of 45 years [1, 2]. Patients at higher risk of presenting endometrial carcinoma are overweight women and those with polycystic ovarian syndrome (PCOS) [50]. The standard treatment of endometrial cancer involves hysterectomy and bilateral salpingo-oophorectomy, due to the hormonal sensitivity of endometrial tumors [51]. In endometrial cancer IA without infiltration to the myometrium and no extrauterine involvement, conservative treatment can be offered to women who wish to maintain fertility. To counsel a women wishing fertility-sparing treatment options properly, myometrial evaluation by MRI should be performed [52].

For women with early-stage endometrial cancer, treatments involving use of progesterone either orally (600 mg medroxyprogesterone acetate daily or 160 mg megestrol acetate daily) or delivered by an intrauterine device (levonorgestrel-releasing IUD) have been described. The combination of IUD and oral progesterone treatment has also been proposed [53]. In retrospective studies a 72 % positive response rate to treatment has been reported [54–56]. In prospective studies, the treatment of complex endometrial hyperplasia using a levonorgestrel IUD has been shown to achieve greater regression in histology, and lower relapse rates than treatment with oral progesterone [57–59]. Lower rates of hysterectomy have also been reported after treatment with levonorgestrel IUDs [57–59].

Generally, relapses are frequent and occur in up to 50 % of cases that undergo conservative treatment [60]. Standard conservative treatments should be followed-up by hysteroscopic examinations every third month and endometrial sampling [61]. In cases of recurrence a second cycle of progesterone treatment has been associated with response rates of up to 89 % [62].

The combination of surgical resection and progesterone treatment has been associated with good oncologic and pregnancy outcomes in a small number of patients (Table 1) [63].

In women free of relapse, pregnancy should be achieved within the shortest period of time, and assisted reproductive treatments may have a place in reducing time to conception, thus reducing the time at risk of recurrence. Ovarian stimulation in cases of endometrial cancer has been an issue because of the supraphysiological estrogen levels attained during hormone treatments required for recovery of oocytes for IVF, and possible tumor stimulation. A few cases of successful live-births after IVF in women with previous endometrial cancer have been reported [64–71]. In these patients infertility treatment was not associated with an increased cancer recurrence rate [72].

The addition of letrozole to standard gonadotropin protocols has been proposed for ovarian stimulation among women with estrogen-sensitive tumors [73, 74]. The protocols, initially developed for women with breast cancer, could also be used in patients with endometrial cancers [75]. The performance of ovarian stimulation with a levonorgestrel IUD in situ has also been found to minimize the effect of estrogenic stimulation on the endometrium [76].

Whenever the desired family size has been reached, patients should undergo hysterectomy and bilateral salpingo-oophorectomy as a result of the persistent relapse risk [77].

A proportion of women treated for cancer might achieve pregnancy by surrogacy agreement, which is the carrying of a pregnancy by a third party (surrogate), a procedure that is allowed in some countries. Surrogacy gives the possibility of having biologically related children if gametes have been previously cryopreserved [76, 78].

As regards the QoL of women who have undergone fertility-sparing treatments in connection with early-stage endometrial cancer, the results of a meta-analysis indicated improved outcomes after treatment with levonorgestrel IUDs compared with oral progesterone, with reduced weight gain, sleep disorders, headaches, mood and libido disorders [79, 80].

### Ovarian cancer

Ovarian cancers make up 2.6 % of all female cancers. In 2015 around 21 300 new cases of ovarian cancer were diagnosed in the US. The median age at diagnosis is 63 years, with 12 % of patients under the age of 44 years [1, 2]. The different approaches in fertility-sparing surgery in cases of ovarian cancer and borderline ovarian tumors are summarized in Table 2.

#### Epithelial ovarian cancer

Most cases of epithelial ovarian cancer are diagnosed at an advanced stage, making it the most lethal tumor of all gynecological malignancies. Standard treatment consists of bilateral salpingo-oophorectomy, hysterectomy, omentectomy as well as pelvic and para-aortic lymphadenectomy [81].

In women presenting with epithelial ovarian cancer diagnosed at an early stage (typically FIGO stage IA) who wish to preserve fertility, unilateral salpingo-oophorectomy together with appropriate staging, omentectomy, pelvic and para-aortic lymphadenectomy can be performed to preserve the uterus and one healthy ovary [82]. If the contralateral ovary appears macroscopically normal, most authors discourage sampling of it due to impairment of ovarian reserve and causation of additional adhesions by performing the biopsies [82]. In cases of epithelial ovarian cancer with bilateral ovarian involvement a conservative approach should not be applied [83].

Laparoscopic fertility-sparing surgery has been shown to be a feasible approach in cancers of FIGO stage IA and the 3-year survival rate is about 95 % [84]. In patients presenting with a higher-risk early-stage ovarian cancer (IAG3 or higher) some authors have described fertility-sparing procedures in connection with non-impaired survival rates. However, the level of evidence regarding fertility-sparing surgery in high-risk ovarian cancer is limited due to the very small number of cases published [85]. In one study, if recurrence after fertility-sparing surgery occurred, long-term survival was 87 % as regards ovarian and 48 % as regards extra-ovarian relapse [82]. Data are still insufficient as regards other tumor types such as clear-cell carcinoma, but no differences in survival rates after fertility-sparing surgery have been reported in these patients when compared with women who have undergone radical surgery or fertility-sparing surgery in connection with non-clear-cell carcinoma [86]. Overall 5-year survival rates have been reported to be as high as 87 %, with approximately 12 % of patients suffering cancer recurrence after fertility-sparing surgery, when combining both low- and high-risk cancers [17].

The use of platinum-based adjuvant chemotherapy has been proposed for patients with high-risk ovarian cancer (IAG2 or higher) as well as clear-cell carcinoma after fertility-sparing surgery [85, 87].

Some authors have suggested the addition of assisted reproductive techniques using gonadotropic ovarian stimulation for egg retrieval after the performance of fertility-sparing unilateral oophorectomy. These procedures are aimed at safeguarding fertility potential by cryopreservation of embryos or oocytes for the future. The patient, thereafter, may undergo adnexectomy of the remnant ovary in a subsequent operation [88]. Reduced ovarian reserve may be a concern in women with previous ovarian operations [89]. Up to now, data are lacking on ovarian cancer relapse rates after gonadotropic stimulation. However, data on women at high risk of ovarian cancer as a result of BRCA mutations are reassuring and no association between gonadotropic ovarian stimulation and ovarian cancer has been observed in these patients [74, 90].

Ovarian tissue cryopreservation in patients with early ovarian cancers or borderline tumors is highly controversial but has been described by some authors [32]. As autotransplantation of the retrieved ovarian tissue is not feasible due to the risk of reintroducing malignant cells, alternatives have been discussed, such as culture and maturation of oocytes gained from the tissue in vitro, a procedure still under development which could be used in the future [91].

As regards QoL, available data indicate no major differences in sexual satisfaction or sexual concerns in women who have undergone fertility-sparing surgery compared with women who have undergone radical surgery [46].

#### Borderline ovarian tumors

Borderline ovarian tumors (BOTs) comprise 10–20 % of ovarian epithelial tumors [92]. In one study, among patients younger than 40 years, one third of ovarian cancer cases had borderline ovarian tumors [92]. Survival rates are about 99 %, with 70-month disease-free survival in cases of stage I tumors, and the survival rate in cases of stage III tumors is about 89 % [3].

**Table 2** Fertility-sparing interventions in women with borderline ovarian tumors or ovarian cancer

| Diagnosis | Type of Surgery | Description | Reproductive and Obstetric Outcomes | Oncologic Outcome | Quality of Life |
|---|---|---|---|---|---|
| Borderline Ovarian Tumor FIGO Stage Ia | Unilateral oophorectomy/ bilateral cystectomy | Removing the affected ovary only, keeping in place the unaffected one and the uterus | Spontaneous pregnancies have been reported with favorable obstetric outcome [99] | Higher recurrence rates in fertility-sparing surgery compared with radical surgery, with no difference in mortality [97, 98]. Recurrence 0 %–20 % versus 12 %–58 % when only cystectomy was performed [6] | High quality of life and higher sexual satisfaction scores after fertility-sparing surgery [103] |
| Borderline Ovarian Tumor FIGO Stages Ic–III | Unilateral oophorectomy/ bilateral cystectomy, peritoneal staging, pelvic & para-aortic lymphadenectomy, omentectomy | Removing the affected ovary only, thorough oncological staging | Pregnancy rate of 86 %, more than half of the patients required fertility treatment [99] | No difference in recurrence or survival compared with radical surgery removing both ovaries and the uterus [6, 99]. | Lack of data |
| Ovarian Epithelial Cancer FIGO Stage IA, grade 1 | Unilateral oophorectomy, peritoneal staging, pelvic & para-aortic lymphadenectomy and omentectomy | Removing the affected ovary only, thorough oncological staging | Pregnancy rates of >60 % Pregnancies have been reported with favorable obstetric outcome [145] | 5-year survival 87 %, recurrence 7–12 % [6, 17] | No difference in quality of life aspects or sexual satisfaction scores compared with radical surgery [46] |
| Ovarian Epithelial Cancer – FIGO Stage IA, grade 2–3 or Clear Cell Carcinoma | Unilateral oophorectomy, peritoneal staging, pelvic & para-aortic lymphadenectomy, omentectomy and adjuvant chemotherapy | Removing the affected ovary only, thorough oncological staging Adjuvant platinum-based chemotherapy | Pregnancy rate of 80 % with live-birth rate of 65 % in women presenting with cancer grades 1–3. Higher number of women with cancer grades 1–2 attempting pregnancy in comparison with women with grade 3 cancers [87] | No difference in recurrence or survival compared with radical surgery [86] | Lack of data |
| Malignant Germ Cell Cancers grade I | Unilateral oophorectomy, peritoneal staging, omentectomy, pelvic & para-aortic lymphadenectomy and adjuvant chemotherapy | Removing the affected ovary only, adjuvant BEP chemotherapy has been recommended, or expectant management | 76 % pregnancy rate. Pregnancies have been reported with favorable obstetric outcome [147, 148] | Fertility-sparing surgery has not been associated with impaired oncological outcome [108] | Good quality of life reported with good psychological health and sexual function [129] |

Modified from: Rodriguez-Wallberg KA, Oktay K. Fertility preservation during cancer treatment: clinical guidelines. Cancer management and research. 2014;6:105-17
Abbreviations: *FIGO* International Federation of Gynecology and Obstetrics, *BEP* bleomycin, etoposide and cisplatin

Because of relatively young age and good prognosis of the disease, conservative surgery can be performed in most BOT patients. Usually, adnexectomy on the affected side is performed, since cystectomy of the tumor has been associated with higher recurrence rates [3]. In case of bilateral BOTs, unilateral adnexectomy and contralateral cystectomy can be performed in women who wish to maintain reproductive potential. Even though fertility outcomes are uncertain, oncological prognoses similar to those of patients treated by means of radical surgery have been described [93, 94]. Surgical staging and histological subtypes (micropapillary and stromal micro-invasion) of BOTs have had no impact on recurrence [95]. Although associated with good prognosis overall, a higher level of lethal recurrence has been reported in cases of micopapillary serous BOT [96].

In general, conservative treatment of BOTs is associated with higher recurrence rates compared with radical treatment [3, 97]. However, after a follow-up period of seven years mortality has been reported to be very low and most authors regard conservative surgery as safe [98]. In a recent study on 59 patients concerning the role of fertility-sparing surgery in cases of advanced borderline tumors (FIGO stages IC–FIGO III) it was concluded that fertility-sparing surgery was not associated with relapse or mortality [99].

After conservative treatment of BOTs, patients should be counseled about the risk of diminished ovarian reserve following repeated conservative ovarian surgery or adnexectomy, and fertility counseling should be provided. Oocyte cryopreservation for future use can be an option for many of those women who do not have the intention to attempt pregnancy in the short term [89]. Due to the limited amount of data available it is not clear whether ovarian stimulation affects relapse time [100, 101]. In in vitro models no detrimental stimulatory effects of FSH or estradiol (E2) were found in BOT cells [102].

After suffering BOTs patients report a good quality of life and good sexual function. Fertility-sparing surgery is not associated with a higher QoL, but patients after such surgery showed higher-level sexual activity than patients treated radically [103].

### Germ cell tumors

Malignant ovarian germ cell tumors are rare (3–5 % of ovarian tumors), but are the most common ovarian tumors in very young women (< 20 years of age) [104, 105].

The majority of patients with malignant ovarian germ cell tumors are diagnosed with stage 1 disease as a result of the rapidly growing character of this kind of tumor [105]. Overall survival rates in cases of germ cell tumors are encouraging and fertility-sparing surgery is not associated with worsening of outcome [106–108].

Ovarian germ cell tumors are relatively heterogeneous, and there is great variation in management. In cases of immature teratoma, 5-year survival rates at stages I and II have been described as being as high as > 93 %, with higher recurrence rates in cases of grade 2–3 tumors and advanced-stage tumors [109, 110]. In yolk-sac tumors after fertility-sparing surgery and standard neoadjuvant chemotherapy 5-year survival has been found to be > 90 % and a fertility-sparing approach has been suggested irrespective of cancer stage [111–113]. In pure dysgerminoma, 10-year disease-free survival was > 90 %, with overall survival around 100 % [114, 115]. Due to this excellent long-term outcome, several authors suggest fertility-sparing treatment at all stages of ovarian dysgerminoma [116]. The usual treatment of ovarian germ cell tumors consists of unilateral adnexectomy, peritoneal staging and omentectomy [117]. However, some authors have described less invasive surgical procedures involving unilateral adnexectomy, cytology and peritoneal sampling in cases of dysgerminoma and immature teratoma limited to the ovary [110, 114]. In yolk-sac tumors, however, complete staging has been associated with a favorable outcome as a result of different adjuvant treatment at advanced stages [111, 113].

Bilateral disease is uncommon in cases of germ cell tumors and if the contralateral ovary appears macroscopically normal no biopsy is advised owing to the risk of extra adhesions and impairment of ovarian reserve [118, 119]. After fertility-sparing surgery, chemotherapy with bleomycin, etoposide and cisplatin (BEP) has been associated with improved disease-free survival [120]. However, recently a surveillance approach has been suggested for 50 % of patients with early stage I tumors [121]. In cases of early-stage yolk-sac tumors (stage I) surgery patients (with chemotherapy limited only to cases of relapse) showed higher recurrence rates but no difference in overall survival, saving 77 % of patients from chemotherapy [122]. However, in cases of higher-stage yolk-sac tumors standard-dose BEP chemotherapy has been associated with favorable overall survival rates and no apparent compromise of fertility rates [113, 123]. In early-stage pure dysgerminoma also, chemotherapy is only recommended in cases of relapse, according to several authors [114, 115]. In patients with immature ovarian teratoma, stage I, grade 2–3, adjuvant chemotherapy has been recommended by some authors, while the results of several studies suggest that an expectant approach with chemotherapy only in relapse situations in these patients may be more appropriate [124–126]. This is important because germ-cell cancer survivors treated with chemotherapy have shown relatively high chemotherapy-related secondary malignancy rates later in life [127]. Reproductive function, on the other hand, has been reported to be relatively good, with more than 80 % of patients retaining reproductive function after chemotherapy and surgery [116, 119]. IVF treatment in patients after germ-cell tumor therapy has been described in only a few cases [128].

Overall quality of life scores in germ-cell tumor survivors are good, with fertility preservation playing an important part [129].

## Reproductive outcomes after fertility-sparing surgery in cases of gynecological cancer

Gestation in women treated for gynecological cancer may require specialized surveillance, in particular if the treatment has resulted in anatomic disturbance of the cervix or the uterus due to operative procedures or radiation therapy.

In one study, in cases of early-stage cervical cancer, after LLETZ resection no impairment of fertility was observed. However, depending on the depth of resection, patients showed a higher risk of preterm delivery (OR 1.7) and premature rupture of the membranes (OR 2.69), with no effect on neonatal outcome [130]. Many spontaneous conceptions have been reported after radical trachelectomy, with rates of over 80 % when robot-assisted trachelectomy was performed [131]. Pregnancy rates of up to 60 % have been reported after abdominal and vaginal trachelectomy [132, 133]. Interestingly, even after neoadjuvant chemotherapy and vaginal trachelectomy in cases of IB1 cancer, a pregnancy rate of 86 % has been reported in women who attempted to conceive [134]. Performance of assisted reproductive techniques to achieve pregnancy has been reported to be necessary in up to 50 % of cases [135].

In general, rates of pregnancy loss after trachelectomy are higher than in the general population [133]. As a result of amputation of the cervix, high risks of preterm delivery and premature rupture of the membranes have been described [136, 137]. Recent data indicate relatively favorable outcomes, with more than 90 % of patients delivering in the third trimester [131]. However, the data are conflicting and whereas one study group reported 65 % of infants prematurely born (< 37 weeks) but only 4 % at less than 32 weeks of gestation [44], a recent review reported 28 % of premature children born before the 32nd week of gestation in a large population of > 300 live-births after trachelectomy [17]. Routine performance of cerclage is still a matter of controversy, and cerclage-related complications have been described [133, 138]. Several studies describe higher delivery rates achieved at term or during the third trimester after cerclage [139, 140]. In any case, the risk of prematurity should be considered as well as access to a center with specialized neonatal care. Frequent vaginal ultrasonography should be performed to assess the risk of prematurity associated with shortness of the cervix, and fetal lung maturation should be induced when necessary [141].

As a result of postoperative scar tissue after trachelectomy, elective cesarean section after 37 weeks of gestation is recommended [136].

Pregnancies in women with previous endometrial cancer have been reported, with success rates of over 60 % in women who attempted pregnancy [63, 72]. Pregnancy is achieved faster after treatments involving assisted reproductive techniques and miscarriage rates seem to be comparable to those in the general population [72, 142]. Overall, no adverse outcomes related to cancer treatment have been observed in over 75 live-births reported after endometrial cancer [17, 72].

In women with fertility-sparing surgery for ovarian cancer, use of assisted reproductive treatments involving IVF is indicated in many cases owing to a reduced ovarian reserve after repeated ovarian surgery or unilateral adnexectomy [143]. In series of cases reported, over 60 % of women who actively attempted pregnancy conceived, and miscarriage rates were low (< 30 %) [144, 145]. At present more than 220 pregnancies after ovarian cancer have been reported, with an overall miscarriage rate of 17 % [17]. Similar data have been reported for women treated for BOTs [99]. Interestingly, adjuvant chemotherapy has not been associated with infertility, but young age at the time of chemotherapy has been associated with premature menopause later in life [145, 146]. After fertility-sparing surgery in connection with germ-cell tumors, 76 % of patients who sought pregnancy conceived naturally [147], and pregnancies in patients after fertility-sparing surgery and germ-cell tumor treatment did not show any complications [148].

International guidelines for fertility preservation have been published and access to fertility preservation for young female cancer patients encouraged, in particular by use of assisted reproductive methods globally available and regarded as clinical routines, such as cryopreservation of oocytes or embryos after emergency IVF [6, 30–33, 149]. As regards fertility-sparing surgery for fertility preservation among women with gynecological cancer, global utilization of the methods available is currently unknown. In a recent European study, data was collected from several countries, demonstrating a low incidence of fertility-preserving surgery and it raised concerns as regards the need to centralize such treatments at accredited units, to ensure a sufficient number of patients at each center, with maintenance of good healthcare quality [150].

## Risk-reducing salpingo-oophorectomy in women at high risk of ovarian cancer who wish to preserve fertility

Women who are carriers of BRCA1 mutations present with a 39–46 % lifetime risk of developing ovarian cancer, and for carriers of BRCA2 mutations the lifetime risk is 12–20 %. The ovarian cancers that predominantly develop in BRCA1 and BRCA2 mutation-carriers are of serous or endometrioid histology and of high grade. In women with known BRCA mutations, periodic screening for ovarian cancer by way of assay of CA125 and transvaginal ultrasonography is recommended after the age of 30–35 years, or 5–10 years before the youngest age at which ovarian cancer was first diagnosed in the family [151].

Risk-reducing salpingo-oophorectomy has been shown to reduce the risk of ovarian cancer by 85–90 % and it should be offered to women with a BRCA mutation by age 40, or after the conclusion of childbearing [151].

Women who are carriers of BRCA mutations may have not yet built their families at the recommended age of risk-reducing salpingo-oophorectomy, and some of them may wish to undergo procedures to preserve fertility. Data on fertility preservation for BRCA mutation-carriers are largely linked to their concomitant risk of breast cancer, and in that respect reports are reassuring, as the ovarian stimulation and IVF procedures required to cryopreserve embryos or oocytes have not been shown to negatively affect the risks of breast cancer or breast cancer relapse in reported patient series [74, 90, 152]. Although pregnancy appears to be safe for BRCA mutation-carriers after breast cancer, specific studies on women with BRCA mutations are lacking. Such women may elect to utilize preimplantation genetic diagnosis during IVF to avoid transmitting the mutation to their children, but this option may create additional psychological distress, and, therefore, thorough counseling and psychosocial evaluation are essential [153]. Additionally, it has been noted that carriers of BRCA mutations may have lower ovarian reserves and can experience earlier menopause than non-mutation carriers, and thus the reproductive span of BRCA carriers may be 2–4 years shorter than that in the general population [74, 154].

## Conclusions

Current data on fertility-preservation options for women with early-stage gynecological cancer indicate oncological safety and high efficacy of fertility-sparing surgery. Some women presenting with sub-fertility may need to undergo assisted reproductive treatments to achieve pregnancy, which has not been shown to affect the oncologic outcome negatively. International guidelines for fertility preservation have been published and these underline the importance of timely discussion of the impact of cancer treatment on future fertility, and options for fertility preservation in all patients of reproductive age. The role of fertility-sparing treatment at more advanced stages of gynecological cancer has to be analyzed in further studies as a result of scarce data in this field.

## Abbreviations

BEP, bleomycin, etoposide and cisplatin; BOT, borderline ovarian tumor; BRCA, breast cancer 1/2 mutation; E2, estradiol; FSH, follicle-stimulating hormone; IUD, intrauterine device; IVF, in vitro fertilization; LLETZ, large loop excision of the transformation zone; OR, odds ratio; PCOS, polycystic ovary syndrome; QoL, quality of life

## Acknowledgements
None.

## Funding
This work has been supported by grants from The Swedish Society of Medicine, and Karolinska Institutet (KAR-W). Dr Rodriguez-Wallberg is supported by a Clinical Investigator Grant from Stockholm County Council.

## Authors' contributions
MF and KAR-W equally contributed to the writing and revision of the manuscript. Both authors read and approved the final manuscript.

## Competing interests
The authors declare that they have no competing interest.

## Author details
[1]Department of Obstetrics and Gynecology, Division of Gynecological Endocrinology and Reproductive Medicine, Medical University of Vienna, Vienna, Austria. [2]Wunschbaby Institut Feichtinger, Vienna, Austria. [3]Department of Oncology – Pathology, Karolinska Institutet, Stockholm, Sweden. [4]Department of Obstetrics and Gynecology, Section of Reproductive Medicine, Karolinska University Hospital, Novumhuset Plan 4, SE-141 86 Stockholm, Sweden.

## References
1. Siegel RL, Miller KD, Jemal A. Cancer statistics, 2016. CA Cancer J Clin. 2016; 66:7–30.
2. Howlader N, Noone AM, Krapcho M, Garshell J, Miller D, Altekruse SF, Kosary CL, Yu M, Ruhl J, Tatalovich Z, Mariotto A, Lewis DR, Chen HS, Feuer EJ, Cronin KA (eds). SEER Cancer Statistics Review, 1975-2012, National Cancer Institute. Bethesda, MD, http://seer.cancer.gov/csr/1975_2012/, based on November 2014 SEER data submission, posted to the SEER web site, April 2015.
3. Zanetta G, Rota S, Chiari S, Bonazzi C, Bratina G, Mangioni C. Behavior of borderline tumors with particular interest to persistence, recurrence, and progression to invasive carcinoma: a prospective study. J Clin Oncol. 2001; 19:2658–64.
4. Rosen A, Rodriguez-Wallberg KA, Rosenzweig L. Psychosocial distress in young cancer survivors. Semin Oncol Nurs. 2009;25:268–77.
5. Howard-Anderson J, Ganz PA, Bower JE, Stanton AL. Quality of life, fertility concerns, and behavioral health outcomes in younger breast cancer survivors: a systematic review. J Natl Cancer Inst. 2012;104:386–405.
6. Rodriguez-Wallberg KA, Oktay K. Fertility preservation during cancer treatment: clinical guidelines. Cancer Manag Res. 2014;6:105–17.
7. Rodriguez-Wallberg KA. Principles of cancer treatment: impact on reproduction. Adv Exp Med Biol. 2012;732:1–8.
8. Thibaud E, Rodriguez-Macias K, Trivin C, Esperou H, Michon J, Brauner R. Ovarian function after bone marrow transplantation during childhood. Bone Marrow Transplant. 1998;21:287–90.
9. Wallberg KA, Keros V, Hovatta O. Clinical aspects of fertility preservation in female patients. Pediatr Blood Cancer. 2009;53:254–60.
10. Wright JD, NathavithArana R, Lewin SN, Sun X, Deutsch I, Burke WM, et al. Fertility-conserving surgery for young women with stage IA1 cervical cancer: safety and access. Obstet Gynecol. 2010;115:585–90.

11. Spoozak L, Lewin SN, Burke WM, Deutsch I, Sun X, Herzog TJ, et al. Microinvasive adenocarcinoma of the cervix. Am J Obstet Gynecol. 2012;206:80:e1-6.

12. Marchiole P, Benchaib M, Buenerd A, Lazlo E, Dargent D, Mathevet P. Oncological safety of laparoscopic-assisted vaginal radical trachelectomy (LARVT or Dargent's operation): a comparative study with laparoscopic-assisted vaginal radical hysterectomy (LARVH). Gynecol Oncol. 2007;106:132–41.

13. Gien LT, Covens A. Fertility-sparing options for early stage cervical cancer. Gynecol Oncol. 2010;117:350–7.

14. Dargent DBJ, Remy I. Pregnancies following radical trachelectomy for invasive cervical cancer. Society of Gynecologic Oncologists—Abstracts. Gynecol Oncol. 1994;52:105–8.

15. Helpman L, Grisaru D, Covens A. Early adenocarcinoma of the cervix: is radical vaginal trachelectomy safe? Gynecol Oncol. 2011;123:95–8.

16. Xu L, Sun FQ, Wang ZH. Radical trachelectomy versus radical hysterectomy for the treatment of early cervical cancer: a systematic review. Acta Obstet Gynecol Scand. 2011;90:1200–9.

17. Zapardiel I, Cruz M, Diestro MD, Requena A, Garcia-Velasco JA. Assisted reproductive techniques after fertility-sparing treatments in gynaecological cancers. Hum Reprod Update 2016 [Epub ahead of print].

18. Hoogendam JP, Zweemer RP, Hobbelink MG, van den Bosch MA, Verheijen RH, Veldhuis WB. 99mTc-Nanocolloid SPECT/MRI Fusion for the Selective Assessment of Nonenlarged Sentinel Lymph Nodes in Patients with Early-Stage Cervical Cancer. J Nucl Med. 2016;57:551–6.

19. Shepherd JH, Spencer C, Herod J, Ind TE. Radical vaginal trachelectomy as a fertility-sparing procedure in women with early-stage cervical cancer-cumulative pregnancy rate in a series of 123 women. BJOG. 2006;113:719–24.

20. Fagotti A, Gagliardi ML, Moruzzi C, Carone V, Scambia G, Fanfani F. Excisional cone as fertility-sparing treatment in early-stage cervical cancer. Fertil Steril. 2011;95:1109–12.

21. Maneo A, Sideri M, Scambia G, Boveri S, Dell'anna T, Villa M, et al. Simple conization and lymphadenectomy for the conservative treatment of stage IB1 cervical cancer. An Italian experience. Gynecol Oncol. 2011;123:557–60.

22. Plante M, Lau S, Brydon L, Swenerton K, LeBlanc R, Roy M. Neoadjuvant chemotherapy followed by vaginal radical trachelectomy in bulky stage IB1 cervical cancer: case report. Gynecol Oncol. 2006;101:367–70.

23. Robova H, Halaska MJ, Pluta M, Skapa P, Matecha J, Lisy J, et al. Oncological and pregnancy outcomes after high-dose density neoadjuvant chemotherapy and fertility-sparing surgery in cervical cancer. Gynecol Oncol. 2014;135:213–6.

24. Pareja R, Rendon GJ, Vasquez M, Echeverri L, Sanz-Lomana CM, Ramirez PT. Immediate radical trachelectomy versus neoadjuvant chemotherapy followed by conservative surgery for patients with stage IB1 cervical cancer with tumors 2cm or larger: A literature review and analysis of oncological and obstetrical outcomes. Gynecol Oncol. 2015;137:574–80.

25. Morice P, Castaigne D, Haie-Meder C, Pautier P, El Hassan J, Duvillard P, et al. Laparoscopic ovarian transposition for pelvic malignancies: indications and functional outcomes. Fertil Steril. 1998;70:956–60.

26. Morice P, Juncker L, Rey A, El-Hassan J, Haie-Meder C, Castaigne D. Ovarian transposition for patients with cervical carcinoma treated by radiosurgical combination. Fertil Steril. 2000;74:743–8.

27. Ghadjar P, Budach V, Kohler C, Jantke A, Marnitz S. Modern radiation therapy and potential fertility preservation strategies in patients with cervical cancer undergoing chemoradiation. Radiat Oncol. 2015;10:50.

28. Feeney DD, Moore DH, Look KY, Stehman FB, Sutton GP. The fate of the ovaries after radical hysterectomy and ovarian transposition. Gynecol Oncol. 1995;56:3–7.

29. Wo JY, Viswanathan AN. Impact of radiotherapy on fertility, pregnancy, and neonatal outcomes in female cancer patients. Int J Radiat Oncol Biol Phys. 2009;73:1304–12.

30. von Wolff M, Thaler CJ, Frambach T, Zeeb C, Lawrenz B, Popovici RM, et al. Ovarian stimulation to cryopreserve fertilized oocytes in cancer patients can be started in the luteal phase. Fertil Steril. 2009;92:1360–5.

31. Bedoschi G, Oktay K. Current approach to fertility preservation by embryo cryopreservation. Fertil Steril. 2013;99:1496–502.

32. Donnez J, Dolmans MM. Fertility preservation in women. Nat Rev Endocrinol. 2013;9:735–49.

33. Garcia-Velasco JA, Domingo J, Cobo A, Martinez M, Carmona L, Pellicer A. Five years' experience using oocyte vitrification to preserve fertility for medical and nonmedical indications. Fertil Steril. 2013;99:1994–9.

34. Dahhan T, Dancet EA, Miedema DV, van der Veen F, Goddijn M. Reproductive choices and outcomes after freezing oocytes for medical reasons: a follow-up study. Hum Reprod. 2014;29:1925–30.

35. Rodriguez-Wallberg KA, Karlstrom PO, Rezapour M, Castellanos E, Hreinsson J, Rasmussen C, et al. Full-term newborn after repeated ovarian tissue transplants in a patient treated for Ewing sarcoma by sterilizing pelvic irradiation and chemotherapy. Acta Obstet Gynecol Scand. 2015;94:324–8.

36. Green DM, Sklar CA, Boice Jr JD, Mulvihill JJ, Whitton JA, Stovall M, et al. Ovarian failure and reproductive outcomes after childhood cancer treatment: results from the Childhood Cancer Survivor Study. J Clin Oncol. 2009;27:2374–81.

37. Kim SS, Lee WS, Chung MK, Lee HC, Lee HH, Hill D. Long-term ovarian function and fertility after heterotopic autotransplantation of cryobanked human ovarian tissue: 8-year experience in cancer patients. Fertil Steril. 2009;91:2349–54.

38. Donnez J, Dolmans MM, Pellicer A, Diaz-Garcia C, Sanchez Serrano M, Schmidt KT, et al. Restoration of ovarian activity and pregnancy after transplantation of cryopreserved ovarian tissue: a review of 60 cases of reimplantation. Fertil Steril. 2013;99:1503–13.

39. Rodriguez-Wallberg KA, Tanbo T, Tinkanen H, Thurin-Kjellberg A, Nedstrand E, et al. Current practice and clinical achievements in cryopreservation of ovarian tissue for fertility preservation in the Nordic Countries – Compilation of 20 years of multicentre experience. Acta Obstetricia et Gynecologica Scandinavica 2016, in press.

40. Donnez J, Dolmans MM. Ovarian cortex transplantation: 60 reported live births brings the success and worldwide expansion of the technique towards routine clinical practice. J Assist Reprod Genet. 2015;32:1167–70.

41. Nakanishi T, Wakai K, Ishikawa H, Nawa A, Suzuki Y, Nakamura S, et al. A comparison of ovarian metastasis between squamous cell carcinoma and adenocarcinoma of the uterine cervix. Gynecol Oncol. 2001;82:504–9.

42. Brannstrom M, Johannesson L, Bokstrom H, Kvarnstrom N, Molne J, Dahm-Kahler P, et al. Livebirth after uterus transplantation. Lancet. 2015;385:607–16.

43. Pondrom S. US to Offer Uterus Transplants. Am J Transplant. 2016;16:375–6.

44. Plante M, Gregoire J, Renaud MC, Roy M. The vaginal radical trachelectomy: an update of a series of 125 cases and 106 pregnancies. Gynecol Oncol. 2011;121:290–7.

45. Aust T, Herod J, Macdonald R, Gazvani R. Infertility after fertility-preserving surgery for cervical carcinoma: the next challenge for reproductive medicine? Hum Fertil (Camb). 2007;10:21–4.

46. Chan JL, Letourneau J, Salem W, Cil AP, Chan SW, Chen LM, et al. Sexual satisfaction and quality of life in survivors of localized cervical and ovarian cancers following fertility-sparing surgery. Gynecol Oncol. 2015;139:141–7.

47. Froeding LP, Ottosen C, Rung-Hansen H, Svane D, Mosgaard BJ, Jensen PT. Sexual functioning and vaginal changes after radical vaginal trachelectomy in early stage cervical cancer patients: a longitudinal study. J Sex Med. 2014;11:595–604.

48. Froding LP, Ottosen C, Mosgaard BJ, Jensen PT. Quality of life, urogynecological morbidity, and lymphedema after radical vaginal trachelectomy for early-stage cervical cancer. Int J Gynecol Cancer. 2015;25:699–706.

49. Fanfani F, Landoni F, Gagliardi ML, Fagotti A, Preti E, Moruzzi MC, et al. Sexual and Reproductive Outcomes in Early Stage Cervical Cancer Patients after Excisional Cone as a Fertility-sparing Surgery: An Italian Experience. J Reprod infertility. 2014;15:29–34.

50. Haoula Z, Salman M, Atiomo W. Evaluating the association between endometrial cancer and polycystic ovary syndrome. Hum Reprod. 2012;27:1327–31.

51. Amant F, Moerman P, Neven P, Timmerman D, Van Limbergen E, Vergote I. Endometrial cancer. Lancet. 2005;366:491–505.

52. Ben-Shachar I, Vitellas KM, Cohn DE. The role of MRI in the conservative management of endometrial cancer. Gynecol Oncol. 2004;93:233–7.

53. Kim MK, Seong SJ, Kim YS, Song T, Kim ML, Yoon BS, et al. Combined medroxyprogesterone acetate/levonorgestrel-intrauterine system treatment in young women with early-stage endometrial cancer. Am J Obstet Gynecol. 2013;209:358. e1-4.

54. Minig L, Franchi D, Boveri S, Casadio C, Bocciolone L, Sideri M. Progestin intrauterine device and GnRH analogue for uterus sparing treatment of endometrial precancers and well-differentiated early endometrial carcinoma in young women. Ann Oncol. 2011;22:643–9.

55. Baker J, Obermair A, Gebski V, Janda M. Efficacy of oral or intrauterine device-delivered progestin in patients with complex endometrial hyperplasia with atypia or early endometrial adenocarcinoma: a meta-analysis and systematic review of the literature. Gynecol Oncol. 2012; 125:263–70.

56. Hubbs JL, Saig RM, Abaid LN, Bae-Jump VL, Gehrig PA. Systemic and local hormone therapy for endometrial hyperplasia and early adenocarcinoma. Obstet Gynecol. 2013;121:1172–80.

57. Gallos ID, Krishan P, Shehmar M, Ganesan R, Gupta JK. LNG-IUS versus oral progestogen treatment for endometrial hyperplasia: a long-term comparative cohort study. Hum Reprod. 2013;28:2966–71.

58. Gallos ID, Krishan P, Shehmar M, Ganesan R, Gupta JK. Relapse of endometrial hyperplasia after conservative treatment: a cohort study with long-term follow-up. Hum Reprod. 2013;28:1231–6.

59. Abu Hashim H, Ghayaty E, El Rakhawy M. Levonorgestrel-releasing intrauterine system vs oral progestins for non-atypical endometrial hyperplasia: a systematic review and metaanalysis of randomized trials. Am J Obstet Gynecol. 2015;213: 469–78.

60. Ushijima K, Yahata H, Yoshikawa H, Konishi I, Yasugi T, Saito T, et al. Multicenter phase II study of fertility-sparing treatment with medroxyprogesterone acetate for endometrial carcinoma and atypical hyperplasia in young women. J Clin Oncol. 2007;25:2798–803.

61. Gunderson CC, Fader AN, Carson KA, Bristow RE. Oncologic and reproductive outcomes with progestin therapy in women with endometrial hyperplasia and grade 1 adenocarcinoma: a systematic review. Gynecol Oncol. 2012;125:477–82.

62. Park JY, Lee SH, Seong SJ, Kim DY, Kim TJ, Kim JW, et al. Progestin re-treatment in patients with recurrent endometrial adenocarcinoma after successful fertility-sparing management using progestin. Gynecol Oncol. 2013;129:7–11.

63. Mazzon I, Corrado G, Masciullo V, Morricone D, Ferrandina G, Scambia G. Conservative surgical management of stage IA endometrial carcinoma for fertility preservation. Fertil Steril. 2010;93:1286–9.

64. Paulson RJ, Sauer MV, Lobo RA. Pregnancy after in vitro fertilization in a patient with stage I endometrial carcinoma treated with progestins. Fertil Steril. 1990;54:735–6.

65. Sardi J, Anchezar Henry JP, Paniceres G, Gomez Rueda N, Vighi S. Primary hormonal treatment for early endometrial carcinoma. Eur J Gynaecol Oncol. 1998;19:565–8.

66. Shibahara H, Shigeta M, Toji H, Wakimoto E, Adachi S, Ogasawara T, et al. Successful pregnancy in an infertile patient with conservatively treated endometrial adenocarcinoma after transfer of embryos obtained by intracytoplasmic sperm injection. Hum Reprod. 1999;14:1908–11.

67. Ogawa S, Koike T, Shibahara H, Ohwada M, Suzuki M, Araki S, et al. Assisted reproductive technologies in conjunction with conservatively treated endometrial adenocarcinoma. A case report. Gynecol Obstet Investig. 2001;51:214–6.

68. Pinto AB, Gopal M, Herzog TJ, Pfeifer JD, Williams DB. Successful in vitro fertilization pregnancy after conservative management of endometrial cancer. Fertil Steril. 2001;76:826–9.

69. Lowe MP, Cooper BC, Sood AK, Davis WA, Syrop CH, Sorosky JI. Implementation of assisted reproductive technologies following conservative management of FIGO grade I endometrial adenocarcinoma and/or complex hyperplasia with atypia. Gynecol Oncol. 2003;91:569–72.

70. Nakao Y, Nomiyama M, Kojima K, Matsumoto Y, Yamasaki F, Iwasaka T. Successful pregnancies in 2 infertile patients with endometrial adenocarcinoma. Gynecol Obstet Investig. 2004;58:68–71.

71. Yarali H, Bozdag G, Aksu T, Ayhan A. A successful pregnancy after intracytoplasmic sperm injection and embryo transfer in a patient with endometrial cancer who was treated conservatively. Fertil Steril. 2004;81: 214–6.

72. Park JY, Seong SJ, Kim TJ, Kim JW, Kim SM, Bae DS, et al. Pregnancy outcomes after fertility-sparing management in young women with early endometrial cancer. Obstet Gynecol. 2013;121:136–42.

73. Oktay K, Turkcuoglu I, Rodriguez-Wallberg KA. GnRH agonist trigger for women with breast cancer undergoing fertility preservation by aromatase inhibitor/FSH stimulation. Reprod Biomed Online. 2010;20:783–8.

74. Rodriguez-Wallberg KA, Oktay K. Fertility preservation and pregnancy in women with and without BRCA mutation-positive breast cancer. Oncologist. 2012;17:1409–17.

75. Azim A, Oktay K. Letrozole for ovulation induction and fertility preservation by embryo cryopreservation in young women with endometrial carcinoma. Fertil Steril. 2007;88:657–64.

76. Juretzka MM, O'Hanlan KA, Katz SL, El-Danasouri I, Westphal LM. Embryo cryopreservation after diagnosis of stage IIB endometrial cancer and subsequent pregnancy in a gestational carrier. Fertil Steril. 2005;83:1041.

77. Niwa K, Tagami K, Lian Z, Onogi K, Mori H, Tamaya T. Outcome of fertility-preserving treatment in young women with endometrial carcinomas. BJOG. 2005;112:317–20.

78. Lavery S, Ng C, Kyrgiou M, Farthing A. Gestational surrogacy after intra-operative oocyte collection in a hysterectomised woman diagnosed with endometrial cancer. BJOG. 2011;118:1669–71.

79. Gallos ID, Shehmar M, Thangaratinam S, Papapostolou TK, Coomarasamy A, Gupta JK. Oral progestogens vs levonorgestrel-releasing intrauterine system for endometrial hyperplasia: a systematic review and metaanalysis. Am J Obstet Gynecol. 2010;203:547. e1-10.

80. Tomao F, Peccatori F, Pup LD, Franchi D, Zanagnolo V, Panici PB, et al. Special issues in fertility preservation for gynecologic malignancies. Crit Rev Oncol Hematol. 2016;97:206–19.

81. Redman C, Duffy S, Bromham N, Francis K, Guideline Development G. Recognition and initial management of ovarian cancer: summary of NICE guidance. BMJ. 2011;342:d2073.

82. Bentivegna E, Fruscio R, Roussin S, Ceppi L, Satoh T, Kajiyama H, et al. Long-term follow-up of patients with an isolated ovarian recurrence after conservative treatment of epithelial ovarian cancer: review of the results of an international multicenter study comprising 545 patients. Fertil Steril. 2015;104:1319–24.

83. Morice P, Leblanc E, Rey A, Baron M, Querleu D, Blanchot J, et al. Conservative treatment in epithelial ovarian cancer: results of a multicentre study of the GCCLCC (Groupe des Chirurgiens de Centre de Lutte Contre le Cancer) and SFOG (Societe Francaise d'Oncologie Gynecologique). Hum Reprod. 2005;20: 1379–85.

84. Ghezzi F, Cromi A, Fanfani F, Malzoni M, Ditto A, Pierandrea I, et al. Laparoscopic fertility-sparing surgery for early ovarian epithelial cancer: a multi-institutional experience. Gynecol Oncol. 2016. Epub ahead of print.

85. Ditto A, Martinelli F, Bogani G, Lorusso D, Carcangiu M, Chiappa V, et al. Long-term safety of fertility sparing surgery in early stage ovarian cancer: comparison to standard radical surgical procedures. Gynecol Oncol. 2015; 138:78–82.

86. Kajiyama H, Shibata K, Mizuno M, Hosono S, Kawai M, Nagasaka T, et al. Fertility-sparing surgery in patients with clear-cell carcinoma of the ovary: is it possible? Hum Reprod. 2011;26:3297–302.

87. Fruscio R, Corso S, Ceppi L, Garavaglia D, Garbi A, Floriani I, et al. Conservative management of early-stage epithelial ovarian cancer: results of a large retrospective series. Ann Oncol. 2013;24:138–44.

88. Alvarez M, Sole M, Devesa M, Fabregas R, Boada M, Tur R, et al. Live birth using vitrified–warmed oocytes in invasive ovarian cancer: case report and literature review. Reprod Biomed Online. 2014;28:663–8.

89. Druckenmiller S, Goldman KN, Labella PA, Fino ME, Bazzocchi A, Noyes N. Successful Oocyte Cryopreservation in Reproductive-Aged Cancer Survivors. Obstet Gynecol. 2016;127:474–80.

90. Perri T, Lifshitz D, Sadetzki S, Oberman B, Meirow D, Ben-Baruch G, et al. Fertility treatments and invasive epithelial ovarian cancer risk in Jewish Israeli BRCA1 or BRCA2 mutation carriers. Fertil Steril. 2015;103:1305–12.

91. Abir R, Ben-Aharon I, Garor R, Yaniv I, Ash S, Stemmer SM, et al. Cryopreservation of in vitro matured oocytes in addition to ovarian tissue freezing for fertility preservation in paediatric female cancer patients before and after cancer therapy. Hum Reprod. 2016;31:750–62.

92. Skirnisdottir I, Garmo H, Wilander E, Holmberg L. Borderline ovarian tumors in Sweden 1960-2005: trends in incidence and age at diagnosis compared to ovarian cancer. Int J Cancer. 2008;123:1897–901.

93. Faluyi O, Mackean M, Gourley C, Bryant A, Dickinson HO. Interventions for the treatment of borderline ovarian tumours. Cochrane Database Syst Rev. 2010;(9). Art. No.: CD007696. doi:10.1002/14651858.CD007696.pub2.

94. Vasconcelos I, de Sousa Mendes M. Conservative surgery in ovarian borderline tumours: a meta-analysis with emphasis on recurrence risk. Eur J Cancer. 2015; 51:620–31.

95. Uzan C, Muller E, Kane A, Rey A, Gouy S, Bendiffallah S, et al. Prognostic factors for recurrence after conservative treatment in a series of 119 patients with stage I serous borderline tumors of the ovary. Ann Oncol. 2014;25:166–71.

96. Vasconcelos I, Darb-Esfahani S, Sehouli J. Serous and mucinous borderline ovarian tumours: differences in clinical presentation, high-risk histopathological features, and lethal recurrence rates. BJOG. 2016;123:498–508.

97. Fauvet R, Boccara J, Dufournet C, David-Montefiore E, Poncelet C, Darai E. Restaging surgery for women with borderline ovarian tumors: results of a French multicenter study. Cancer. 2004;100:1145–51.

98. Suh-Burgmann E. Long-term outcomes following conservative surgery for borderline tumor of the ovary: a large population-based study. Gynecol Oncol. 2006;103:841–7.

99. Helpman L, Beiner ME, Aviel-Ronen S, Perri T, Hogen L, Jakobson-Setton A, et al. Safety of ovarian conservation and fertility preservation in advanced borderline ovarian tumors. Fertil Steril. 2015;104:138–44.

100. Denschlag D, von Wolff M, Amant F, Kesic V, Reed N, Schneider A, et al. Clinical recommendation on fertility preservation in borderline ovarian neoplasm: ovarian stimulation and oocyte retrieval after conservative surgery. Gynecol Obstet Investig. 2010;70:160–5.

101. Darai E, Fauvet R, Uzan C, Gouy S, Duvillard P, Morice P. Fertility and borderline ovarian tumor: a systematic review of conservative management, risk of recurrence and alternative options. Hum Reprod Update. 2013;19:151–66.

102. Basille C, Olivennes F, Le Calvez J, Beron-Gaillard N, Meduri G, Lhomme C, et al. Impact of gonadotrophins and steroid hormones on tumour cells derived from borderline ovarian tumours. Hum Reprod. 2006;21:3241–5.

103. Farthmann J, Hasenburg A, Weil M, Fotopoulou C, Ewald-Riegler N, du Bois O, et al. Quality of life and sexual function in patients with borderline tumors of the ovary. A substudy of the Arbeitsgemeinschaft Gynaekologische Onkologie (AGO) study group ROBOT study. Support Care Cancer. 2015;23:117–23.

104. Quirk JT, Natarajan N, Mettlin CJ. Age-specific ovarian cancer incidence rate patterns in the United States. Gynecol Oncol. 2005;99:248–50.

105. Smith HO, Berwick M, Verschraegen CF, Wiggins C, Lansing L, Muller CY, et al. Incidence and survival rates for female malignant germ cell tumors. Obstet Gynecol. 2006;107:1075–85.

106. Chan JK, Tewari KS, Waller S, Cheung MK, Shin JY, Osann K, et al. The influence of conservative surgical practices for malignant ovarian germ cell tumors. J Surg Oncol. 2008;98:111–6.

107. Mangili G, Sigismondi C, Gadducci A, Cormio G, Scollo P, Tateo S, et al. Outcome and risk factors for recurrence in malignant ovarian germ cell tumors: a MITO-9 retrospective study. Int J Gynecol Cancer. 2011;21:1414–21.

108. Park JY, Kim DY, Suh DS, Kim JH, Kim YM, Kim YT, et al. Outcomes of pediatric and adolescent girls with malignant ovarian germ cell tumors. Gynecol Oncol. 2015;137:418–22.

109. Weinberg LE, Lurain JR, Singh DK, Schink JC. Survival and reproductive outcomes in women treated for malignant ovarian germ cell tumors. Gynecol Oncol. 2011;121:285–9.

110. Jorge S, Jones NL, Chen L, Hou JY, Tergas AI, Burke WM et al. Characteristics, treatment and outcomes of women with immature ovarian Teratoma, 1998-2012. Gynecologic oncology 2016 [Epub ahead of print].

111. Nawa A, Obata N, Kikkawa F, Kawai M, Nagasaka T, Goto S, et al. Prognostic factors of patients with yolk sac tumors of the ovary. Am J Obstet Gynecol. 2001;184:1182–8.

112. Kang H, Kim TJ, Kim WY, Choi CH, Lee JW, Kim BG, et al. Outcome and reproductive function after cumulative high-dose combination chemotherapy with bleomycin, etoposide and cisplatin (BEP) for patients with ovarian endodermal sinus tumor. Gynecol Oncol. 2008;111:106–10.

113. de La Motte RT, Pautier P, Duvillard P, Rey A, Morice P, Haie-Meder C, et al. Survival and reproductive function of 52 women treated with surgery and bleomycin, etoposide, cisplatin (BEP) chemotherapy for ovarian yolk sac tumor. AnnOncol. 2008;19:1435–41.

114. Vicus D, Beiner ME, Klachook S, Le LW, Laframboise S, Mackay H. Pure dysgerminoma of the ovary 35 years on: a single institutional experience. Gynecol Oncol. 2010;117:23–6.

115. Mangili G, Sigismondi C, Lorusso D, Cormio G, Scollo P, Vigano R, et al. Is surgical restaging indicated in apparent stage IA pure ovarian dysgerminoma? The MITO group retrospective experience. Gynecol Oncol. 2011;121:280–4.

116. Brewer M, Gershenson DM, Herzog CE, Mitchell MF, Silva EG, Wharton JT. Outcome and reproductive function after chemotherapy for ovarian dysgerminoma. J Clin Oncol. 1999;17:2670–5.

117. Pectasides D, Pectasides E, Kassanos D. Germ cell tumors of the ovary. Cancer Treat Rev. 2008;34:427–41.

118. Kurman RJ, Norris HJ. Malignant germ cell tumors of the ovary. Hum Pathol. 1977;8:551–64.

119. Gershenson DM. Management of ovarian germ cell tumors. J Clin Oncol. 2007;25:2938–43.

120. Cushing B, Giller R, Cullen JW, Marina NM, Lauer SJ, Olson TA, et al. Randomized comparison of combination chemotherapy with etoposide, bleomycin, and either high-dose or standard-dose cisplatin in children and adolescents with high-risk malignant germ cell tumors: a pediatric

intergroup study–Pediatric Oncology Group 9049 and Children's Cancer Group 8882. J Clin Oncol. 2004;22:2691–700.

121. Billmire DF, Cullen JW, Rescorla FJ, Davis M, Schlatter MG, Olson TA, et al. Surveillance after initial surgery for pediatric and adolescent girls with stage I ovarian germ cell tumors: report from the Children's Oncology Group. J Clin Oncol. 2014;32:465–70.

122. Park JY, Kim DY, Suh DS, Kim JH, Kim YM, Kim YT, et al. Outcomes of surgery alone and surveillance strategy in young women with stage I malignant ovarian germ cell tumors. Int J Gynecol Cancer. 2016;26:859–64.

123. Satoh T, Aoki Y, Kasamatsu T, Ochiai K, Takano M, Watanabe Y, et al. Administration of standard-dose BEP regimen (bleomycin + etoposide + cisplatin) is essential for treatment of ovarian yolk sac tumour. Eur J Cancer. 2015;51:340–51.

124. Cushing B, Giller R, Ablin A, Cohen L, Cullen J, Hawkins E, et al. Surgical resection alone is effective treatment for ovarian immature teratoma in children and adolescents: a report of the pediatric oncology group and the children's cancer group. Am J Obstet Gynecol. 1999;181:353–8.

125. Mangili G, Scarfone G, Gadducci A, Sigismondi C, Ferrandina G, Scibilia G, et al. Is adjuvant chemotherapy indicated in stage I pure immature ovarian teratoma (IT)? A multicentre Italian trial in ovarian cancer (MITO-9). Gynecol Oncol. 2010;119:48–52.

126. Vicus D, Beiner ME, Clarke B, Klachook S, Le LW, Laframboise S, et al. Ovarian immature teratoma: treatment and outcome in a single institutional cohort. Gynecol Oncol. 2011;123:50–3.

127. Travis LB, Beard C, Allan JM, Dahl AA, Feldman DR, Oldenburg J, et al. Testicular cancer survivorship: research strategies and recommendations. J Natl Cancer Inst. 2010;102:1114–30.

128. Kitajima Y, Endo T, Hayashi T, Ishioka S, Baba T, Honnma H, et al. A successful IVF-pregnancy in a patient who underwent conservative surgery followed by a regimen of cisplatin, vinblastine and peplomycin to treat an advanced ovarian mixed germ cell tumour: a case report. Hum Reprod. 2007;22:850–2.

129. Champion V, Williams SD, Miller A, Reuille KM, Wagler-Ziner K, Monahan PO, et al. Quality of life in long-term survivors of ovarian germ cell tumors: a Gynecologic Oncology Group study. Gynecol Oncol. 2007;105:687–94.

130. Kyrgiou M, Koliopoulos G, Martin-Hirsch P, Arbyn M, Prendiville W, Paraskevaidis E. Obstetric outcomes after conservative treatment for intraepithelial or early invasive cervical lesions: systematic review and meta-analysis. Lancet. 2006;367:489–98.

131. Johansen G, Lonnerfors C, Falconer H, Persson J. Reproductive and oncologic outcome following robot-assisted laparoscopic radical trachelectomy for early stage cervical cancer. Gynecol Oncol. 2016;141:160–5.

132. Beiner ME, Covens A. Surgery insight: radical vaginal trachelectomy as a method of fertility preservation for cervical cancer. Nat Clin Pract Oncol. 2007;4:353–61.

133. Pareja R, Rendon GJ, Sanz-Lomana CM, Monzon O, Ramirez PT. Surgical, oncological, and obstetrical outcomes after abdominal radical trachelectomy - a systematic literature review. Gynecol Oncol. 2013;131:77–82.

134. Yan H, Liu Z, Fu X, Li Y, Che H, Mo R, et al. Long-term outcomes of radical vaginal trachelectomy and laparoscopic pelvic lymphadenectomy after neoadjuvant chemotherapy for the IB1 cervical cancer: A series of 60 cases. Int J Surg. 2016;29:38–42.

135. Hauerberg L, Hogdall C, Loft A, Ottosen C, Bjoern SF, Mosgaard BJ, et al. Vaginal radical trachelectomy for early stage cervical cancer. Results of the Danish National Single Center Strategy. Gynecol Oncol. 2015;138:304–10.

136. Ebisawa K, Takano M, Fukuda M, Fujiwara K, Hada T, Ota Y, et al. Obstetric outcomes of patients undergoing total laparoscopic radical trachelectomy for early stage cervical cancer. Gynecol Oncol. 2013;131:83–6.

137. Park JY, Kim DY, Suh DS, Kim JH, Kim YM, Kim YT, et al. Reproductive outcomes after laparoscopic radical trachelectomy for early-stage cervical cancer. J Gynecol Oncol. 2014;25:9–13.

138. Olawaiye A, Del Carmen M, Tambouret R, Goodman A, Fuller A, Duska LR. Abdominal radical trachelectomy: Success and pitfalls in a general gynecologic oncology practice. Gynecol Oncol. 2009;112:506–10.

139. Jolley JA, Battista L, Wing DA. Management of pregnancy after radical trachelectomy: case reports and systematic review of the literature. Am J Perinatol. 2007;24:531–9.

140. Kim CH, Abu-Rustum NR, Chi DS, Gardner GJ, Leitao Jr MM, Carter J, et al. Reproductive outcomes of patients undergoing radical trachelectomy for early-stage cervical cancer. Gynecol Oncol. 2012;125:585–8.

141. Pils S, Eppel W, Seemann R, Natter C, Ott J. Sequential cervical length screening in pregnancies after loop excision of the transformation zone conisation: a retrospective analysis. BJOG. 2014;121:457–62.

142. Gallos ID, Yap J, Rajkhowa M, Luesley DM, Coomarasamy A, Gupta JK. Regression, relapse, and live birth rates with fertility-sparing therapy for endometrial cancer and atypical complex endometrial hyperplasia: a systematic review and metaanalysis. Am J Obstet Gynecol. 2012;207:266:e1-12.

143. Park JY, Heo EJ, Lee JW, Lee YY, Kim TJ, Kim BG, et al. Outcomes of laparoscopic fertility-sparing surgery in clinically early-stage epithelial ovarian cancer. J Gynecol Oncol. 2016;27:e20.

144. Fotopoulou C, Braicu I, Sehouli J. Fertility-sparing surgery in early epithelial ovarian cancer: a viable option? Obstet Gynecol Int. 2012;2012:238061.

145. Zapardiel I, Diestro MD, Aletti G. Conservative treatment of early stage ovarian cancer: oncological and fertility outcomes. Eur J Surg Oncol. 2014; 40:387–93.

146. Letourneau J, Chan J, Salem W, Chan SW, Shah M, Ebbel E, et al. Fertility sparing surgery for localized ovarian cancers maintains an ability to conceive, but is Associated with diminished reproductive potential. J Surg Oncol. 2015;112:26–30.

147. Ertas IE, Taskin S, Goklu R, Bilgin M, Goc G, Yildirim Y, et al. Long-term oncological and reproductive outcomes of fertility-sparing cytoreductive surgery in females aged 25 years and younger with malignant ovarian germ cell tumors. J Obstet Gynaecol Res. 2014;40:797–805.

148. Boran N, Tulunay G, Caliskan E, Kose MF, Haberal A. Pregnancy outcomes and menstrual function after fertility sparing surgery for pure ovarian dysgerminomas. Arch Gynecol Obstet. 2005;271:104–8.

149. Loren AW, Mangu PB, Beck LN, Brennan L, Magdalinski AJ, Partridge AH, et al. Fertility preservation for patients with cancer: American Society of Clinical Oncology clinical practice guideline update. J Clin Oncol. 2013;31:2500–10.

150. Kesic V, Rodolakis A, Denschlag D, Schneider A, Morice P, Amant F, et al. Fertility preserving management in gynecologic cancer patients: the need for centralization. Int J Gynecol Cancer. 2010;20:1613–9.

151. Routine Screening for Hereditary Breast and Ovarian Cancer Recommended. American Congress of Obstetricians and Gynecologists. March 23, 2009. Available at: http://www.acog.org/About-ACOG/News-Room/News-Releases/2009/Routine-Screening-for-Hereditary-Breast-and-Ovarian-Cancer-Recommended. Accessed Apr 2015.

152. Kim J, Turan V, Oktay K. Long-term safety of letrozole and gonadotropin stimulation for fertility preservation in women with breast cancer. J Clin Endocrinol Metab. 2016;101:1364–71.

153. Quinn GP, Vadaparampil ST, Bower B, Friedman S, Keefe DL. Decisions and ethical issues among BRCA carriers and the use of preimplantation genetic diagnosis. Minerva Med. 2009;100:371–83.

154. Oktay K, Kim JY, Barad D, Babayev SN. Association of BRCA1 mutations with occult primary ovarian insufficiency: a possible explanation for the link between infertility and breast/ovarian cancer risks. J Clin Oncol. 2010;28:240–4.

# 9

# Clinical features and treatment of vulvar Merkel cell carcinoma

Austin Huy Nguyen[1*], Ahmed I. Tahseen[1], Adam M. Vaudreuil[1], Gabriel C. Caponetti[2] and Christopher J. Huerter[3]

## Abstract

**Background:** Merkel cell carcinoma is a rare and aggressive neoplasm originating from mechanoreceptor Merkel cells of the stratum basale of the epidermis. Cases affecting the vulva are exceedingly rare, with the currently available literature primarily in case report form.

**Body:** Systematic review of the PubMed database returned 17 cases of Merkel cell carcinoma affecting the vulva. Patients presented at a mean age of 59.6 years with a firm, mobile vulvar mass. Symptoms of pain, erythema, pruritus, edema, and ulceration have been reported. Tumor histology is consistent with that of neuroendocrine tumors and typical Merkel cell carcinomas. Neuroendocrine and cytokeratin immunostains are frequently utilized in histopathological workup. Surgical management was the unanimous first-line therapy with adjuvant radiation in most cases. Recurrence occurred in 70.6% of patients at a mean follow-up of 6.3 months. Mortality was at 47.0% at a mean of 7.8 months after initial operation.

**Conclusion:** Merkel cell carcinoma affecting the vulva is an extremely rare and highly aggressive neoplasm. The present review of published cases serves to comprehensively describe the clinical course and treatment approaches for vulvar Merkel cell carcinoma.

**Keywords:** Vulvar neoplasms, Skin neoplasms, Merkel tumor, Neuroendocrine tumors

## Background

Merkel cell carcinoma (MCC) is a rare and aggressive neoplasm first described in 1972 by Toker [1]. The tumor is thought to originate from the Merkel cell mechanoreceptors located in the stratum basale of the epidermis [2]. Although rare, the incidence of this neoplasm is increasing due to the advancing age of the population, higher rates of sun exposure, and a growing proportion of immunocompromised individuals [2]. MCC occurs predominately in the elderly with an average age of onset at 69 years old and a slightly higher prevalence in males (1.56:1 Male:Female) [3]. Additional risk factors include Caucasian race (incidence of 0.23 per 100,000) [2] and immunosuppression, with a younger age at presentation for immunocompromised individuals [4]. The neoplasm is predominately found in the head and neck (41–50%), followed by the extremities (32–38%), and then the trunk (12–14%) [2]. Regarding the etiology of the

tumor, a recent study [5] described a polyomavirus detected in 43 to 100% of MCC tissue samples. The pathogenesis of this Merkel cell polyomavirus, however, still requires further investigation.

The primary lesion of MCC typically presents as a solitary, painless, rapidly growing, red to bluish nodule [2, 6]. Definitive diagnosis requires histopathologic analysis of a biopsy. Upon hematoxylin and eosin staining, the lesion will appear similar to other neuroendocrine tumors consisting of small round cells, hyperchromic nuclei, frequent mitosis, and variable architecture [2]. With hematoxylin and eosin staining alone it is difficult to differentiate MCC from other small cell tumors, especially metastatic small cell cancer of the lung. Accordingly, immunohistochemical evaluation is recommended [2, 7]. An immunopanel including cytokeratin 20 (CK20) and thyroid transcription factor-1 (TTF-1) allows the greatest sensitivity and specificity for excluding small cell lung cancer [7]. CK20 is highly sensitive for MCC (positive in 89 to 100% of cases) while TTF-1 is sensitive for small cell lung cancer (positive in 83 to 100% of cases), and consistently negative in MCC [7].

* Correspondence: AHN30605@creighton.edu
[1]Creighton University School of Medicine, 2500 California Plaza, Omaha, NE 68102, USA
Full list of author information is available at the end of the article

While various staging guidelines have been proposed historically, the most recent and widely accepted staging guideline is the AJCC staging system [7, 8], which draws upon evidence from the analysis of 5823 cases in the National Cancer Database with a median follow-up of 64 months [3, 7]. Staging affects an individual's prognosis, with 5-year survivals rates of 79% at stage IA to only 18% at stage IV [3]. Additionally, 50 to 70% of patients will develop lymph node metastases and 33 to 70% of those will go on to develop distant disease [2]. The most common sites of metastasis are as follows: brain (18%), liver (13%), lung (10–23%), bone (10–15%), distant skin (9–30%), and distant lymph node (9%) [2]. Due to this high rate of metastasis, patients with a primary MCC should be screened for nodal metastases with sentinel lymph node biopsy. Additionally, other imaging modalities are gaining importance during diagnostic workup. For example, PET/CT may be useful in identifying distant metastases [7]. In one article reviewing 102 patients, PET/CT altered the stage and treatment course in 22% of the cases [9].

Treatment of MCC varies by stage, with the main categories being treatment of the primary lesion, treatment of regional disease, and treatment of distant metastasis. Surgical excision is the treatment of choice for primary lesions [2, 6, 7]. The two surgical approaches are wide local excision with 1 to 2 cm margins and depth to the investing fascia or Mohs surgery. These approaches have equal efficacy if they attain tumor-free margins [2]. In addition to surgery, adjuvant radiotherapy is often recommended. Postoperative radiation has shown to lower the risk of local and regional recurrences and has been associated with a longer overall survival [7]. In the case of a positive node, adjuvant therapy to the nodal basin is recommended and associated with longer disease-free survival [2, 6]. Adjuvant therapy often consists of surgical removal of the basin nodes or regional radiotherapy, or a combination of the two. It is recommended to get a multidisciplinary tumor board consultation in metastatic disease, and to consider any combination of additional surgery, radiotherapy, and chemotherapy [7]. Recommendations concerning follow up for patients after MCC treatment are broad [7]. This allows for individualization based on patient factors and physician preference. The standard regimen is routine physical and skin exam every 3 to 6 months for the first 2 years, followed by every 6 to 12 months thereafter. This recommendation takes into consideration that the median time to recurrence is 8 months with 90% of recurrences happening within 2 years [7].

While MCC is rare, a primary lesion affecting the vulva is extremely rare. The vulvar location of primary tumors is especially unique as cutaneous MCC is characteristically more frequent in men [3]. A study of 3870 MCC cases from the National Cancer Institute's Surveillance, Epidemiology, and End Results Program database found only two cases (0.05%) affecting the vulva [10]. Currently, all data on vulvar MCC is found in "case report and literature review" form. The present study seeks to comprehensively review the available patient data to accurately describe the clinical course and treatment approaches for vulvar MCC.

## Main text
### Search strategy
The National Library of Medicine's PubMed database was systematically searched to December 2016 without date restrictions using the following search terms: "vulva" and "vulvar" combined with "Merkel cell carcinoma," "cutaneous apudoma," "neuroendocrine carcinoma," "trabecular carcinoma." Titles and abstracts were screened for possible inclusion, followed by full text of potentially relevant studies. Included studies were original studies discussing the clinical course (including presentation, diagnostic workup, treatment, and outcome) of patients with MCC affecting the vulva. Studies were excluded if not written in English, not of primary human subjects, or not malignancies of the vulva.

Initial PubMed search (see Fig. 1) returned 146 potentially relevant articles. After screening of titles and abstracts, the full text of 18 studies was retrieved for review [11–27]. Upon full text review, one study was excluded for providing insufficient clinical data on patient-level clinical course (i.e. this study was a large cancer database study of general MCC with minimal summary statistics provided specifically for vulvar MCC). Ultimately, 17 case reports

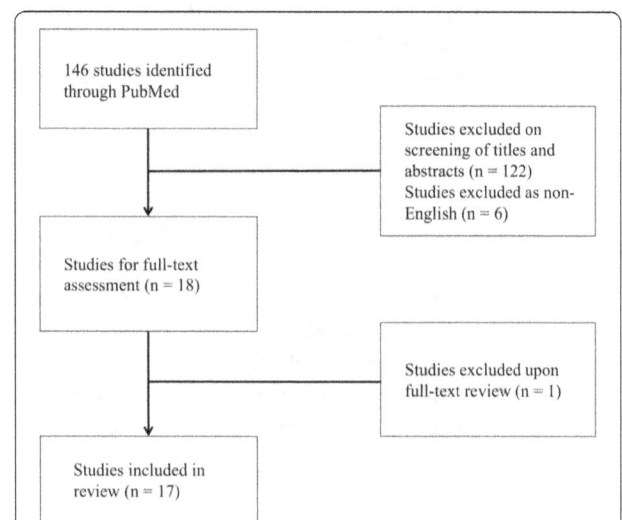

**Fig. 1** Initial PubMed search returned 146 studies. Screening by title and abstract left 18 studies, of which full text was reviewed. Ultimately, 17 cases were included in this review

were included in this review. The greatest number of cases were reported in the United States (7 cases), followed by Spain (2 cases).

## Clinical presentation

Patients presented at a mean age of 59.6 years (range 28–79 years). The clinical presentation of the 17 included cases are summarized in Table 1. Lesions were most commonly located on the labia majora ($n = 9$, 52.9%) with no distinct predilection for side (left, $n = 9$; right: $n = 7$; unreported: $n = 1$). 23.5% of cases ($n = 4$) extended to affect the vaginal wall, while other affected anatomical locations included the labia minora, paraclitoral or the bartholin gland. Patients generally complained of a rapidly growing mass (average history of 4.7 months, range of 1–18 months) that was 7.5 cm (range 1.75–47.5 cm) on average at presentation. The lesions was described as a firm, painless ($n = 3$, 17.6%) or tender ($n = 5$, 29.4%) nodule that was mobile. Cases reported associated pruritus ($n = 2$, 11.8%), swelling or edema ($n = 3$, 17.6%), ulceration ($n = 4$, 23.5%), and erythema ($n = 2$, 11.8%). Bleeding and purulent discharge was reported in a fraction of cases (each, $n = 2$, 11.8%). Discoloration ($n = 3$, 17.6%) was reported as yellow, purple or brown.

**Table 1** Clinical presentation of vulvar merkel cell carcinoma ($n = 17$)

| Characteristic | n (% or range) |
| --- | --- |
| Mean age (years) | 59.6 (28–79) |
| Mean tumor diameter (cm) | 7.5 (1.8–47.5) |
| Mean disease duration (months) | 4.7 (1–18) |
| Location[a] | |
| Labia majora | 9 (52.9) |
| Labia minora | 3 (17.6) |
| Paraclitoral | 1 (5.9) |
| Bartholin gland | 3 (17.6) |
| Intravaginal extension | 4 (23.5) |
| Inguinal | 1 (5.9) |
| Vulva, Unspecified | 1 (5.9) |
| Clinical findings[a] | |
| Firm | 2 (11.8) |
| Painless | 3 (17.6) |
| Tender | 5 (29.4) |
| Mobile | 2 (11.8) |
| Pruritus | 2 (11.8) |
| Swelling/edema | 3 (17.6) |
| Ulceration | 4 (23.5) |
| Erythema | 2 (11.8) |

[a]Sum exceeds 100% due to non-mutually exclusive categories

## Workup

Blood and urine chemistries were unremarkable in the few cases reporting values, excepting occasional comorbidities that did not impact vulvar MCC diagnostics. Histopathological evaluation (Table 2) was the primary diagnostic modality, performed using needle biopsy ($n = 5$, 29.4%), incisional or excisional biopsy ($n = 5$, 29.4%), evaluation following tumor resection ($n = 1$, 5.9%), or unspecified ($n = 6$, 35.3%). Histologically, vulvar MCC is

**Table 2** Histopathological evaluation of vulvar merkel cell carcinomas

| Characteristic | n (%) |
| --- | --- |
| Histologic finding ($n = 17$) | |
| Small cells | 12 (70.6) |
| High N/C ratio, scant cytoplasm | 12 (70.6) |
| Nests, islands, trabecular | 11 (64.7) |
| Hyperchromatic | 10 (58.8) |
| High mitotic index | 8 (47.1) |
| Necrosis | 6 (35.3) |
| Irregular nuclei | 4 (23.5) |
| Fibrous | 4 (23.5) |
| Apoptosis | 4 (23.5) |
| Sheets | 3 (17.6) |
| Hemorrhage | 2 (11.8) |
| Ulceration | 2 (11.8) |
| Electron microscopy ($n = 7$)[a] | |
| Dense core granules | 6 (85.7) |
| Intermediate filaments | 5 (71.4) |
| Immunostaining ($n = 14$)[a] | |
| Neuroendocrine markers | |
| Chromogranin | 7 (50) |
| NSE | 7 (50) |
| Synaptophysin | 6 (42.9) |
| PGP 9.5 | 2 (14.3) |
| Keratin stains ($n = 13$)[a] | |
| Pancytokeratin AE1/AE3 | 7 (53.8) |
| CAM5.2 | 4 (30.8) |
| Low molecular weight CK | 3 (23.1) |
| CK7 | 1 (7.7) |
| CK8 | 2 (15.4) |
| CK18 | 3 (23.1) |
| CK19 | 1 (7.7) |
| CK20 | 4 (30.8) |
| Perinuclear dot/granular | 7 (53.8) |

*Abbreviations: CK* cytokeratin, *N/C ratio* nuclear/cytoplasmic ratio, *NSE* neuron specific enolase, *PGP* protein gene product
[a]Total n, reflected in percentages, is less than 17 due to inconsistent reporting of electron microscopy or positive and negative immunostains

typical of neuroendocrine tumors and traditional MCC (see Fig. 2). Routine evaluation with hematoxylin and eosin demonstrated small, undifferentiated, hyperchromatic cells with a high N/C ratio and scanty cytoplasm. Cells were arranged in nested, trabecular pattern ($n = 11$, 64.7%) separated by fibrous connective bands and/or were in sheets ($n = 3$, 17.6%). Indicators of aggressive malignancy were common, including high mitotic index ($n = 8$, 47.1%), irregular nuclei ($n = 4$, 23.5%), necrotic and apoptotic cells ($n = 6$ and 4, respectively), hemorrhage ($n = 2$, 11.8%) and ulcerated dermis ($n = 2$, 11.8%). Electron microscopy was reported in 7 cases (41.2%). In these cases, tumor cells exhibited cytoplasmic membrane-bound dense core neurosecretory granules ($n = 6$, 85,7%) and intermediate filaments ($N = 5$, 71.4%).

Immunostain results were reported in all but 2 cases and are summarized in Table 2. Neuroendocrine and keratin stains were the most commonly used for histopathological diagnostic workup. Cases commonly stained positive for neuron specific enolase ($n = 7$), chromogranin ($n = 7$), and synaptophysin ($n = 6$). Keratin stains included pancytokeratin AE1/AE3 ($n = 7$), CAM5.2 ($n = 4$), and low molecular weight cytokeratins ($n = 3$). Generally, cytokeratin immunoreactivity patterns demonstrated perinuclear dots and/or cytoplasmic granularity. Other immunostains with two or fewer positives included CD56, Ki-67, endomysial antibody, carcinoembryonic antigen, and S100. Stains with no positives included CD45, TTF-1, HMB45, desmin, vimentin, smooth muscle actin, CA125, CD31, and CD34.

Ultrasound was performed in 4 cases. While three reports demonstrated no tumor findings on ultrasound, one case [11] reported ultrasound to detect a well circumscribed, heterogeneous, cystic mass with irregular vascularity. Plain chest radiographs were unremarkable in all 9 cases reporting use of X-ray imaging, except one case [20] in which extensive lung metastases were shown. CT scans, performed in 10 cases, appeared to be the most sensitive for detection of metastases.

### Management and outcome

All patients received surgical excision as first line therapy. Vulvectomy was performed in ten patients (58.8%). Wide local excision was performed in 4 cases (23.5%)

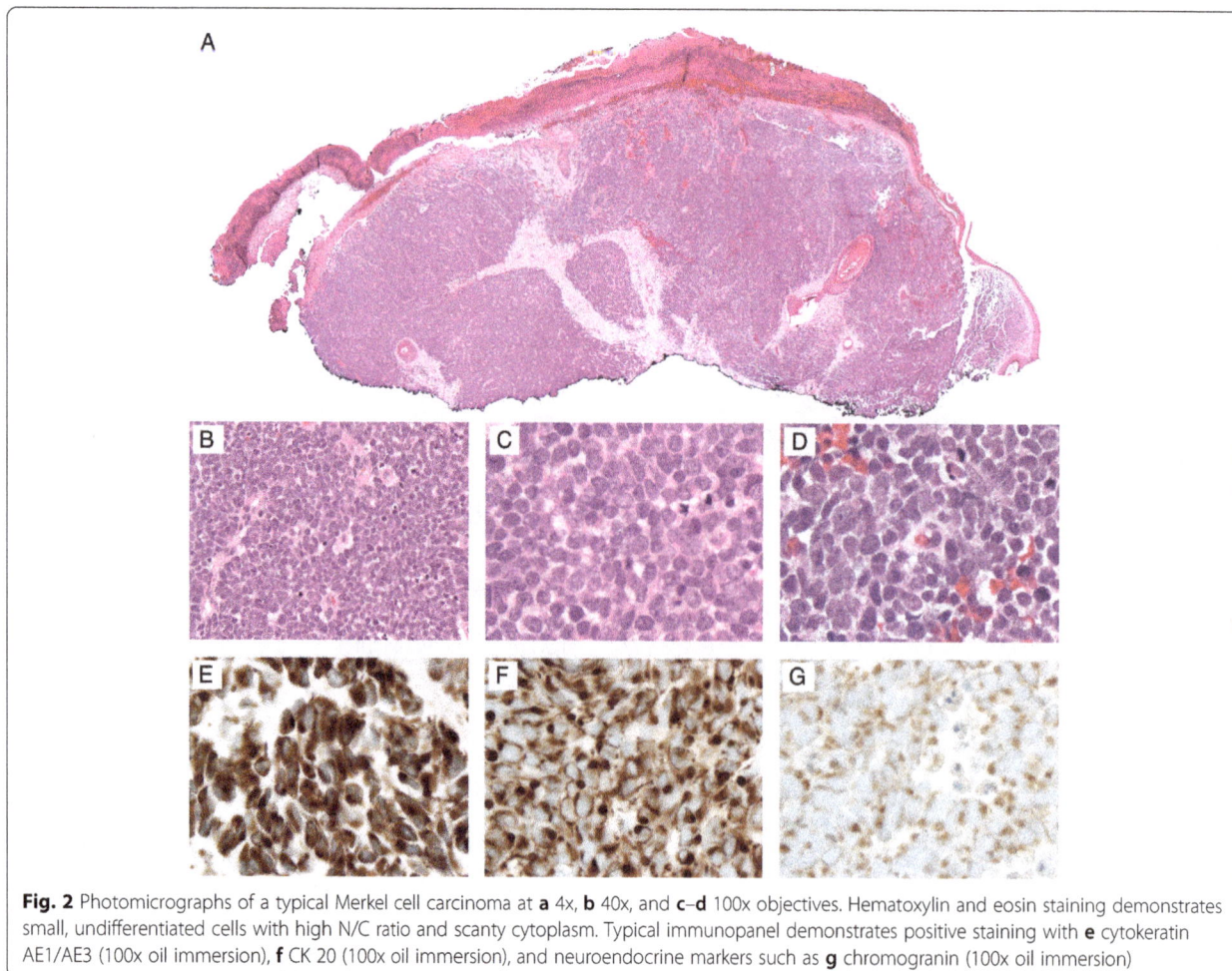

**Fig. 2** Photomicrographs of a typical Merkel cell carcinoma at **a** 4x, **b** 40x, and **c–d** 100x objectives. Hematoxylin and eosin staining demonstrates small, undifferentiated cells with high N/C ratio and scanty cytoplasm. Typical immunopanel demonstrates positive staining with **e** cytokeratin AE1/AE3 (100x oil immersion), **f** CK 20 (100x oil immersion), and neuroendocrine markers such as **g** chromogranin (100x oil immersion)

with 2 cm margins, where reported. Excision was unable to be completed in one case due to inaccessibility of the lesion, and surgical approach was not reported in another case until recurrence. Inguinal lymph node dissection was reported in 10 cases (58.8%). Some form of adjuvant radiotherapy was administered in 11 cases (64.7%). Of those reporting sufficient data, radiation dosage was 400 to 6500 cGy at first dose of adjuvant radiotherapy, with additional courses at varied doses. Radiation was administered locally in the pelvic region, with some cases administering radiation at inguinal or even para-aortic lymph nodes. 11 cases reported radiation as a part of the treatment regimen, however three did not provide follow-up results for the patient, as radiotherapy had not been performed at the time the cases were written [11, 12, 15]. Of the eight patients with reported follow up, six patients experienced recurrence at an average of 5.8 months after treatment [14, 17, 21, 24–26]. Five of these cases reported the amount of radiation therapy, with an average of 6008 cGy [14, 21, 24–26]. Six patients had recurrent disease after radiation therapy, three died after 0 [14], 3 [25], and 4 months [26] post-radiotherapy. Three patients with recurrence were still alive at 0 [24], 0 [21], and 8 months [17] post-radiotherapy. Of the two patients who did not experience recurrence, one patient received 5940 cGy and died at 8 months post-radiotherapy due to sepsis [18], while the other received 5000 cGy plus an additional 5000 cGy targeted at original mass location and was still alive at 24 months post-radiotherapy [16].

Patient prognosis was poor. Recurrence occurred in 11 patients (64.7%) at a mean follow-up of 4.7 months (range 2–9 months). Two patients were disease-free at 13 and 24 months follow-up, respectively (three patients lost to follow-up or outcome not reported). Recurrent lesions were managed surgically or with cisplatin and etoposide combination chemotherapy (n = 5; 2 cases did not specify regimen). Eight patients (47.0%) succumbed to advanced disease, with death at an average of 9.6 months after initial surgical operation (range 0.36–20 months post-operation). The clinical course of all included cases is summarized in Table 3.

## Discussion

The overall histopathological picture of vulvar MCC is fairly consistent with typical MCC. Histological evaluation remains the primary diagnostic modality, including a hematoxylin and eosin section along with an appropriate immunopanel. National Comprehensive Cancer Network guidelines for general MCC [7] recommend immunopanels to include CK20 and TTF-1. Most low-molecular-weight cytokeratin markers and CK20 will be positive in a perinuclear dot-like pattern, while CK7 and TTF-1 (immunoreactive in >80% of small cell lung cancers) are typically negative [7]. Neuroendocrine markers are recommended in only equivocal cases. Of the presently reviewed vulvar MCC cases, 76.5% (n = 13) of cases were evaluated using neuroendocrine markers, with NSE as the most commonly used (n = 7). While 76.5% (n = 13) of cases also included some sort of cytokeratin staining, only five cases were stained for CK20 and two cases were stained for CK7 (with 80% and 50% of cases positive, respectively). Histopathological workup of vulvar MCC appears to consistently include both neuroendocrine and cytokeratin markers.

A study histopathologically evaluating 21 cases [28] demonstrated MCC to express B cell lineage markers, including terminal deoxynucleotidyl transferase (TdT) and the paired box gene 5 (PAX 5). Additionally, most of the MCCs evaluated in this study expressed one or more immunoglobulin subclasses as well as kappa or lambda chains. The TdT and PAX5 coexpression is suggestive of a pro/pre- or pre-B cell origin for MCC, rather than postmitotic Merkel cells in select tumors. This disparity may aid in understanding why Merkel cell polyoma viral infection is not present in all cases. Additionally, this may have implications for therapy. Subclassification of MCC tumors by immunophenotype could create a paradigm of individualized treatment dictated by cellular origin (i.e. pre-B cell-derived tumors versus postmitotic Merkel cell tumors). However, further investigation is required to substantiate this model of MCC origin. Additionally, extensive clinical trials would be required to validate treatment regimens based on origin.

Surgical excision is the first line approach to primary MCC tumors. All reports received vulvectomy or wide local excision with 2 cm margins. National Comprehensive Cancer Network guidelines for general MCC [7] recommend sentinel lymph node biopsy followed by surgical removal using wide excision with 1–2 cm margins. Removal to investing fascia of muscle or pericranium is recommended, when clinically feasible. Additionally, physicians may consider techniques that allow more exhaustive histologic margin assessment, such as Mohs technique, modified Mohs with permanent sections for final margin assessment, or complete circumferential and peripheral deep margin assessment. No cases of vulvar MCC reported more exhaustive margin assessment such as Mohs techniques. Considering the high recurrence rate and the limits in accessibility for excision of vulvar MCC, Mohs techniques could be of potential value in the management of this condition. Such technique could improve margin control and possibly increase tissue preservation. A multi-institutional retrospective study [29] of 240 MCC cases not limited by anatomic location reported use of Mohs micrographic surgery in 13.8% of patients, most commonly with stage I disease. While overall survival of stage I/II patients did not differ with

**Table 3** Summary of Clinical Presentation, Treatment, and Outcome of Vulvar Merkel Cell Carcinoma Cases

| Case | Age | Location/Size | Presentation | Treatment | Outcome + Survival |
|------|-----|---------------|--------------|-----------|--------------------|
| Bottles et al. 1984 [27] | 73 | Left labia majora. | Minute ulcer w/chronic ulceration | Initial: Testosterone + hydrocortisone cream to heal initial ulcer. 10 months, 3 weeks: Vulvectomy + Left Inguinal lymphadenectomy | 9 Months: Local raised, nodular, erythematous tumor 3 x 2 cm + Left Inguinal LN metastases 11 months (11 days post operation): death due to acute MI + cardiopulmonary failure. Inguinal and paraaortic nodes, bone, liver, pulmonary vessel metastases. |
| Copeland et al. 1985 [26] | 59 | Left labium majus 6 x 8 cm | 18 month history of painful lump + Local tumor + Left Inguinal LN metastases | Initial: Left hemivulvectomy + lymphadenectomy + Radiotherapy 8 months: Vulvar lesion excision. | 8 months: Vulvar + several pulmonary metastases. 12 months: Death |
| Husseinzadeh et al. 1988 [25] | 47 | Right labium majus + vaginal introit. 4.2 x 3 cm | 3 month history of right labial/groin swelling with brown vaginal discharge and pain on sitting. Local tumor + bilateral inguinal LN metastases | Initial: Vulvectomy + Bilateral lymphadenectomy + Radiotherapy 3 months: Excision + Chemotherapy | 3 months: right thigh nodule, forehead nodule, single nodular lesion in left hilar region. 6 months: Death. Autopsy: hilar, lung, liver, pancreas metastases. |
| Chandeying et al. 1989 [24] | 28 | Right labium majus 4 cm | 1 month history of painless lump. Local tumor + bilateral inguinal LN metastases | Initial: Vulvectomy + bilateral lymphadenectomy + radiotherapy | 3 months: Right leg pain improved with symptomatic treatment. 4 months out: Alive. No subsequent follow up. |
| Loret de Mola et al. 1993 [23] | 28 | Left fourchette 1.5 x 2 cm | 3 month history of Vulvar growth and irritation. Local tumor | Initial: local excision. 2 months: Wide local excision + left inguinal lymphadenectomy 8 months: chemotherapy | 8 months: liver metastases. 20 months: Death. |
| Chen 1994 [22] | 68 | Left paraclitoral 3 x 2.5 cm | 1 month history of mass. Local tumor. | Initial: Local excision 10 months: Chemotherapy. | 9 months: bilateral Inguinal LN and liver metastases. 10 months = Vulva, scalp, bone and paraaortic LN. 17 months: Death. |
| Scurry et al. 1996 [21] | 68 | Left labium minus + fourchette 4 x 3 cm. | 5 month history of painless lump with rapid growth in last 2 weeks. Local tumor + overlying discolored purplish skin. bilateral inguinal LN metastases | Initial: Vulvectomy + bilateral inguinal and Left pelvic Lymphadenectomy 2 months: Radiotherapy | Residual pelvic nodes post treatment. 2 months: para aortic LN. 5 months: Alive with residual disease. |
| Gil et al. 1997 [19] | 74 | Right labium majus 9 cm | 3–4 month history of local tumor | Initial: Wide Local excision | 13 months: free of disease |
| Fawzi et al. 1997 [20] | 78 | Right vulvar mass 5.5 x 4 cm | 1 month history of perineal itching and discomfort. Pulmonary LN metastases. | Initial: Radical vulvectomy + bilateral inguinal LN dissection | 20 days postoperative: break down of right groin site and subsequent death due to bleeding. No autopsy. |
| Hierro et al. 2000 [18] | 79 | Left labium minus 2.5 cm | Local tumor | Initial: local excision. 2 months: Radiotherapy | 2 months local recurrence and regional LN metastases. 10 months: Death |
| Nuciforo et al. 2004 [17] | 62 | Right labia majora 20 mm | Local painful tumor. | Initial: local excision. 3 months: Radical vulvectomy + Radiotherapy. | 3 months: bilateral inguinal LN metastases. 11 months: abdominal and mediastinal LN. 19 months: Alive with Several abdominal and thoracic metastases. |
| Khoury et al. 2005 [16] | 49 | Right vulvar mass 2 cm | Spontaneously ruptured Bartholin's gland abscess with small induration at the site. | Initial: Drained abscess + wide local excision + bilateral LN dissection + Radiation therapy | 24 months: Alive with no evidence of recurrence. |
| Pawar et al. 2005 [15] | 35 | Left labium majus 4 x 6 cm | One week history of painful swelling of the vulva + purulent discharge + LN mass | Initial: Drained abscess + antibiotics + partial excision | No follow up, patient planned to receive radiotherapy in her home country. |

**Table 3** Summary of Clinical Presentation, Treatment, and Outcome of Vulvar Merkel Cell Carcinoma Cases *(Continued)*

| Mohit et al. 2009 [14] | 50 | Left labia majora 3–4 cm | 3 month history of palpable mass. | Initial: local excision 2 months: Radiotherapy 2 months, 3 weeks: radical vulvectomy 9 months: Chemotherapy | 2 months: Recurrent mass 10 x 12 cm w/spontaneously bleeding ulcerations 9 months: left hip pain 10 months: no evidence of metastases 11 months: death due to Pulmonary embolism secondary to DVT of LLE. |
|---|---|---|---|---|---|
| Sheikh et al. 2010 [13] | 63 | Right labium majus 5 x 7 cm | Post menopausal bleeding with fungating primary lesion. | Initial: wide local excision. | 2 months: local + distant recurrence with multiple firm inguinal LN bilaterally + death before follow up treatment |
| Iavazzo et al. 2011 [12] | 63 | Left Labium 9 cm | 6 month history of pruritus treated w/corticosteroid cream. 5 cm inguinal LN metastases. | Initial: radical vulvectomy + radiotherapy | No follow up |
| Winer et al. 2012 [11] | 69 | Right inguinal 3–4 cm | Patient noted Inguinal lesion. | Initial: Surgical excision Future plans for adjuvant chemotherapy + radiotherapy | No follow up |

use of Mohs versus wide excision, recurrence rates and tissue preservation in these cohorts were not compared. Further evaluation of the utility of Mohs technique in vulvar MCC is warranted.

The high recurrence rate of MCC in spite of the emphasis on wide local excision and margin clearance suggests surgical management of this condition to be inadequate. In light of this poor clinical response to surgical excision, further development of medical therapies is paramount. Medical management in the available published cases was limited to cisplatin and etoposide combination therapy. With current medical management consisting only of cytotoxic chemotherapy and radiation (which causes many adverse side effects and is not mechanism-based, disease-specific therapy) there is a need for more effective and targeted treatment agents. Newer developed agents, such as TKI's, show encouraging efficacy in other cancers and in some case reports when used for MCC. Additionally they have low toxicity and lack immune suppression due to the nature of their targeting aberrantly expressed genes commonly mutated in human cancers. A case report of metastatic MCC in a 69-year-old female demonstrated partial response to pazopanib, a tyrosine kinase inhibitor (TKI) [30]. Multiple clinical trials are underway investigating the efficacy of TKIs in MCC. These include MLN0128 (mTOR, NCT02514824), cabozantinib (c-Met and VEGFR2, NCT02036476), imatinib (NCT00068783), temsirolimus (mTOR, NCT01155258), and everolimus and vatalnib combination therapy (NCT00655655). Other biologicals are also under investigation for treatment of patients with MCC, including adjuvant ipilimumab (NCT02196961), avelumab (NCT02155647), tremelimumab and durvalumab combination therapy (NCT02643303). The age of biological and targeted therapy is rapidly changing clinical oncology, as a whole, and is promising for treatment of advanced MCC.

## Conclusion

Merkel cell carcinoma affecting the vulva is a rare and aggressive neoplasm that presents as a firm, mobile mass at a mean age of 59.6 years. Pain, ulceration, edema, and erythema may also be present. The lesion is histopathologically consistent with MCC, appearing as small hyperchromatic cells with high nucleus to cytoplasm ratio distributed in nested, trabecular patterns. Electron microscopy demonstrates cells with dense core granules and intermediate filaments. Neuroendocrine immunostain markers aid in histopathological evaluation, especially chromogranin, synaptophysin, and neuron-specific enolase. Additionally, cytokeratin stains are commonly immunoreactive, including pancytokeratin stains and CAM5.2, which will generally demonstrate a perinuclear dot or cytoplasmic granularity. Surgical management is the primary treatment modality, and adjuvant radiotherapy may be considered. However, recurrence and tumor progression are very common problems. Metastatic disease may be managed with cisplatin and etoposide combination therapy. This condition has high mortality (47.0% of 17 cases) at a mean follow-up of 7.8 months (range, 0.6–16 months) after first surgical operation. Continued investigation of targeted therapy is warranted for improved treatment in this highly aggressive disease.

**Abbreviations**
AJCC: American Joint Commission of Cancer; CK20: Cytokeratin 20; MCC: Merkel cell carcinoma; TTF-1: Thyroid transcription factor-1

**Acknowledgements**
None.

**Funding**
This work is supported in part by the Creighton University School of Medicine, Office of Medical Education. The funding body played no role in the design of the study and collection, analysis, and interpretation of data and in writing the manuscript.

**Authors' contributions**
AHN and AMV conceived and designed the study. AHN, AIT, and AMV helped in acquisition, analysis and interpretation of data. All authors participated in drafting the manuscript or revising it critically for important intellectual content. All authors read and approved the final manuscript. As corresponding author, AHN is accountable for all aspects of the work in ensuring that questions related to the accuracy or integrity of any part of the work are appropriately investigated and resolved.

**Competing interests**
The authors declare that they have no competing interests.

**Author details**
[1]Creighton University School of Medicine, 2500 California Plaza, Omaha, NE 68102, USA. [2]Department of Pathology and Laboratory Medicine, Perelman School of Medicine, University of Pennsylvania, 3400 Spruce Street, Philadelphia, PA, USA. [3]Division of Dermatology, Creighton University School of Medicine, 2500 California Plaza, Omaha, NE 68102, USA.

**References**
1. Toker C. Trabecular carcinoma of the skin. Arch Dermatol. 1972;105(1):107–10.
2. Duprat JP, Landman G, Salvajoli JV, Brechtbuhl ER. A review of the epidemiology and treatment of Merkel cell carcinoma. Clinics (Sao Paulo). 2011;66(10):1817–23.
3. Lemos BD, Storer BE, Iyer JG, et al. Pathologic nodal evaluation improves prognostic accuracy in Merkel cell carcinoma: analysis of 5823 cases as the basis of the first consensus staging system. J Am Acad Dermatol. 2010;63(5): 751–61. doi:10.1016/j.jaad.2010.02.056.
4. Schwartz JL, Bichakjian CK, Lowe L, et al. Clinicopathologic features of primary Merkel cell carcinoma: a detailed descriptive analysis of a large contemporary cohort. Dermatol Surg. 2013;39(7):1009–16. doi:10.1111/dsu.12194.
5. Feng H, Shuda M, Chang Y, Moore PS. Clonal integration of a polyomavirus in human Merkel cell carcinoma. Science. 2008;319(5866):1096–100. doi:10.1126/science.1152586.
6. Henness S, Vereecken P. Management of Merkel tumours: an evidence-based review. Curr Opin Oncol. 2008;20(3):280–6. doi:10.1097/CCO. 0b013e3282fe6ad8.
7. National Comprehensive Cancer Network. NCCN clinical practice guidelines in oncology: Merkel cell carcinoma. 2016.
8. American Joint Committee on Cancer. AJCC cancer staging manual. 2010.
9. Siva S, Byrne K, Seel M, et al. 18 F-FDG PET provides high-impact and powerful prognostic stratification in the staging of Merkel cell carcinoma: a 15-year institutional experience. J Nucl Med. 2013;54(8):1223–9. doi:10.2967/jnumed. 112.116814.
10. Albores-Saavedra J, Batich K, Chable-Montero F, Sagy N, Schwartz AM, Henson DE. Merkel cell carcinoma demographics, morphology, and survival based on 3870 cases: a population based study. J Cutan Pathol. 2010;37(1): 20–7. doi:10.1111/j.1600-0560.2009.01370.x.
11. Winer IS, Lonardo F, Johnson SC, Deppe G. Merkel cell carcinoma in a patient with noninvasive vulvar Paget's disease. Am J Obstet Gynecol. 2012; 207(1):e9–e11. doi:10.1016/j.ajog.2012.03.028.
12. Iavazzo C, Terzi M, Arapantoni-Dadioti P, Dertimas V, Vorgias G. Vulvar merkel carcinoma: a case report. Case Rep Med. 2011;2011:546972. doi:10.1155/2011/546972.
13. Sheikh ZA, Nair I, Vijaykumar DK, Jojo A, Nandeesh M. Neuroendocrine tumor of vulva: a case report and review of literature. J Cancer Res Ther. 2010;6(3):365–6. doi:10.4103/0973-1482.73370.
14. Mohit M, Mosallai A, Monabbati A, Mortazavi H. Merkel cell carcinoma of the vulva. Saudi Med J. 2009;30(5):717–8. doi:10.1111/j.1526-4610.2008.01139.x.
15. Pawar R, Vijayalakshmy AR, Khan S, al Lawati FAR. Primary neuroendocrine carcinoma (Merkel's cell carcinoma) of the vulva mimicking as a Bartholin's gland abscess. Ann Saudi Med. 2005;25(2):161–4.
16. Khoury-Collado F, Elliott KS, Lee YC, Chen PC, Abulafia O. Merkel cell carcinoma of the Bartholin's gland. Gynecol Oncol. 2005;97(3):928–31. doi:10.1016/j.ygyno.2004.12.064.
17. Nuciforo PG, Fraggetta F, Fasani R, Braidotti P, Nuciforo G. Neuroendocrine carcinoma of the vulva with paraganglioma-like features. Histopathology. 2004;44(3):304–6. doi:10.1111/j.1365-2559.2004.01778.x.
18. Hierro I, Blanes A, Matilla A, Muñoz S, Vicioso L, Nogales FF. Merkel cell (neuroendocrine) carcinoma of the vulva. A case report with immunohistochemical and ultrastructural findings and review of the literature. Pathol Res Pract. 2000;196(7):503–9. doi:10.1016/S0344-0338(00)80052-7.
19. Gil-Moreno A, Garcia-Jiménez A, González-Bosquet J, et al. Merkel cell carcinoma of the vulva. Gynecol Oncol. 1997;64(3):526–32.
20. Fawzi HW, Cross PA, Buckley CH, Monaghan JM. Neuroendocrine (Merkel cell) carcinoma of the vulva. J Obstet Gynaecol. 1997;17(1):100–1. doi:10.1080/01443619750114310.
21. Scurry J, Brand A, Planner R, Dowling J, Rode J. Vulvar Merkel Cell Tumor with Glandular and Squamous Differentiation. Gynecol Oncol. 1996;62(2): 292–7. doi:10.1006/gyno.1996.0229.
22. Chen KT. Merkel's cell (neuroendocrine) carcinoma of the vulva. Cancer. 1994;73(8):2186–91.
23. de Mola JR L, Hudock PA, Steinetz C, Jacobs G, Macfee M, Abdul-Karim FW. Merkel cell carcinoma of the vulva. Gynecol Oncol. 1993;51(2):272–6.
24. Chandeying V, Sutthijumroon S, Tungphaisal S. Merkel cell carcinoma of the vulva: a case report. Asia Oceania J Obstet Gynaecol. 1989;15(3):261–5.
25. Husseinzadeh N, Wesseler T, Newman N, Shbaro I, Ho P. Neuroendocrine (Merkel cell) carcinoma of the vulva. Gynecol Oncol. 1988;29(1):105–12.
26. Copeland LJ, Cleary K, Sneige N, Edwards CL. Neuroendocrine (Merkel cell) carcinoma of the vulva: a case report and review of the literature. Gynecol Oncol. 1985;22(3):367–78.
27. Bottles K, Lacey CG, Goldberg J, Lanner-Cusin K, Hom J, Miller TR. Merkel cell carcinoma of the vulva. Obstet Gynecol. 1984;63(3 Suppl):61S–5S.
28. Zur HA, Rennspiess D, Winnepenninckx V, Speel EJ, Kurz AK. Early B-cell differentiation in Merkel cell carcinomas: clues to cellular ancestry. Cancer Res. 2013;73(16):4982–7. doi:10.1158/0008-5472.CAN-13-0616.
29. Tarantola TI, Vallow LA, Halyard MY, et al. Prognostic factors in Merkel cell carcinoma: analysis of 240 cases. J Am Acad Dermatol. 2013;68(3):425–32. doi:10.1016/j.jaad.2012.09.036.
30. Davids MS, Charlton A, Ng S-S, et al. Response to a novel multitargeted tyrosine kinase inhibitor pazopanib in metastatic Merkel cell carcinoma. J Clin Oncol. 2009;27(26):e97–100. doi:10.1200/JCO.2009.21.8149.

# 10

# Safety and efficacy of salvage nano-particle albumin bound paclitaxel in recurrent cervical cancer

Lindsey E. Minion[1], Dana M. Chase[2], John H. Farley[2], Lyndsay J. Willmott[2] and Bradley J. Monk[2*]

## Abstract

**Background:** After platinum and taxane chemotherapy, with or without bevacizumab, active regimens for advanced or recurrent cervical cancer are lacking. Our objective was to review a single institution experience in treating recurrent, refractory cervical cancer with nano-particle albumin bound (NAB) paclitaxel with or without bevacizumab.

**Methods:** This retrospective case series was conducted in accordance with the regulations set forth by the Institutional Review Board at St. Joseph's Hospital and Medical center. The chemotherapy log at the outpatient infusion center at the University of Arizona Cancer Center was reviewed to identify all advanced cervical cancer patients treated with NAB-paclitaxel from November 2011 until February 2015. The following data points were extracted from patient charts: demographic information, number of cycles, progression free survival (PFS), overall survival (OS), dose reductions and dose-limiting toxicities. In addition the average number of treatment cycles and age at recurrence were calculated.

**Results:** A total of 12 subjects were identified as receiving treatment with NAB-paclitaxel. Mean age at time of recurrence was 47.2 years (36–55). Nine subjects had squamous cell histology and three subjects had adenocarcinoma histology. All subjects had failed treatment with platinum and taxane, or platinum and topotecan chemotherapy. Two subjects were lost to follow up. The Median number of cycles of NAB-paclitaxel was 6.5 (2–19). The total number of cycles of NAB-paclitaxel in the study population was 65. Seven subjects were treated in combination with bevacizumab. Of these, three subjects are still alive and one subject is currently receiving active treatment with NAB-paclitaxel. The median PFS and OS for all subjects that met mortality endpoint was 4.8 months and 8.9 months ($n = 7$), respectively. One subject discontinued NAB-paclitaxel secondary to peripheral neuropathy, and one subject developed a vesicovaginal fistula while obtaining combination NAB-paclitaxel and bevacizumab therapy.

**Conclusions:** NAB-paclitaxel with or without bevacizumab is tolerable and potentially active in treating recurrent cervical cancer after failing platinum-taxane or topotecan chemotherapy. This small case series deserves confirmation through prospective clinical trials.

**Keywords:** Nano-particle albumin bound paclitaxel, Recurrent cervical cancer, Metronomic chemotherapy

* Correspondence: bradley.monk@dignityhealth.org
[2]Division of Gynecologic Oncology, Department of Obstetrics and Gynecology, University of Arizona Cancer Center at Dignity Health St. Joseph's Hospital and Medical Center, 500 West Thomas Road, Suite 660, Phoenix, AZ 85013, USA
Full list of author information is available at the end of the article

## Background

Hallmarks of recurrent cervical cancer continue to be poor prognosis, and limited treatment options. In this heavily pre-treated population with prior radiation, where disease is not amenable to surgical excision, there has been an evolution in cytotoxic chemotherapy regimens [1]. Gynecologic Oncology Group (GOG) protocol 204 established double therapy of cisplatin and paclitaxel as the standard of care. This combination had an overall response rate of 29.1 % [2]. Then, GOG-240 demonstrated an improvement in both PFS, and OS endpoints from this doublet with the addition of bevacizumab. By harnessing this anti-angiogenic agent, there was an addition of 3.4 months to OS [3]. However, if a GOG-240 treatment regimen fails, there are no established treatment options in recurrent cervical cancer.

Nano-particle albumin bound (NAB) paclitaxel is a 130-nanimeter, chremophor-free preparation of paclitaxel. This preparation eliminates the need for pre-medication, has a shorten infusion time, and increase tumor concentration as compared to standard preparation [4, 5].

NAB-paclitaxel was evaluated in recurrent cervical cancer a phase II trial as a part of the GOG-127 queue. For this trial all 35 subjects were taxane naïve. Subjects were treated with 125 mg/m$^2$ on days 1, 8 and 15 of a 28-day cycle. Results demonstrated moderate activity with a median PFS, and OS was 5.0 and 9.4 months, respectively. Ten subjects had a partial response, and additional 15 subjects had stable disease [6].

Targeting angiogenesis, the phenotypic driver of cervical cancer, is central to effective therapy of this disease [7]. In addition to agents that directly inhibit vascular growth pathways, there is significant data corroborating that the administration of chemotherapy in reduced doses with a more frequent schedule produces an anti-angiogenic effect. So-called metronomic chemotherapy reduces endothelial repair time, endothelial cell proliferation, migration and circulating levels of endothelial progenitor cells [8–10].

Thus, based on a prior positive phase II evaluation of NAB-paclitaxel, and anti-angiogenic induced properties with metronomic administration we treated recurrent cervical cancer patient that failed prior chemotherapy with NAB-paclitaxel with or without bevacizumab.

## Methods

### Patients

This retrospective chart review was conducted in accordance with the regulations set forth by the Institutional Review Board of The Dignity Health at St. Joseph's Hospital and Medical Center. The pharmacy chemotherapy log was review at the University of Arizona Cancer Center Chemotherapy Infusion Suite at Dignity Health at St. Joseph's Hospital and Medical Center from to identify all patients that received nab-paclitaxel. Charts were review

for patients that had the diagnoses of cervical carcinoma. All subjects were assigned a subject number, and information was de-identified during data collection. The data points collected included: demographic, tumor history, prior therapies, adverse events and treatment response.

### Statistical considerations

The primary endpoint of this series was PFS defined as initiation of nab-paclitaxel to discontinuation of treatment. Secondary endpoint included: dose reductions, completed cycles, adverse events, time to progression, time to death and indication for discontinuation of therapy. Adverse events were categorized using the Common Terminology Criteria for Adverse Events (CTCAE – version 4.0) [11]. The median number of cycles, PFS and OS were calculated.

## Results

From November 2011 to February of 2015 time period, 12 patients with the diagnoses of recurrent cervical carcinoma received NAB-paclitaxel. Two subjects were lost to follow up; one patient relocated out-of-state. The remaining 10 patients had the average age of 43.5 (range 36–55). Seven subjects were self-identified as non-Hispanic white, 4 subjects Hispanic and one other. Table 1 displays the demographic characteristic of the study group.

**Table 1** Patient demographics

| Characteristic | Category | n |
|---|---|---|
| Age Group | 35–40 | 3 |
| | 41–45 | 4 |
| | 46–50 | 1 |
| | 51–55 | 3 |
| | >56 | 1 |
| Ethnicity | Non-Hispanic | 7 |
| | Hispanic | 4 |
| | Other | 1 |
| Cell Type | Squamous Cell Carcinoma | 7 |
| | Adenocarcinoma | 3 |
| Lines of Prior Therapy | 1 | 8 |
| | 2 | 2 |
| Prior Radiation | Yes | 9 |
| | No | 1 |
| Prior Surgery | Yes | 5 |
| | No | 5 |
| Prior Paclitaxel | Yes | 9 |
| | No | 1 |
| Prior Bevacizumab | Yes | 6 |
| | No | 4 |

All subjects had recurrent cervical cancer. Of note, prior to NAB-paclitaxel therapy all subjects had failed prior cytotoxic chemotherapy. Two subjects failed 2 prior lines of chemotherapy. Chemotherapy administered in conjunction with primary radiation, as a radio-sensitizer, was not counted as a systemic chemotherapy regimen. Nine subjects had prior radiation therapy. Of the prior chemotherapy, 9 subjects had prior paclitaxel, and 6 had prior bevacizumab treatment. The only subject not treated with prior paclitaxel had failed prior topotecan. The majority of the subjects had prior pelvic radiation therapy ($n = 9$).

Subjects were treated with nab-paclitaxel with a dose of 60 mg/m$^2$ to 100 mg/m$^2$. There were 5 dose reductions, and 7 dose delays. Most common indication for treatment alterations was myleosuppression. Eight subjects were treated concomitantly with bevacizumab. A total of 65 cycles were completed; mean cycles completed 6.5 (range 2–19).

There were no grade 4 or 5 adverse events. The only grade 3 adverse events were anemia-requiring transfusion of packed red blood cells. One subject was diagnosed with a vesicovaginal fistula during NAB-paclitaxel therapy. For a complete list of adverse events please see Table 2.

Three subjects are still alive; one subject is currently receiving active treatment with NAB-paclitaxel. Median PFS and OS for all subjects that met mortality endpoint were 4.8 and 8.9 months ($n = 7$), respectively (Figs. 1 and 2). Median PFS and OS for the subjects treated with NAB-paclitaxel and bevacizumab that meet mortality endpoint was 6.9 and 14.02 months ($n = 6$), respectively. One subject discontinued NAB-paclitaxel secondary to peripheral neuropathy.

**Table 2** Adverse Events

|  | Grade 1–2 | Grade 3–4 |
| --- | --- | --- |
| Anemia | 4 | 6 |
| Thrombocytopenia | 1 | 0 |
| Leukopenia | 4 | 0 |
| Fatigue | 7 | 0 |
| Insomnia | 1 | 0 |
| Weight Loss | 3 | 0 |
| Neuropathy | 2 | 0 |
| Constipation | 4 | 0 |
| Diarrhea | 3 | 0 |
| Nausea & Vomiting | 5 | 0 |
| Hypertension | 1 | 0 |
| Epistasis | 1 | 0 |
| Vesicovaginal Fistula | 1 | 0 |
| Pleural Effusion | 2 | 0 |
| Small Bowel Obstruction | 1 | 0 |
| Atrial fibrillation | 1 | 0 |

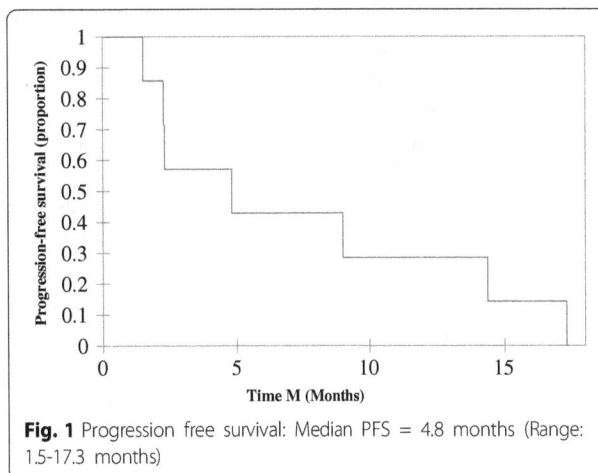

**Fig. 1** Progression free survival: Median PFS = 4.8 months (Range: 1.5-17.3 months)

## Discussion

NAB-paclitaxel has three Food and Drug Administration (FDA) approved indications: locally advanced or metastatic non-small cell lung cancer, metastatic adenocarcinoma of the pancreas, and metastatic breast cancer after failure of combination chemotherapy or relapse within 6 months of adjuvant therapy [12, 13]. There have been limited evaluations of NAB-paclitaxel in cervical cancer. Here we review our experience in treating heavily pre-treated recurrent cervical cancer patients that have failed prior cytotoxic chemotherapy.

NAB-paclitaxel was previously reviewed in the 127 series. This phase II study queue was launched in the 1990's by the GOG to evaluate recurrent squamous cell cervical cancer. Most agents studied were not effective with overall response rates ranged from 0 to 22 %. In this series, NAB-paclitaxel was the most effective agent demonstrating a partial response in 10 of 35 subjects (28.6 %). An additional 15 subjects experienced stable disease (42.9 %) [14, 15].

In comparison, within the prior phase II evaluation of NAB-paclitaxel in cervical cancer, our subjects were heavily pre-treated, versus the paclitaxel naïve status of the prior study.

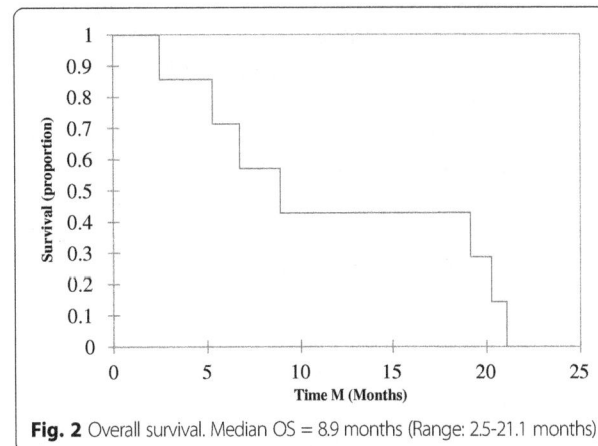

**Fig. 2** Overall survival. Median OS = 8.9 months (Range: 2.5-21.1 months)

While that data supported further investigation of NAB-paclitaxel, it is important to not disregard this significant limitation. Furthermore, data here supports the metronomic administration of this agent and this is the first report of such a dosing schedule in the setting of recurrent cervical cancer.

One subject was diagnosed with a vesicovaginal fistula during NAB-paclitaxel therapy. This subject was a 35 year old initially diagnosed with stage IIA2 adenocarcinoma. Nineteen months after her primary treatment of cisplatin and radiation, she experienced her first recurrence, and was treated with carboplatin and paclitaxel doublet therapy. Biopsy proven recurrent disease was noted during surveillance. The patient's exam was notable for "thickened area palpable inferior to the urethra". This subject completed 11 cycles of NAB-paclitaxel at 80 mg/m$^2$ and bevacizumab 10 mg/kg, and after eleventh cycle the fistula was detected on exam.

While this subject represents 10 % of our study population, the authors argue that this is more likely a representation of a pretreated-patient with extensive pelvic disease. Furthermore, the occurrence of this complication is more likely due to the administered bevacizumab with the known complication of fistula formation. This is supported by the lack of fistulas that occurred in the phase II study of NAB-paclitaxel. As this was a limited study population, future studies will need to address the incidence of fistulas during NAB-paclitaxel therapy.

While this study provides evidence for the feasibility and tolerability of NAB-paclitaxel in the setting of recurrent cervical cancer, there are several limitations to this data including: lack of patient reported outcomes, Response Evaluation Criteria In Solid Tumors (RECIST) response, and small study population.

## Conclusions

In conclusion, anti-angiogenic therapy has proven pivotal in the treatment of recurrent, metastatic and persistent cervical cancer, however if a GOG-240 treatment regimen fails, there are no established treatment options in recurrent cervical cancer. Metronomic-chemotherapy maybe another treatment option as this administration schedule produces anti-angiogenic properties by effecting endothelial repair time, endothelial cell proliferation, migration, and circulating levels of endothelial progenitor cells. NAB-paclitaxel was overall well tolerated with no grade 4 or 5 adverse events. NAB-paclitaxel with or without bevacizumab is feasible and potentially active in treating recurrent cervical cancer after failing platinum-taxane or topotecan chemotherapy. This small case series deserves confirmation through prospective clinical trials.

## Abbreviations

CTCAE: common terminology criteria for adverse events; FDA: Food and Drug Administration; GOG: Gynecologic Oncology Group; mg/kg: milligram per kilogram; mg/m$^2$: milligram per meters-square; NAB: nano-particle albumin bound; OS: overall survival; PFS: progression free survival; RECIST: response evaluation criteria in solid tumors.

## Competing interests

Lindsey E. Minion, Dana M. Chase, John H. Farley and Lyndsay J. Willmott, have nothing to disclose related to the content of this study. Bradley J. Monk's institution has received per capita funding from Genentech/Roche for clinical trials. Bradley J. Monk has also received honoraria from Genentech/Roche for consulting and is a part of their speaker's bureau.

## Authors' contributions

BM was responsible for study conception and design. LM was responsible for data collection. All authors were involved in data interpretation, manuscript writing and figure creation. All authors gave final approval of final manuscript.

## Author details

$^1$Dignity Health St. Joseph's Hospital and Medical Center, 500 West Thomas Road, Suite 660, Phoenix, AZ 85013, USA. $^2$Division of Gynecologic Oncology, Department of Obstetrics and Gynecology, University of Arizona Cancer Center at Dignity Health St. Joseph's Hospital and Medical Center, 500 West Thomas Road, Suite 660, Phoenix, AZ 85013, USA.

## References

1. Tewari K, Monk B. Chemotherapy for metastatic and recurrent cervical cancer. Curr Oncol Rep. 2005;7:419–34.
2. Monk BJ, Sill MW, McMeekin DS, Cohn DE, et al. Phase III trial of four cisplatin containing doublet combinations in stage IVB, recurrent, or persistent cervical carcinoma: a Gynecologic Oncology Group study. J Clin Oncol. 2009;27:4649–55.
3. Tewari KS, Sill MW, Long III HJ, et al. Improved survival with bevacizumab in advanced cervical cancer. N Engl J Med. 2014;370:734–43.
4. Gardner ER, Dahut WL, Scripture CD, et al. Randomized crossover pharmacokinetic study of solvent based paclitaxel and nab-paclitaxel. Clin Cancer Res. 2008;14(13):4200–5.
5. Desai N, Trieu V, Yao Z, et al. Increased antitumor activity, intratumor paclitaxel concentration and endothelial cell transport of cremophor-free, albumin-bound paclitaxel, ABI-007, compared with cremophor-based paclitaxel. Clin Cancer Res. 2006;12(4):1317–24.
6. Alberts DS, Blessing JA, Landrum LM, et al. Phase II trial of nab-paclitaxel in the treatment of recurrent or persistent advanced cervix cancer: A gynecologic oncology group study. Gynecol Oncol. 2012;127(3):451–5.
7. Willmott LJ, Monk BJ. Cervical cancer therapy: current, future and anti-angiogensis targeted treatment. Expert Rev Anticancer Ther. 2009;9(7):895–903.
8. Pasquier E, Honore S, Braguer D. Microtubule-targeting agents in angiogensis. Where do we stand? Drug Resist Updat. 2006;9(1–2):74–86.
9. Kerbel SK, Kamen BA. The anti-angiogenic basis of metronomic chemotherapy. Nat Rev Cancer. 2004;4(6):423–36.
10. Ng SS, Figg WD, Sparreboom A. Taxane-mediated antiangiogenesis in vitro: influence of formulation vehicles and binding proteins. Cancer Res. 2004; 64(3):821–4.
11. National Cancer Institute: Common Terminology Criteria for Adverse Events v4.0. NCI, NIH, DHHS. May 29, 2009, NIH publication # 09-7473. http://evs.nci. nih.gov/ftp1/CTCAE/CTCAE_4.03_2010-06-14_QuickReference_5x7.pdf
12. Gradishar WJ, Tjudlandin S, Davidson N, et al. Phase III Trial of Nanoparticle Albumin-Bound Paclitaxel Compared With Polyethylated Castor Oil–Based Paclitaxel in Women With Breast Cancer. J Clin Oncol. 2005;23(31):7794–803.
13. Abraxane [package insert]. Summitt, NJ: Celgene Coporation; 2014.
14. Tewari K, Monk B. Gynecologic oncology group trials of chemotherapy for metastatic and recurrent cervical cancer. Curr Oncol Rep. 2005;7(6):419–34.
15. Brewer CA, Blessing JA, Nagourney RA, McMeekin DS, Lele S, Zweizig SL. Cisplatin plus gemcitabine in previously treated squamous cell carcinoma of the cervix: a phase II study of the Gynecologic Oncology Group. Gynecol Oncol. 2006; 100(2):385–8.

# 11

# Adenocarcinoma of Mullerian origin: review of pathogenesis, molecular biology, and emerging treatment paradigms

Lauren Patterson Cobb[1*], Stephanie Gaillard[2], Yihong Wang[3], Ie-Ming Shih[3] and Angeles Alvarez Secord[1]

## Abstract

Traditionally, epithelial ovarian, tubal, and peritoneal cancers have been viewed as separate entities with disparate origins, pathogenesis, clinical features, and outcomes. Additionally, previous classification systems for ovarian cancer have proposed two primary histologic groups that encompass the standard histologic subtypes. Recent data suggest that these groupings no longer accurately reflect our knowledge surrounding these cancers. In this review, we propose that epithelial ovarian, tubal, and peritoneal carcinomas represent a spectrum of disease that originates in the Mullerian compartment. We will discuss the incidence, classification, origin, molecular determinants, and pathologic analysis of these cancers that support the conclusion they should be collectively referred to as adenocarcinomas of Mullerian origin. As our understanding of the molecular and pathologic profiling of adenocarcinomas of Mullerian origin advances, we anticipate treatment paradigms will shift towards genomic driven therapeutic interventions.

Keywords: Adenocarcinoma, Mullerian origin, Epithelial ovarian carcinoma, Fallopian tube carcinoma, Peritoneal carcinoma

## Introduction

Adenocarcinoma of Mullerian origin was first described by Dr. Swerdlow in 1959 [1]. The original manuscript entitled, "Mesothelioma of the pelvic peritoneum resembling papillary cystadenocarcinoma of the ovary," described a patient with a malignant left-sided pelvic mass. The mass surrounded the left fallopian tube without mucosal involvement; bilateral ovaries and the right tube were negative for disease. Histologically, the tumor closely resembled a papillary ovarian cystadenocarcinoma. Dr. Swerdlow theorized that while ovarian or tubal carcinoma was unlikely, the tumor probably developed from tissue with a similar embryological origin as the ovary (specifically, the pelvic peritoneum, fallopian tubes, or uterus). He ultimately concluded that the cancer arose from the pelvic peritoneum [1]. In retrospect, this case represents the earliest documentation of adenocarcinoma of Mullerian origin. There is a growing body of evidence that suggests this terminology applies to epithelial ovarian,

peritoneal, and tubal cancers, as well as select cancers previously designated as "cancers of unknown primary" (CUP). Select endometrial cancers may also be included in future classifications, but as the treatment paradigms are different, we chose not to include them in this review.

Recent data regarding the genetics and histopathology of epithelial ovarian cancer (EOC) has improved our understanding of ovarian carcinogenesis. These results and current hypotheses indicate that epithelial ovarian, peritoneal, and tubal cancers are not distinct entities but represent a spectrum of disease that originates in the Mullerian compartment. Due to this new information, the FIGO staging classification for ovarian, tubal, and peritoneal cancers was revised (Table 1) [2]. Tubal and peritoneal cancers are now included in the ovarian cancer staging classification, and the primary site designated when possible [2,3]. This new staging exemplifies our current understanding of the relationship between these disease entities and challenges our previous classification of ovarian, peritoneal, and tubal cancers. We and others assert that this group of gynecologic cancers should be collectively designated as adenocarcinomas of Mullerian origin. In this review, we will focus on the incidence,

* Correspondence: lauren.cobb@duke.edu
[1]Division of Gynecologic Oncology, Department of Obstetrics and Gynecology, Duke Cancer Institute, Duke University Medical Center, Durham, NC 27710, USA
Full list of author information is available at the end of the article

**Table 1 Ovarian cancer staging (FIGO 2013 vs. FIGO 1988)**

| FIGO (1988) | FIGO (2013) |
| --- | --- |
| I: Tumor limited to the ovaries | I: Tumor confined to ovaries or fallopian tube(s)[a] |
| IA: Tumor limited to 1 ovary (capsule intact), no tumor on ovarian surface, no malignant cells in ascites or peritoneal washings | IA: Tumor limited to 1 ovary (capsule intact) or fallopian tube; no tumor on ovarian or fallopian tube surface; no malignant cells in the ascites or peritoneal washings |
| IB: Tumor limited to both ovaries (capsules intact), no tumor on ovarian surface, no malignant cells in ascites or peritoneal washings | IB: Tumor limited to both ovaries (capsules intact) or fallopian tubes; no tumor on ovarian or fallopian tube surface; no malignant cells in the ascites or peritoneal washings |
| IC: Tumor limited to 1 or both ovaries with any of the following: capsule ruptured, tumor on ovarian surface, malignant cells in ascites or peritoneal washings | IC: Tumor limited to 1 or both ovaries or fallopian tube(s) with any of the following: |
|  | IC1: Surgical spill intraoperatively |
|  | IC2: Capsule ruptured before surgery or tumor on ovarian or fallopian tube surface |
|  | IC3: Malignant cells in the ascites or peritoneal washings |
| II: Tumor involves 1 or both ovaries with pelvic extension | II: Tumor involves 1 or both ovaries or fallopian tubes with pelvic extension (below pelvic brim) or primary peritoneal cancer[b] |
| IIA: Extension and/or implants on uterus and/or tube(s); no malignant cells in ascites or peritoneal washings | IIA: Extension and/or implants on uterus and/or fallopian tubes and/or ovaries |
| IIB: Extension to other pelvic tissues; no malignant cells in ascites or peritoneal washings | IIB: Extension to other pelvic intra-peritoneal tissues |
| IIC: Pelvic extension (IIA or IIB) with malignant cells in ascites or peritoneal washings |  |
| III: Tumor involves 1 or both ovaries with microscopically confirmed peritoneal metastases outside the pelvis and/or regional lymph node metastasis | III: Tumor involves 1 or both ovaries or fallopian tubes, or primary peritoneal cancer, with cytologically or histologically confirmed spread to the peritoneum outside the pelvis and/or metastasis to the retroperitoneal lymph nodes |
| IIIA: Microscopic peritoneal metastasis beyond pelvis | IIIA1: Positive retroperitoneal lymph nodes only (cytologically or histologically proven) |
|  | IIIA1(i): Metastasis up to 10 mm in greatest dimension |
|  | IIIA1(ii): Metastasis more than 10 mm in greatest dimension |
|  | IIIA2: Microscopic extra-pelvic (above the pelvic brim) peritoneal involvement with or without positive retroperitoneal lymph nodes |
| IIIB: Macroscopic peritoneal metastasis beyond pelvis, 2 cm or less in greatest dimension | IIIB: Macroscopic peritoneal metastasis beyond the pelvis up to 2 cm in greatest dimension, with or without metastasis to the retro-peritoneal lymph nodes (includes extension of tumor to capsule of liver and spleen without parenchymal involvement of either organ) |
| IIIC: Peritoneal metastasis beyond pelvis more than 2 cm in greatest dimension and/or regional lymph node metastasis | IIIC: Macroscopic peritoneal metastasis beyond the pelvis more than 2 cm in greatest dimension, with or without metastasis to the retro-peritoneal lymph nodes (includes extension of tumor to capsule of liver and spleen without parenchymal involvement of either organ) |
| IV: Distant metastasis (excludes peritoneal metastasis) | IV: Distant metastasis excluding peritoneal metastases |
|  | IVA: Pleural effusion with positive cytology |
|  | IVB: Parenchymal metastases and metastases to extra-abdominal organs (including inguinal lymph nodes and lymph nodes outside of the abdominal cavity)[c] |

[a]It is not possible to have stage I peritoneal cancer.
[b]Dense adhesions with histologically proven tumor cells justify upgrading apparent stage I tumors to stage II.
[c]Extra-abdominal metastases include transmural bowel infiltration and umbilical deposits.
Adapted from Zeppernick F, Meinhold-Heerlein I. The new FIGO staging system for ovarian, fallopian tube, and primary peritoneal cancer. *Archives of gynecology and obstetrics.* Aug 1 2014.

classification, and origin of Mullerian adenocarcinomas. We will also review the molecular and pathologic profiling that support the concept of adenocarcinomas of Mullerian origin as a unified entity and will assist in diagnostic and treatment paradigms.

## Review

### Incidence

It is difficult to discern how many annual deaths occur due to adenocarcinomas of Mullerian origin. While EOC caused approximately 14,030 deaths in the United States in 2013 [4] and 151,905 deaths worldwide in 2012 [5], it is unclear exactly how many deaths were caused by peritoneal and tubal cancers. Peritoneal and tubal carcinomas have been considered rare malignancies and separate entities from ovarian carcinomas; thus, epidemiologic studies have proven difficult [6]. Tubal carcinomas account for only 0.14-1.8% of gynecologic malignancies [7,8]. In the United States, from 1995–2004, the age adjusted incidence rates for tubal and peritoneal carcinomas were 3.7 and 6.8 per million, respectively [6]. Newer theories indicate that the number of peritoneal and tubal cancers may be grossly underestimated.

Additionally, CUP accounts for 3-5% of malignant epithelial cancers [9] and in 2012, there were an estimated 31,000 new cases of CUP in the United States [10]. Potentially 5% of CUP may originate in the female reproductive system based on data from post mortem autopsy studies [9,11]. It is important to recognize the adenocarcinoma of Mullerian origin subset of CUP when it occurs, because these cancers will typically have a more favorable prognosis and sensitivity to platinum-based chemotherapeutic regimens [12]. Identification of adenocarcinoma of Mullerian origin, specifically in patients with CUP, will guide appropriate treatment options, and provide information regarding prognosis [9,12].

## Current classification

### Epithelial ovarian cancer classification

EOC classification has changed significantly over the past decade. The most recent proposed division of EOC includes two distinct histologic groups: type I and type II cancers. It should be noted that the type I and type II classification is generally used to broadly classify ovarian neoplasms for research purposes based on their unique clinical and molecular genetic features [13]. The classification was not meant to be used for clinical purposes. Type I tumors include low-grade serous and low-grade endometrioid cancers, as well as mucinous, clear cell, and transitional cell carcinomas. Tumors in this category typically develop from atypical proliferative borderline tumors, benign cystic lesions, or endometriosis. Transitional cell tumors and mucinous tumors do not typically have Mullerian features, but may develop from cortical inclusion cysts and Walthard cell nests [14]. However, there is an uncommon subtype of mucinous tumors which does demonstrate Mullerian (endocervical) characteristics [15,16]. Generally, type I tumors are more indolent, present at an earlier stage, are confined to the ovary, and are often large. When type I tumors, specifically clear cell and mucinous cancers, are not detected early, they usually have a worse prognosis than type II cancers [14].

Type II cancers account for approximately 75% of EOC and the vast majority of ovarian cancer deaths. These include high-grade serous and high-grade endometrioid carcinomas, as well as carcinosarcomas and undifferentiated carcinomas. These cancers are typically aggressive and diagnosed at a later stage [13,14,17]. Until recently the origin or precursor lesion for the type II cancers was unknown [18]. However, it is now recognized that the precursor lesion exists in the fallopian tube, as discussed later in this review [14,17,19-21].

### Fallopian tube cancer classification

As mentioned above, per the 2014 FIGO staging classification, tubal and peritoneal cancers are now considered collectively with ovarian cancer [2]. Regarding histologic classification, serous tubal carcinomas are most frequent (49.5-83.3%), followed by endometrioid (8.3%-50%), mixed (3.9-16.7%), transitional (11.7%), undifferentiated (7.8-11.3%), mucinous (3%-7.6%), and clear cell (1.9%) cancers [7]. These histologic subtypes are similar to the proportions seen in EOC; however, clear cell histology is more common in EOC, while transitional cell and undifferentiated histology is more frequent in tubal cancers [7,8]. In the past, the diagnosis of tubal carcinoma was made based on pathologic criteria with at least one the following: 1) the primary tumor arises from the endosalpinx in the fallopian tube 2) the histologic pattern resembles epithelial mucosa and is often papillary in nature 3) there is a clear transition between benign and malignant epithelium if the wall is involved, and 4) there is no evidence of malignancy in the ovaries or endometrium, or if tumor is present, there is less tumor than is present in the fallopian tube [7].

### Peritoneal cancer classification

Peritoneal carcinomas have been called multiple names including peritoneal papillary serous carcinoma, peritoneal mesothelioma, primary peritoneal carcinoma, and normal-sized ovary carcinoma syndrome. In 1993, the Gynecologic Oncology Group established specific guidelines for the diagnosis of peritoneal carcinoma: 1) ovaries are of normal size or enlarged only as a result of a benign process 2) extraovarian involvement is greater than surface ovarian involvement 3) ovarian involvement does not show evidence of cortical invasion, is confined to the ovarian surface epithelium and cortical stroma and is less than 5×5 mm, and 4) histologically, the cancer is primarily of serous type, appearing similar or identical to ovarian serous adenocarcinoma of any grade [22]. Historically, peritoneal cancers have been reported to be more frequently multifocal with diffuse micronodular spread and more difficult to cytoreduce compared to EOC [23]. In 1994, Fowler et al. characterized the natural history of peritoneal adenocarcinoma of Mullerian origin. He reported that most were classified as serous histology and had either omental disease or diffuse carcinomatosis [12]. Currently, while viewed as separate entities, patients with peritoneal carcinoma are commonly included in ovarian cancer trials, treated similarly to ovarian cancer with cytoreductive surgery and platinum-based chemotherapy [24], and now considered collectively with ovarian and tubal cancer in the staging guidelines [2].

### Theories regarding adenocarcinoma of Mullerian origin

Comprehension of the embryologic origin of the Mullerian system is critical to understanding the theories surrounding the origin of ovarian, peritoneal, and tubal cancers. Ovarian surface epithelium (OSE) is derived from the coelomic epithelium in early development. The coelomic epithelium is derived from the mesoderm, consists of the epithelial lining of the intraembryonic body cavity or coelom, and overlies the intraembryonic body cavity (which will become the peritoneum), including the area that will develop into the gonadal structures. During fetal development, near the area that will form the gonadal structures, the coelomic epithelium invaginates to give rise to the Mullerian (paramesonephric) ducts (which will ultimately differentiate to become the fallopian tubes, uterus, cervix, and upper vagina). Therefore, while the reproductive organs and peritoneum originate from distinct pathways, the Mullerian epithelia, OSE, and peritoneal (coelomic) epithelium have a close developmental relationship (Figure 1) [25].

Ovarian carcinogenesis was previously thought to occur through the invagination of the OSE into the underlying stroma to form inclusion cysts. Metaplasia of the epithelium on the wall of these cysts was proposed to transform the OSE into the aforementioned cell types and their corresponding tumors: serous, mucinous, clear cell, endometrioid and transitional cell carcinomas. This theory

seems unlikely for two reasons: (1) the normal ovary does not bear resemblance to the morphologic phenotype of any of these tumors, and (2) it suggests that ovarian cancers develop de novo. However, cancers typically develop in a stepwise fashion from a benign lesion to a malignancy [14]. An alternate theory proposed that ovarian tumors develop from nearby paraovarian and paratubal cysts consisting of Mullerian-type epithelium, called the "secondary Mullerian system." As the tumors grow from these cysts, they infringe upon the ovary, compress it, and eventually obliterate it, making it appear as though it is ovarian in origin [14,26]. This theory seems unlikely as well, given that paratubal and paraovarian cysts rarely contain precursor lesions resembling serous, clear cell, or endometrioid carcinomas [14]. However, the secondary Mullerian system may also include endosalpingiosis, endometriosis, and endocerviocosis. Metaplasia from these tissues are commonly observed in ovarian malignancies [27]; thus, this theory may account for the development of some ovarian cancers [27]. The most recent theory proposes that the majority of serous, endometrioid, and clear cell "primary ovarian" cancers actually develop from the fallopian tube and endometrium, the "primary Mullerian system" and will be discussed further in this review [14,27].

### Origin of type I EOC

In type I EOC, there is considerable evidence that clear cell and endometrioid carcinomas may originate from endometriosis. The pathogenesis of endometriosis is complex and theories include retrograde menstruation as well as metaplasia of extrauterine cells. Retrograde menstruation would indicate that endometrioid and

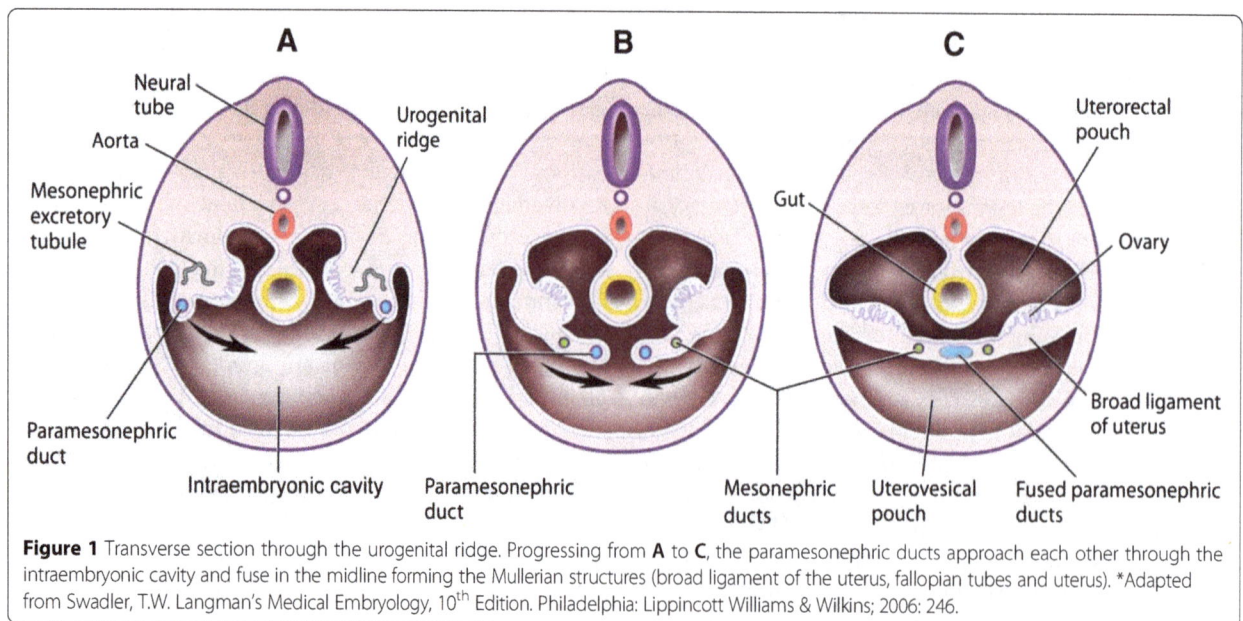

**Figure 1** Transverse section through the urogenital ridge. Progressing from **A** to **C**, the paramesonephric ducts approach each other through the intraembryonic cavity and fuse in the midline forming the Mullerian structures (broad ligament of the uterus, fallopian tubes and uterus). *Adapted from Swadler, T.W. Langman's Medical Embryology, 10th Edition. Philadelphia: Lippincott Williams & Wilkins; 2006: 246.

clear cell cancers develop from endometrial tissue, the primary Mullerian system, which secondarily involves the ovary [14]. Several studies have demonstrated an increased risk of ovarian cancer in the setting of endometriosis [28-30]. A meta-analysis of endometriosis in EOC concluded that the prevalence of endometriosis was significantly higher in women with clear cell cancers (35.9%) and endometrioid carcinomas (19%), compared to those with serous (4.5%), and mucinous (1.4%) cancers [31].

The origin of mucinous carcinoma is unclear. It is commonly accepted that a majority of mucinous cancers involving the reproductive tract are actually metastases from extraovarian sites, usually gastrointestinal in origin. True primary ovarian mucinous carcinomas are uncommon, accounting for only 3% of ovarian carcinomas, although one recent theory includes mucinous metaplasia of Brenner (transitional cell) tumors [32]. Brenner tumors and mucinous carcinomas (intestinal type) may share similar histogenesis at the tubal peritoneal junction from transitional cell nests that exist there [13]. As mentioned previously, an uncommon subtype of mucinous tumors does demonstrate Mullerian (endocervical) characteristics [15,16]. Most advanced mucinous cancers are likely metastatic gastrointestinal and pancreaticobilliary cancers that involve the ovary and peritoneum.

With regard to low-grade serous carcinoma (LGSC), multiple studies support the step-wise progression of serous cystadenoma or adenofibroma to atypical proliferative serous tumor (atypical serous borderline tumor), to noninvasive micropapillary serous borderline tumor, to invasive LGSC (Figure 2) [33]. Previously, we reported identical hallmark *KRAS* mutations in serous borderline ovarian tumors and their associated Mullerian inclusion cysts, suggesting a relationship between the two. It is unclear if Mullerian inclusion cysts represent a precursor lesion, signify metastatic disease from the primary borderline tumor, or develop due to a metaplastic field effect [34]. While *KRAS* and *BRAF* mutations are common in borderline tumors, *NRAS* mutations are only seen in carcinomas and may represent the requisite oncogenic switch to invasive serous cancer [35]. There is also evidence to support the development of LGSC from fallopian tube precursors or papillary tubal hyperplasia [14,27,36,37].

### Origin of type II EOC

An observation by Piek et al. would eventually revolutionize hypotheses regarding the origin of high-grade serous carcinoma (HGSC). In 2001, Piek and colleagues examined specimens from women who had undergone a risk reducing bilateral salpingo-oophorectomy who were either BRCA mutation carriers or had a strong family history of ovarian cancer. Fifty percent of the specimens had preinvasive dysplastic lesions (later coined "serous tubal intraepithelial carcinoma" (STIC)) that resembled HGSC. Almost all specimens had high levels of p53 protein accumulation (indicating accumulation of a nonfunctional p53 protein due to a *TP53* genetic mutation). Initially this new information was interpreted to mean that tubal carcinoma should be included in the in the spectrum of BRCA-associated disease [38]. In 2003, Piek et al.

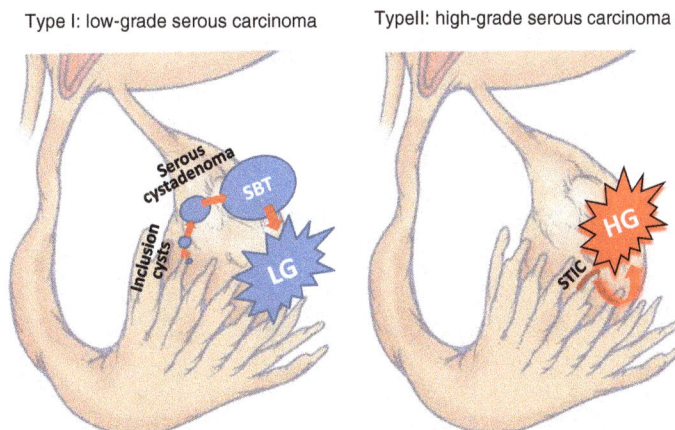

**Figure 2** The dualistic pathways in developing low-grade and high-grade "ovarian" serous carcinoma. The Type I pathway develops from the presumed fallopian tube epithelial stem cells that disseminated into the ovulation site where those stem cells form surface inclusion cysts. Those cysts may continue to grow into serous cystadenomas and clonally develop into serous borderline tumors, which represent the precursor lesions of low-grade serous carcinomas. In contrast to the step-wise tumor progression pathway as observed in Type I serous tumors, in the Type 2 pathway, many high-grade serous carcinomas arise as a result of dissemination of their precursor lesions, serous tubal intraepithelial carcinomas (STICs), in the fallopian tube fimbriated ends.

reevaluated their findings and hypothesized that lesions in the fallopian tube epithelium are the precursor lesions for hereditary and *BRCA*-mutated ovarian cancer [19]. Further studies performed in *BRCA* mutation carriers revealed that benign areas of the tubal epithelium overexpressing p53 nonfunctional protein may represent a precursor to STIC in the pathway to the development of HGSC [21,39]. STICs are present in the majority of serous ovarian (59-67%), peritoneal (67%), and tubal (100%) carcinomas [17,21,25]. In contrast, STICs were not identified in mucinous, endometrioid, or carcinosarcoma histologic subtypes [40]. In addition, further studies have reported identical *TP53* mutations in paired STIC and the concurrent HGSC indicating a clonal relationship between them [20]. While most HGSCs arise from STICs, alternative pathways in developing HGSC also exist. For instance, a small number of HGSCs appear to arise from serous borderline tumors or LGSCs (Figure 3) [27,41].

While it is not clear how STIC is related to the development of peritoneal cancers, some have hypothesized that sloughed tubal cancer cells disseminate into the peritoneal cavity and implant accordingly. While Sood et al. proposed hematogenous spread of ovarian cancer cells with a predilection for implantation in the omentum [42], perhaps both modes of metastasis (peritoneal and hematogenous dissemination) play a role in Mullerian carcinogenesis.

Overall, contemporary data indicate that endometrioid and clear cell cancers arise from endometrial tissue with the fallopian tube as a conduit between the uterus, ovary,

and peritoneum; serous cancers from STICs in the fallopian tube [36]; Brenner and mucinous cancers from transitional-type epithelium found at the tubal-peritoneal junction that secondarily implant or metastasize to the ovary and peritoneal surfaces; and rare mucinous cancers from endocervical mucinous neoplasms. Therefore, while historically documented as separate processes, we would argue that ovarian, tubal, and peritoneal cancers should be uniformly referred to as adenocarcinomas of Mullerian origin given their similar pathogenesis.

### Disease outcomes for adenocarcinoma of Mullerian origin

In a recent meta-analysis, Sørensen et al. compared serous peritoneal, tubal and ovarian cancer with regards to risk factors, epidemiology, clinicopathology, and molecular biology to address whether these diseases should be considered separately. When comparing peritoneal cancers with ovarian cancers, even though most of these studies were limited by small sample sizes, nine studies showed no significant difference in survival [43-51]. Only three studies showed poorer survival for peritoneal cancers [52-54]; however, two of these studies had a small number of patients with peritoneal cancer [52,53]. When comparing tubal cancers to ovarian cancers, Sørensen et al. sited three studies showing similar survival between these two disease entities [54-56] and two showing improved survival for tubal cancers [57,58]. The studies by Usach et al. [57] and Wethington et al. [58] were large studies using the SEER database and did not

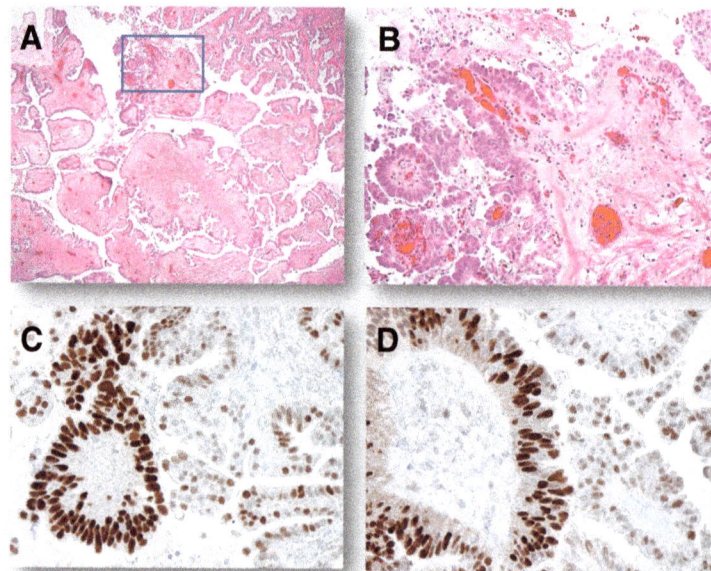

**Figure 3** A high-grade serous carcinoma arises from a serous borderline tumor. **A**. A low-magnification view shows a focal high-grade serous carcinoma developing from the papillae (square) in a background of a typical serous borderline tumor. **B**. A higher magnification demonstrates enlarged and atypical high-grade serous carcinoma cells that organize in a papillary architecture. **C** and **D**. Immunohistochemistry of p53 shows that high-grade serous carcinoma cells are diffusely positive for p53, a pattern consistent with a missense *TP53* mutation while the adjacent epithelial cells from the background serous borderline tumor are only focally and weakly positive, a pattern consistent with a wild-type *TP53* sequence.

include information on residual disease after debulking surgery. All of the aforementioned studies had limitations. Most of these studies included small sample sizes, utilized differing definitions of optimal cytoreduction, and failed to include detailed information regarding pathology, surgery, treatment regimens, recurrences, and confounding risk factors, making them difficult to compare and then generalize their findings. Despite an extensive literature search by Sørensen and colleagues, the small number of studies as well as their limitations preclude definitive conclusions regarding survival outcomes between ovarian, tubal, and peritoneal cancers.

## Biomarkers and pathologic assessment for adenocarcinoma of Mullerian origin

Serum biomarkers are useful for the detection, response assessment, and prognosis in a variety of solid tumors, including adenocarcinomas of Mullerian origin. Cancer antigen 125 (CA125) is the only biomarker commonly used for monitoring treatment response and cancer progression in EOC [59], as well as tubal and peritoneal cancers [60]. CA125 is a glycoprotein encoded by the gene MUC16. In patients with advanced EOC, CA125 is elevated (greater than 35 u/mL) approximately 90% of the time. However, in patients with early stage EOC, CA125 is elevated only 50-60% of the time. CA125 is an excellent marker for ovarian cancer, but is nonspecific and can be abnormal in other benign and malignant indications. CA125 expression levels also vary by histology and are elevated in 85% of serous, 65% of endometrioid, 40% of clear cell, and 36% of undifferentiated adenocarcinomas [59].

There are additional markers that are useful to distinguish between various solid tumors. These include carbohydrate antigen 19–9 (CA19-9), carcinoembryonic antigen (CEA), and human epididymis protein 4 (HE4). CA19-9 is member of the Lewis blood group antigens and is elevated in 27% and 76% of serous and mucinous ovarian cancers, respectively. CEA is a glycoprotein that is expressed in 25-50% of women with EOC and over 80% of patients with colorectal carcinomas. Human epididymis protein 4 (HE4) is overexpressed in serous and endometrioid carcinomas. Unlike CA125, HE4 is more specific to ovarian malignancy and serum levels are usually not elevated with nonmalignant processes [59]. A subset analysis of premenopausal patients enrolled in a prospective clinical trial (NCT00315692) demonstrated that HE4 had a sensitivity of 88.9% and a specificity of 91.8% for the detection of malignancy. In this analysis, invasive malignancy was ruled out for 98% of premenopausal women with an elevated CA-125 and a normal HE4 level [61]. There are other additional markers that have been used in combination with CA125, including cancer antigen 15–3 (CA15-3) and tumor associated glycoprotein 72 (TAG-72). Although CA15-3 is elevated in 57-71% of ovarian malignancies (versus 2-6% of benign ovarian processes), it has a low specificity for ovarian cancer and is primarily used for the diagnosis of breast malignancies. TAG-72 is expressed more commonly in gastrointestinal and pancreatic tumors as well as mucinous ovarian carcinomas [59]. Biomarkers can be useful for identifying adenocarcinomas of Mullerian origin in women with CUP, as well as following response to treatment.

## Pathological analysis of adenocarcinoma of Mullerian origin

Ovarian, tubal, and peritoneal cancers have similar pathologic findings which vary based on histologic subtype, but not by primary site of origin. We describe common histopathologic and immunophenotype findings for adenocarcinomas of Mullerian origin stratified by the various subtypes. Pathologic findings support a clear link between serous ovarian, tubal, and peritoneal cancers. However, information regarding pathologic similarities between tubal and peritoneal clear cell, mucinous, and endometrioid carcinomas is minimal given the relatively rare frequency of these histologic subtypes.

### High-grade serous carcinoma

**Histopathology** HGSCs of the ovary, fallopian tube, and peritoneum are almost identical in histopathology. Microscopically, the architecture could vary from glandular to complex papillary to solid pattern, with the tumor cells infiltrating or replacing the surrounding normal tissues. The papillae are usually large, irregularly branching, and highly cellular. Psammoma bodies may be present in varying numbers, but are rarely as numerous as in LGSC. The marked cytologic atypia and frequent mitotic figures (including atypical ones) characterize HGSC. The tumor cells are enlarged, with high nuclear/cytoplasmic ratio and great variation in size. Tumor giant cells are commonly seen. The nuclei are of high-grade with vesicular chromatin and prominent nucleoli [33].

**Immunophenotype** Immunophenotypically, ovarian and tubal HGSCs strongly and diffusely express p16, and CK7; express WT-1, PAX-8, estrogen receptor, CA125 and E-cadherin in most cases; do not express Her-2, calretinin, or CK20; and have a high Ki67 proliferative index (Figure 4) [33,62-65]. The staining pattern for p53 protein is usually consistent with either a missense mutation (diffusely and intensely positive) or nonsense/deletion type mutation (completely negative) [33]. Overall, peritoneal serous carcinomas almost always demonstrate the same immunohistochemistry pattern as ovarian and tubal HGSCs, with minor and inconsistent differences in WT-1, b-catenin, vimentin and CK20 expression [62,66-69].

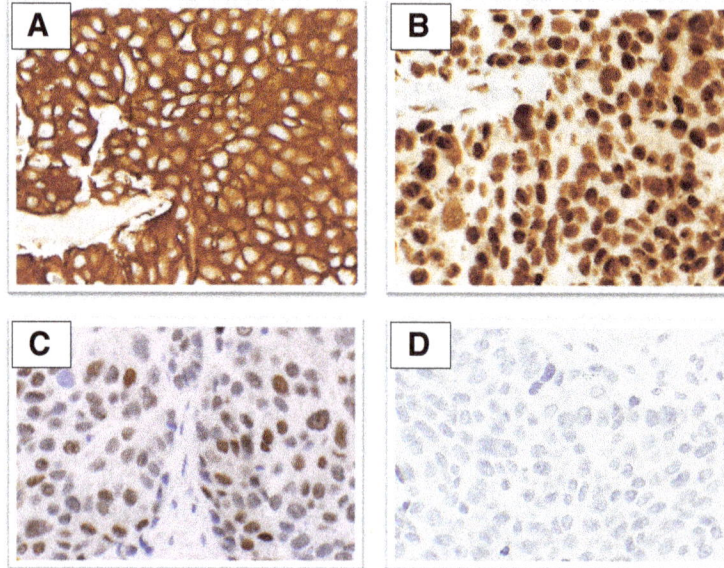

**Figure 4** Representative microscopic sections of high-grade serous adenocarcinoma of Mullerian origin demonstrating positive immunostaining for **(A)** CK-7, **(B)** WT-1, **(C)** PAX-8, and **(D)** negative immunostaining for CK-20.

### Low-grade serous carcinoma

**Histopathology** Similar to HGSC, there is strong evidence to support the tubal origin of LGSC [36]. In general, LGSC is characterized by micropapillae and small round nests of neoplastic cells that infiltrate the stroma in a haphazard pattern, with infrequent mitoses and only mild variation in tumor cell size and shape of nuclei. The nuclear/cytoplasmic ratio may be high but the nuclei are uniform, small, and round to oval. Psammoma bodies are common and may be numerous. Necrosis or multinucleated tumor giant cells are not features of LGSC. In contrast to HGSC, LGSC is usually associated with a non-invasive serous borderline component [33].

**Immunophenotype** As previously discussed, the precursor lesions for LGSC are presumed to be epithelial inclusion cysts (leading to serous cystadenoma/adenofibroma, to atypical serous borderline tumor, to noninvasive micropapillary serous borderline tumor, to invasive LGSCs). These epithelial inclusion cysts were previously thought to arise from invaginations of the OSE that undergo metaplasia; however, the inclusion cysts may originate from tubal epithelia that secondarily implant on disrupted OSE and invaginate [36]. Li et al. demonstrated that OSE primarily has a mesothelial phenotype (calretinin(+)/PAX8(−)), while the majority of epithelial inclusion cysts demonstrate a tubal phenotype (calretinin(−)/PAX8(+)) [37]. It is not surprising then that LGSCs also express PAX8. Additionally, they express ER and WT-1, similar to HGSC. In contrast to HGSC, LGSC is characterized by decreased expression of p53 and p16 (usually negative, scattered, or patchy), and a lower Ki67 proliferative index [33].

Low-grade serous peritoneal carcinoma is a rare entity; and therefore, available information about this disease is minimal. Schmeler et al. were the first to clinically describe low-grade serous peritoneal cancer. Patients were confirmed to have low-grade serous carcinomas with destructive invasion. Microscopically the cancers had relatively uniform round to oval nuclei, mild to moderate atypia, evenly distributed chromatin, and no more than 12 mitoses per 10 high-power fields (HPF). Additionally, these patients met the previously described GOG criteria for peritoneal carcinoma. Specific immunostaining was not described [70].

### Mucinous carcinoma

**Histopathology** The majority of primary mucinous tumors of the ovary mimic features of gastric or pancreaticobilliary mucinous neoplasms, while another much less common subtype harbor Mullerian (endocervical) characteristics. A spectrum of morphologic changes from cystadenoma to atypical proliferative mucinous tumor (mucinous borderline tumor) to invasive mucinous carcinoma can often be appreciated. They are usually large unilateral neoplasms with a smooth capsule and confined to the ovary at diagnosis (stage I). Stromal invasion may be infiltrative or expansile [15,16]. Mucinous tumors of the fallopian tube and peritoneum are rare, but have been reported [7,8,24,71].

**Immunophenotype** Ovarian mucinous carcinomas display predominance of CK7 over CK20. PAX-8 staining is much less frequent (40%) despite that it is almost universally positive (95–100%) in ovarian serous, endometrioid, and clear cell carcinomas [72]. WT1, ER, PR and p16 are not expressed in primary mucinous carcinomas. p53 protein may be present in 30% of cases, but strong and diffuse overexpression (as found in HGSC) is not characteristic [33,73-75].

### Clear cell carcinoma

**Histopathology** Clear cell carcinoma has also been associated with endometriosis and displays the following architectural and cytological features: papillary, tubulocystic or solid architecture; hobnail tumor cells with clear cytoplasm; and large, atypical nuclei with conspicuous nucleoli and only moderate polymorphism. Clear cell carcinoma papillae are distinguishable from those of serous carcinoma in that they are short and round, may show eosinophilic and hyalinized stroma, and are generally lined with only one or two layers of cells. Hyaline bodies are present in approximately 25% of cases. Mitoses are less frequent than in other types of ovarian carcinomas (usually < 5 per 10 HPF) [15,16]. While most literature focuses on "ovarian" clear cell carcinoma, there are published case reports of peritoneal and tubal clear cell cancers [76-79]. The histopathologic findings are similar to ovarian clear cell carcinomas, but immunostaining is not consistently available [76-78].

**Immunophenotype** Generally, clear cell carcinomas display a CK7(+)/CK20(-) phenotype; express PAX-8; and lack expression of ER and WT-1. p53 and p16 are usually negative, weak, focal or patchy. Hepatocyte nuclear factor-1β (HNF-1β) is a specific and sensitive marker for ovarian clear cell carcinomas that is not expressed in HGSC [80-82].

### Endometrioid carcinoma

**Histopathology** Endometrioid carcinomas of the ovary highly resemble endometrioid carcinomas of the uterus in morphology. These cancers may coexist with endometriosis and arise from endometriotic cysts. They are mostly low-grade adenocarcinomas demonstrating a confluent glandular growth pattern with stromal disappearance, or evidence of stromal invasion and squamous metaplasia to varied degrees. Fifteen to thirty percent of patients have concurrent endometrial hyperplasia or carcinoma [83]. Similar histopathologic descriptions have been detailed in few case reports and case series of endometrioid carcinoma of the fallopian tube, but immunostaining was not described in detail [76,84-87]. The even rarer entity of endometrioid carcinoma of the peritoneum has been described in reference to extraovarian endometriosis-associated malignancy [88-90], however specific immunostaining has not been described.

**Immunophenotype** Endometrioid carcinomas typically demonstrate CK7(+)/CK20(-) phenotype; express ER, PR and PAX-8; but lack WT-1 and p16 expression, as well as p53 overexpression. Exceptions to these patterns have been reported in poorly differentiated varieties, which overlap with HGSC in morphology [33,91].

### Molecular determinants of adenocarcinoma of Mullerian origin

The data regarding the molecular determinants of adenocarcinoma of Mullerian origin is primarily based on genomic studies of EOC [92]. However, some studies do include tubal and peritoneal cancers. Tothill et al. reported that serous and endometrioid cancers demonstrate a high degree of molecular heterogeneity and could be categorized into six subgroups based on gene expression profiling. Importantly, the primary site of disease could not be used as a classification parameter [93]. Tothill and colleagues reported six distinct subtypes referred to as C1-C6. C3 primarily consisted of serous low malignant potential tumors, while C6 primarily consisted of low-grade, early stage endometrial cancers. C1, C2, C4, and C5 mainly contained high-grade serous and high-grade endometrial cancers. Notably, C5 demonstrated a mesenchymal profile which was associated with relatively poor overall survival [93]. This finding is consistent with our understanding of cells acquiring the mesenchymal phenotype as they acquire invasiveness in the process of epithelial to mesenchymal transition (EMT). However, in the TCGA data set, a correlation between the mesenchymal subtype and survival was not seen [92]. Further evaluation is needed to confirm the associations between gene expression classifications and clinical outcome.

In 2013, Yang and colleagues took an integrated approach (as opposed to the previous transcriptome approach) to analyze serous cancers in the TCGA database and categorize the transcriptional subtypes into integrated mesenchymal and integrated epithelial subtypes. This new approach integrated mRNA expression with associated alterations in genomic, epigenetic, and miRNA systems. With this approach, Yang et al. were able to uncover a master miRNA regulatory network that consistently associated the integrated mesenchymal subtype of serous cancer with poor overall survival [94].

Additionally, intense interest has focused on using microarray data to identify molecularly-defined subgroups of women with HGSC who may benefit from anti-angiogenic therapy with bevacizumab. Gourley et al. evaluated a cohort of HGSC samples from the ICON7 study and identified three major subgroups; two with upregulation of angiogenic gene expression and one with upregulation of immune genes (and concurrent downregulation of angiogenic genes). Women in the immune subgroup had improved overall and progression-free survival (PFS) over the other two angiogenic subgroups. However, with the incorporation of bevacizumab, the immune subgroup had worse PFS (Hazard ratio (HR) = 1.73 (1.12-2.68)) and overall survival (HR, 2.00 (1.11-3.61)) compared to those treated with chemotherapy alone. In contrast, the pro-angiogenic subgroup treated with bevacizumab had a trend toward improved PFS [95]. Winterhoff and colleagues examined another subgroup of the ICON7 trial and reported that the greatest benefit from bevacizumab appeared in patients with serous carcinomas with the mesenchymal subtype (median PFS increased 9.5 months (25.5 [95%CI 21.1, NA] vs. 16 [95%CI 10.5, NA] months, p = 0.053)) [96]. The results from these studies suggest that bevacizumab therapy may be directed based on molecular subtypes. However, further assessment in a phase III integral biomarker trial is needed to determine if tumor-derived molecular classifications can direct individualized treatment with bevacizumab.

These studies all suggest possible new directions for therapies in serous ovarian cancer and may ultimately redefine our concept of ovarian cancer subtypes in an integrated molecular manner. While integral and integrated molecular biomarkers are critical to our understanding of cancer and new therapeutic strategies, our discussion of the molecular determinants of adenocarcinomas of Mullerian origin will be based on the dualistic Type I and II ovarian cancer model, recognizing that this model represents a simplistic categorization. We will also focus primarily on molecular findings in epithelial ovarian cancer, as detailed molecular data for tubal and peritoneal carcinomas is unavailable (Table 2).

### High-grade serous ovarian, tubal, and peritoneal carcinoma
High-grade Mullerian cancers display predominantly serous histology, but also include some endometrial carcinomas, carcinosarcomas, and undifferentiated cancers. While less is known about the molecular profile of undifferentiated Mullerian tumors and carcinosarcomas, it appears that gene expression profiles and genetic alterations are very similar to those found in serous carcinomas [97,98]. These tumors exhibit a high level of genetic instability and are characterized by extensive chromosomal alterations and mutation of the tumor suppressor gene, TP53 [99,100]. Mutation of TP53 is an early event in the pathogenesis of HGSC and is found in STICs [20,101]. The presence of TP53 mutations is nearly ubiquitous (>95%) in HGSC, thus it is not a useful prognostic or predictive biomarker [100].

The Cancer Genome Atlas (TCGA) Project recently analyzed mRNA and microRNA expression, exome sequencing of entire coding regions, copy number alterations, and methylation of 489 HGSC [92]. The high degree of genomic instability in these cancers is notable with 30 regional chromosomal aberrations (8 recurrent gains and 22 losses), 63 focal areas of amplification, and 50 focal deletions. By comparison, there were few mutations in individual genes identified. TP53 was mutated in nearly all cases (>95%) and the next most commonly mutated genes were BRCA1 and BRCA2 (germline mutations present in 9% and 8% respectively, with somatic mutations in an additional 3% of cases). BRCA inactivation leads to defective repair of double stranded DNA breaks by homologous recombination. Although germline and somatic mutations of BRCA1 and

**Table 2 Subtypes of adenocarcinomas of Mullerian origin**

|  | High-grade serous | Low-grade serous | Mucinous | Clear cell | Endometrioid |
|---|---|---|---|---|---|
| **Precursor lesion** | Tubal intraepithelial carcinoma | Atypical serous borderline tumor | Metaplasia of transitional cells or metastasis from GI primary tumor* | Atypical Endometriosis | Atypical Endometriosis |
| **Histologic features** | Positive: p16, CK7, WT-1, PAX-8, ER, CA125, E-cadherin (in most cases), p53 | Positive: PAX8, ER, WT-1, | Positive: CK7, PAX-8 (40%), p53 (30%) | Positive: CK7, PAX-8, HNF-1β | Positive: CK7, ER, PR, PAX-8 |
|  | Negative: Her-2, calretinin, CK20 | Negative: p53 and p16 (negative, scattered or patchy) | Negative: WT-1, ER, PR and p16 | Negative: CK20, ER, WT-1, p53 and p16 (negative, weak, focal or patchy) | Negative: WT-1, p16, CK 20, p53 |
| **Molecular aberrations** | TP53 mutations | BRAF, KRAS, NRAS mutations | KRAS mutation | PTEN loss | PTEN loss |
|  | BRCA1/2 mutations |  | HER2 amplification | PIK3CA mutation | PIK3CA mutation |
|  | Chromosomal instability |  |  | ARID1A mutation | ARID1A mutation |
| **Risk factors** | Inherited BRCA1/2 mutation |  |  | Endometriosis | Endometriosis |
|  |  |  |  |  | Lynch syndrome |

*Origin of Mullerian mucinous tumors is not definitively known.

*BRCA2* account for <15% of cases, it was estimated that defects in homologous recombination genes, such as *EMSY, PTEN, RAD51C, ATM/ATR*, and Fanconi anemia genes, are present in 50% of all HGSC [92]. This may indicate that a large proportion of HGSC may be sensitive to treatments targeting DNA repair, such as PARP1 inhibitors.

Significant alterations have also been identified in the PI3K-AKT pathway. However, unlike type I cancers (such as clear cell or low-grade endometrioid cancers, which exhibit mutations in *PTEN* and *PIK3CA*), the pathway alterations in HGSCs are characterized by deletions (*PTEN*) and amplifications (*PIK3CA, KRAS,* and *AKT1/2*). Mutations in each individual gene account for <1% of the alterations. Similarly the retinoblastoma (Rb) signaling pathway is altered in 67% of cases with frequent down-regulation of *CDKN2A* (30%), deletion of *RB1* (8%), and amplification of *CCNE1* (20%), with few mutations found in these genes [92,102]. These data further support the finding that HGSC are characterized by generalized genomic instability rather than point mutations of driver genes.

Molecular signatures have been identified that are prognostic and/or predictive of response to therapy [103,104]. Whether or how these molecular signatures could guide clinical care is unclear. Confirmation of the initial results as well as biomarker-directed therapeutic trials are needed to determine if molecular signatures can be used to guide therapy in women with HGSC.

### Low-grade serous carcinoma

Unlike HGSC, LGSCs do not exhibit chromosomal instability and are not associated with *TP53* or *BRCA* mutations [105,106]. Instead, mutations in the MAP kinase pathway are common with mutations in *BRAF* (38%) and *KRAS* (19%) the most frequent [107-109] as well as NRAS mutations [35]. These mutations also appear to be mutually exclusive [35,107]. In addition to the MAPK pathway mutations, LGSCs are more likely to exhibit increased expression of ER/PR, E-cadherin, PAX2, and IGF-1 compared to HGSC [110]. LGSC typically responds poorly to cytotoxic chemotherapy with an average response rate of only 4% in women with recurrent disease [111]. Based on studies suggesting that mutations in MAPK pathway genes act as driver mutations, inhibitors of the MAPK pathway, and in particular MEK inhibitors, are of great interest. Indeed, this has led to the trial of MAPK inhibitors for the treatment of women with recurrent LGSC. In a phase II trial of selumetinib, a MEK1/2 inhibitor, 15% of patients had an objective response to therapy and 65% had stable disease [112]. Further trials are ongoing, but these results present the potential of targeted individualized therapy based on a molecular understanding of the disease.

### Mucinous carcinoma

Unlike HGSCs, in which *TP53* and *BRCA* mutations are most common, these mutations are relatively rare in mucinous tumors. Instead, the majority of mucinous tumors exhibit either *HER2* amplification or *KRAS* mutation [113]. The *KRAS* gene encodes the K-Ras protein, a key member of the RAS/RAF/MEK/ERK/MAP kinase signaling pathway that transduces various growth signals from the cell surface to the nucleus. *KRAS* mutations resulting in constitutive activation of the G protein are commonly found in codons 12, 13, and 61 and have been identified in a number of solid tumors [114]. *KRAS* mutations have been described in up to 68% of cases of mucinous ovarian cancer, while present in only 5% of non-mucinous tumors [113,115,116]. The large majority of mutations were identified in codon 12 (94%) [117]. *KRAS* mutations are thought to occur early in the development of these cancers as they are found in benign, low malignant potential, and borderline tumors of mucinous histology [117,118]. The high level of *KRAS* mutations in mucinous ovarian cancer may have treatment implications as targeted agents are being developed to target *KRAS* mutated tumors.

Overexpression/amplification of *HER2 (ERBB2)*, a member of the epidermal growth factor receptor family that acts upstream of *KRAS*, has been identified in up to 35% of mucinous ovarian cancer cases [113,119-121]. Ethnic differences may exist as *HER2* positivity was higher in Asian cohorts [119-121]. While no association was identified between *HER2* status and outcomes, responses of *HER2* amplified mucinous ovarian tumors to HER2 directed therapy have been reported [120-123].

### Clear cell carcinoma

Similar to the other type I Mullerian carcinomas, clear cell carcinomas are not associated with chromosomal instability or mutations in *TP53* or *BRCA*. Notably, clear cell carcinomas of Mullerian origin exhibit distinctive gene expression profiles from other Mullerian histologies, while sharing significant expression patterns with clear cell tumors of the kidney and endometrium [124,125]. Ovarian clear cell carcinomas show increased activation of angiogenic, hypoxic cell growth, and glucose metabolic pathways and demonstrate increased sensitivity to anti-angiogenic therapies [126]. Clinical trials using anti-angiogenic tyrosine kinase inhibitors are currently in progress.

Nearly 50% of clear cell ovarian carcinomas were found to harbor *ARID1A* mutations resulting in loss of its encoded protein, BAF250a, a subunit of the SWI-SNF chromatin remodeling complex [127]. Loss of BAF250a expression is thought to be an early event in the pathogenesis of clear cell tumors as endometriotic cyst epithelium in direct contact with the tumor also exhibited loss of expression while cyst epithelium remote to the tumor did not [128]. Studies have shown that ARID1A acts as a tumor suppressor and coordinates with p53 protein to regulate cellular growth [129]. However, inactivating mutations of ARID1A alone do not appear to be sufficient for tumor formation, but likely require additional genetic alterations resulting in activation of the PI3K-Akt pathway [130,131]. Activating mutations in PIK3CA are found in 33% of cases, PTEN loss in 12%, with alterations in PI3K-Akt pathway occurring in 62% [131,132]. Preclinical studies suggest that targeting the PI3K-Akt pathway inhibits clear cell carcinoma tumor growth in a mouse model and that loss of ARID1A further sensitizes cells to PI3K- and Akt-inhibition [133,134]. Clinical trials of agents targeting the PI3K-Akt pathway are ongoing (NCT02142803, NCT01196429).

### Endometrioid carcinoma

Similar to the dualistic pathway of pathogenesis of serous carcinomas, molecular profiling of high-grade endometrioid carcinomas are notable for mutations in TP53 with the absence of other molecular alterations, while low-grade endometrioid carcinomas were strongly associated with microsatellite instability (20%), CTNNB1 mutations (~50%), and KRAS mutations (up to 35%) [135-137]. High-grade endometrioid carcinomas were found to have a gene expression profile similar to HGSC [93]. Low-grade endometrioid carcinomas, however, are similar to clear cell adenocarcinomas in their association with endometriosis, expression of ARID1A mutations, and activation of the PI3K-Akt pathway. Ovarian endometrioid carcinomas are characterized by frequent somatic ARID1A inactivating mutations (30-55% of cases) [127,137,138]. Mutations typically are deletion or nonsense mutations which result in loss of protein expression [139]. ARID1A loss is associated with loss of PTEN and mutations in PIK3CA resulting in increased activation of the PI3K-Akt pathway [140]. It has been demonstrated in a genetically engineered mouse model that co-deletion of ARID1A and PTEN results in the formation of ovarian carcinoma with morphological and molecular features resembling human ovarian endometrioid carcinoma [130]. Activating mutations of PIK3CA are found in 20% of endometrioid carcinomas, while mutations in PTEN are present in 14-20%, and loss of heterozygosity of PTEN was present in 42% [136,137,141,142]. Loss of ARID1A has also been identified in endometrial hyperplasia with atypia, the precursor lesion of endometrioid carcinoma, and appears to be an early event in its pathogenesis [143]. However, despite the similarities between clear cell carcinomas and endometrioid carcinomas in ARID1A and PI3K-Akt pathway aberrations, protein array analysis showed differential expression between the two subtypes with endometrioid carcinomas expressing higher levels of steroid hormone receptors (ER and PR), and clear cell carcinomas expressing higher levels of Cyclin E, SMAD3, and e-cadherin [140]. Similarly, BRAF mutations were identified in 24% of endometrioid carcinomas, but were not identified in any case of clear cell carcinoma [107].

Other mutations frequently found in low-grade endometrioid carcinomas include mutations in CTNNB1 (the gene that encodes beta-catenin) and mutations in mismatch repair genes. Mutations in CTNNB1 are found in up to 50% of endometrioid ovarian tumors and are associated with improved outcomes [135-137]. Mutations typically result in over-expression of nuclear beta-catenin and increased transcription of down-stream target genes, such as the proto-oncogene MYC. These changes are present in a majority of borderline endometrioid ovarian tumors suggesting it is an early event in tumorigenesis [144]. Patients with Lynch syndrome are also at risk for developing EOC, most commonly the endometrioid subtype. Microsatellite instability has been detected in up to 20% of endometrioid tumors [136]. Similar to other Lynch-associated tumors, these tumors often exhibit abnormal mismatch repair protein expression with complete loss of MLH1, MSH2, MSH6, and/or PMS2 [145].

## Conclusions

Our review of the molecular, genetic, and histopathologic data supports the comprehensive inclusion of epithelial ovarian, tubal, and peritoneal cancers, as well as select CUP, as adenocarcinomas of Mullerian origin. While the dualistic Type I and II model of epithelial ovarian cancer suggests two main categories, it is unclear if this model can be extended to adenocarcinomas of Mullerian origin. However, it is clear that the different histologic subtypes within these categories are distinct with regard to clinical outcome, pathophysiologic, and molecular features which may have therapeutic implications. In light of the aforementioned advancements in genomics we propose a new nomenclature for this set of diseases. The terminology may include adenocarcinoma of Mullerian origin, followed by presumed primary site (ovary, fallopian tube, peritoneum), histologic subtype, and mutation status (if relevant). This type of nomenclature would appropriately capture the similarities among adenocarcinomas of Mullerian origin in both origin and histology, but recognize the unique molecular differences between them, all of which inform treatment decisions and prognosis. An example of such a classification could be "adenocarcinoma of Mullerian origin, fallopian tube primary, high-grade serous histology, BRCA1 mutation." Currently, the standard treatment of adenocarcinomas of Mullerian origin includes cytoreductive surgery and multi-agent platinum-based chemotherapy. The advances made in understanding the underlying molecular determinants of adenocarcinomas of Mullerian origin, as well as development of targeted therapeutics, will enable the implementation of genomic-driven treatment decisions in the future, elucidation of novel targets that can be used in preventive strategies, and better identification of precursor lesions that will yield improved survival outcomes.

## Competing interests
Dr. Secord reports grant support from Precision Therapeutics, Sanofi-Aventis, Genentech, Astellas Pharma Inc., Astex Pharmaceuticals Inc., Bristol-Myers Squibb (BMS), Incyte, Boerhinger Ingelheim, Tesaro, Eisai-Morphotek, Endocyte/Merck, Amgen, and Astra-Zeneca. She also discloses that she has served as a consultant for Precision Therapeutics, Genentech, GSK, and Boerhinger Ingelheim. All other authors report no competing interests.

## Authors' contributions
AAS, LPC, SG, YW, and IS all provided substantial contributions to conception and drafting of this review. AAS and LPC were primarily responsible for drafting sections regarding background, incidence, classification and origin; YW and IS were primarily responsible for drafting the section regarding pathological analysis; SG was primarily responsible for drafting the section regarding molecular determinants. All authors read and approved the final version of the manuscript.

## Acknowledgements
We'd like to thank Rex Bentley, MD in the Duke Department of Pathology for providing the additional pathologic images used in Figure 4.

## Author details
[1]Division of Gynecologic Oncology, Department of Obstetrics and Gynecology, Duke Cancer Institute, Duke University Medical Center, Durham, NC 27710, USA. [2]Division of Medical Oncology, Department of Internal Medicine, Duke University Medical Center, Durham, NC 27710, USA. [3]Department of Gynecology and Obstetrics, Johns Hopkins University School of Medicine, Baltimore, MD 21205, USA.

## References
1. Swerdlow M. Mesothelioma of the pelvic peritoneum resembling papillary cystadenocarcinoma of the ovary; case report. Am J Obstet Gynecol. 1959;77(1):197–200.
2. Prat J. Staging classification for cancer of the ovary, fallopian tube, and peritoneum. Int J Gynaecol Obstet. 2014;124(1):1–5. doi:10.1016/j.ijgo.2013.10.001.
3. Zeppernick F, Meinhold-Heerlein I. The new FIGO staging system for ovarian, fallopian tube, and primary peritoneal cancer. Arch Gynecol Obstet. 2014. doi:10.1007/s00404-014-3364-8.
4. Siegel R, Naishadham D, Jemal A. Cancer statistics, 2013. CA Cancer J Clin. 2013;63(1):11–30. doi:10.3322/caac.21166.
5. Ferlay J SI, Ervik M, Dikshit R, Eser S, Mathers C, Rebelo M, Parkin DM, Forman D, Bray, F., 2012 G. Cancer Incidence and Mortality Worldwide: IARC CancerBase No. 11 [Internet]. In: Lyon FIAfRoC, editor. Internet. Lyon, France2012.
6. Goodman MT, Shvetsov YB. Incidence of ovarian, peritoneal, and fallopian tube carcinomas in the United States, 1995–2004. Cancer Epidemiol Biomarkers Prev. 2009;18(1):132–9. doi:10.1158/1055-9965.epi-08-0771.
7. Pectasides D, Pectasides E, Economopoulos T. Fallopian tube carcinoma: a review. Oncologist. 2006;11(8):902–12. doi:10.1634/theoncologist.11-8-902.
8. Kalampokas E, Kalampokas T, Tourountous I. Primary fallopian tube carcinoma. Eur J Obstet Gynecol Reprod Biol. 2013;169(2):155–61. doi:10.1016/j.ejogrb.2013.03.023.
9. Pavlidis N, Pentheroudakis G. Cancer of unknown primary site. Lancet. 2012;379(9824):1428–35. doi:10.1016/s0140-6736(11)61178-1.
10. Kim KW, Krajewski KM, Jagannathan JP, Nishino M, Shinagare AB, Hornick JL, et al. Cancer of unknown primary sites: what radiologists need to know and what oncologists want to know. AJR Am J Roentgenol. 2013;200(3):484–92. doi:10.2214/ajr.12.9363.
11. Pentheroudakis G, Golfinopoulos V, Pavlidis N. Switching benchmarks in cancer of unknown primary: from autopsy to microarray. Eur J Cancer. 2007;43(14):2026–36. doi:10.1016/j.ejca.2007.06.023.
12. Fowler JM, Nieberg RK, Schooler TA, Berek JS. Peritoneal adenocarcinoma (serous) of Mullerian type: a subgroup of women presenting with peritoneal carcinomatosis. Int J Gynecol Cancer. 1994;4(1):43–51.
13. Koshiyama M, Matsumura N. Recent concepts of ovarian carcinogenesis: type I and type II. 2014;2014:934261. doi:10.1155/2014/934261.
14. Kurman RJ, Shih IM. The origin and pathogenesis of epithelial ovarian cancer: a proposed unifying theory. Am J Surg Pathol. 2010;34(3):433–43. doi:10.1097/PAS.0b013e3181cf3d79.
15. Prat J. New insights into ovarian cancer pathology. Ann Oncol. 2012;23 suppl 10:x111–x7. doi:10.1093/annonc/mds300.
16. Soslow RA. Histologic Subtypes of Ovarian Carcinoma: An Overview. Int J Gynecol Pathol. 2008;27(2):161–74. doi:10.1097/PGP.0b013e31815ea812.
17. Erickson BK, Conner MG, Landen Jr CN. The role of the fallopian tube in the origin of ovarian cancer. Am J Obstet Gynecol. 2013;209(5):409–14. doi:10.1016/j.ajog.2013.04.019.
18. Turner N, Tutt A, Ashworth A. Hallmarks of 'BRCAness' in sporadic cancers. Nat Rev Cancer. 2004;4(10):814–9. doi:10.1038/nrc1457.
19. Piek JM, Verheijen RH, Kenemans P, Massuger LF, Bulten H, van Diest PJ. BRCA1/2-related ovarian cancers are of tubal origin: a hypothesis. Gynecol Oncol. 2003;90(2):491.
20. Kuhn E, Kurman RJ, Vang R, Sehdev AS, Han G, Soslow R, et al. TP53 mutations in serous tubal intraepithelial carcinoma and concurrent pelvic high-grade serous carcinoma–evidence supporting the clonal relationship of the two lesions. J Pathol. 2012;226(3):421–6. doi:10.1002/path.3023.
21. Kindelberger DW, Lee Y, Miron A, Hirsch MS, Feltmate C, Medeiros F, et al. Intraepithelial carcinoma of the fimbria and pelvic serous carcinoma: Evidence for a causal relationship. Am J Surg Pathol. 2007;31(2):161–9. doi:10.1097/01.pas.0000213335.40358.47.
22. C Nay Fellay MF, Delaloye FF, Bauer J. Extraovarian Primary Peritoneal Carcinoma. Management of Rare Adult Tumours. Paris: Springer Publishing Company; 2010. p. 279–92.
23. Pentheroudakis G, Pavlidis N. Serous papillary peritoneal carcinoma: unknown primary tumour, ovarian cancer counterpart or a distinct entity? A systematic review. Crit Rev Oncol Hematol. 2010;75(1):27–42. doi:10.1016/j.critrevonc.2009.10.003.
24. Roh SY, Hong SH, Ko YH, Kim TH, Lee MA, Shim BY, et al. Clinical characteristics of primary peritoneal carcinoma. Cancer Res Treat. 2007;39(2):65–8. doi:10.4143/crt.2007.39.2.65.
25. Auersperg N, Wong AS, Choi KC, Kang SK, Leung PC. Ovarian surface epithelium: biology, endocrinology, and pathology. Endocr Rev. 2001;22(2):255–88. doi:10.1210/edrv.22.2.0422.
26. Lauchlan SC. The secondary Mullerian system. Obstet Gynecol Surv. 1972;27(3):133–46.
27. Li J, Fadare O, Xiang L, Kong B, Zheng W. Ovarian serous carcinoma: recent concepts on its origin and carcinogenesis. J Hematol Oncol. 2012;5:8. doi:10.1186/1756-8722-5-8.
28. Kobayashi H, Sumimoto K, Moniwa N, Imai M, Takakura K, Kuromaki T, et al. Risk of developing ovarian cancer among women with ovarian endometrioma: a cohort study in Shizuoka, Japan. Int J Gynecol Cancer. 2007;17(1):37–43. doi:10.1111/j.1525-1438.2006.00754.x.
29. Brinton LA, Gridley G, Persson I, Baron J, Bergqvist A. Cancer risk after a hospital discharge diagnosis of endometriosis. Am J Obstet Gynecol. 1997;176(3):572–9.
30. Brinton LA, Lamb EJ, Moghissi KS, Scoccia B, Althuis MD, Mabie JE, et al. Ovarian cancer risk associated with varying causes of infertility. Fertil Steril. 2004;82(2):405–14. doi:10.1016/j.fertnstert.2004.02.109.
31. Van Gorp T, Amant F, Neven P, Vergote I, Moerman P. Endometriosis and the development of malignant tumours of the pelvis. A review of literature. Best Pract Res Clin Obstet Gynaecol. 2004;18(2):349–71. doi:10.1016/j.bpobgyn.2003.03.001.
32. Lim D, Oliva E. Precursors and pathogenesis of ovarian carcinoma. Pathology. 2013;45(3):229–42. doi:10.1097/PAT.0b013e32835f2264.
33. Vang R, Shih Ie M, Kurman RJ. Ovarian low-grade and high-grade serous carcinoma: pathogenesis, clinicopathologic and molecular biologic features, and diagnostic problems. Adv Anat Pathol. 2009;16(5):267–82. doi:10.1097/PAP.0b013e3181b4fffa.
34. Alvarez AA, Moore WF, Robboy SJ, Bentley RC, Gumbs C, Futreal PA, et al. K-ras mutations in Mullerian inclusion cysts associated with serous borderline

tumors of the ovary. Gynecol Oncol. 2001;80(2):201–6. doi:10.1006/gyno.2000.6066.

35. Emmanuel C, Chiew YE, George J, Etemadmoghadam D, Sharma R, Russell P et al. Genomic classification of serous ovarian cancer with adjacent borderline differentiates RAS-pathway and TP53-mutant tumors and identifies NRAS as an oncogenic driver. Clin Cancer Res. 2014. doi:10.1158/1078-0432.ccr-14-1292.

36. Vang R, Shih Ie M, Kurman RJ. Fallopian tube precursors of ovarian low- and high-grade serous neoplasms. Histopathology. 2013;62(1):44–58. doi:10.1111/his.12046.

37. Li J, Abushahin N, Pang S, Xiang L, Chambers SK, Fadare O, et al. Tubal origin of 'ovarian' low-grade serous carcinoma. Mod Pathol. 2011;24(11):1488–99. doi:10.1038/modpathol.2011.106.

38. Piek JM, van Diest PJ, Zweemer RP, Jansen JW, Poort-Keesom RJ, Menko FH, et al. Dysplastic changes in prophylactically removed Fallopian tubes of women predisposed to developing ovarian cancer. J Pathol. 2001;195(4):451–6. doi:10.1002/path.1000.

39. Lee Y, Miron A, Drapkin R, Nucci MR, Medeiros F, Saleemuddin A, et al. A candidate precursor to serous carcinoma that originates in the distal fallopian tube. J Pathol. 2007;211(1):26–35. doi:10.1002/path.2091.

40. Przybycin CG, Kurman RJ, Ronnett BM, Shih Ie M, Vang R. Are all pelvic (nonuterine) serous carcinomas of tubal origin? Am J Surg Pathol. 2010;34(10):1407–16. doi:10.1097/PAS.0b013e3181ef7b16.

41. Dehari R, Kurman RJ, Logani S, Shih IM. The development of high-grade serous carcinoma from atypical proliferative (borderline) serous tumors and low-grade micropapillary serous carcinoma: a morphologic and molecular genetic analysis. Am J Surg Pathol. 2007;31(7):1007–12. doi:10.1097/PAS.0b013e31802cbbe9.

42. Pradeep S, Kim SW, Wu SY, Nishimura M, Chaluvally-Raghavan P, Miyake T, et al. Hematogenous metastasis of ovarian cancer: rethinking mode of spread. Cancer Cell. 2014;26(1):77–91. doi:10.1016/j.ccr.2014.05.002.

43. Bloss JD, Liao SY, Buller RE, Manetta A, Berman ML, McMeekin S, et al. Extraovarian peritoneal serous papillary carcinoma: a case–control retrospective comparison to papillary adenocarcinoma of the ovary. Gynecol Oncol. 1993;50(3):347–51. doi:10.1006/gyno.1993.1223.

44. Bloss JD, Brady MF, Liao SY, Rocereto T, Partridge EE, Clarke-Pearson DL. Extraovarian peritoneal serous papillary carcinoma: a phase II trial of cisplatin and cyclophosphamide with comparison to a cohort with papillary serous ovarian carcinoma—a Gynecologic Oncology Group Study. Gynecol Oncol. 2003;89(1):148–54. doi:http://dx.doi.org/10.1016/S0090-8258(03)00068-4.

45. Khalifeh I, Munkarah AR, Lonardo F, Malone JM, Morris R, Lawrence WD, et al. Expression of Cox-2, CD34, Bcl-2, and p53 and survival in patients with primary peritoneal serous carcinoma and primary ovarian serous carcinoma. Int J Gynecol Pathol. 2004;23(2):162–9.

46. Killackey MA, Davis AR. Papillary Serous Carcinoma of the Peritoneal Surface: Matched-Case Comparison with Papillary Serous Ovarian Carcinoma. Gynecol Oncol. 1993;51(2):171–4. doi:http://dx.doi.org/10.1006/gyno.1993.1267.

47. Barda G, Menczer J, Chetrit A, Lubin F, Beck D, Piura B, et al. Comparison between primary peritoneal and epithelial ovarian carcinoma: a population-based study. Am J Obstet Gynecol. 2004;190(4):1039–45. doi:10.1016/j.ajog.2003.09.073.

48. Ayhan A, Taskiran C, Yigit-Celik N, Bozdag G, Gultekin M, Usubutun A, et al. Long-term survival after paclitaxel plus platinum-based combination chemotherapy for extraovarian peritoneal serous papillary carcinoma: is it different from that for ovarian serous papillary cancer? Int J Gynecol Cancer. 2006;16(2):484–9. doi:10.1111/j.1525-1438.2006.00590.x.

49. Dubernard G, Morice P, Rey A, Camatte S, Fourchotte V, Thoury A, et al. Prognosis of stage III or IV primary peritoneal serous papillary carcinoma. Eur J Surg Oncol. 2004;30(9):976–81. doi:http://dx.doi.org/10.1016/j.ejso.2004.08.005.

50. Dalrymple JC, Bannatyne P, Russell P, Solomon HJ, Tattersall MHN, Atkinson K, et al. Extraovarian peritoneal serous papillary carcinoma. A clinicopathologic study of 31 cases. Cancer. 1989;64(1):110–5. doi:10.1002/1097-0142(19890701)64:1<110::AID-CNCR2820640120>3.0.CO;2-5.

51. Schorge JO, Miller YB, Qi L-J, Muto MG, Welch WR, Berkowitz RS, et al. Genetic Alterations of the WT1 Gene in Papillary Serous Carcinoma of the Peritoneum. Gynecol Oncol. 2000;76(3):369–72. doi:http://dx.doi.org/10.1006/gyno.1999.5711.

52. Halperin R, Zehavi S, Langer R, Hadas E, Bukovsky I, Schneider D. Primary peritoneal serous papillary carcinoma: a new epidemiologic trend? A matched-case comparison with ovarian serous papillary cancer. Int J Gynecol Cancer. 2001;11(5):403–8.

53. Eisenhauer EL, Sonoda Y, Levine DA, Abu-Rustum NR, Gemignani ML, Sabbatini PJ, et al. Platinum resistance and impaired survival in patients with advanced primary peritoneal carcinoma: matched-case comparison with patients with epithelial ovarian carcinoma. Am J Obstet Gynecol. 2008;198(2):213.e1–e7. doi:http://dx.doi.org/10.1016/j.ajog.2007.07.003.

54. Schnack TH, Sorensen RD, Nedergaard L, Hogdall C. Demographic clinical and prognostic characteristics of primary ovarian, peritoneal and tubal adenocarcinomas of serous histology–a prospective comparative study. Gynecol Oncol. 2014;135(2):278–84. doi:10.1016/j.ygyno.2014.08.020.

55. Dunn MS, Manahan KJ, Geisler JP. Primary carcinoma of the fallopian tube and epithelial ovarian carcinoma: A case–control analysis. J Reprod Med. 2008;53(9):691–4.

56. Moore KN, Moxley KM, Fader AN, Axtell AE, Rocconi RP, Abaid LN, et al. Serous fallopian tube carcinoma: A retrospective, multi-institutional case–control comparison to serous adenocarcinoma of the ovary. Gynecol Oncol. 2007;107(3):398–403. doi:http://dx.doi.org/10.1016/j.ygyno.2007.09.027.

57. Usach I, Blansit K, Chen LM, Ueda S, Brooks R, Kapp DS, et al. Survival differences in women with serous tubal, ovarian, peritoneal, and uterine carcinomas. Am J Obstet Gynecol. 2015;212(2):188.e1–6. doi:10.1016/j.ajog.2014.08.016.

58. Wethington SL, Herzog TJ, Seshan VE, Bansal N, Schiff PB, Burke WM, et al. Improved survival for fallopian tube cancer. Cancer. 2008;113(12):3298–306. doi:10.1002/cncr.23957.

59. Tanyi JL, Scholler N. Oncology biomarkers for gynecologic malignancies. Front Biosci. 2012;4:1097–110.

60. Levy T, Weiser R, Boaz M, Ben Shem E, Golan A, Menczer J. The significance of the pattern of serum CA125 level ascent to above the normal range in epithelial ovarian, primary peritoneal and tubal carcinoma patients. Gynecol Oncol. 2013;129(1):165–8. doi:http://dx.doi.org/10.1016/j.ygyno.2012.12.024.

61. Holcomb K, Vucetic Z, Miller MC, Knapp RC. Human epididymis protein 4 offers superior specificity in the differentiation of benign and malignant adnexal masses in premenopausal women. Am J Obstet Gynecol. 2011;205(4):358.e1–6. doi:10.1016/j.ajog.2011.05.017.

62. Nofech-Mozes S, Khalifa MA, Ismiil N, Saad RS, Hanna WM, Covens A, et al. Immunophenotyping of serous carcinoma of the female genital tract. Mod Pathol. 2008;21(9):1147–55.

63. Kobel M, Kalloger SE, Carrick J, Huntsman D, Asad H, Oliva E, et al. A limited panel of immunomarkers can reliably distinguish between clear cell and high-grade serous carcinoma of the ovary. Am J Surg Pathol. 2009;33(1):14–21. doi:10.1097/PAS.0b013e3181788546.

64. Laury AR, Hornick JL, Perets R, Krane JF, Corson J, Drapkin R, et al. PAX8 reliably distinguishes ovarian serous tumors from malignant mesothelioma. Am J Surg Pathol. 2010;34(5):627–35. doi:10.1097/PAS.0b013e3181da7687.

65. Cathro HP, Stoler MH. Expression of cytokeratins 7 and 20 in ovarian neoplasia. Am J Clin Pathol. 2002;117(6):944–51. doi:10.1309/2t1y-7bb7-dape-pq6l.

66. Wiseman W, Michael CW, Roh MH. Diagnostic utility of PAX8 and PAX2 immunohistochemistry in the identification of metastatic Mullerian carcinoma in effusions. Diagn Cytopathol. 2011;39(9):651–6. doi:10.1002/dc.21442.

67. Hou T, Liang D, He J, Chen X, Zhang Y. Primary peritoneal serous carcinoma: a clinicopathological and immunohistochemical study of six cases. Int J Clin Exp Pathol. 2012;5(8):762–9.

68. Liu Q, Lin JX, Shi QL, Wu B, Ma HH, Sun GQ. Primary peritoneal serous papillary carcinoma: a clinical and pathological study. Pathol Oncol Res. 2011;17(3):713–9. doi:10.1007/s12253-011-9375-x.

69. Attanoos RL, Webb R, Dojcinov SD, Gibbs AR. Value of mesothelial and epithelial antibodies in distinguishing diffuse peritoneal mesothelioma in females from serous papillary carcinoma of the ovary and peritoneum. Histopathology. 2002;40(3):237–44.

70. Schmeler KM, Sun CC, Malpica A, Deavers MT, Bodurka DC, Gershenson DM. Low-grade serous primary peritoneal carcinoma. Gynecol Oncol. 2011;121(3):482–6. doi:10.1016/j.ygyno.2011.02.017.

71. Seidman JD. Mucinous lesions of the fallopian tube. A report of seven cases. Am J Surg Pathol. 1994;18(12):1205–12.

72. Ozcan A, Shen SS, Hamilton C, Anjana K, Coffey D, Krishnan B, et al. PAX 8 expression in non-neoplastic tissues, primary tumors, and metastatic tumors: a comprehensive immunohistochemical study. Mod Pathol. 2011;24(6):751–64. doi:10.1038/modpathol.2011.3.

73. Kmet LM, Cook LS, Magliocco AM. A review of p53 expression and mutation in human benign, low malignant potential, and invasive epithelial ovarian tumors. Cancer. 2003;97(2):389–404. doi:10.1002/cncr.11064.

74. Kamal CK, Simionescu CE, Margaritescu C, Stepan A. P53 and Ki67 immunoexpression in mucinous malignant ovarian tumors. Rom J Morphol Embryol. 2012;53(3 Suppl):799–803.

75. Acs G, Pasha T, Zhang PJ. WT1 is differentially expressed in serous, endometrioid, clear cell, and mucinous carcinomas of the peritoneum, fallopian tube, ovary, and endometrium. Int J Gynecol Pathol. 2004;23(2):110–8.

76. Alvarado-Cabrero I, Young RH, Vamvakas EC, Scully RE. Carcinoma of the fallopian tube: a clinicopathological study of 105 cases with observations on staging and prognostic factors. Gynecol Oncol. 1999;72(3):367–79. doi:10.1006/gyno.1998.5267.

77. de la Torre FJ, Rojo F, Garcia A. Clear cells carcinoma of fallopian tubes associated with tubal endometriosis. Case report and review. Arch Gynecol Obstet. 2002;266(3):172–4.

78. Ryuko K, Iwanari O, Abu-Musa A, Fujiwaki R, Kitao M. Primary clear cell adenocarcinoma of the fallopian tube with brain metastasis: a case report. Asia-Oceania J Obstet Gynaecol. 1994;20(2):135–40.

79. Wuntakal R, Lawrence A. Are oestrogens and genetic predisposition etiologic factors in the development of clear cell carcinoma of the peritoneum? Med Hypotheses. 2013;80(2):167–71. doi:10.1016/j.mehy.2012.11.021.

80. Phillips V, Kelly P, McCluggage WG. Increased p16 expression in high-grade serous and undifferentiated carcinoma compared with other morphologic types of ovarian carcinoma. Int J Gynecol Pathol. 2009;28(2):179–86. doi:10.1097/PGP.0b013e318182c2d2.

81. DeLair D, Oliva E, Kobel M, Macias A, Gilks CB, Soslow RA. Morphologic spectrum of immunohistochemically characterized clear cell carcinoma of the ovary: a study of 155 cases. Am J Surg Pathol. 2011;35(1):36–44. doi:10.1097/PAS.0b013e3181ff400e.

82. Cameron RI, Ashe P, O'Rourke DM, Foster H, McCluggage WG. A panel of immunohistochemical stains assists in the distinction between ovarian and renal clear cell carcinoma. Int J Gynecol Pathol. 2003;22(3):272–6. doi:10.1097/01.pgp.0000071044.12278.43.

83. Irving JA, Catasus L, Gallardo A, Bussaglia E, Romero M, Matias-Guiu X, et al. Synchronous endometrioid carcinomas of the uterine corpus and ovary: alterations in the beta-catenin (CTNNB1) pathway are associated with independent primary tumors and favorable prognosis. Hum Pathol. 2005;36(6):605–19. doi:10.1016/j.humpath.2005.03.005.

84. Fujiwaki R, Takahashi K, Ryuko K, Watanabe Y, Nishiki Y, Kitao M. Primary endometrioid carcinoma of the fallopian tube. Acta Obstet Gynecol Scand. 1996;75(5):508–10.

85. Navani SS, Alvarado-Cabrero I, Young RH, Scully RE. Endometrioid carcinoma of the fallopian tube: a clinicopathologic analysis of 26 cases. Gynecol Oncol. 1996;63(3):371–8. doi:10.1006/gyno.1996.0338.

86. Rabczynski J, Ziolkowski P. Primary endometrioid carcinoma of fallopian tube. Clinicomorphologic study. Pathol Oncol Res. 1999;5(1):61–6.

87. Alvarado-Cabrero I, Navani SS, Young RH, Scully RE. Tumors of the fimbriated end of the fallopian tube: a clinicopathologic analysis of 20 cases, including nine carcinomas. Int J Gynecol Pathol. 1997;16(3):189–96.

88. Modesitt SC, Tortolero-Luna G, Robinson JB, Gershenson DM, Wolf JK. Ovarian and extraovarian endometriosis-associated cancer. Obstet Gynecol. 2002;100(4):788–95.

89. Heaps JM, Nieberg RK, Berek JS. Malignant neoplasms arising in endometriosis. Obstet Gynecol. 1990;75(6):1023–8.

90. Stern RC, Dash R, Bentley RC, Snyder MJ, Haney AF, Robboy SJ. Malignancy in endometriosis: frequency and comparison of ovarian and extraovarian types. Int J Gynecol Pathol. 2001;20(2):133–9.

91. Caduff RF, Svoboda-Newman SM, Bartos RE, Ferguson AW, Frank TS. Comparative analysis of histologic homologues of endometrial and ovarian carcinoma. Am J Surg Pathol. 1998;22(3):319–26.

92. Integrated genomic analyses of ovarian carcinoma. Nature. 2011;474(7353):609–15. doi:10.1038/nature10166.

93. Tothill RW, Tinker AV, George J, Brown R, Fox SB, Lade S, et al. Novel molecular subtypes of serous and endometrioid ovarian cancer linked to clinical outcome. Clin Cancer Res. 2008;14(16):5198–208. doi:10.1158/1078-0432.ccr-08-0196.

94. Yang D, Sun Y, Hu L, Zheng H, Ji P, Pecot Chad V, et al. Integrated Analyses Identify a Master MicroRNA Regulatory Network for the Mesenchymal Subtype in Serous Ovarian Cancer. Cancer Cell. 2013;23(2):186–99. doi:http://dx.doi.org/10.1016/j.ccr.2012.12.020.

95. Gourley C, McCavigan A, Perren T, Paul J, Michie CO, Churchman M, et al. Molecular subgroup of high-grade serous ovarian cancer (HGSOC) as a predictor of outcome following bevacizumab. J Clin Oncol. 2014;32(5s):(suppl; abstr 5502).

96. Boris JN, Winterhoff SK, Oberg AL, Wang C, Riska SM, Konecny GE, et al. Bevacizumab and improvement of progression-free survival (PFS) for patients with the mesenchymal molecular subtype of ovarian cancer. J Clin Oncol. 2014;32(5s):(suppl; abstr 5509).

97. Lisowska KM, Olbryt M, Dudaladava V, Pamula-Pilat J, Kujawa K, Grzybowska E, et al. Gene expression analysis in ovarian cancer - faults and hints from DNA microarray study. Front Oncol. 2014;4:6. doi:10.3389/fonc.2014.00006.

98. Schipf A, Mayr D, Kirchner T, Diebold J. Molecular genetic aberrations of ovarian and uterine carcinosarcomas–a CGH and FISH study. Virchows Arch. 2008;452(3):259–68. doi:10.1007/s00428-007-0557-6.

99. Gorringe KL, George J, Anglesio MS, Ramakrishna M, Etemadmoghadam D, Cowin P et al. Copy number analysis identifies novel interactions between genomic loci in ovarian cancer. PloS One. 2010;5(9). doi:10.1371/journal.pone.0011408.

100. Ahmed AA, Etemadmoghadam D, Temple J, Lynch AG, Riad M, Sharma R, et al. Driver mutations in TP53 are ubiquitous in high grade serous carcinoma of the ovary. J Pathol. 2010;221(1):49–56. doi:10.1002/path.2696.

101. Mehra K, Mehrad M, Ning G, Drapkin R, McKeon FD, Xian W, et al. STICS, SCOUTs and p53 signatures; a new language for pelvic serous carcinogenesis. Front Biosci. 2011;3:625–34.

102. Espinosa I, Catasus L, Canet B, D'Angelo E, Munoz J, Prat J. Gene expression analysis identifies two groups of ovarian high-grade serous carcinomas with different prognosis. Mod Pathol. 2011;24(6):846–54. doi:10.1038/modpathol.2011.12.

103. Spentzos D, Levine DA, Kolia S, Otu H, Boyd J, Libermann TA, et al. Unique gene expression profile based on pathologic response in epithelial ovarian cancer. J Clin Oncol. 2005;23(31):7911–8. doi:10.1200/JCO.2005.02.9363.

104. Berchuck A, Iversen ES, Lancaster JM, Pittman J, Luo J, Lee P, et al. Patterns of gene expression that characterize long-term survival in advanced stage serous ovarian cancers. Clin Cancer Res. 2005;11(10):3686–96. doi:10.1158/1078-0432.CCR-04-2398.

105. O'Neill CJ, Deavers MT, Malpica A, Foster H, McCluggage WG. An immunohistochemical comparison between low-grade and high-grade ovarian serous carcinomas: significantly higher expression of p53, MIB1, BCL2, HER-2/neu, and C-KIT in high-grade neoplasms. Am J Surg Pathol. 2005;29(8):1034–41.

106. Singer G, Stohr R, Cope L, Dehari R, Hartmann A, Cao DF, et al. Patterns of p53 mutations separate ovarian serous borderline tumors and low- and high-grade carcinomas and provide support for a new model of ovarian carcinogenesis: a mutational analysis with immunohistochemical correlation. Am J Surg Pathol. 2005;29(2):218–24.

107. Singer G, Oldt 3rd R, Cohen Y, Wang BG, Sidransky D, Kurman RJ, et al. Mutations in BRAF and KRAS characterize the development of low-grade ovarian serous carcinoma. J Natl Cancer Inst. 2003;95(6):484–6.

108. Jones S, Wang TL, Kurman RJ, Nakayama K, Velculescu VE, Vogelstein B, et al. Low-grade serous carcinomas of the ovary contain very few point mutations. J Pathol. 2012;226(3):413–20. doi:10.1002/path.3967.

109. Prat J. Ovarian carcinomas: five distinct diseases with different origins, genetic alterations, and clinicopathological features. Virchows Arch. 2012;460(3):237–49. doi:10.1007/s00428-012-1203-5.

110. Gershenson DM. The life and times of low-grade serous carcinoma of the ovary. Am Soc Clin Oncol Educ Book. 2013. doi:10.1200/EdBook_AM.2013.33.e195.

111. Gershenson DM, Sun CC, Bodurka D, Coleman RL, Lu KH, Sood AK, et al. Recurrent low-grade serous ovarian carcinoma is relatively chemoresistant. Gynecol Oncol. 2009;114(1):48–52. doi:10.1016/j.ygyno.2009.03.001.

112. Farley J, Brady WE, Vathipadiekal V, Lankes HA, Coleman R, Morgan MA, et al. Selumetinib in women with recurrent low-grade serous carcinoma of the ovary or peritoneum: an open-label, single-arm, phase 2 study. Lancet Oncol. 2013;14(2):134–40. doi:10.1016/s1470-2045(12)70572-7.

113. Anglesio MS, Kommoss S, Tolcher MC, Clarke B, Galletta L, Porter H, et al. Molecular characterization of mucinous ovarian tumours supports a stratified treatment approach with HER2 targeting in 19% of carcinomas. J Pathol. 2013;229(1):111–20. doi:10.1002/path.4088.

114. Bos JL. ras oncogenes in human cancer: a review. Cancer Res. 1989;49(17):4682–9.

115. Cuatrecasas M, Villanueva A, Matias-Guiu X, Prat J. K-ras mutations in mucinous ovarian tumors: a clinicopathologic and molecular study of 95 cases. Cancer. 1997;79(8):1581–6.

116. Gemignani ML, Schlaerth AC, Bogomolniy F, Barakat RR, Lin O, Soslow R, et al. Role of KRAS and BRAF gene mutations in mucinous ovarian carcinoma. Gynecol Oncol. 2003;90(2):378–81.

117. Nodin B, Zendehrokh N, Sundstrom M, Jirstrom K. Clinicopathological correlates and prognostic significance of KRAS mutation status in a pooled prospective cohort of epithelial ovarian cancer. Diagnostic Pathol. 2013;8:106. doi:10.1186/1746-1596-8-106.

118. Brown J, Frumovitz M. Mucinous tumors of the ovary: current thoughts on diagnosis and management. Curr Oncol Rep. 2014;16(6):389. doi:10.1007/s11912-014-0389-x.

119. Yan B, Choo SN, Mulyadi P, Srivastava S, Ong CW, Yong KJ, et al. Dual-colour HER2/chromosome 17 chromogenic in situ hybridisation enables accurate assessment of HER2 genomic status in ovarian tumours. J Clin Pathol. 2011;64(12):1097–101. doi:10.1136/jclinpath-2011-200082.

120. Chay WY, Chew SH, Ong WS, Busmanis I, Li X, Thung S, et al. HER2 amplification and clinicopathological characteristics in a large Asian cohort of rare mucinous ovarian cancer. PLoS One. 2013;8(4), e61565. doi:10.1371/journal.pone.0061565.

121. Huang RY, Chen GB, Matsumura N, Lai HC, Mori S, Li J, et al. Histotype-specific copy-number alterations in ovarian cancer. BMC Med Genom. 2012;5:47. doi:10.1186/1755-8794-5-47.

122. McAlpine JN, Wiegand KC, Vang R, Ronnett BM, Adamiak A, Kobel M, et al. HER2 overexpression and amplification is present in a subset of ovarian mucinous carcinomas and can be targeted with trastuzumab therapy. BMC Cancer. 2009;9:433. doi:10.1186/1471-2407-9-433.

123. Jain A, Ryan PD, Seiden MV. Metastatic mucinous ovarian cancer and treatment decisions based on histology and molecular markers rather than the primary location. J Natl Compr Canc Netw. 2012;10(9):1076–80.

124. Zorn KK, Bonome T, Gangi L, Chandramouli GV, Awtrey CS, Gardner GJ, et al. Gene expression profiles of serous, endometrioid, and clear cell subtypes of ovarian and endometrial cancer. Clin Cancer Res. 2005;11(18):6422–30. doi:10.1158/1078-0432.ccr-05-0508.

125. Schwartz DR, Kardia SL, Shedden KA, Kuick R, Michailidis G, Taylor JM, et al. Gene expression in ovarian cancer reflects both morphology and biological behavior, distinguishing clear cell from other poor-prognosis ovarian carcinomas. Cancer Res. 2002;62(16):4722–9.

126. Stany MP, Vathipadiekal V, Ozbun L, Stone RL, Mok SC, Xue H, et al. Identification of novel therapeutic targets in microdissected clear cell ovarian cancers. PLoS One. 2011;6(7), e21121. doi:10.1371/journal.pone.0021121.

127. Wiegand KC, Shah SP, Al-Agha OM, Zhao Y, Tse K, Zeng T, et al. ARID1A Mutations in Endometriosis-Associated Ovarian Carcinomas. N Engl J Med. 2010;363(16):1532–43. doi:doi:10.1056/NEJMoa1008433.

128. Ayhan A, Mao TL, Seckin T, Wu CH, Guan B, Ogawa H, et al. Loss of ARID1A expression is an early molecular event in tumor progression from ovarian endometriotic cyst to clear cell and endometrioid carcinoma. Int J Gynecol Cancer. 2012;22(8):1310–5. doi:10.1097/IGC.0b013e31826b5dcc.

129. Guan B, Wang TL, Shih IM. ARID1A, a factor that promotes formation of SWI/SNF-mediated chromatin remodeling, is a tumor suppressor in gynecologic cancers. Cancer Res. 2011;71(21):6718–27. doi:10.1158/0008-5472.can-11-1562.

130. Guan B, Rahmanto YS, Wu RC, Wang Y, Wang Z, Wang TL et al. Roles of deletion of Arid1a, a tumor suppressor, in mouse ovarian tumorigenesis. J Nat Cancer Inst. 2014;106(7). doi:10.1093/jnci/dju146.

131. Huang HN, Lin MC, Huang WC, Chiang YC, Kuo KT. Loss of ARID1A expression and its relationship with PI3K-Akt pathway alterations and ZNF217 amplification in ovarian clear cell carcinoma. Mod Pathol. 2014;27(7):983–90. doi:10.1038/modpathol.2013.216.

132. Kuo KT, Mao TL, Jones S, Veras E, Ayhan A, Wang TL, et al. Frequent activating mutations of PIK3CA in ovarian clear cell carcinoma. Am J Pathol. 2009;174(5):1597–601. doi:10.2353/ajpath.2009.081000.

133. Oishi T, Itamochi H, Kudoh A, Nonaka M, Kato M, Nishimura M, et al. The PI3K/mTOR dual inhibitor NVP-BEZ235 reduces the growth of ovarian clear cell carcinoma. Oncol Rep. 2014;32(2):553–8. doi:10.3892/or.2014.3268.

134. Samartzis EP, Gutsche K, Dedes KJ, Fink D, Stucki M, Imesch P. Loss of ARID1A expression sensitizes cancer cells to PI3K- and AKT-inhibition. Oncotarget. 2014;5(14):5295–303.

135. Sarrio D, Moreno-Bueno G, Sanchez-Estevez C, Banon-Rodriguez I, Hernandez-Cortes G, Hardisson D, et al. Expression of cadherins and catenins correlates with distinct histologic types of ovarian carcinomas. Hum Pathol. 2006;37(8):1042–9. doi:10.1016/j.humpath.2006.03.003.

136. Geyer JT, Lopez-Garcia MA, Sanchez-Estevez C, Sarrio D, Moreno-Bueno G, Franceschetti I, et al. Pathogenetic pathways in ovarian endometrioid adenocarcinoma: a molecular study of 29 cases. Am J Surg Pathol. 2009;33(8):1157–63. doi:10.1097/PAS.0b013e3181a902e1.

137. Gadducci A, Lanfredini N, Tana R. Novel insights on the malignant transformation of endometriosis into ovarian carcinoma. Gynecol Endocrinol. 2014;30(9):612–7. doi:10.3109/09513590.2014.926325.

138. Guan B, Mao TL, Panuganti PK, Kuhn E, Kurman RJ, Maeda D, et al. Mutation and loss of expression of ARID1A in uterine low-grade endometrioid carcinoma. Am J Surg Pathol. 2011;35(5):625–32. doi:10.1097/PAS.0b013e318212782a.

139. Wu RC, Wang TL, Shih IM. The emerging roles of ARID1A in tumor suppression. Canc Biol Ther. 2014;15(6):655–64. doi:10.4161/cbt.28411.

140. Wiegand KC, Hennessy BT, Leung S, Wang Y, Ju Z, McGahren M, et al. A functional proteogenomic analysis of endometrioid and clear cell carcinomas using reverse phase protein array and mutation analysis: protein expression is histotype-specific and loss of ARID1A/BAF250a is associated with AKT phosphorylation. BMC Cancer. 2014;14:120. doi:10.1186/1471-2407-14-120.

141. Sato N, Tsunoda H, Nishida M, Morishita Y, Takimoto Y, Kubo T, et al. Loss of heterozygosity on 10q23.3 and mutation of the tumor suppressor gene PTEN in benign endometrial cyst of the ovary: possible sequence progression from benign endometrial cyst to endometrioid carcinoma and clear cell carcinoma of the ovary. Cancer Res. 2000;60(24):7052–6.

142. Campbell IG, Russell SE, Choong DY, Montgomery KG, Ciavarella ML, Hooi CS, et al. Mutation of the PIK3CA gene in ovarian and breast cancer. Cancer Res. 2004;64(21):7678–81. doi:10.1158/0008-5472.can-04-2933.

143. Werner HM, Berg A, Wik E, Birkeland E, Krakstad C, Kusonmano K, et al. ARID1A loss is prevalent in endometrial hyperplasia with atypia and low-grade endometrioid carcinomas. Mod Pathol. 2013;26(3):428–34. doi:10.1038/modpathol.2012.174.

144. Oliva E, Sarrio D, Brachtel EF, Sanchez-Estevez C, Soslow RA, Moreno-Bueno G, et al. High frequency of beta-catenin mutations in borderline endometrioid tumours of the ovary. J Pathol. 2006;208(5):708–13. doi:10.1002/path.1923.

145. Aysal A, Karnezis A, Medhi I, Grenert JP, Zaloudek CJ, Rabban JT. Ovarian endometrioid adenocarcinoma: incidence and clinical significance of the morphologic and immunohistochemical markers of mismatch repair protein defects and tumor microsatellite instability. Am J Surg Pathol. 2012;36(2):163–72. doi:10.1097/PAS.0b013e31823bc434.

# 12

# Will bevacizumab biosimilars impact the value of systemic therapy in gynecologic cancers?

Bradley J. Monk[1], Warner K. Huh[2], Julie Ann Rosenberg[3] and Ira Jacobs[4*]

**Abstract**

**Objective:** Bevacizumab is an important component in the treatment of various cancers, and despite guidelines recommending its use in both ovarian and cervical cancer, patient access to bevacizumab and other angiogenesis inhibitors is limited. Biosimilars are large, structurally complex molecules that are intended to be highly similar to, and treat the same condition(s) as, an existing licensed or approved (reference) biologic, with no clinically meaningful differences in purity, potency and safety. This article summarizes the role of bevacizumab in the treatment paradigm of ovarian and cervical cancer. We also discuss the potential role of biosimilars to bevacizumab, which may offer more affordable options in the future treatment of gynecologic cancers.

**Methods:** Literature searches of PubMed and ClinicalTrials.gov databases were conducted. Regulatory and individual pharmaceutical company web pages were also reviewed. Search terms included "biosimilar" and "bevacizumab," and these were used to identify information regarding biosimilar development, reporting results of biosimilar studies or biosimilars in development.

**Results:** At present, four bevacizumab biosimilar candidates are undergoing comparative clinical assessment, with the potential to increase access and offer efficiencies across healthcare systems.

**Conclusions:** It is anticipated that biologics such as bevacizumab will continue to play a key role in the treatment of an array of gynecologic cancers. Biosimilars to bevacizumab are currently in development and have the potential to increase access to medicines in a variety of settings, including gynecologic cancers.

**Keywords:** Bevacizumab, Biosimilar, Ovarian cancer, Cervical cancer

## Introduction

Bevacizumab (Avastin®) is a recombinant humanized monoclonal immunoglobulin G1 antibody that binds to the human vascular endothelial growth factor and blocks its activity and angiogenesis [1]. Bevacizumab is the only complex biologic therapy indicated for the treatment of patients with cervical, epithelial ovarian and fallopian tube cancer in the United States (Table 1) and Europe. Bevacizumab is also approved for the treatment of patients with metastatic colorectal cancer, non-small-cell lung cancer (NSCLC) and metastatic renal cell cancer [1, 2]. Additionally, it is indicated for the treatment of

patients with glioblastoma in the United States [1] and for use in metastatic breast cancer in Europe [2].

It is expected that the use of bevacizumab in gynecologic cancers will increase, given the recent approval (in combination with carboplatin and gemcitabine) in platinum-sensitive ovarian cancer in the United States [3] and Canada [4]. However, patient access to bevacizumab and other angiogenesis inhibitors is limited [5]. This is due to several factors, including insurance coverage, drug availability, supply and manufacturing, and concerns regarding the cost-effectiveness of bevacizumab for some patients [5].

Biologics are large, structurally complex medicinal products. Their active ingredients are created by biological processes rather than chemical synthesis. Although biologics cannot be replicated, it is possible to

* Correspondence: ira.jacobs@pfizer.com
[4]Early Oncology Development and Clinical Research, Pfizer, 219 East 42nd Street, New York, NY 10017-5755, USA
Full list of author information is available at the end of the article

**Table 1** Bevacizumab: approved indications in the United States [1]

| Clinical indication | Combination regimen | Treatment setting |
| --- | --- | --- |
| Metastatic colorectal cancer | Intravenous 5-fluorouracil–based chemotherapy | First- or second-line treatment |
| Metastatic colorectal cancer | Fluoropyrimidine-irinotecan– or fluoropyrimidine-oxaliplatin–based chemotherapy | Second-line treatment in patients who have progressed on a first-line bevacizumab-containing regimen |
| Non-squamous non-small-cell lung cancer | Carboplatin and paclitaxel | First-line treatment of unresectable, locally advanced, recurrent or metastatic disease |
| Glioblastoma | Monotherapy | Adult patients with progressive disease following prior therapy[a] |
| Metastatic renal cell carcinoma | Interferon alfa | Adult patients |
| Cervical cancer | Paclitaxel and cisplatin or paclitaxel and topotecan | Persistent, recurrent or metastatic disease |
| Platinum-resistant recurrent epithelial ovarian, fallopian tube or primary peritoneal cancer | Paclitaxel, pegylated liposomal doxorubicin or topotecan | Adult patients |
| Platinum-sensitive recurrent epithelial ovarian, fallopian tube or primary peritoneal cancer[b] | Carboplatin and paclitaxel or carboplatin and gemcitabine chemotherapy (followed by bevacizumab) | Adult patients who have relapsed ≥6 months following last treatment with platinum-based chemotherapy |

[a]Effectiveness based on improvement in objective response rate. No data available demonstrating improvement in disease-related symptoms or survival with bevacizumab
[b]FDA approval granted on 6 Dec 2016 [3]

create a version (termed "biosimilar") that is highly similar to an already licensed or approved reference biologic in terms of purity, safety and efficacy [6, 7]. Biosimilars have the potential to increase patient access to biologic medicines, such as bevacizumab, and this may subsequently improve clinical outcomes.

This article reviews the role of bevacizumab in the treatment paradigm of ovarian and cervical cancer. We also discuss the potential role of biosimilars to bevacizumab, which may offer more affordable options in the future treatment of gynecologic cancers.

## Review

Literature searches of PubMed and ClinicalTrials.gov databases were conducted. Regulatory and individual pharmaceutical company web pages were also reviewed. Search terms included "biosimilar" and "bevacizumab," and these were used to identify information pertaining to biosimilar development, reporting results of biosimilar studies, or biosimilars in development.

### Bevacizumab in the treatment of gynecologic cancers: an overview

Bevacizumab, in combination with chemotherapy, is an important component of treatment of ovarian cancer. Approval of combination bevacizumab for the treatment of platinum-resistant recurrent epithelial ovarian or fallopian tube cancer was based on the results of an international, open-label, randomized study, AURELIA (Avastin Use in Platinum-Resistant Epithelial Ovarian Cancer), in patients with measurable ovarian cancer that had progressed <6 months following platinum-based

treatment [8]. Median progression-free survival (PFS) was 6.7 months with bevacizumab (10 mg/kg every 2 weeks or 15 mg/kg every 3 weeks) plus chemotherapy (weekly paclitaxel, pegylated liposomal doxorubicin or topotecan) vs 3.4 months with chemotherapy alone ($P < 0.001$). Objective response rate was 27.3% with bevacizumab plus chemotherapy vs 11.8% with chemotherapy alone ($P = 0.001$). No statistically significant difference in overall survival (OS) was observed between the two treatment regimens. Hypertension and proteinuria were common adverse events in patients treated with bevacizumab plus chemotherapy [8].

The United States Food and Drug Administration (FDA) recently granted approval of bevacizumab for the treatment of platinum-sensitive recurrent epithelial ovarian, fallopian tube or primary peritoneal cancer [3]. Approval was based on the results of two randomized Phase 3 studies. The Gynecologic Oncology Group (GOG) -0213 study showed that median OS was 42.6 months with bevacizumab plus chemotherapy vs 37.3 months with chemotherapy alone ($P = 0.056$). The GOG-0213 study also showed improvement in PFS with bevacizumab plus chemotherapy (13.8 months) compared with chemotherapy alone (10.4 months; $P < 0.0001$). In the OCEANS (Ovarian Cancer Study Comparing Efficacy and Safety of Chemotherapy and Anti-Angiogenic Therapy in Platinum-Sensitive Recurrent Disease) study, median PFS was 12.4 months with bevacizumab plus chemotherapy vs 8.4 months with chemotherapy plus placebo ($P < 0.0001$). However, no statistically significant difference in OS was observed between the two treatment groups. The adverse events associated with bevacizumab in the GOG-0213 and OCEANS studies were consistent with those observed in previous studies, and included fatigue, low white blood cell count with fever, low sodium, pain in extremity, low platelet count, elevated protein in the urine, high blood pressure and headache [3]. Bevacizumab, in combination with a chemotherapy backbone, is also a key component in the treatment of cervical cancer. Approval of combination bevacizumab for the treatment of persistent, recurrent or metastatic cervical cancer was granted on the results of an international Phase 2 randomized trial [9]. Results from this study showed that bevacizumab plus chemotherapy (cisplatin plus paclitaxel or topotecan) was associated with increased OS (17.0 months) compared with chemotherapy alone (13.3 months) (P = 0.004). Significantly higher response rates were observed with bevacizumab plus chemotherapy (48%) compared with chemotherapy alone (36%) (P = 0.008). In addition, bevacizumab plus chemotherapy was associated with a higher frequency of hypertension, thromboembolic events and gastrointestinal fistulas, compared with chemotherapy alone [9]. In summary, bevacizumab in combination with chemotherapy is the mainstay of treatment for a variety of gynecologic cancers.

## Challenges and barriers to the use of bevacizumab in clinical practice

A recent retrospective population-based study using the Surveillance, Epidemiology, and End Results (SEER)-Medicare database of 9491 women with epithelial ovarian cancer showed that, despite strong evidence of improved survival associated with therapy recommended by National Comprehensive Cancer Network (NCCN) guidelines, [10] over 70% of women receiving initial treatment for epithelial ovarian cancer did not receive treatment consistent with NCCN recommendations [11]. Ultimately, this may adversely affect patient care and is a serious global concern.

Despite the clinical success of bevacizumab in cancers with a large global incidence, such as lung and colorectal cancers, and clear guidelines recommending its use in both ovarian [10] and cervical cancer, [12] there is a notable lack of patient access to bevacizumab. Disparities in access to bevacizumab and other targeted therapies have been reported in Europe, with some countries reporting only occasional access to bevacizumab, or access for only 50% of patients with ovarian cancer [5]. Therefore, it is important to identify areas of inefficiencies and to understand barriers to patient access.

Several factors, including healthcare system infrastructure, stage at diagnosis, population health and lifestyle and availability of anticancer agents, can influence access to cancer therapy. Issues related to insurance coverage, treatment cost, drug availability, supply and manufacturing may create barriers to the use of bevacizumab in many countries worldwide. A survey conducted by the European

Society of Medical Oncology (ESMO) Consortium reported budget and affordability issues, and problems with the manufacture and supply of bevacizumab as the most common factors leading to suboptimal access to bevacizumab in a variety of cancers [5].

Clinical trials demonstrated bevacizumab improves PFS in patients with ovarian cancer [8] and OS in cervical cancer [9]. Although bevacizumab with chemotherapy is more effective with regard to PFS than chemotherapy alone, it is not a cost-effective, front-line treatment regimen in the overall population of patients with ovarian cancer (Table 2) [13]. Furthermore, approximately three-quarters of US oncologists do not consider bevacizumab a "good value" treatment option [14]. However, a recent analysis utilized results from the AURELIA study of bevacizumab plus chemotherapy versus chemotherapy alone in patients with platinum-resistant recurrent ovarian cancer [8]. This analysis concluded that bevacizumab was cost-effective in this setting [15]. Taken together, it is clear that further studies are needed to determine the cost-effectiveness of bevacizumab in the real-world setting.

Bevacizumab will continue to remain an important component in the treatment of gynecologic cancers as well as other settings. In light of the limited access to bevacizumab worldwide, additional treatment options for gynecologic cancers are eagerly awaited.

## Development of biosimilars and their potential benefits

Patents for bevacizumab will shortly expire in the United States and Europe [16]. Biosimilars are large, structurally complex molecules that are intended to be highly similar to, and treat the same condition(s) as, an existing licensed or approved (reference) biologic [6, 7]. Biosimilars may offer increased treatment options for patients and physicians and have the potential to optimize efficiencies across healthcare systems worldwide. Additionally, biosimilars may provide lower cost alternatives and therefore increase access to biologics and allow greater use of biologic therapies, which may facilitate improved clinical outcomes.

The aim of biosimilar development is not to re-establish efficacy and safety, but to demonstrate similarity to the reference biologic in terms of quality, safety and efficacy (Fig. 1) [6, 7]. The development of biosimilars involves biochemical, biophysical and functional comparative studies, and detailed characterization of the potential biosimilar. Together with comparative nonclinical, pharmacokinetic (PK), and comparative clinical trials, these data comprise the "totality of the evidence" [6].

Biosimilars must have an identical primary amino acid sequence and the same route of administration, strength and type of administration as the reference biologic [6, 7]. Biosimilars are manufactured through a process of reverse

**Table 2** Cost-effectiveness of bevacizumab in the front-line treatment of ovarian cancer [13]

| Citation | Treatment regimen | Total/Incremental costs (USD) | Effectiveness/Incremental effectiveness | ICER | Key findings |
|---|---|---|---|---|---|
| Cohn et al. 2011 | PAC + CAR | 2.5 million[a] | 10.3 months[b] | Referent | Addition of BEV and maintenance BEV was not cost-effective |
| | PAC + CAR + BEV | 21.4 million[a] | 11.2 months[b] | USD479,712 per PFLY gained | |
| | (PAC + CAR + BEV) + maintenance BEV | 78.3 million[a] | 14.1 months[b] | USD401,088 per PFLY gained | |
| Barnett et al. 2013 | PAC + CAR | 6220[c] | 2.80[d] | Referent | Use of BEV with standard first-line taxane was not cost-effective in stage III/IV ovarian cancer. May be suitable in high-risk patients although ICER exceeded thresholds |
| | PAC + CAR + BEV | 20,751[c] | 2.89[d] | USD168,610 per QALY | |
| | PAC + CAR + BEV for high-risk patients | 56,351[c] | 2.88[d] | Dominated | |
| Chan et al. 2014 | PAC + CAR | 535[e] | 10.5[b] | Referent | For high-risk, advanced ovarian cancer patients, ICER was almost USD170,000 per life-year saved |
| | PAC + CAR + BEV plus maintenance BEV | 3760 (3225 for maintenance)[e] | 15.9[b] | USD167,771 per LYG | |

*BEV* bevacizumab; *CAR* carboplatin; *ICER* incremental cost-effectiveness ratio; *LYG* life-year gained; *PAC* paclitaxel; *PFLY* progression-free life-year; *QALY* quality-adjusted life-year; *USD* United States dollars
[a]Total cost for 600 patients
[b]Median progression-free survival
[c]Mean cost
[d]QALY
[e]Total cost per cycle
Dominated: BEV was more costly and less effective

engineering and must undergo extensive comparative structural and functional characterization using state-of-the-art technology and highly specialized techniques to identify any differences between the proposed biosimilar and the reference biologic, particularly those that may alter the mechanism of action [17].

A series of analytical similarity assessments are conducted to confirm identical amino acid sequences, similar post-translational modifications and highly similar biologic activity between the proposed biosimilar and the reference biologic. Analytical similarity forms the foundation for similarity in safety and efficacy. In addition, a

comprehensive assessment of the structural and functional similarity of the potential biosimilar and the reference biologic is conducted using state-of-the-art techniques, physicochemical methods and functional assays [17].

Regulatory agencies do not typically require extensive nonclinical studies for the approval of biosimilars, although this is assessed on a case-by-case basis [6, 7]. A comparative clinical study is generally conducted in one therapeutic indication to demonstrate that there are no clinically meaningful differences in PK, pharmacodynamics (PD), efficacy or safety, including immunogenicity, between the potential biosimilar and the reference biologic. The goal of a

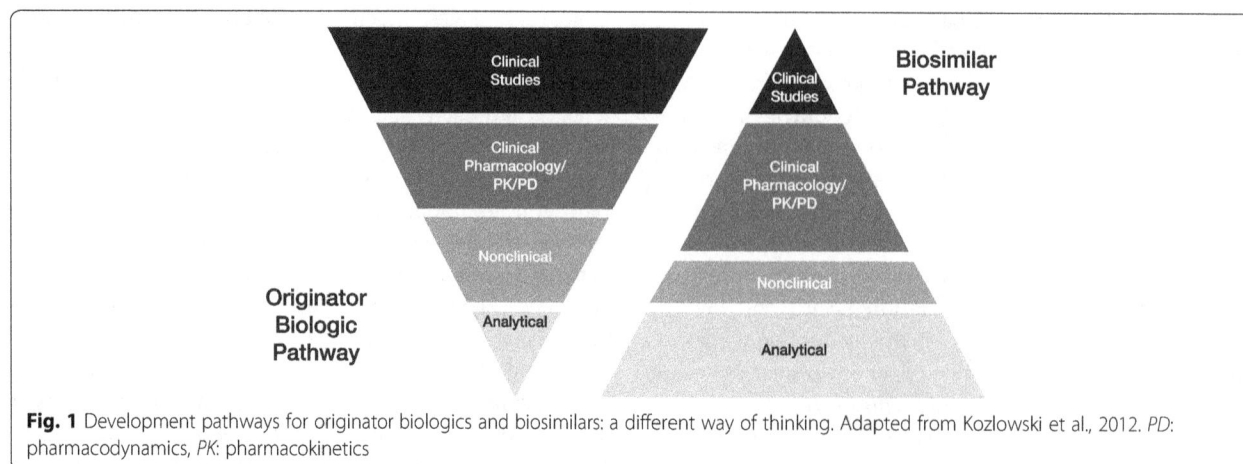

**Fig. 1** Development pathways for originator biologics and biosimilars: a different way of thinking. Adapted from Kozlowski et al., 2012. *PD*: pharmacodynamics, *PK*: pharmacokinetics

**Table 3** Bevacizumab biosimilars in late-stage clinical development

| Sponsor | Biosimilar candidate | Patient population | Study objectives | Key findings |
|---|---|---|---|---|
| Amgen | ABP 215 | NSCLC | Functional similarity and PK equivalence | •Similar functional characteristics<br>•Equivalent PK [26] |
| | | NSCLC | Clinical equivalence of objective response rate | •Clinical equivalence<br>•Similar safety and immunogenic profiles to bevacizumab [20] |
| Biocad | BCD-021 | NSCLC | PK and safety | •Similar PK and safety [21] |
| | | NSCLC | Overall response rate | •Similar efficacy, safety and immunogenicity [22] |
| Boehringer Ingelheim | BI 695502 | NSCLC | Efficacy and safety | •Recruiting (NCT02272413) |
| | | mCRC | Efficacy and safety | •Recruiting (NCT02776683) |
| Pfizer | PF-06439535 | NSCLC | Nonclinical evaluation | •Similar structure and in vitro biological activity [24]<br>•Similar in vivo toxicology [24] |
| | | NSCLC | PK and safety | •PK similarity [25]<br>•Comparable safety profile [25] |
| | | NSCLC | Comparative efficacy and safety | •Ongoing (NCT02364999) |

*NSCLC* non-small-cell lung cancer; *PK* pharmacokinetics

comparative clinical study is to address any residual uncertainty between the proposed biosimilar and the reference biologic [6, 7]. Because all biologics, including biosimilars, have the potential to trigger an immunogenic response, which may alter the PK, efficacy or safety properties, [18] the formation of antidrug antibodies is carefully monitored throughout development and during postmarketing surveillance.

### Biosimilars and the scientific basis of extrapolation across indications

Extrapolation is a scientific and regulatory principle that describes the approval of a biosimilar for use in an indication held by the reference biologic, which is not directly studied in a comparative clinical trial with a biosimilar. Extrapolation is key to the concept of biosimilarity and is based on establishing a similar mechanism of action for the biosimilar in various disease indications [6]. As well as reducing or eliminating the need for studies in multiple indications, extrapolation can potentially allow greater access to biosimilars, with minimal delays in treatment. The concept of extrapolation is supported by the US FDA and the European Medicines Agency (EMA) regulatory guidelines [6, 7]. However, the decision to extrapolate data from one indication to another is made on a case-by-case basis, with strong scientific justification and the totality of evidence.

The mechanism of action of bevacizumab involves the inhibition of vascular endothelial growth factor (VEGF), which has an important role in tumor angiogenesis and vascularization [1, 2]. Bevacizumab is an effective treatment for a number of tumors and its mechanism of action is independent of tumor site [1]. This forms the basis of the scientific rationale for extrapolation of similarity data across indications and may support the approval of bevacizumab biosimilars in indications held by the reference biologic without clinical studies in gynecologic indications.

### Bevacizumab biosimilar candidates in development

Four bevacizumab biosimilar candidates have completed preclinical assessments and, based on the totality of evidence, are currently undergoing comparative clinical assessments (Table 3). ABP 215 (Amgen) showed similar in vitro functional characteristics and equivalent human PK to bevacizumab [19] and demonstrated clinical equivalence and similar safety and immunogenic profiles as bevacizumab in patients with non-squamous NSCLC [20]. BCD-021 (Biocad) showed similar PK and safety to bevacizumab in patients with NSCLC [21]. BCD-021 also demonstrated similar efficacy, safety and immunogenicity to bevacizumab in patients with advanced non-squamous NSCLC [22]. A multicenter, randomized, double-blind clinical trial is ongoing to evaluate the efficacy and safety of BI 695502 (Boehringer Ingelheim) compared with bevacizumab (in combination with chemotherapy) in patients with advanced non-squamous NSCLC (ClinicalTrials.gov, NCT02272413). PF-06439535 (Pfizer) showed a similar structure and in vitro biological activity, and a similar in vivo toxicologic and toxicokinetic profile as bevacizumab [23, 24]. PF-06439535 also demonstrated PK similarity and comparable safety profiles to bevacizumab in healthy male volunteers [25]. A trial of PF-06439535 vs bevacizumab sourced in the EU in patients with advanced non-squamous NSCLC who have not received prior chemotherapy is ongoing.

### Conclusions

It is anticipated that biologics such as bevacizumab will continue to play a key role in the treatment of an array of gynecologic cancers. Limited access to bevacizumab and the lack of cost-effectiveness in some patients has driven the need to develop safe and effective biosimilars to bevacizumab, which have the potential to increase access to medicines and offer efficiencies across health-care systems.

## Abbreviations
AURELIA: Avastin Use in Platinum-Resistant Epithelial Ovarian Cancer; EMA: European Medicines Agency; ESMO: European Society of Medical Oncology; FDA: Food and Drug Administration; GOG: Gynecologic Oncology Group; NCCN: National Comprehensive Cancer Network; NSCLC: non-small-cell lung cancer; OCEANS: Ovarian Cancer Study Comparing Efficacy and Safety of Chemotherapy and Anti-Angiogenic Therapy in Platinum-Sensitive Recurrent Disease; OS: Overall survival; PFS: Progression-free survival; SEER: Surveillance, Epidemiology, and End Results; VEGF: Vascular endothelial growth factor.

## Acknowledgments
Medical writing support was provided by Neel Misra, MSc, of Engage Scientific Solutions and was funded by Pfizer.

## Funding
This report is supported by Pfizer Inc.

## Authors' contributions
All authors were involved in drafting the article or revising it critically for important intellectual content, and all authors approved the final version to be submitted for publication.

## Authors' information
Not applicable

## Competing interests
Dr Monk discloses that St. Joseph's Hospital institution has received research grants from Novartis, Amgen, Lilly, Genentech, Janssen/Johnson & Johnson, Array, TESARO and Morphotek. He has received honoraria for speaker bureaus from Roche/Genentech, AstraZeneca, Janssen/Johnson & Johnson, and Myriad. Additionally, Dr Monk has been a consultant for Roche/Genentech, Merck, TESARO, AstraZeneca, Gradalis, Advaxis, Cerulean, Amgen, Vemillion, ImmunoGen, Pfizer, Bayer, NuCana, Insys, GlaxoSmithKline, Verastem, Mateon (formerly OxiGENE), PPD and Clovis. Dr Warner K. Huh declared no conflicts of interest. Dr Julie Ann Rosenberg and Dr Ira Jacobs are full-time employees of Pfizer Inc.

## Author details
[1]Arizona Oncology (US Oncology Network), University of Arizona College of Medicine, Creighton University School of Medicine at St. Joseph's Hospital, Phoenix, AZ, USA. [2]University of Alabama at Birmingham, Birmingham, AL, USA. [3]Pfizer, Groton, CT, USA. [4]Early Oncology Development and Clinical Research, Pfizer, 219 East 42nd Street, New York, NY 10017-5755, USA.

## References
1. Genentech Inc. Avastin (bevacizumab) injection prescribing information. 2004. http://www.gene.com/download/pdf/avastin_prescribing.pdf. Accessed 18 Oct 2016.
2. European Medicines Agency. Summary of product characteristics: Avastin (bevacizumab) 25 mg/ml concentrate for solution for infusion. http://www. ema.europa.eu/docs/en_GB/document_library/EPAR_-_Product_ Information/human/000582/WC500029271.pdf. Accessed 18 Oct 2016.
3. Wire B. FDA approves Genentech's Avastin® (Bevacizumab) plus chemotherapy for a specific type of advanced ovarian cancer. 2016. http:// www.businesswire.com/news/home/20161206006296/en/FDA-Approves-Genentech%E2%80%99s-Avastin%C2%AE-Bevacizumab-Chemotherapy-Specific. Accessed 17 Jan 2016.
4. Hoffmann-La Roche Limited. Avastin (bevacizumab) 100 mg and 400 mg vials (25 mg/mL solution for injection) Product monograph. 2016. http:// www.rochecanada.com/content/dam/roche_canada/en_CA/documents/ Research/ClinicalTrialsForms/Products/ConsumerInformation/Monograph sandPublicAdvisories/Avastin/Avastin_PM_E.pdf. Accessed 17 Jan 2016.
5. Cherny N, Sullivan R, Torode J, Saar M, Eniu A. ESMO European Consortium Study on the availability, out-of-pocket costs and accessibility of antineoplastic medicines in Europe. Ann Oncol. 2016;27:1423–43.
6. US Food and Drug Administration. Scientific considerations in demonstrating biosimilarity to a reference product: guidance for industry. 2015. http://www.fda.gov/downloads/DrugsGuidanceComplianceRegulatory Information/Guidances/UCM291128.pdf. Accessed 18 Oct 2016.
7. European Medicines Agency. Guideline on similar biological medicinal products containing biotechnology-derived proteins as active substance: non-clinical and clinical issues. 2015. http://www.ema.europa.eu/docs/en_ GB/document_library/Scientific_guideline/2015/01/WC500180219.pdf. Accessed 25 Aug 2015.
8. Pujade-Lauraine E, Hilpert F, Weber B, Reuss A, Poveda A, Kristensen G, et al. Bevacizumab combined with chemotherapy for platinum-resistant recurrent ovarian cancer: The AURELIA open-label randomized phase III trial. J Clin Oncol. 2014;32:1302–8.
9. Tewari KS, Sill MW, Long 3rd HJ, Penson RT, Huang H, Ramondetta LM, et al. Improved survival with bevacizumab in advanced cervical cancer. N Engl J Med. 2014;370:734–43.
10. National Comprehensive Cancer Network. NCCN clinical practice guidelines in oncology: ovarian cancer. 2016. https://www.nccn.org/professionals/ physician_gls/pdf/ovarian.pdf. Accessed 18 Oct 2016.
11. Urban RR, He H, Alfonso-Cristancho R, Hardesty MM, Goff BA. The cost of initial care for Medicare patients with advanced ovarian cancer. J Natl Compr Canc Netw. 2016;14:429–37.
12. National Comprehensive Cancer Network. NCCN clinical practice guidelines in oncology: cervical cancer. 2016. https://www.nccn.org/professionals/ physician_gls/pdf/cervical.pdf. Accessed 18 Oct 2016.
13. Poonawalla IB, Parikh RC, Du XL, VonVille HM, Lairson DR. Cost effectiveness of chemotherapeutic agents and targeted biologics in ovarian cancer: a systematic review. Pharmacoeconomics. 2015;33:1155–85.
14. Nadler E, Eckert B, Neumann PJ. Do oncologists believe new cancer drugs offer good value? Oncologist. 2006;11:90–5.
15. Chappell NP, Miller C, Barnett J, Fielden A. Is FDA approved bevacizumab cost-effective in the setting of platinum-resistant recurrent ovarian cancer? Obstet Gynecol. 2016;127:6–7.
16. Genetic Engineering & Biotechnology News. Biosimilars: 11 Drugs to watch. 2014. http://www.genengnews.com/insight-and-intelligence/biosimilars-11-drugs-to-watch/77900135. Accessed 14 Mar 2017.
17. Bui LA, Hurst S, Finch GL, Ingram B, Jacobs IA, Kirchhoff CF, et al. Key considerations in the preclinical development of biosimilars. Drug Discov Today. 2015;20(Suppl 1):3–15.
18. Bendtzen K. Anti-TNF-alpha biotherapies: perspectives for evidence-based personalized medicine. Immunotherapy. 2012;4:1169–79.
19. Born TL, Huynh Q, Mathur A, Velayudhan J, Canon J, Reynhardt K, et al. Functional similarity assessment results comparing bevacizumab to biosimilar candidate ABP 215. Ann Oncol. 2014;25(Suppl 4):v163.
20. Thatcher N, Thomas M, Paz-Ares Rodriguez L, Ostoros G, Pan J, Goldschmidt JH, et al. Randomized, double-blind, phase 3 study evaluating efficacy and safety of ABP 215 compared with bevacizumab in patients with non squamous non-small-cell lung cancer. Paper presented at: 2016 Annual Meeting of the American Society of Clinical Oncology (ASCO); June 3–7, 2016; Chicago, IL, USA.
21. Orlov S, Burdaeva O, Nechaeva MP, Kopp MV, Kotiv BN, Sheveleva LP, et al. Pharmacokinetics and safety of BCD-021, bevacizumab biosimilar candidate, compared to Avastin in patients. J Thorac Oncol. 2014;32(Suppl):e13500.
22. Filon O, Orlov S, Burdaeva O, Kopp MV, Kotiv BN, Alekseev S, et al. Efficacy and safety of BCD-021, bevacizumab biosimilar candidate, compared to Avastin: Results of international multicenter randomized double blind phase

Will bevacizumab biosimilars impact the value of systemic therapy in gynecologic...

103

III study in patients with advanced non-squamous NSCLC. J Clin Oncol. 2015; 33(Suppl):8057.

23. Rule K, Peraza M, Shiue M, Finch G, Thibault S, Rosenberg JA, et al. Nonclinical development of PF 06439535, a potential biosimilar to bevacizumab. J Thorac Oncol. 2015;10:S485.

24. Peraza M, Shiue M, Phenix S. Comparative nonclinical assessment of the potential biosimilar PF-06439535 and bevacizumab. Paper presented at: 54th Annual Meeting and ToxExpo of Society of Toxicology (SOT); March 22–26, 2015; San Diego, CA, USA.

25. Knight B, Rassam D, Liao S, Ewesuedo R. A phase I pharmacokinetics study comparing PF-06439535 (a potential biosimilar) with bevacizumab in healthy male volunteers. Cancer Chemother Pharmacol. 2016;77:839–46.

26. Markus R, Born T, Chow V, Zhang N, Huynh Q, Maher G. Functional similarity and human pharmacokinetic (PK) equivalence of ABP 215 and bevacizumab. J Clin Oncol. 2015;33:15.

# 13

# A long-term surviving patient with recurrent low-grade serous ovarian carcinoma treated with the MEK1/2 inhibitor, selumetinib

Munetaka Takekuma[1], Kwong K. Wong[2] and Robert L. Coleman[2*]

## Abstract

**Background:** Selumetinib is a potent, selective, orally available, and non-ATP competitive small molecule inhibitor of mitogen-activated protein kinase kinase 1/2 (MEK1/2) that has demonstrated single agent activity in a number of solid tumor including recurrent low-grade serous ovarian carcinoma (LGSOC). However, the long-term prognosis of patients who receive selumetinib, as well as the late toxicity of the agent, have not yet been described.

**Case Presentation:** In this case report, we present a patient with recurrent LGSOC with KRAS mutation whose tumor has not progressed and who has maintained a good general condition without severe toxicities following treatment with selumetinib for more than 7 years. Next generation sequencing of her tumor revealed a G12V mutation in KRAS. MAPK signaling inhibition plays a role in the biology of LGSOC.

**Conclusions:** Although biomarkers have yet to definitively define patients with LGSOC who are likely to respond to therapy, exploration of specific alterations should be pursued in an excersie to develop a reliable companion diagnostic test.

**Keywords:** Low-grade serous ovarian cancer, MEK inhibitor, Selumetinib, *KRAS* mutation

## Background

Serous carcinoma is the most common histological type of ovarian cancer accounting for 70–80 % of all new diagnoses. Evaluation of the molecular biology of high-grade serous ovarian cancer (HGSOC) describes a disease associated with frequent P53 alterations, including hemizygous loss, mutation, or amplification. The natural history of HGSOC has been well documented and despite significant improvements in surgical and adjuvant treatment options, the number of patients cured has altered very little over the last two decades. International Federation of Gynecology and Obstetrics (FIGO) grading (grades 1, 2, and 3) has also been a well-documented prognostic factor for many of its histological subtypes. However, investigation in the early 1990's suggested that

low-grade serous ovarian cancer (LGSOC) could be most reliably identified through a bivariate classification (low and high). Further, patients with LGSOC appeared to have a much different natural history. [1] For instance, several studies have documented that LGSOC is not as sensitive to cytotoxic chemotherapy relative to its HGSOC counterpart but it is associated with much longer expected overall survival [2, 3]. In addition, molecular and genomic studies have shown that LGSOC appears to have a higher frequency of functional estrogen (ER) and progesterone receptor (PR) expression, *KRAS* or *BRAF* mutations, a higher frequency of expression of active mitogen-activated protein kinase (MAPK), and a lower frequency of *TP53* mutations than does HGSOC [4–7].

Selumetinib is a potent, selective, orally available, and non-ATP competitive small molecule inhibitor of mitogen-activated protein kinase kinase 1/2 (MEK1/2) that has demonstrated single agent activity (objective responses) in a number of solid tumor including recurrent

* Correspondence: rcoleman@mdanderson.org
[2]Department of Gynecologic Oncology & Reproductive Medicine, University of Texas, M.D. Anderson Cancer Center, 1155 Herman Pressler Dr., CPB6.3590, Houston, TX 77030, USA
Full list of author information is available at the end of the article

LGSOC [8, 9]. Herein, we present the clinical experience of a woman with chemo- and hormonally-refractory recurrent LGSOC associated with a *KRAS* mutation whose tumor has continually responded to selumetinib for more than 7 years.

## Case presentation

A 40-year-old woman with bilateral ovarian masses was found at laparotomy to have a suspected ovarian malignancy in October 1997. Surgical extirpation included supracervical hysterectomy, bilateral salpingo-oophorectomy, appendectomy, and staging biopsies. The pathology was confirmed as a low-grade papillary serous carcinoma of the ovary arising from a tumor of low malignant potential in both ovaries with microscopic metastatic implants in the omentum and peritoneal surfaces. She was staged as FIGO Stage IIIA and was treated with post-operative intravenous paclitaxel (175 mg/m$^2$) and carboplatin (AUC 5, PC) for six cycles.

She did well until October 2005, when the patient's serum cancer antigen 125 (CA125) level was found to be increased and imaging studies showed recurrent peritoneal tumor. Biopsy confirmed recurrent LGSOC and she underwent a secondary cytoreduction. Final pathology also revealed ER and PR expression. Unfortunately, the distribution of her recurrent disease precluded complete surgical resection, leaving measurable disease in the small bowel mesentery. She was treated adjuvantly with nine cycles of PC achieving stable disease as her best response. Due to neuropathy, fatigue and marrow exhaustion she was not able to undergo further PC treatment. She was then treated with letrozole, an aromatase inhibitor, at a dose of 2.5 mg daily for 19 months. In May 2008, the patient's imaging studies showed unequivocal progression of a left upper quadrant lesion, and the letrozole was discontinued.

In consideration of additional therapeutic options and clinical trials, we performed a mutational analysis of the recurrent tumor by next generation sequencing (NGS) [10]. This revealed a *KRAS* mutation (Fig. 1). Fortunately, GOG-239, a phase II clinical trial of selumetinib in patients with LGSOC became available at this time, to which she enrolled in June 2008. Selumetinib was administered orally at a dose of 50 mg twice daily. A computerized tomography (CT) scan was performed in February 2009, and no new implants, ascites, masses or adenopathy were seen in the abdomen or pelvis. The impression was that there were stable implants. An implant close to the hepatic flexure of the colon had a measurement of 1.8 cm (Fig. 2a). Subsequent CT imaging scan done in June 2009 showed sufficient change in her measurable disease, including the previous hepatic flexure implant (0.9 cm, Fig. 2b) to register a partial

response. She has continued on this therapy nearly uninterrupted since. Most of her multiple recurrent lesions, which were frequently associated with calcific deposits have lost their soft tissue component and/or cystic nature. Concern for lack of active disease, she has subsequently undergone several PET-CT images reveal FDG-avid implants. In addition, tumor growth was observed following two treatment breaks required for care of other medical issues unrelated to disease or therapy. Remarkably, reinitiation of selumetinib resulted in tumor implant size reduction and for one lesion, resolution.

Our patient has experienced mild adverse events over the many years of therapy. Most notable were intermittent rashes (maximum grade 2) at anatomically disparate areas, such as the trunk, chest, and eyelids, each of which were treated conservatively with antibiotic ointments and topical antihistamines. She has also experienced grade 1 stomatits, intermittently. Of most notable effect, she experienced de-pigmentation of her hair (now blonde) and a birthmark on her right arm (no longer visible). During the duration of her treatment the formulation of selumetinib administered was changed from a daily sachet ("mix and drink", 100 mg BID) to tablets (50 mg BID). Initially, this patient's adverse events did increase in frequency and intensity during the transition, although they did not require discontinuation of the therapy and further administration was not compromised. Continuous monitoring for MEK-related cardiovascular, ophthalmological and metabolic dysfunctions are ongoing.

## Discussion

We present an unusual patient with recurrent LGSOC with a *KRAS* mutation (G12V) whose tumor has not progressed and who has maintained a good general condition without severe toxicities by means of treatment with selumetinib, a MEK inhibitor, for more than 7 years. We believe she is the longest continuously treated patient with MEK-therapy under any indication.

As mentioned, this patient continues to participate in GOG-239, a phase II trial of selumetinib in women with recurrent, measurable LGSOC. Farley et al. recently reported the results from this trial, and demonstrated an overall response rate was 15 %, median progression-free survival was 11 months (interquartile range [IQR] 3.6–15.9) [9], and the median follow-up time in patients who survived was 21 months (IQR 17–30). At the time of the publication (reflecting information gathered until database lock), nine patients (17 %) had been on therapy for more than 15 months.

LGSOCs typically have an indolent course with recurrences developing over many years, but eventually these tumors develop intra-abdominal carcinomatosis, which proves to be fatal, and LGSOC has been recognized as

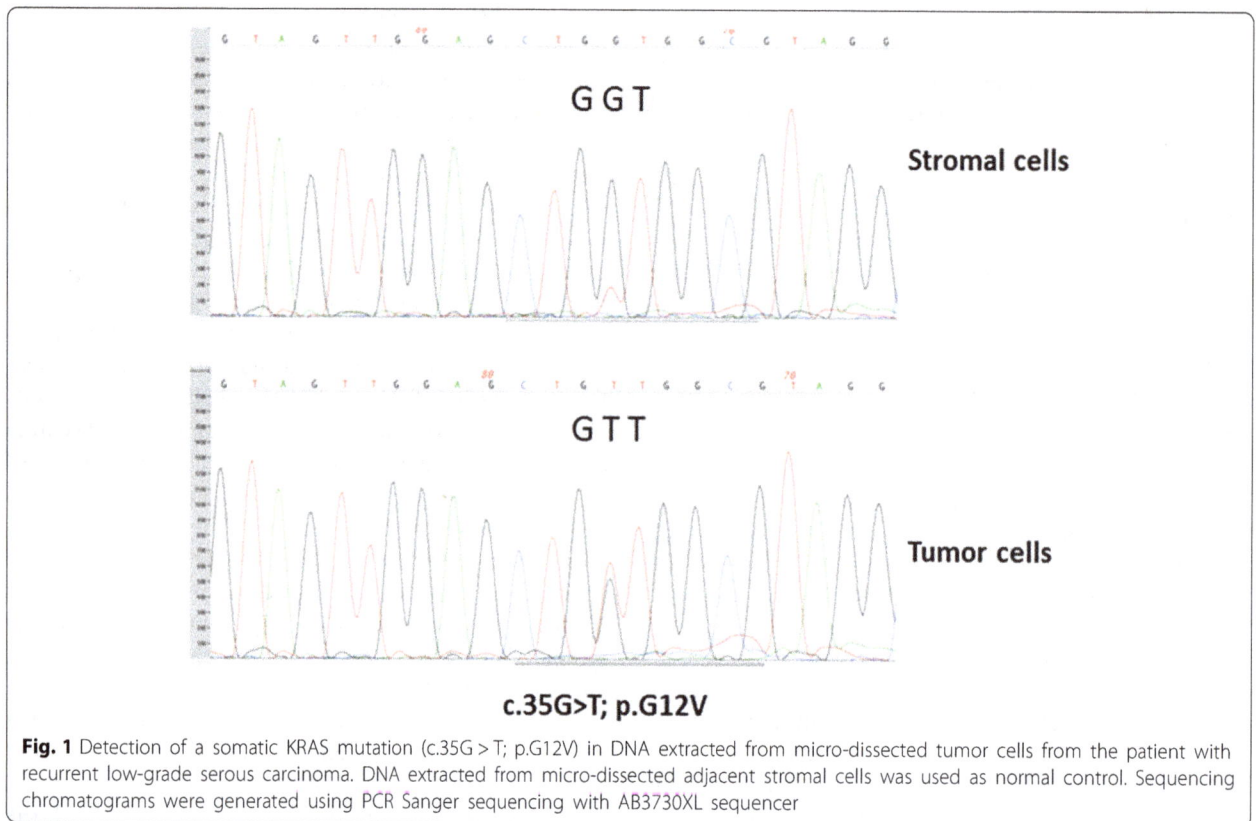

**Fig. 1** Detection of a somatic KRAS mutation (c.35G > T; p.G12V) in DNA extracted from micro-dissected tumor cells from the patient with recurrent low-grade serous carcinoma. DNA extracted from micro-dissected adjacent stromal cells was used as normal control. Sequencing chromatograms were generated using PCR Sanger sequencing with AB3730XL sequencer

more chemoresistant than HGSOC [2, 3]. In 2008, Schmeler et al. reported their experience with 25 patients with LGSOC treated with neoadjuvant chemotherapy for inoperable disease at diagnosis; all patients were treated with a platinum-based regimen, and only one (4 %) experienced a complete response, while none had a partial response, 21 had stable disease, and two (8 %) had progressive disease [2]. In 2009, Gershenson et al. published an analysis of 58 patients with recurrent LGSOC in which the overall response rate was 3.7 %; dividing the regimens by platinum-status, the response rate was 4.9 % in platinum-sensitive tumors and 2.1 % in platinum-resistant tumors, but that difference did not reach statistical significance ($p = 0.63$) [3]. Since the response rate of LGSOC to conventional treatment is extremely poor, investigation into new therapeutic approach is urgently needed.

The clinical efficacy of hormonal therapy for LGSOC is modest. A 2012 report from the M.D. Anderson Cancer Center documented an overall response rate and stable disease rate of 9 and 62 %, respectively [11]. There was a statistically significant relationship

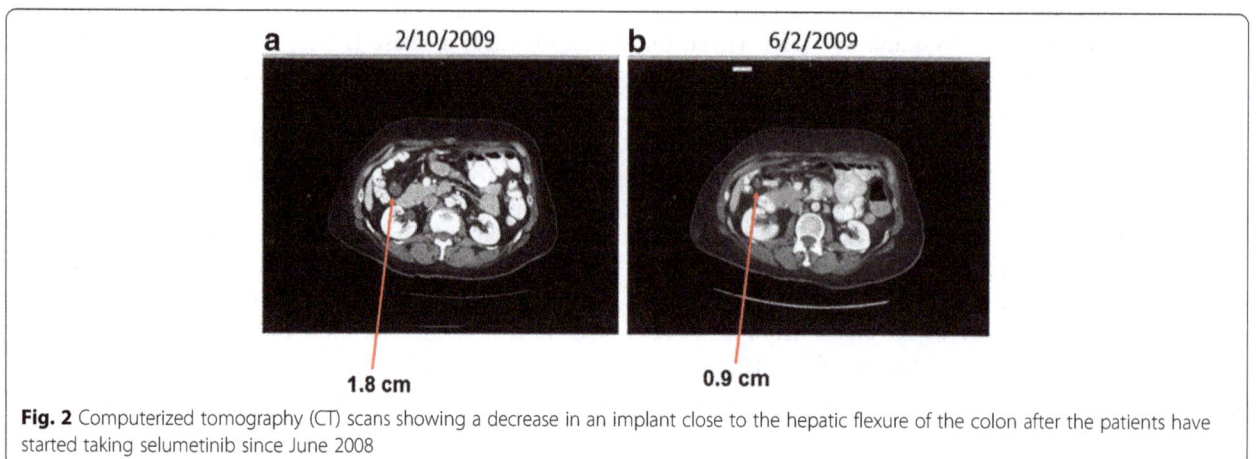

**Fig. 2** Computerized tomography (CT) scans showing a decrease in an implant close to the hepatic flexure of the colon after the patients have started taking selumetinib since June 2008

**Table 1** Low 185 passage whole genome sequencing

| Gene | Amino acid change | Tumor DNA | | | Blood DNA | | | Functional impact |
|------|-------------------|-----------|---|---|-----------|---|---|---------|
| | | Mutant allele reads | Wild-type allele reads | Frequency of mutant allele | Mutant allele reads | Wild-type allele reads | Frequency of mutant allele | |
| CCDC110 | P209Q | 7 | 9 | 44 | 0 | 8 | 0 | Neutral |
| FAT1 | Q2933P | 6 | 6 | 50 | 0 | 6 | 0 | Neutral |
| PCDHGA1 | A443T | 7 | 6 | 54 | 0 | 5 | 0 | Neutral |
| USP45 | K67E | 6 | 6 | 50 | 0 | 5 | 0 | Medium |
| RP1L1 | Q1861P | 5 | 7 | 42 | 0 | 9 | 0 | Neutral |
| PLBD1 | L25delL | 7 | 7 | 50 | 0 | 9 | 0 | Neutral |
| KRAS | G12V | 8 | 11 | 42 | 0 | 9 | 0 | Medium |
| KRT84 | I206V | 11 | 4 | 73 | 0 | 3 | 0 | Neutral |
| ADAMTS17 | N1094S | 6 | 7 | 46 | 0 | 8 | 0 | Neutral |
| ADAM33 | M764T | 7 | 9 | 44 | 0 | 4 | 0 | Low |

between response and platinum-status in terms of both overall response rate (ORR, 13.5 % vs 2.7 %) and time to progression (TPP, 8.9 vs 5.7 months, $P = 0.003$).

The mitogen-activated protein kinase (MAPK), also known as extracellular signal-regulated protein kinase (ERK), is a downstream target of RAS, RAF, and MAP/ERK kinase and is crucial for transduction of growth signals from several key growth factors, cytokines, and proto-oncogenes [12]. Mutations or overexpression of components, including *KRAS* and *BRAF*, in the MAPK pathway leads to constitutive activation of MAPK by phosphorylation. Activation of MAPK in turn activates downstream protein kinases, nuclear proteins, and transcription factors [13], which may contribute to the development of various tumors [14].

MEK is an attractive therapeutic target, as it lies downstream of multiple activators of the pathway. As such, selumetinib would be considered to have its greatest effects on tumors harboring *RAS* or *BRAF* activating mutations. While activating *RAS* mutations have been documented as a frequent event in serous borderline tumors and LGSOC, [14–16] there has been poor correlation between response to selumetinib and *RAS* or *BRAF* mutation. Of interest, G12D and G12V are the two most common *KRAS* mutations. However, their downstream signaling is not completely the same. G12D variant signals primarily through PI3K, JNK, p38, and FAK signaling pathways [17, 18] but signals less through the RAF/ERK pathway. Furthermore, G12D causes constitutive PI3K/mTOR activity [18]. One the other hand, the G12V variant signals predominantly through MAPK signaling cascade but has lost the ability to bind to and signal through PI3K [18]. Thus, we speculate that tumor cells with G12V mutation will be more sensitive to MEK inhibitor while those with G12D will require inhibitors targeting both MEK and PI3K pathways. Alternatively, additional mutation(s) in the tumor cells may contribute

to the sensitivity to selumetinib. Using low passage (10X) whole genome sequencing, we have identified 9 additional potential somatic missense mutations (Table 1). Most of the amino acid changes have no predictive functional impact on the protein function except *USP45* gene. USP45 encodes an ubiquitin-specific protease, which may modulate the MAPK pathway [19]. Thus, further investigation is warranted. In addition, despite intensive studies, the genetic and molecular basis for resistance to selumetinib remains poorly understood. Grasso et al. reported that p70 S6 kinase and its downstream target ribosomal protein S6 may be biomarkers of resistance to selumetinib in colorectal cancer [20].

## Conclusions

Treatment of LGSOC continues to evolve as new targets emerge with functional consequence. Our case report and others point to MAPK signaling as one pathway with therapeutic viability. Currently, two prospective, randomized phase III clinical trials of single agent MEK inhibitors (binimetinib and trametinib, both versus physician's choice chemotherapy or hormones) are being conducted in women with LGSOC (NCT01849874, NCT02101788). Both trials require central pathology review to confirm the diagnosis and allow MEK inhibitor cross-over on progression of control therapy. Although recruitment to the former, using binimetinib, was recently halted due to an unfavorable planned futility assessment, a comprehensive review of the final results from these trials will be important to determine the role MEK inhibitors in this rare disease.

## Patient consent

Written informed consent was obtained from the patient for publication of this Case Report and any accompanying images. A copy of the written consent is available for review by the Editor-in-Chief of this journal.

## Competing interests

RLC has received clinical trial research grants from AstraZeneca. KKW and MT declare no competing interests.

## Authors' contributions

All authors contributed to the design, data acquisition, data analysis and interpretation and manuscript preparation (writing and assembly). All authors read and approved the final manuscript.

## Author details

[1]The Division of Gynecology, Shizuoka Cancer Center, Shizuoka 411-8777, Japan. [2]Department of Gynecologic Oncology & Reproductive Medicine, University of Texas, M.D. Anderson Cancer Center, 1155 Herman Pressler Dr., CPB6.3590, Houston, TX 77030, USA.

## References

1. Shvartsman HS, Sun CC, Bodurka DC, Mahajan V, Crispens M, Lu KH, et al. Comparison of the clinical behavior of newly diagnosed stages II-IV low-grade serous 213 carcinoma of the ovary with that of serous ovarian tumors of low malignant potential that recur as low-grade serous carcinoma. Gynecol Oncol. 2007;105:625–29.
2. Schmeler KM, Sun CC, Bodurka DC, Deavers MT, Malpica A, Coleman RL, et al. Neoadjuvant chemotherapy for low-grade serous carcinoma of the ovary or peritoneum. Gynecol Oncol. 2008;108:510–4.
3. Gershenson DM, Sun CC, Bodurka D, Coleman RL, Lu KH, Sood AK, et al. Recurrent low-grade serous ovarian carcinoma is relatively chemoresistant. Gynecol Oncol. 2009;114:48–52.
4. Singer G, Oldt III R, Cohen Y, Wang BG, Sidransky D, Kurman RJ, et al. Mutations in BRAF and KRAS characterize the development of low-grade ovarian serous carcinoma. J Natl Cancer Inst. 2003;95:484–6.
5. Singer G, Kurman RJ, Chang HW, Cho S, Shih IM. Diverse tumorigenic pathways in ovarian serous carcinoma. Am J Pathol. 2002;160:1223–8.
6. Hsu CY, Bristow R, Cha M, Wang B, Ho CL, Kurman RJ, et al. Characterization of active mitogen-activated protein kinase in ovarian serous carcinomas. Clin Cancer Res. 2004;10:6432–6.
7. Singer G, Stohr R, Cope L, Dehari R, Hartmann A, Cao DF, et al. Patterns of p53 mutations separate ovarian serous borderline tumors and low- and high-grade carcinomas and provide support for a new model of ovarian carcinogenesis: a mutational analysis with immunohistochemical correlation. Am J Surg Pathol. 2005;29:218–24.
8. Della Pepa C, Tonini G, Santini D, Losito S, Pisano C, Di Napoli M, et al. Low grade serous ovarian carcinoma: from the molecular characterization to the best therapeutic strategy. Cancer Treatment Rev. 2015;41:136–43.
9. Farley J, Brady WE, Vathipadiekal V, Lankes HA, Coleman R, Morgan MA, et al. Selumetinib in women with recurrent low-grade serous carcinoma of the ovary or peritoneum: an open-label, single-arm, phase 2 study. Lancet Oncol. 2013;14:134–40.
10. Wong KK, Tsang YT, Deavers MT, Mok SC, Zu Z, Sun C, Malpica A, Wolf JK, Lu KH, Gershenson DM. BRAF mutation is rare in advanced-stage low-grade ovarian serous carcinomas. Am J Pathol. 2010;177(4):1611–7.
11. Gershenson DM, Sun CC, Lyer RB, Malpica AL, Kavanagh JJ, Bodurka DC, et al. Hormonal therapy for recurrent low-grade serous carcinoma of the ovary or peritoneum. Gynecol Oncol. 2012;125:661–66.
12. Olson JM, Hallahan AR. p38 MAP kinase: a convergence point in cancer therapy. Trends Mol Med. 2004;10:125–9.
13. Peyssonnaux C, Eychene A. The Raf/MEK/ERK pathway: new concepts of activation. Biol Cell. 2001;93:53–62.
14. Allen LF, Sebolt-Leopold J, Meyer MB. CI-1040 (PD184352), a targeted signal transduction inhibitor of MEK (MAPKK). Semin Oncol. 2003;30(5 Suppl 16):105–16.
15. Cuatrecasas M, Erill N, Musulen E, et al. K-ras mutations in nonmucinous ovarian epithelial tumors: a molecular analysis and clinicopathological study of 144 patients. Cancer. 1998;82:1088–95.
16. Cuatrecasas M, Villanueva A, Matias-Guiu X, Prat J. K-ras mutations in mucinous ovarian tumors. Cancer. 1997;79:1581–6.
17. Cespedes MV, Sancho FJ, Guerrero S, et al. K-ras Asp12 mutant neither interacts with Raf, nor signals through Erk and is less tumorigenic than K-ras Val12. Carcinogenesis. 2006;27(11):2190–200.
18. Ihle NT, Byers LA, Kim ES, et al. Effect of KRAS oncogene substitutions on protein behavior: implications for signaling and clinical outcome. J Natl Cancer Inst. 2012;104(3):228–39.
19. Yamashita M, Shinnakasu R, Asou H, Kimura M, Hasegawa A, Hashimoto K, Hatano N, Ogata M, Nakayama T. Ras-ERK MAPK cascade regulates GATA3 stability and Th2 differentiation through ubiquitin-proteasome pathway. J Biol Chem. 2005;280(33):29409–19.
20. Grasso S, Tristante E, Saceda M, Carbonell P, Mayor-Lopez L, Carballo-Santana M, et al. Resistance to selumetinib (AZD6244) in colorectal cancer cell lines is mediated by p70S6K and RPS6 activation. Neoplasia. 2014;16:845–60.

# 14

# Breaking down the evidence for bevacizumab in advanced cervical cancer: past, present and future

Victor Rodriguez-Freixinos and Helen J. Mackay[*]

## Abstract

Despite the introduction of screening and, latterly, vaccination programs in the developed world, globally cervical cancer remains a significant health problem. For those diagnosed with advanced or recurrent disease even within resource rich communities, prognosis remains poor with an overall survival (OS) of just over 12 months. New therapeutic interventions are urgently required. Advances in our understanding of the mechanisms underlying tumor growth and the downstream effects of human papilloma virus (HPV) infection identified angiogenesis as a rational target for therapeutic intervention in cervical cancer. Anti-angiogenic agents showed promising activity in early phase clinical trials culminating in a randomized phase III study of the humanized monoclonal antibody to vascular endothelial growth factor (VEGF), bevacizumab, in combination with chemotherapy. This pivotal study, the Gynecologic Oncology Group protocol 240, met its primary endpoint demonstrating a significant improvement in OS. Bevacizumab became the first targeted agent to be granted regulatory approval by the United States Food and Drug Administration for use alongside chemotherapy in adults with persistent, recurrent or metastatic carcinoma of the cervix. This review outlines the rationale for targeting angiogenesis in cervical cancer focusing on the current indications for the use of bevacizumab in this disease and future directions.

**Keywords:** Angiogenesis, Bevacizumab, Recurrent and metastatic cervical cancer, Target therapy, Human papilloma virus

## Introduction

Following the introduction of population based screening, the incidence of cervical cancer has been declining in the developed world a trend that is expected to continue with the increased availability and implementation of HPV vaccination programs. Globally, however, cervical cancer remains a major health issue and is the third most common cancer affecting women with 85 % of the diagnoses and 88 % of deaths due to this disease occurring in resource poor regions of the world [1]. Even within the United States (US), despite the availability of screening programs, in 2015 over 12,000 women will be diagnosed with cervical cancer with approximately 4000 women expected to die from their disease. Furthermore, between 2000 and 2012 the proportion of women diagnosed with stage IV cervical cancer in the US rose [2]. Advanced cervical cancer disproportionately affects women from lower socio-economic groups, those who are under or uninsured, women of African American or Hispanic ethnicity and those from medically underserved communities [3].

Early-stage cervical cancer is a potentially curable disease either by surgery (for those diagnosed with International Federation of Gynecology and Obstetrics (FIGO) stage IA/B1 disease) or by a combination of low dose chemotherapy administered concurrently with radiotherapy followed by intracavitary brachytherapy. For those not suitable for local control, who recur or who are diagnosed with metastatic disease outcomes are poor with 5-year survival rates between 5 and 15 % [4]. In this setting any treatment is palliative and the goals of care are to prolong survival but also, and perhaps more importantly, to maintain and/or improve quality of life (QoL). A number of first line, cisplatin based, doublet, combination

* Correspondence: Helen.Mackay@uhn.ca
Division of Medical Oncology and Hematology, Princess Margaret Hospital, University of Toronto, 610 University Avenue, Toronto, Ontario M5G 2 M9, Canada

chemotherapy regimens have been investigated in prospective randomized clinical trials conducted by the Gynecologic Oncology Group (GOG). These culminated in GOG 204, a four-arm study that compared cisplatin in combination with paclitaxel, vinorelbine, gemcitabine or topotecan [5]. Outcomes were similar in all arms with a non-significant trend in favor of cisplatin/paclitaxel (overall survival (OS) 12.9 months) compared to the other three arms (OS 10–10.3 months) and similar overall response rates (ORR). In a further randomized phase III clinical trial conducted by the Japanese GOG (JGOG) carboplatin in combination with paclitaxel was found to be non-inferior to cisplatin/paclitaxel [6]. For women with poor prognostic features including poor performance status, prior treatment with chemoradiation or recurrence within 1 year, response duration can be short at less than 6 months in some cases. Response to treatment is also influenced by the site of recurrence with disease control in previously irradiated areas proving particularly challenging [7]. There are no standard of care second line options for these women when their cancer progresses. New therapeutic approaches are, therefore, urgently required. However, the cervical cancer patient demographic also poses unique challenges in terms of sustainable drug development where cost effectiveness and access to new treatments for those in need are key issues. Furthermore, conducting clinical trials in this patient group can also pose difficulties as women diagnosed with advanced cervical cancer frequently come from sections of society where, historically, engagement in clinical research has been low.

Targeting angiogenesis is one of the most promising therapeutic strategies to emerge in recent years in the treatment of cervical cancer. Angiogenesis is a critical process in cervical carcinogenesis and tumor progression. Following the publication in 2014 of the randomized phase III study GOG 240, the US Food and Drug Administration (FDA) approved the first anti-angiogenic agent, bevacizumab (Avastin, Genentech/Roche), in combination with chemotherapy for use in women with advanced cervical cancer [8]. This article will review the rationale for studying anti-angiogenic therapy in cervical cancer, focus on the clinical use of bevacizumab and finally highlight potential future directions.

## Review
### Angiogenesis in cervical cancer and rationale for targeting
*Angiogenesis*

Angiogenesis is a physiologic and highly ordered process that involves the regulation of multiple signaling pathways and requiring interaction between different cell types, including endothelial cells, stromal cells (fibroblasts), and their interaction with the extracellular matrix, cytokines and growth factors, which leads to the effective formation of new blood vessels. Hypoxia and the mechanisms that mediate hypoxic response are key drivers of physiologic angiogenesis. Under hypoxic conditions expression of hypoxia inducible factor, (HIF- 1$\alpha$) is induced in endothelial cells, resulting in VEGF-A, and vascular endothelial growth factor receptor 2 (VEGFR-2) expression [9]. Although numerous proangiogenic factors have been described there is universal agreement that the VEGF family of ligands, (VEGF-A, to -D and placental growth factor [PLGF]) and their associated receptor tyrosine kinases (VEGFR)-1, 2 and 3 are the most important regulators of angiogenesis. VEGF-A, usually referred to as VEGF, binds to VEGFR-1 and VEGFR-2; the stimulation of endothelial cell mitogenesis and vascular permeability is mediated by its interaction with VEGFR-2 [10]. PLGF and VEGF-B selectively bind to VEGFR-1 and stimulate vessel growth and maturation and recruit proangiogenic bone marrow-derived progenitors [11, 12]. VEGF-C and VEGF-D primarily interact with VEGFR-3 stimulating lymphangiogenesis [13]. Other crucial steps in physiologic angiogenesis involve the recruitment of pericytes. Pericytes, recruited primarily by platelet-derived growth factor (PDGF), secreted by endothelial cells, are essential for the stabilization, maturation and support of new vessels [14]. Angiopoietins (Angs) 1 and 2 are expressed on the surface of pericytes and are ligands of the endothelial cell receptor Tie-2. Thus, the angiopoietin/Tie pathway is involved in the stability of mature vessels and proliferation of endothelial cells. However, the contribution of Ang-1 and Ang-2 to the angiogenesis process is distinct. Ang-1 functions as a Tie2 receptor agonist when it binds to TIE-2 receptors expressed on the surface of endothelial cells, maintaining the integrity of existing vessels. In contrast, Ang-2 is mainly secreted by endothelial cells at sites of active vascular remodeling. Ang-2 acts antagonistically to Ang1, promoting sprouting angiogenesis facilitating the effects of VEGF [15, 16], whilst VEGF also upregulates Ang-2 in endothelial cells [17].

Many cancers exploit aberrant angiogenic mechanisms to stimulate tumor growth and metastasis. Tumor angiogenesis was established as a potentially attractive therapeutic target for the treatment of cancer with the publication of Folkman's hypothesis in 1971 [18]. Angiogenesis is required for tumor growth beyond 1-2 mm$^3$, when the tumor demand for oxygen and nutrients surpasses the local supply and the hypoxic microenvironment, through the expression of HIFs leads to the activation of angiogenesis. Tumor related angiogenesis, in contrast to physiologic angiogenesis, leads to a more disorganized vasculature, which is also more permeable, limiting the delivery of drugs to tumor cells. Anti-angiogenic agents have been shown to transiently 'normalize' the tumor vasculature, resulting in an increased delivery of oxygen and drugs into the tumor microenvironment [19].

Many cancers induce VEGF-A expression promoting the formation of new tumor blood vessels, rapid tumor growth, and facilitation of metastatic potential [20]. Other mechanisms also contribute to tumor related angiogenesis, such as overexpression of VEGF receptors, especially VEGFR-1. Several multi-target tyrosine-kinase inhibitors (TKIs) of VEGFR have recently been evaluated showing encouraging results [21]. In addition, constitutive activation in a number of oncogenes such as *ras*, *PI3k* and *src*, or the loss of tumor suppressor function, for example through mutations in the tumor suppressor gene von Hippel Lindau which enhances the activity of HIF1α, have the capacity to induce proangiogenic factors and growth factors, promoting tumor angiogenesis [22–24].

VEGF-A potentiates proliferation of endothelial cells by activating the C-Raf-MAPK/ERK kinase signaling pathway [25]. Furthermore, there is interplay between other proangiogenic pathways, which are upregulated in tumors. These include Angs, fibroblast growth factor (FGF)/fibroblast growth factor receptor (FGFR), PDGF/platelet-derived growth factor receptor (PDGFR), hepatocyte growth factor (HGF)/MET and the PI3K/Akt/mTOR signaling pathways. The Ang–TIE2 pathway is of particular interest, as Ang-1 and 2 are upregulated in many cancer subtypes. Research on this signaling system has also provided evidence on the role of pericyte cells, which secrete ang-1 and express PDGF receptors, and explains the anti angiogenic action of some of the multi-targeted TKI inhibitors [26, 27]. The PDGF family consists of PDGF-A to -D polypeptide homodimers and the PDGF-AB heterodimer ligands and their binding tyrosine kinase receptors, PDGFR-α and −β. Aberrant activation of this pathway is implicated in pericyte recruitment to vessels; secretion of proangiogenic factors; stimulation of endothelial cell proliferation, and promotion of lymphangiogenesis among others [28]. The FGF/FGFR family compromises a total of 23 members, 18 of which function as ligands for four receptor tyrosine kinases (FGFR-1 to −4), regulating normal cell growth and differentiation and angiogenesis [29]. Overexpression of FGF, mainly FGF1 and FGF2, and FGFR contribute to different mechanisms, such as activating mutations, gene amplification and translocations, among others, leading to enhanced angiogenesis through the stimulation and release of other proangiogenic factors [30]. In addition, a collaborative interplay between FGF and VEGF signaling has also been demonstrated to be important for angiogenic and metastatic processes [31]. The inhibition of these alternate pathways (PDGF, FGF) may mediate resistance and potentiate VEGF inhibition, supporting a multitargeted approach inhibiting both VEGFR and PDGFR [32]. The HGF/MET binding also mediates tumor angiogenesis and growth in a variety of epithelial malignancies. The HGF/MET axis is responsible for the cell-scattering phenotype

and increases angiogenesis by direct activation of endothelial cells or via downstream stimulation of pro-angiogenic pathways, including PI3K/Akt and Src and production of proangiogenic factors, such as VEGF [33–35]. The PI3K/Akt/mTOR cascade is also involved in angiogenesis through the interaction of the mTOR complex 1 and 2 with the VEGF pathway, and moreover, Akt has shown importance for endothelial cell survival [36, 37].

Greater understanding of these pathways continues to provide valuable insights into the molecular mechanisms that underlie tumor angiogenesis and provide a foundation for the development of novel anti-angiogenic therapeutic strategies.

### Angiogenesis in cervical cancer

High-risk HPV subtypes 16 and 18 (although other subtypes have also been implicated) are responsible for approximately 70 % of invasive cervical cancers [38]. Emerging data suggest that viral integration into the host cell genome results in overexpression of a number of host genes, which are potential drivers of carcinogenesis [39]. However, the HPV oncoproteins E5, E6, and E7 are the primary viral factors responsible for initiation and progression of cervical cancer. E6, E7 and to a lesser extent E5 play key roles in upregulating angiogenesis through the VEGF pathway through their effects on p53 degradation, HIF-1α and inactivation of retinoblastoma protein (pRb). HPV E6 promotes p53 ubiquitination and degradation after E6-p53 binding. Degradation of p53 promotes angiogenesis by down regulating thrombospondin-1 and by increased production of VEGF. HPV E7 results in abrogation of pRb function resulting in p21-RB pathway dysregulation thereby increasing VEGF. In addition, HPV E6 (in a p53 independent manner) and E7 also enhance the induction of HIF-1α, thus increasing VEGF through a second mechanism [40–43] (Fig. 1).

Over the past decade, the relationship between HPV-16 and 18 associated cervical tumors, hypoxia, markers of tumor angiogenesis and prognosis has emerged. Initial descriptions of high risk HPV related premalignant cervical lesions seen on colposcopy included atypical angiogenic proliferation along the basement membrane and suggested a role for angiogenesis in the transition from premalignant lesions to invasive cervical carcinoma. Microvessel density (MVD) has been reported to increase with the grade of pre-malignant lesions [44]. High intratumoral microvessel density (MVD) in cervical cancer has been associated with poorer prognosis, advanced stage at presentation, and greater risk of nodal involvement [45]. However, this data is controversial with some studies showing a poor prognosis, others a better prognosis and some no effect on outcome. In an analysis

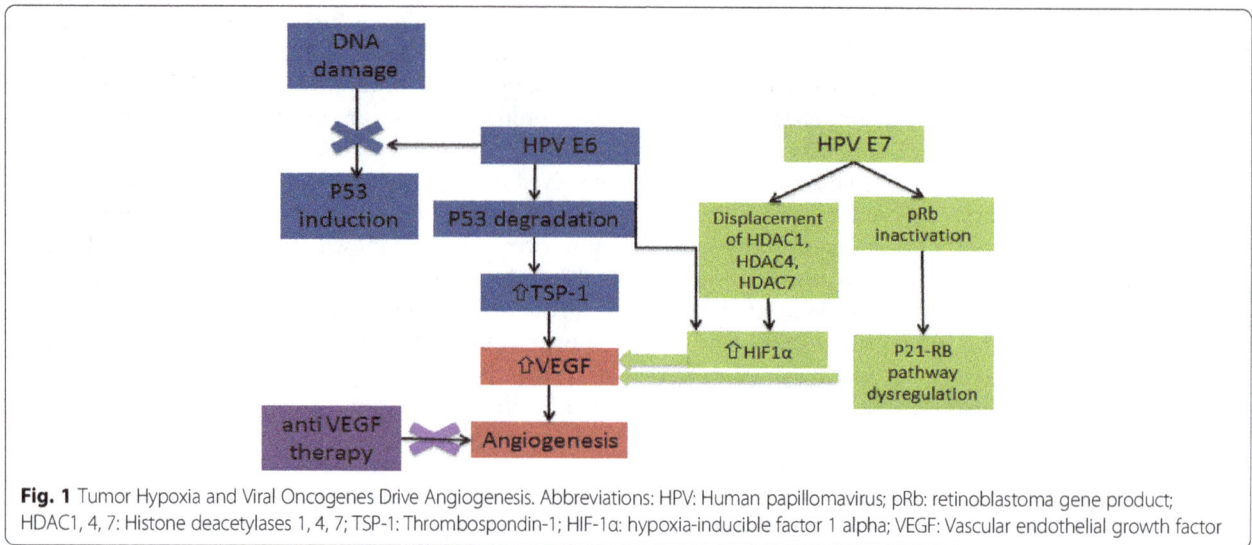

**Fig. 1** Tumor Hypoxia and Viral Oncogenes Drive Angiogenesis. Abbreviations: HPV: Human papillomavirus; pRb: retinoblastoma gene product; HDAC1, 4, 7: Histone deacetylases 1, 4, 7; TSP-1: Thrombospondin-1; HIF-1α: hypoxia-inducible factor 1 alpha; VEGF: Vascular endothelial growth factor

performed on tumor specimens from the phase III study GOG 109 [45], which investigated the addition of cisplatin chemotherapy to adjuvant radiation following radical hysterectomy, MVD was an independent prognostic marker for improved progression-free survival (PFS) and OS [hazard ratio (HR) = 0.36, 95 % CI: 0.17–0.79, $p = 0.010$]. In an ad hoc analysis of GOG 109 [46], specimens were assessed for expression of markers of tumor angiogenesis including VEGF, TSP-1 (anti-angiogenesis factor), cluster of differentiation 31 (CD31) and CD105 (tumor-specific endothelial marker). CD31 was used in the GOG 109 analysis to measure MVD and predicted for a good outcome. In contrast, the presence of CD105-positive vessels in cervical cancer samples has shown an association with risk of lymph node metastasis, and worse PFS and OS [47]. The differences in outcome observed in these studies may relate to the method used to study MVD. Some markers such as CD31, used in GOG109, may reflect "good angiogenesis", with CD31 positive endothelial cells exhibiting organized vasculature, potentially leading to well vascularized and oxygenated tumors, leading to better outcomes, whilst other markers such as CD105 may indicate a more disordered endothelial structure resulting in poorer outcomes. In addition, analysis of VEGF has shown increased VEGF expression in cervical intraepithelial neoplasia grade III and squamous cell carcinoma when compared with control cervical tissue. In the cervical cancer samples higher VEGF levels were associated with advanced stage disease, increase risk of nodal metastasis, and worse PFS and OS [48]. In cervical carcinomas, elevated serum VEGF has been identified as a poor prognostic factor [49, 50].

Angiogenesis plays a pivotal role, not only in initiation of cervical cancer, but also in proliferation and progression of the disease, hence targeting angiogenesis has emerged as a rational therapeutic approach.

**Bevacizumab in advanced and recurrent cervical cancer**

Improving the limited success achieved with traditional cytotoxic chemotherapy in patients with recurrent and metastatic cervical cancer represents a critical unmet medical need. Metastatic cervical cancer patients present a number of challenges including: disease related complications (obstructive uropathy, bleeding); impact of prior therapies (particularly when recurrence occurs in a previously irradiated field), poor performance status and frequent psychosocial issues.

Bevacizumab is a recombinant humanized monoclonal IgG1 antibody directed against VEGF-A which blocks signal transduction through VEGFR-1 and 2 associated pathways. In preclinical models bevacizumab suppressed VEGF-induced tumor growth and reduced tumor MVD. Bevacizumab appeared to normalize primitive tumor vasculature, leading to an increase in tumor oxygenation and potentially enhancing delivery of cytotoxic agents thereby potentiating their efficacy [51]. Bevacizumab has shown clinical activity in different solid tumor types resulting in approval by the FDA for treatment of metastatic colorectal cancer, non-small cell lung cancer, renal cell carcinoma, glioblastoma multiforme and ovarian cancer (Fig. 2).

Wright and colleagues initially reported the clinical utility of bevacizumab in the treatment of persistent or recurrent cervical cancer patients. This small retrospective analysis showed a meaningful clinical benefit rate of 67 % in a heavily pretreated patient population (median of 3 prior regimens), when bevacizumab was combined with chemotherapy [52]. These results catalyzed a phase II trial conducted by the GOG (GOG 227C), which aimed to determine the efficacy and toxicity profile of single agent bevacizumab in advanced cervical cancer patients. This study demonstrated encouraging clinical activity which compared favorably with historical single

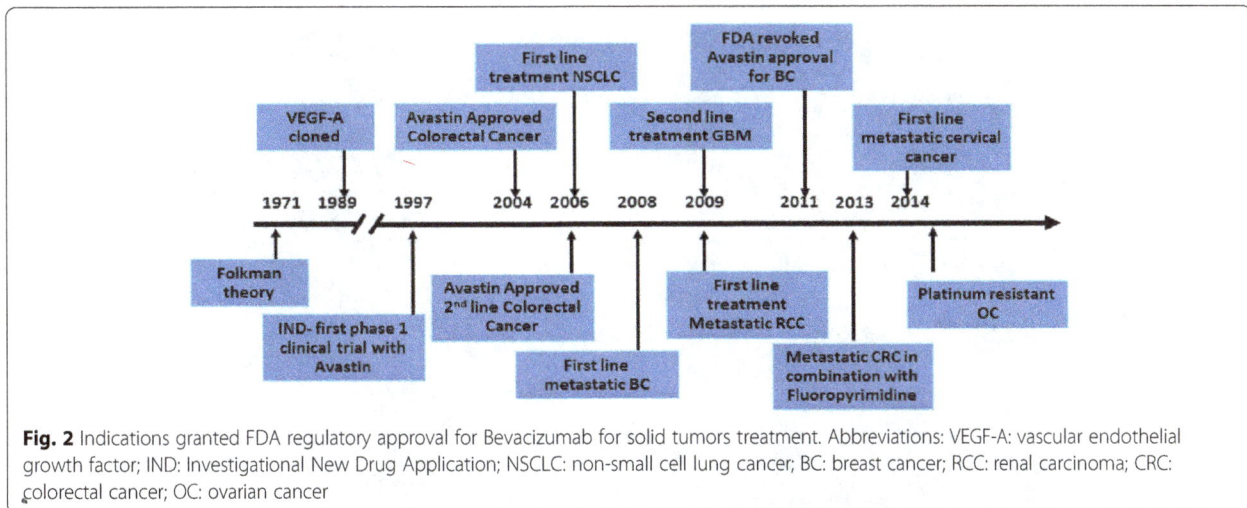

**Fig. 2** Indications granted FDA regulatory approval for Bevacizumab for solid tumors treatment. Abbreviations: VEGF-A: vascular endothelial growth factor; IND: Investigational New Drug Application; NSCLC: non-small cell lung cancer; BC: breast cancer; RCC: renal carcinoma; CRC: colorectal cancer; OC: ovarian cancer

agent cytotoxic phase II studies in similar previously treated patient populations [53]. Among 46 evaluable patients, the ORR was 11 %, with median response duration of 6.21 months (range, 2.83 to 8.28 months), and a median PFS and OS of 3.4 months (95 % CI: 2.53–4.53 months) and 7.3 months (95 % CI, 6.11–10.41 months), respectively. The 6-month PFS rate was 24 %. In this study, almost 83 % of patients had received prior pelvic radiation and 74 % had received at least one prior cytotoxic regimen for recurrent disease (74 %). Bevacizumab was generally well tolerated, fistula occurring in only 2.17 % of patients. Following on from GOG 227C, the combination of bevacizumab with platinum-based chemotherapy was investigated in a further phase II clinical trial. Twenty seven women undergoing first line treatment for locally advanced or recurrent disease received bevacizumab 15 mg/kg combined with cisplatin and topotecan administered on a 21-day cycle. Although the results in median PFS and OS were encouraging (7.1 months and 13.2 months respectively), the toxicity reported from the combination was significant with grade 3–4 hematologic toxicity being common (thrombocytopenia 82 %, anemia 63 %, and neutropenia 56 %) and a significant fistula rate of 26 % [54].

Following on from the promising activity observed in early phase clinical trials, a four-arm prospective, randomized clinical trial, GOG 240, was conducted. The aim of GOG 240 was to demonstrate whether the addition of bevacizumab to chemotherapy lead to an improvement in OS. In addition ORR, PFS, toxicity and health related Quality of Life (HR QoL) end points were also explored. GOG 240 had a 2 × 2 factorial study design that involved randomization to both the standard cisplatin and paclitaxel arm and to a non-platinum containing regimen, paclitaxel and topotecan, with or without Bevacizumab 15 mg/kg intravenously every 21 days (Fig. 3). In the modern era, exploration of a non-platinum based combination was of interest as many

patients receive cisplatin in combination with radiotherapy for their definitive frontline treatment; hence cisplatin may be less effective than previously reported following the introduction of chemotheradiotherapy as a standard of care. Stratification factors included stage IVB vs. recurrent/persistent disease, PS 0–1 and prior concomitant Cisplatin and radiation. Treatment was continued until disease progression (PD), unacceptable toxicity or complete response (CR). In addition, archival diagnostic tissue was collected for correlative studies.

GOG 240 was activated on April 9, 2009 reaching target accrual on January 2, 2012, for a total of 452 patients. Sample size calculation was based on increasing the median OS from 12 to 16 months, detecting with 90 % power, a reduction in the risk of death of at least 30 %, with the one-sided type I error rate limited to 2.5 % for each regimen. Over 220 patients were treated with each of the chemotherapy backbones (225 chemotherapy alone, 227 chemotherapy plus bevacizumab). Clinical characteristics were well distributed between groups receiving the 2 backbones: median age of enrolled patients was 49 years; the majority of patients had squamous cell cancer (70 %) with 20 % having adenocarcinomas. The majority of patients had recurrent disease (73 % chemotherapy arm and 70 % chemotherapy plus bevacizumab arm). The rate of persistent disease was 11 % in both arms and 16 % of patients in each arm presented with advanced disease at diagnosis. The proportion of prior platinum chemotherapy in combination with radiotherapy was also well-balanced between each arm (74 % and 75 % in the chemotherapy and the investigational arm respectively, $p = 0.666$). 55 % of patients had locally recurrent pelvic disease after chemoradiotherapy. Notably, the majority of patients in each chemotherapy group had a PS of 0 (PS 0–1 required for enrollment).

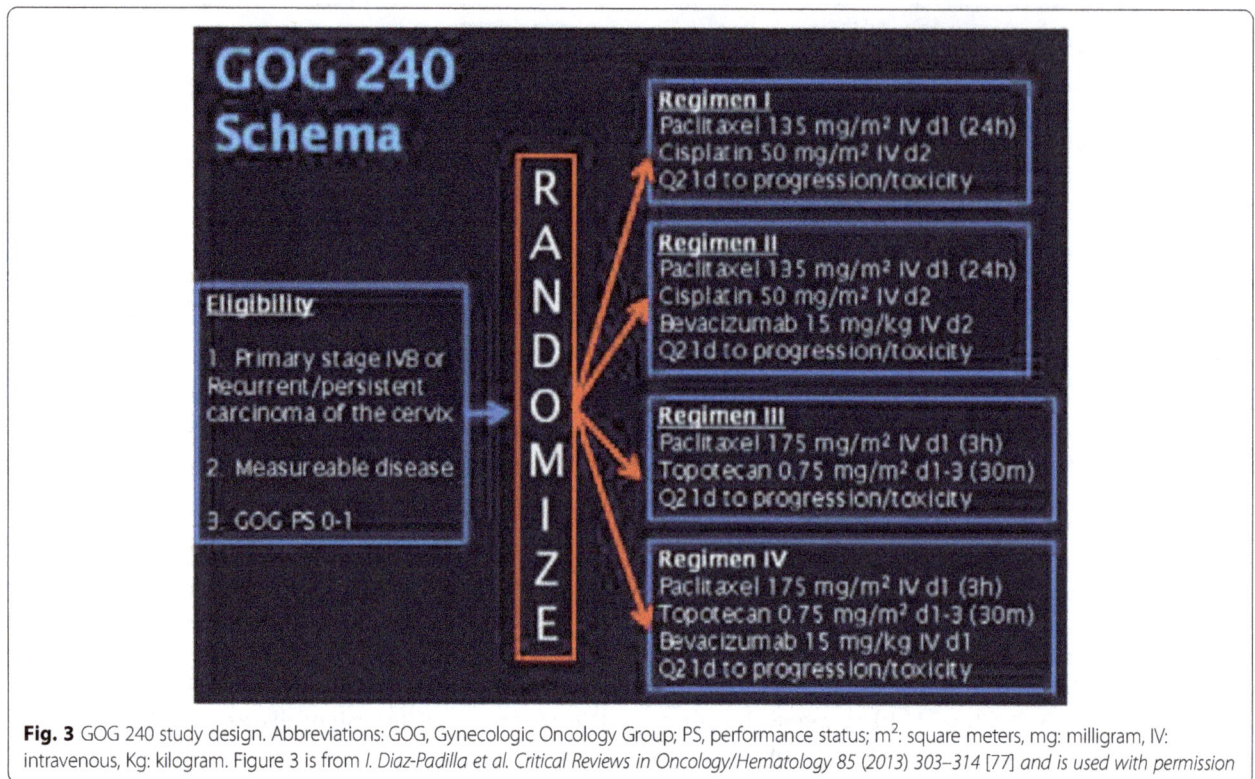

**Fig. 3** GOG 240 study design. Abbreviations: GOG, Gynecologic Oncology Group; PS, performance status; m²: square meters, mg: milligram, IV: intravenous, Kg: kilogram. Figure 3 is from *I. Diaz-Padilla et al. Critical Reviews in Oncology/Hematology 85 (2013) 303–314 [77] and is used with permission*

A pre-planned interim analysis after 174 deaths to determine futility/superiority was conducted on February 6, 2012 and presented at the Society of Gynecologic Oncology (SGO) meeting in 2013 [55]. This demonstrated that the topotecan-paclitaxel arm was not superior or inferior to the cisplatin-paclitaxel arm (median OS 15 vs. 12.5 months respectively, HR 1.20; 95 % CI: 0.82–1.76). Following a second analysis, with a median follow-up of 20.8 months the National Cancer Institute's (NCI) Data Safety Monitoring Board (DSMB) recommended ending the trial and also, due to the data's potential to alter the standard of care, that the results were released into the public domain [56]. The study demonstrated a significant improvement in OS for the addition of bevacizumab to chemotherapy compared to chemotherapy alone (17 months *versus* 13.3 months respectively; HR = 0.71; 95 % CI: 0.54–0.95; $p = 0.0035$). In addition, the benefit of bevacizumab was reported for both chemotherapy regimens—cisplatin-paclitaxel ± bevacizumab median OS 14.3 vs. 17.5 months ($p = 0.03$) and topotecan-paclitaxel ± bevacizumab-median OS 12.7 vs. 16.2 months ($p = 0.08$). The median PFS in the bevacizumab group was 8.2 months compared with 5.9 months in the chemotherapy alone group (HR 0.67; 95 % CI, 0.54–0.82; $p = 0.0002$). Response rate also was higher in the bevacizumab group 48 vs. 36 % ($p = 0.008$). The exploratory subgroup analysis suggested that the effect of bevacizumab was consistent across multiple prognostic subgroups, and that prior platinum

exposure or recurrent disease in the pelvis after prior radiation did not preclude benefit from bevacizumab. These data, published in the New England Journal of Medicine [57], represented the first time a targeted agent showed improvement in OS in patients with cervical cancer. Recent planned subgroup analyses presented in abstract form only, suggested that the addition of bevacizumab was associated with a greater likelihood of CR within the irradiated pelvis (61 %, $N = 11$) compared to chemo alone (39 %, $N = 7$), and that achieving CR (44/452 patients (9.7 %) is associated with prolonged OS (OS 39.3 months while median OS for patients with CR on the cisplatin–paclitaxel–bevacizumab arm has not been reached) [58]. Previously described poor prognostic factors including African American ethnicity, PS, measureable disease within the pelvis, prior cisplatin, and short progression-free interval were also prognostic in GOG 240. However, the investigators questioned their utility at guiding whether to add bevacizumab as high-risk patients did appear to benefit [59].

The addition of bevacizumab to chemotherapy did, however, result in increased toxicity, notably; increased risk of fistula formation and perforation of the gastrointestinal and genitourinary tracts (10.9 vs. 1 %, $p = 0.002$), grade 2 hypertension (25 vs. 2 %, p < 0.001), grade 4 neutropenia (35 vs. 26 %, $p = 0.04$), and thromboembolism (8 vs. 1 %, $p = 0.001$). Gastrointestinal and genitourinary bleeding grade 3–4 was uncommon (2 % vs <1 %, $p = 0.37$

and 3 % vs <1 %, $p = 0.12$, respectively), and clinically relevant central nervous system bleeding did not occur. Fistulae and perforations appeared to occur exclusively in patients who had undergone prior pelvic radiotherapy (reported in abstract form only) [60]. A better understanding of patients at risk is required if we are to minimize fistula/perforation rates in the clinic and adequately advise patients regarding the level of risk. In addition, although differences in HRQoL, assessed using the Functional Assessment of Cancer Therapy—Cervix Trial Outcome Index scale (FACT-Cx TOI scale), did not reach statistical significance on average HRQoL was 1.2 points lower in the bevacizumab containing treatment arm (99 % CI, −4.1 to 1.7; $p = 0.30$) [61].

On August 14, 2014, under the FDA Priority Review program [62] bevacizumab in combination with chemotherapy (both study arms) was granted regulatory approval in the US for treatment of cervical cancer. Following the FDA approval, the National Comprehensive Cancer Network (NCCN) upgraded cisplatin-paclitaxel-bevacizumab to category 1 in August 2014 and listed topotecan-paclitaxel-bevacizumab as category 1 in September 2014 [63]. The final analysis from GOG 240 has confirmed that benefits obtained from the addition of bevacizumab are sustained after 348 events and with a median follow-up of 50 months; bevacizumab-containing regimens continue to demonstrate a significant improvement in OS over chemotherapy alone: 16.8 vs 13.3 months (HR 0.765, 95 % CI: 0.62, 0.95; $p = 0.0068$) [64]. However, survival in the control arms of GOG240 was greater than in previous studies and potentially reflects the higher PS of the clinical trial patient population. How outcome and toxicity translate in the broader non trial patient population is awaited a further area where "real world data" will better inform future clinical practice.

Whilst the data from GOG 240 resulted in a change to the standard of care not all women benefited and that benefit was relatively short lived. Identification of predictive biomarkers both for response and for toxicity is desirable if we are to optimize the use of this drug. Initial reports from correlative studies evaluated the impact of pretreatment circulating tumor cells (CTCs) on OS showing a correlation between high pretreatment CTC counts, and greater declines of CTC during treatment, with lower risk of death (HR 0.87; 95 % CI 0.79, 0.95) upon addition of bevacizumab [65]. Data from this and from other correlative studies are required and validation is essential if predictive biomarkers are to become clinically useful. There are potentially opportunities to explore predictive biomarkers across tumor types and data sets which may benefit a larger number of patients, particularly in relation to prediction of toxicity.

Whilst the addition of bevacizumab to chemotherapy has become a new standard of care for women in resource rich communities it remains inaccessible to those at greatest need. The cost implications and generalizability of incorporating bevacizumab in poorly resourced countries and communities is a significant issue, however questions around cost-effectiveness have also risen even in resource rich regions. An initial cost-effectiveness analysis reported by Phippen et al. showed an incremental cost-effectiveness ratio (ICER) of $155 K/quality adjusted life year (QALY) [66]. However, an updated analysis using a Markov decision tree model that incorporated the final OS and toxicity data (improvement of 3.9 months and fistula rate of 8.6 %) showed the cost of the addition of bevacizumab was $53,784 compared to $5688 for the chemotherapy alone arm. Thus, the addition of bevacizumab represents an increase of 13.2 times the cost for chemotherapy alone, adding $73,791 per 3.5 months of life gained and an incremental ICER of $21,083 per month of added life, mostly due to the cost of bevacizumab rather than related with the management of related toxicity [67]. Further exploratory analysis also suggested that adding Bevacizumab would become cost-effective, with a significant decline in the ICER, by either reducing the dose of bevacizumab from 15 to 7.5 mg/kg, or diminishing the costs of bevacizumab. Whether the benefit conferred by bevacizumab is worthwhile or not from a cost-effectiveness perspective, remains a societal and clinical dilemma. Further cost-effective analyses based on real world experience, are warranted. In addition the introduction of generic drugs into the market may in time reduce the cost of targeting angiogenesis using this approach. However, this will not remove the need to advocate on a global level for accessible health care for our most economically vulnerable patient populations.

### Summary and future directions

Angiogenesis is central to cervical cancer development and progression. Publication of GOG 240 showing a significant improvement in OS, PFS and ORR, without a concomitant deterioration of HRQoL, demonstrated proof of concept concerning integration of anti-angiogenesis therapy for advanced cervical cancer patients, and represents a practice-changing clinical trial. The significance of 3.7 months improvement in OS is most clear when placed in context with prior clinical trials in this setting (Fig. 4) [57, 68–71], (Table 1) [5, 6, 57, 70, 71]. Targeting angiogenesis is therefore a successful strategy that should be further investigated in the next generation of clinical trials.

Several questions remain around optimal use of bevacizumab. The JGOG 0505 clinical trial [6] established non-inferiority of the better tolerated combination of carboplatin and paclitaxel compared to cisplatin-paclitaxel. Extrapolating from other gynecologic cancers, bevacizumab should be safe in combination with this regimen

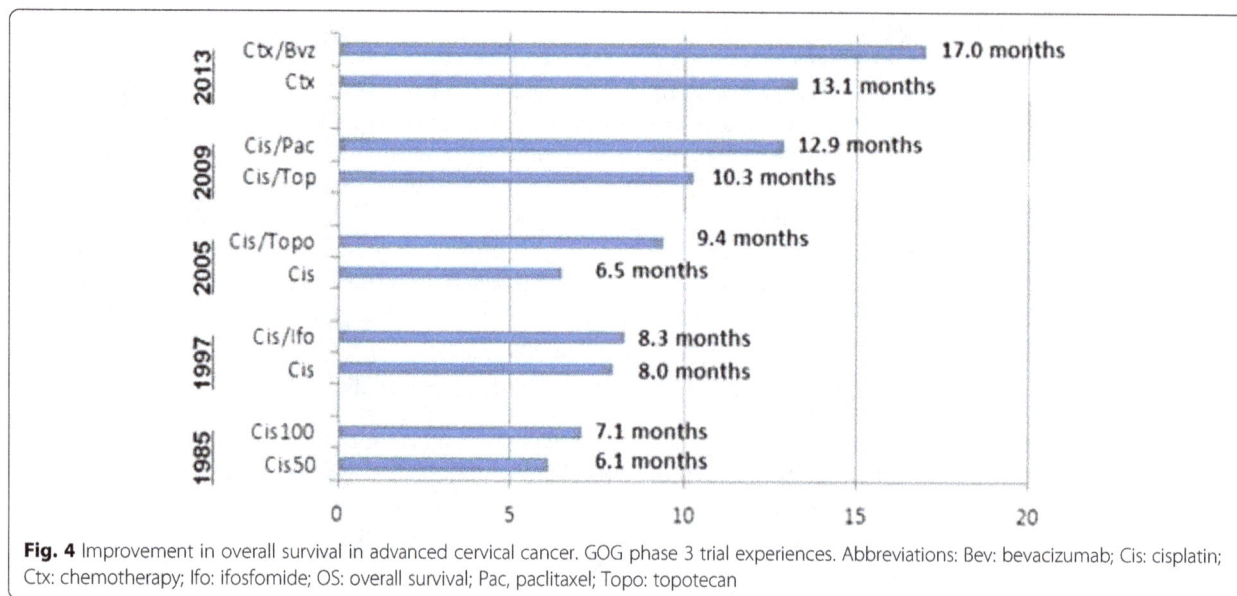

**Fig. 4** Improvement in overall survival in advanced cervical cancer. GOG phase 3 trial experiences. Abbreviations: Bev: bevacizumab; Cis: cisplatin; Ctx: chemotherapy; Ifo: ifosfomide; OS: overall survival; Pac, paclitaxel; Topo: topotecan

in women with cervical cancer, however its efficacy has not been evaluated in a prospective randomized trial. In addition, extrapolating from ovarian cancer, in the real world setting there may be a role for continuing bevacizumab alone following discontinuation of chemotherapy especially given the potential improvement in quality of life from discontinuing cytotoxic agents. More data is required in order to endorse this approach.

Evidence from the GOG 109 [5] and a number of other studies showed that improved oxygenation and tumors with higher MVD can lead to better outcomes with chemoradiotherapy. The combination of an anti-angiogenic agent, that promotes vascular normalization and improved

oxygenation combined with multimodality therapy could potentially lead to better outcomes. However, data concerning anti-angiogenic agent/radiotherapy combinations in other tumor types suggest increased risk of fistula formation [72], already a concern in women receiving bevacizumab in recurrent and metastatic disease. Radiation Therapy Oncology Group (RTOG) 1704 evaluated the safety and toxicity profile of adding bevacizumab (10 mg/kg every 2 weeks) for three cycles to pelvic chemoradiotherapy and brachytherapy. In 49 untreated patients with locally advanced cervical cancer (stage IB–IIIB), with a median follow-up of 3.8 years, the 3-year OS was 81.3 % (95 % [CI], 67.2–89.8 %) and the 3-year locoregional

**Table 1** Comparison of GOG phases 3 randomized clinical trials for women with recurrent or advanced cervical cancer. GOG Protocols 169, 179, 204, 240 and JGOG 0505

|  | GOG 169 [70] | GOG 179 [71] | GOG 204 [5] | GOG 240 [57] | JGOG 0505 [6] |
|---|---|---|---|---|---|
| Modalities | Cis ± Pac | Cis ± Topo | Cis-Pac<br>vs Cis- Topo<br>vs Cis- GC<br>vs Cis-VR | Ctx vs Ctx + bevacizumab | CDDP-Pac vs CB-Pac |
| Stage | IVB, recurrent, or persistent SCC | IVB, recurrent, or persistent SCC | IVB, recurrent, or persistent SCC, ACA, or ASC | IVB, recurrent, or persistent SCC, ACA, or ASC | IVB, recurrent, or persistent SCC, ACA, or ASC |
| N | 264 | 293 | 513 | 452 | 253 |
| PS | 0–2 | 0–2 | 0–1 | 0–1 | 0–2 |
| ORR | 19 vs 36 % | 13 vs 27 % | 29.1 vs 23.4 vs 22.3 vs 25.9 % | 36 vs 48 % | - |
| PFS | 2.8 vs 4.8 mo | 2.9 vs 4.6 mo | 5.8 vs 4.6 vs 4.7 vs 3.9 mo | 5.9 vs 8.2 mo | 6.9 vs 6.21 |
| P value | <001 | NS | .06 vs .04 vs .19 | .002 | .004 |
| OS | 8.8 vs 9.7 mo | 6.5 vs 9.4 mo | 12.8 vs 10.2 vs 10.3 vs 9.9 mo | 13.3 vs 17 mo | 18.3 vs 17.5 mo |
| P value | NS | .021 | .71 vs .90 vs .89 | .004 | .032 |

*JGOG* Japanese Gynecologic oncology group; *Cis* cisplatin; *Pac* paclitaxel; *Topo* topotecan; *GC* gemcitabine; *VR* vinorelbine; *CB* carboplatin; *SCC* squamous cell carcinoma; *ACA* adenocarcinoma; *ASC* adenosquamous carcinoma; *N* numbers; *PS* performance status; *ORR* overall response rate; *HR* hazard ratio; *mo* months; *PFS* progression free survival; *NS* non significance; *OS* overall survival

failure was 23.2 %. These outcomes compare favorably with historical reports. In addition, the combination was associated with minimal protocol-defined toxicity, the most common toxicity being myelosuppression. Of note, there were no grade 4 gastrointestinal toxicities or gastrointestinal fistulas or perforations [73].

Moving beyond bevacizumab, exploration of novel anti-angiogenic agents targeting parallel angiogenesis related pathways are being undertaken and considered in women with cervical cancer. Single agent, orally administered, multi-TKIs, pazopanib (VEGFR 1, 2, and 3; PDGFR-α and β; and c-KIT inhibitor) and sunitinib (VEGFR 1, 2 and 3; PDGFR, c-KIT, and FLT3 inhibitor) have been investigated. Sunitinib, tested in a phase II clinical trial in patients with unresectable, locally advanced or metastatic cervical carcinoma, was associated with an unacceptably high (26 %) rate of fistula formation combined with only modest activity (no documented objective responses and median time to progression of 3.5 months) therefore further investigation was not warranted [74]. In a second, larger phase II study, 230 patients, with stage IVb persistent/recurrent cervical carcinoma not amenable to curative therapy and at least one prior regimen in the metastatic setting, were randomly assigned to one of three arms: pazopanib alone, lapatinib (a TKI targeting EGFR and HER2/neu) alone, or a combination of the two agents. Pazopanib improved PFS (HR 0.66; 90 % CI, 0.48 to 0.91; $p =$ 0.013) and OS (HR 0.67; 90 % CI, 0.46 to 0.99; $p =$ 0.045) compared with lapatinib alone. Median OS was 50.7 weeks compared with 39.1 weeks for pazopanib and lapatinib, respectively. Pazopanib alone was well tolerated, but the combination of the two drugs lacked efficacy and importantly, the combination arm was terminated at the planned interim analysis for futility due to the significant association with more serious adverse events [75]. Recently, the CIRCCa trial presented in the 2014 ESMO Congress [76] evaluated cediranib (AZD2171), a selective, orally bioavailable TKI of VEGFR-1, 2, and 3, in 69 women with primary metastatic or relapsed cervical cancer. In the CIRCCa trial, patients were randomized (1:1) to receive carboplatin, tri-weekly paclitaxel, for a maximum of 6 cycles plus cediranib (20 mg/day) or placebo concurrently with chemotherapy, and later as maintenance therapy until progression. The addition of cediranib improved median PFS by 5 weeks (8.8 vs 7.5 months; $p = .046$) and response rate by 24 % ($p = .03$). However, as CIRCCa closed prematurely owing to the cessation of commercial production of cediranib, the statistical analysis of the difference in median OS between the two groups was underpowered for comparison (59 vs. 63 weeks; HR, 0.93; 80 % CI, 0.64 to 1.36; $p = 0.401$). However, the addition of cediranib significantly increased the rate

of diarrhea grades 2–4 (50 % compared with 18 % in the placebo group ($p = .005$) and hypertension (34 v 12 %, $p = .038$, respectively). Brivanib, another TKI which targets VEGFR2 and FGFR-1, is currently being evaluated in a phase II study (NCT01267253) conducted by the GOG.

In addition, non-VEGF-dependent therapeutic approaches, including angiopoietin inhibitors, involve other classes of potentially attractive anti-angiogenic drugs and are under investigation in other tumor types. These should also be explored in cervical cancer patients. Furthermore, given that Ang-2 promotes the proangiogenic action of VEGF, the inhibition of Ang-2 and VEGF together could have complementary actions, thus, the combination of an angiopoietin inhibitor, such as Trebananib (AMG386) and an agent such as bevacizumab could be more active than either agent alone. Combining anti-angiogenic agents with drugs which target the PI3K/AKT/mTOR pathway may also offer an unique treatment opportunity. Finally, the role of immunotherapy in the treatment of cervical cancer is under investigation; potentially combining this approach with an anti-angiogenic agent may represent a novel therapeutic opportunity for this patient population.

As more data emerge about the genomic landscape of cervical cancer and its "potentially druggable" mutations rational combinations with anti-angiogenic agents will potentially be identified. However, as with all rare cancers, it is vital that any studies undertaken have a strong underlying rationale and that they are designed to maximize the biological information we can learn from them. Clearly the way forward to improve outcome for advanced cervical cancer is to reduce the rate of recurrence. We have reached the tolerance of the combination of chemotherapy with radiotherapy in the treatment of locally advanced cervical cancer and the coming generation of trials need to explore the role of targeted therapy in combination with chemoradiotherapy in this setting.

## Conclusions

Despite the introduction of screening and vaccination programs cervical cancer remains a significant health problem. The results from the GOG protocol 240 and the FDA approval of bevacizumab in combination with chemotherapy for the treatment of women with advanced stage, persistent, or recurrent cervical cancer has established the role for new target therapies in a population with historically limited options. However in order to optimize the use of this agent we need to learn more about patients at risk of toxicity and explore opportunities for developing predictive biomarkers. Moving forward there is a very strong rationale for further exploration of angiogenesis pathways alone and in combination in cervical cancer. However, globally we need to advocate for affordable and accessible therapeutic options for women affected by this disease.

## Abbreviations

HPV: Human papillomavirus; VEGF: Vascular endothelial growth factor; US: United States; FIGO: International federation of obstetrics and gynecology; QoL: Quality of life; GOG: Gynecologic oncology group; OS: Overall survival; ORR: Overall response rate; JGOG: Japanese gynecologic oncology group; FDA: Food and drug Administration; HIF-1α: Hypoxia-inducible factor 1 alpha; VEGFR: Vascular endothelial growth factor receptor; PLGF: Placental growth factor; PDGF: Platelet derived growth factor; Ang: Angiopoietins; TKIs: Tyrosine-kinase inhibitors; FGF: Fibroblast growth factor; FGFR: Fibroblast growth factor receptor; PDGFR: Platelet-derived growth factor receptor; HGF: Hepatocyte growth factor; pRb: Retinoblastoma protein; HDAC: Histone deacetylases; TSP-1: Thrombospondin-1; MVD: Microvessel density; PFS: Progression free survival; CD: Cluster of differentiation; IND: Investigational New Drug Application; NSCLC: Non-small cell lung cancer; BC: Breast cancer; RCC: Renal carcinoma; CRC: Colorectal cancer; OC: Ovarian cancer; SD: Stable disease; CI: Confidence interval; HRQoL: Health related quality of life; PD: Disease progression; CR: Complete response; PS: Performance status; $m^2$: Square meters; mg: Milligram; iv: Intravenous; Kg: Kilogram; SGO: Society of gynecology oncology (SGO); HR: Hazard ratio; NCI: National Cancer Institute; DSMB: Data Safety Monitoring Board; PFI: Progression-free interval; FACT-Cx TOI: Functional Assessment of Cancer Therapy—Cervix Trial Outcome Index scale; ICER: Cost-effectiveness ratio; NCCN: National Comprehensive Cancer Network; CTCs: Circulating tumor cells; QALY: Quality adjusted life year; Cis: Cisplatin; Ctx: Chemotherapy; Ifo: Ifosfomide; Pac: Paclitaxel; Topo: Topotecan; GC: Gemcitabine; VR: Vinorelbine; CB: Carboplatin; SCC: Squamous cell carcinoma; ACA: Adenocarcinoma; ASC: Adenosquamous carcinoma; N: Numbers; mo: Months; NS: Non significance; FLT3: Fms-like tyrosine kinase 3; EGFR: Epidermal growth factor receptor; HER2: Human epidermal growth factor receptor 2.

## Competing interests

The authors declare that they have no competing interest.

## Authors' contributions

HJM designed the paper and mapped out which subjects should be addressed. VRF performed the literature search, designed the tables and figures and wrote the initial and final drafts of the manuscript, each of which HJM edited. All the authors take responsibility for the accuracy and completeness of the reported data. The corresponding author had final responsibility for the decision to submit for publication. All authors read and approved the final manuscript.

## Authors' information

*Dr. Victor Rodriguez Freixinos* received his Doctor of Medicine (M.D.) in 2006 from University of Murcia, in Murcia, Spain. He completed his medical oncology training in 2011 at University Hospital Vall d' Hebron, Barcelona, Spain. After a few years serving as a junior staff general medical oncologist in Barcelona, Dr. Rodriguez-Freixinos is currently completing a 2-year clinical research fellowship in Drug Development and Gynecologic Oncology at the Princess Margaret Hospital in Toronto, Canada. Dr. Rodriguez-Freixinos' main research interest is directed toward efficient implementation of new molecularly targeted agents into the gynecological cancer treatment armamentarium.

*Dr. Helen Mackay* is a Staff physician in the Division of Medical Oncology and Hematology at Princess Margaret Hospital and an Assistant Professor at the University of Toronto (Department of Medicine). Her research interests are focused toward the development and validation of novel therapeutic strategies and collaborations with translational and basic scientists. She is a principal and co-investigator of a number of Phase I, II and III clinical trials in gynecological malignancy and is currently the co-chair of the NCIC CTG OV 21 a Phase II/III study of intraperitoneal chemotherapy in patients who have undergone neoadjuvant chemotherapy. Other current areas of research include epigenetic therapy and the role of the Hedgehog pathway in gynecological malignancy. She is currently a member of a number of international and national committees including: the ICON 7 Translational Committee (representing NCIC CTG), the Study Committee of the TFRI Ovarian Cancer Biomarker Program, Gynecologic Cancer Steering

Committee Cervical Cancer Task Force: Intergroup/National Cancer Institute (US)/NIH (US), Cervix Working Group (NCIC CTG), Gynecologic Disease Site Group (Cancer Care Ontario) and the GOC CPD Committee.

## References

1. Siegel R, Ma J, Zou Z, Jemal A. Cancer statistics, 2014. CA Cancer J Clin. 2014;64(1):9–29.
2. World Cancer Research Fund International. Cervical cancer statistics. http://www.wcrf.org/int/cancer-facts-figures/data-specific-cancers/cervical-cancer-statistics.
3. Funke M, Gaurav G, Silberstein PT. Demographic and insurance-based disparities in diagnosis of stage IV cervical cancer: A population-based analysis using NCDB. Abstract. ASCO annual meeting 2015. J Clin Oncol. 2015;33(suppl; abstr e17589)
4. Waggoner SE. Cervical cancer. Lancet. 2003;361:2217–25.
5. Monk BJ, Sill MW, McMeekin DS, et al. Phase III trial of four cisplatin-containing doublet combinations in stage IVB, recurrent, or persistent cervical carcinoma: a Gynecologic Oncology Group study. J Clin Oncol. 2009;27(28):4649–55.
6. Kitagawa R, Noriyuki K, Shibata T, et al. Paclitaxel plus carboplatin versus paclitaxel plus cisplatin in metastatic or recurrent cervical Cancer: the open-label randomized phase III trial JCOG0505. J Clin Oncol. 2015;33(19):2129–35.
7. Moore DH, Tian C, Monk BJ, et al. Prognostic factors for response to cisplatin-based chemotherapy in advanced cervical carcinoma: a Gynecologic Oncology Group Study. Gynecol Oncol. 2010;116(1):44–9.
8. FDA News Release. FDA approves Avastin to treat patients with aggressive and late-stage cervical cancer. US Food and Drug Administration. http://www.fda.gov/NewsEvents/Newsroom/PressAnnouncements/ucm410121.htm.
9. Tang N et al. Loss of HIF-1α in endothelial cells disrupts a hypoxia-driven VEGF autocrine loop necessary for tumorigenesis. Cancer Cell. 2004;6:485–95.
10. Ferrara N, Gerber HP, LeCouter J. The biology of VEGF and its receptors. Nature Med. 2003;9:669–76.
11. Park JE, Chen HH, Winer J, Houck KA, Ferrara N. Placenta growth factor. Potentiation of vascular endothelial growth factor bioactivity, in vitro and in vivo, and high affinity binding to Flt-1 but not to Flk-1/KDR. J Biol Chem. 1994;269:25646–54.
12. Olofsson B et al. Vascular endothelial growth factor B (VEGF-B) binds to VEGF receptor-1 and regulates plasminogen activator activity in endothelial cells. Proc Natl Acad Sci U S A. 1998;95:11709–14.
13. Alitalo K, Tammela T, Petrova TV. Lymphangiogenesis in development and human disease. Nature. 2005;438:946–53.
14. Hellstrom M et al. Lack of pericytes leads to endothelial hyperplasia and abnormal vascular morphogenesis. J Cell Biol. 2001;153:543–53.
15. Eklund L, Olsen BR. Tie receptors and their angiopoietin ligands are context-dependent regulators of vascular remodeling. Exp Cell Res. 2006;312:630–41.
16. Adams RH, Alitalo K. Molecular regulation of angiogenesis and lymphangiogenesis. Nature Rev Mol Cell Biol. 2007;8:464–78.
17. Zhang L, Yang N, Park JW, et al. Tumor-derived vascular endothelial growth factor up-regulates angiopoietin-2 in host endothelium and destabilizes host vasculature, supporting angiogenesis in ovarian cancer. Cancer Res. 2003;63:3403–12.
18. Folkman J. Tumor angiogenesis: therapeutic implications. N Engl J Med. 1971;285:1182–6.
19. Jain RK. Normalization of tumor vasculature: an emerging concept in antiangiogenic therapy. Science. 2005;307:58–62.
20. Hicklin DJ, Ellis LM. Role of the vascular endothelial growth factor pathway in tumor growth and angiogenesis. J Clin Oncol. 2005;23:1011–27.
21. Kessler T, Fehrmann F, Bieker R, Berdel WE, Mesters RM. Vascular endothelial growth factor and its receptor as drug targets in hematological malignancies. Curr Drug Targets. 2007;8:257–68.
22. Rak J, Yu JL, Klement G, Kerbel RS. Oncogenes and angiogenesis: signaling three-dimensional tumor growth. J Investig Dermatol Symp Proc. 2000;5:24–33.
23. Pugh CW, Ratcliffe PJ. Regulation of angiogenesis by hypoxia: role of the HIF system. Nature Med. 2003;9:677–84.
24. Hanahan D. Signaling vascular morphogenesis and maintenance. Science. 1997;277:48–50.
25. Gerber HP, McMurtrey A, Kowalski J, et al. Vascular endothelial growth factor regulates endothelial cell survival through the phosphatidylinositol

3'-kinase/Akt signal transduction pathway. Requirement for Flk-1/KDR activation. J Biol Chem. 1998;273:30336–43.

26. Oliner J, Min H, Leal J, et al. Suppression of angiogenesis and tumor growth by selective inhibition of angiopoietin-2. Cancer Cell. 2004;6:507–16.

27. Bergers G, Song S, Meyer-Morse N, Bergsland E, Hanahan D. Benefits of targeting both pericytes and endothelial cells in the tumor vasculature with kinase inhibitors. J Clin Invest. 2003;111:1287–95.

28. Cao Y. Multifarious functions of PDGFs and PDGFRs in tumor growth and metastasis. Trends Mol Med. 2013;19:460–73.

29. Beenken A, Mohammadi M. The FGF family: biology, pathophysiology and therapy. Nat Rev Drug Discov. 2009;8:235–53.

30. Cao Y, Cao R, Hedlund EM. Regulation of tumor angiogenesis and metastasis by FGF and PDGF signaling pathways. J Mol Med (Berl). 2008;86:785–9.

31. Cao R, Ji H, Feng N, et al. Collaborative interplay between FGF-2 and VEGF-C promotes lymphangiogenesis and metastasis. Proc Natl Acad Sci U S A. 2012;109:15894–9.

32. Farhadi M, Capelle H, Erber R. Combined inhibition of vascular endothelial growth factor and platelet-derived growth factor signaling: effects on the angiogenesis, microcirculation, and growth of orthotopic malignant gliomas. J Neurosurg. 2005;102:363–70.

33. You WK, McDonald DM. The hepatocyte growth factor/c-Met signaling pathway as a therapeutic target to inhibit angiogenesis. BMB Rep. 2008;41:833–9.

34. Wojta J, Kaun C, Breuss JM, et al. Hepatocyte growth factor increases expression of vascular endothelial growth factor and plasminogen activator inhibitor-1 in human keratinocytes and the vascular endothelial growth factor receptor flk-1 in human endothelial cells. Lab Invest. 1999;79:427–38.

35. Organ SL, Tsao M. An overview of the c-MET signaling pathway. Ther Adv Med Oncol. 2011;3 suppl 1:S7–S19.

36. Jiang B-H, Liu L-Z. PI3K/PTEN signaling in tumorigenesis and angiogenesis. Biochim Biophys Acta. 1784;2008:150–8.

37. Wang S, Amato KR, Song W, et al. Regulation of endothelial cell proliferation and vascular assembly through distinct mTORC2 signaling pathways. Mol Cell Biol. 2015;35(7):1299–313.

38. IARC monographs on the evaluation of carcinogenic risks to humans. Human papillomaviruses. Lyon (France): International Agency for Research on Cancer; 1995. Vol 64.

39. Ojesina AI, Lichtenstein L, Freeman SS, et al. Landscape of genomic alterations in cervical carcinomas. Nature. 2014;506:371–5.

40. Bosch FX, Lorincz A, Munoz N, Meijer CJ, Shah KV. The causal relation between human papillomavirus and cervical cancer. J Clin Pathol. 2002;55:244–65.

41. Willmott LJ, Monk BJ. Cervical cancer therapy: current, future and anti-angiogensis targeted treatment. Expert Rev Anticancer Ther. 2009;9:895–903.

42. Nakamura M, Bodily JM, Beglin M, Kyo S, Inoue M, Laimins LA. Hypoxia-specific stabilization of HIF-1alpha by human papillomaviruses. Virology. 2009;387:442–8.

43. Bodily JM, Mehta KP, Laimins LA, et al. Human papillomavirus E7 enhances hypoxia-inducible factor 1-mediated transcription by inhibiting binding of histone deacetylases. Cancer Res. 2011;71(3):1187–95.

44. Smith-McCune KK, Weidner N. Demonstration and characterization of the angiogenic properties of cervical dysplasia. Cancer Res. 1994;54:800–4.

45. Cooper RA, Wilks DP, Logue JP, Davidson SE, Hunter RD, Roberts SA, et al. High tumor angiogenesis is associated with poorer survival in carcinoma of the cervix treated with radiotherapy. Clin Cancer Res. 1998;4:2795–800.

46. Randall LM, Monk BJ, Darcy KM, Tian C, Burger RA, Liao SY, et al. Markers of angiogenesis in high-risk, early-stage cervical cancer: a Gynecologic Oncology Group study. Gynecol Oncol. 2009;112:583–9.

47. Zijlmans HJ, Fleuren GJ, Hazelbag S, et al. Expression of endoglin (CD105) in cervical cancer. Br J Cancer. 2009;100:1617–26.

48. Dobbs SP, Hewett PW, Johnson IR, Carmichael J, Murray JC. Angiogenesis is associated with vascular endothelial growth factor expression in cervical intraepithelial neoplasia. Br J Cancer. 1997;76:1410–5.

49. Lebrecht A, Ludwig E, Huber A, Klein M, Schneeberger C, Tempfer C, et al. Serum vascular endothelial growth factor and serum leptin in patients with cervical cancer. Gynecol Oncol. 2002;85:32–5.

50. Loncaster JA, Cooper RA, Logue JP, Davidson SE, Hunter RD, West CM. Vascular endothelial growth factor (VEGF) expression is a prognostic factor for radiotherapy outcome in advanced carcinoma of the cervix. Br J Cancer. 2000;83:620–5.

51. Grothey A, Galanis E. Targeting angiogenesis: progress with anti-VEGF treatment with large molecules. Nat Rev Clin Oncol. 2009;6:507–18.

52. Wright JD, Viviano D, Powell MA, et al. Bevacizumab combination therapy in heavily pretreated, recurrent cervical cancer. Gynecol Oncol. 2006;103(2):489–93.

53. Monk BJ, Sill MW, Burger RA, Gray HJ, Buekers TE, Roman LD. Phase II trial of bevacizumab in the treatment of persistent or recurrent squamous cell carcinoma of the cervix: a Gynecologic Oncology Group study. J Clin Oncol. 2009;27(7):1069–74.

54. Zighelboim I, Wright JD, Gao F, et al. Multicenter phase II trial of topotecan, cisplatin and bevacizumab for recurrent or persistent cervical cancer. Gynecol Oncol. 2013;130:64–8.

55. Tewari KS, Sill MW, Monk BJ, et al. Phase III randomized clinical trial of cisplatin plus paclitaxel vs the non-platinum chemotherapy doublet of topotecan plus paclitaxel in women with recurrent, persistent, or advanced cervical carcinoma: a Gynecologic Oncology Group study [SGO abstract 1]. Gynecol Oncol. 2013;130(1):e2.

56. Bevacizumab significantly improves survival for patients with recurrent and metastatic cervical cancer [press release]. National Cancer Institute. http://www.cancer.gov/news-events/press-releases/2013/GOG240.

57. Tewari KS, Sill MW, Long III HJ, et al. Improved survival with bevacizumab in advanced cervical cancer. N Engl J Med. 2014;370(8):734–43.

58. Eskandera RN, Javab J, Monk BJ, et al. Complete responses in the irradiated field following treatment with chemotherapy with and without bevacizumab in advanced cervical cancer: An NRG Oncology/Gynecologic Oncology Group study. SGO women's health meeting 2014. Abstract 62. Gynecol Oncol. 2015;137:2–91.

59. Tewari KS, Sill M, Moore DH, et al. High-risk patients with recurrent/advanced cervical cancer may derive the most benefit from antiangiogenesis therapy: a Gynecologic Oncology Group (GOG) study. SGO women's health meeting 2014. Abstract 144. Gynecol Oncol. 2014;133:2–207.

60. Willmott LJ, Java JJ, Monk BJ, Shah J, Husain A, Tewari KS. Fistulae in women treated with chemotherapy with and without bevacizumab for persistent, recurrent or metastatic cervical cancer in GOG-240. Melbourne, Australia: International Gynecologic Cancer Society meeting; 2014.

61. Penson RT, Huang HQ, Wenzel LB, et al. Bevacizumab for advanced cervical cancer: patient- reported outcomes of a randomised, phase 3 trial (NRG Oncology–Gynecologic Oncology Group protocol 240. Lancet Oncol. 2015;16:301–11.

62. FDA grants Genentech's Avastin priority review for certain types of cervical cancer [press release]. Genentech. http://www.gene.com/media/press-releases/14569/2014-07-14/fda-grants-genentechs-avastin-priority-r.

63. NCCN Clinical Practice Guidelines in Oncology (NCCN Guidelines). Cervical Cancer. Version 1.2014. NCCN.org. http://www.nccn.org/professionals/physiciangls/pdf/cervical.pdf.

64. Tewari KS, Sill MW, Penson RT, et al. Final overall survival analysis of the phase III randomized trial of chemotherapy with and without bevacizumab for advanced cervical cancer: a NRG Oncology-Gynecologic Oncology Group Study. ESMO congress 2014. Abstract LBA26. Ann Oncol. 2014;25(5):1–41.

65. Tewari KS, Sill M, Monk BJ, et al. Impact of circulating tumor cells (CTCs) on overall survival among patients treated with chemotherapy plus bevacizumab for advanced cervical cancer: An NRG Oncology/Gynecologic Oncology Group study. SGO women's health meeting 2014. Abstract 24. Gynecologic Oncol. 2015;137:2–91.

66. Phippen NT, Leath 3rd CA, Havrilesky LJ, Barnett JC. Bevacizumab in recurrent, persistent, or advanced stage carcinoma of the cervix: is it cost-effective? Gynecol Oncol. 2015;136(1):43–7.

67. Minion L, Bai J, Monk BJ, et al. A Markov model to evaluate cost-effectiveness of antiangiogenesis therapy using bevacizumab in advanced cervical cancer. Gynecol Oncol. 2015;33(8):966.

68. Bonomi P, Blessing JA, Stehman FB, DiSaia PJ, Walton L, Major FJ. Randomized trial of three cisplatin dose schedules in squamous-cell carcinoma of the cervix: a Gynecologic Oncology Group study. J Clin Oncol. 1985;3(8):1079–85.

69. Bloss JD, Blessing JA, Behrens BC, et al. Randomized trial of cisplatin and ifosfamide with or without bleomycin in squamous carcinoma of the cervix: a gynecologic oncology group study. J Clin Oncol. 2002;20:1832–7.

70. Moore DH, Blessing JA, McQuellon RP, et al. Phase III study of cisplatin with or without paclitaxel in stage IVB, recurrent, or persistent squamous cell

carcinoma of the cervix: a Gynecologic Oncology Group study. J Clin Oncol. 2004;22(15):3113–9.

71. Long III HJ, Bundy BN, Grendys Jr EC, et al. Gynecologic Oncology Group Study. Randomized phase III trial of cisplatin with or without topotecan in carcinoma of the uterine cervix: a Gynecologic Oncology Group Study. J Clin Oncol. 2005;23(21):4626–33.

72. Seiwert TY, Haraf DJ, Cohen EE, et al. Phase I study of bevacizumab added to fluorouracil- and hydroxyurea-based concomitant chemoradiotherapy for poor prognosis head and neck Cancer. J Clin Oncol. 2008;26:1732–41.

73. Schefter T, Winter K, Kwon JS, et al. RTOG 0417: Efficacy of Bevacizumab in combination with definitive radiation therapy and cisplatin chemotherapy in untreated patients with locally advanced cervical carcinoma. Int J of Radiat Oncol. 2014;88(1):101–5.

74. Mackay HJ, Tinker A, Winquist E, et al. A phase II study of sunitinib in patients with locally advanced or metastatic cervical carcinoma: NCIC CTG Trial IND.184. Gynecol Oncol. 2010;116:163–7.

75. Monk BJ, Mas Lopez L, Zarba JJ, et al. Phase II, open-label study of pazopanib or lapatinib monotherapy compared with pazopanib plus lapatinib combination therapy in patients with advanced and recurrent cervical cancer. J Clin Oncol. 2010;28:3562–9.

76. Symonds P, Gourley C, Davidson S, West C, Dive C, Paul J, et al. CIRCCA: a randomised double blind phase II trial of carboplatin paclitaxel plus cediranib versus carboplatin-paclitaxel plus placebo in metastatic/recurrent cervical cancer. Ann Oncol. 2014;25 Suppl 4:LBA25-PR.

77. Diaz-Padilla I, Monk BJ, Mackay HJ, Oaknin A. Treatment of metastatic cervical cancer: Future directions involving targeted agents. Crit Rev Oncol Hematol. 2013;85:303–14.

# 15

# The role of immune checkpoint inhibition in the treatment of ovarian cancer

Stéphanie L. Gaillard[1]*, Angeles A. Secord[2] and Bradley Monk[3]

## Abstract

The introduction of immune checkpoint inhibitors has revolutionized treatment of multiple cancers and has bolstered interest in this treatment approach. So far, emerging clinical data show limited clinical efficacy of these agents in ovarian cancer with objective response rates of 10–15% with some durable responses. In this review, we present emerging clinical data of completed trials of immune checkpoint inhibitors and review ongoing studies. In addition we examine the current knowledge of the tumor microenvironment of ovarian cancers with a focus on the significance of PD-L1 expression and tumor-infiltrating lymphocytes on predicting response to immune checkpoint blockade. We evaluate approaches to improve treatment outcomes through the use of predictive biomarkers and patient selection. Finally, we review management considerations including immune related adverse events and response criteria.

**Keywords:** Ovarian cancer, Fallopian tube cancer, Primary peritoneal cancer, Immunotherapy, Immune checkpoint inhibitors, PD-1, PD-L1, CTLA-4

## Background

### Role of immune checkpoints and development of immune checkpoint inhibitors

Ovarian cancer is the most lethal of the gynecologic malignancies. Over 22,000 new cases of ovarian cancer are diagnosed each year in the United States resulting in greater than 14,000 deaths per year [1]. The five year survival rate is less than 25% for women diagnosed with advanced stage disease (stage III or IV) despite aggressive treatment with surgery and adjuvant chemotherapy. Although >80% of patients will have a response to initial therapy, epithelial ovarian cancer ultimately recurs in the majority of patients. Recurrence is associated with a poor prognosis because of the eventual development of chemotherapy-resistant disease. Thus there is a great need, and opportunity, to improve ovarian cancer outcomes by understanding the immune milieu of ovarian cancers and harnessing the power of immunotherapy. This review will focus on the current understanding of the immune microenvironment of ovarian cancers

and the potential role for immunotherapy in the treatment of this disease.

Immunotherapy refers to treatment designed to enhance an individual's own immune function to eradicate malignant cells. While there have been various approaches, from cancer vaccines to adoptive immune cell therapies, immune checkpoint inhibitors have caused a paradigm shift in cancer treatment. These therapies are now FDA-approved for a variety of cancers including melanoma, non-small cell lung cancer (NSCLC), renal cell carcinomas (RCC), bladder cancer, and classical Hodgkin lymphoma. The enthusiasm for this approach stems from evidence of complete and long-lasting tumor regression in malignancies that are often refractory to chemotherapy.

T-cell mediated cancer cell death requires the production of effector T-cells ($T_{eff}$) through the coordinated initiation of a multi-step process involving antigen presentation, priming and activation, T-cell trafficking and infiltration into the tumor, recognition of cancer cells, and cancer cell elimination [2]. This T-cell mediated immune response is regulated by a number of stimulatory and inhibitory signals. Inhibitory signals serve to prevent pathologic over-activation of the immune system, as an uncontrolled inflammatory response could result in the

---

* Correspondence: stephanie.gaillard@duke.edu
[1]Department of Medicine, Division of Medical Oncology, Duke Cancer Institute, 200 Trent Drive, Durham, NC 27710, USA
Full list of author information is available at the end of the article

development of autoimmune or inflammatory disorders. However, inhibition of the $T_{eff}$ response against cancer cells contributes to immune evasion. These inhibitory signals may come from extrinsic sources, such as regulatory T-cells ($T_{regs}$) and inhibitory cytokines, or intrinsic sources, such as immune checkpoint proteins expressed on the surface of $T_{eff}$. It is the balance of these signals that determines the success or failure of the immune system to eliminate cancer cells.

$T_{regs}$ play a critical role in the extrinsic suppression of anti-tumor immunity. When $T_{regs}$ are the dominant T-cell population in the tumor microenvironment, they inhibit tumor-antigen specific immunity and promote tumor growth. Depletion of these $T_{regs}$ can restore anti-tumor immune activity. Similarly, other suppressive immune cells [e.g. myeloid derived suppressor cells (MDSCs), M2 macrophages] influence the balance of regulatory signals.

Immune checkpoint receptors, such as cytotoxic T lymphocyte-associated protein 4 (CTLA-4) and programmed cell death protein 1 (PD-1), have emerged as critical intrinsic modulatory mechanisms impairing natural anti-neoplastic immunity (Fig. 1). These receptors are negative regulators which attenuate normal T-cell activation to prevent pathologic over-activation. Interfering with immune checkpoint signaling has been shown to enhance anti-tumor immune responses through the recovery of T-cell function. The CTLA-4 and PD-1 immune checkpoint proteins function at different points in the process, which may explain their differential activities and toxicities. The CTLA-4 immune checkpoint regulates T-cell priming and activation, activities that occur in the early phases of the immune response. Inhibition of CTLA-4 during the T-cell priming/ activation step leads to dysregulated expansion of auto-reactive T cells, including tumor-specific T-cells. Anti-CTLA-4 inhibitors have been associated with significant immune-related toxicities which are likely a result of the indiscriminate and unselected activation of auto-reactive T-cells.

PD-1 is a cell surface receptor that is upregulated during normal T-cell activation and modulates the activity of antigen-experienced effector T-cells. Interaction of PD-1 with either of its two known ligands, PD-L1 and PD-L2, results in inhibition of T-cell signaling and cytokine production as well as decreased effector T-cell numbers due to limited T-cell proliferation and increased susceptibility to apoptosis. Of the two ligands, PD-L1 appears to be the more relevant in the tumor microenvironment and is expressed on a wide range of tumor cells. Tumor-infiltrating lymphocytes can induce PD-L1 expression on tumor cells leading to reduced anti-tumor immunity [3]. PD-L1 expression may also be regulated through gene amplification or via oncogenic signaling pathways [4–6]. Antibodies directed at either PD-1 or PD-L1 result in abrogation of the negative signal, thus restoring T-cell function.

An important distinction between CTLA-4 and PD-1/ L1 inhibitors is their location of action [7]. Because CTLA-4 regulates T-cell priming and activation, anti-CTLA-4 antibodies lead to activation of T-cells in lymphoid peripheral tissues. Anti-PD-1/L1 effects appear to be limited to the tumor microenvironment without

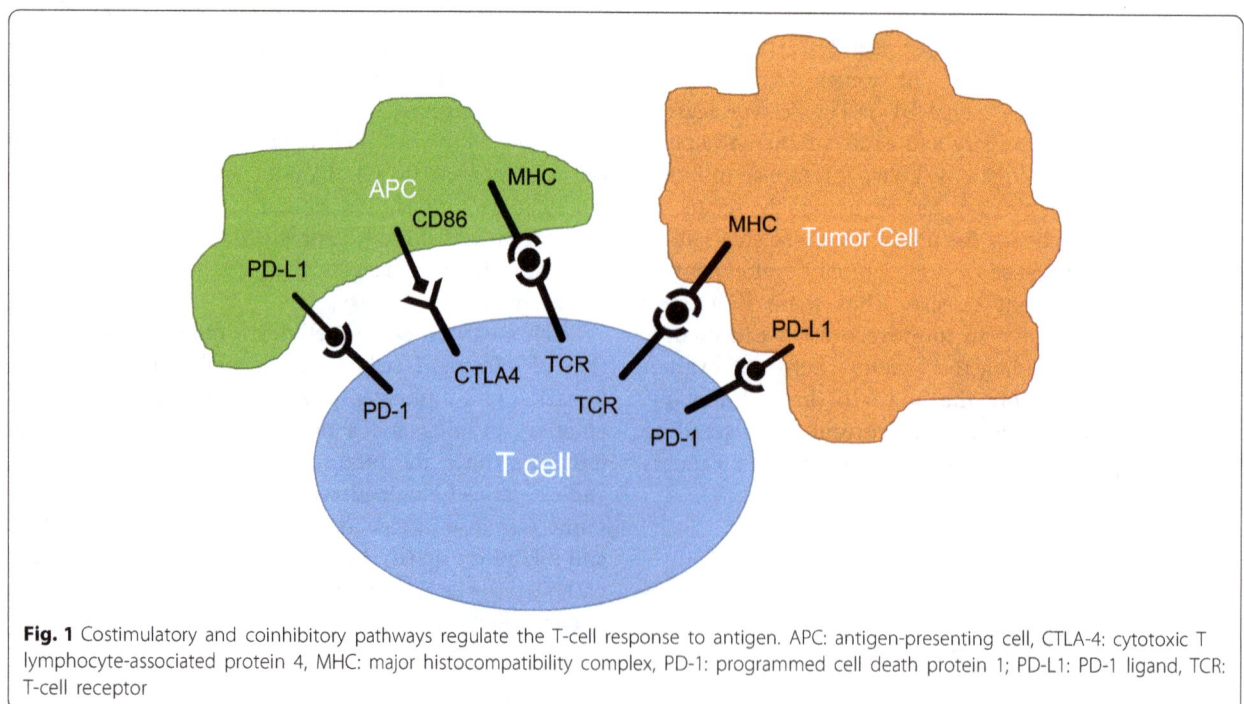

**Fig. 1** Costimulatory and coinhibitory pathways regulate the T-cell response to antigen. APC: antigen-presenting cell, CTLA-4: cytotoxic T lymphocyte-associated protein 4, MHC: major histocompatibility complex, PD-1: programmed cell death protein 1; PD-L1: PD-1 ligand, TCR: T-cell receptor

evidence of recirculation. Thus a number of pharmacodynamic markers for anti-CTLA-4 activity have been identified in the peripheral blood, whereas no biomarkers of PD-1 activity have been isolated from peripheral blood thus far.

### Evidence for using checkpoint inhibitors in ovarian cancer

Two central tenets have emerged to predict effective treatment with immune checkpoint inhibitors: 1) accessibility of the tumor by effector immune cells and 2) dominance of the immune checkpoint pathways as the mechanism suppressing anti-tumor immunity. The first is frequently defined by the presence of tumor-infiltrating lymphocytes or the ratio of effector immune cells [i.e. $T_{eff}$, dendritic cells (DCs), M1 macrophages] to immune suppressive immune cells [i.e. $T_{regs}$, myeloid derived suppressor cells (MDSCs), M2 macrophages]. The second principle is less well defined as no accurate biomarker has been identified, although multiple approaches are being evaluated. Expression of PD-L1 on tumor cells has been suggested as a predictive biomarker to identify cancers that may be more responsive to PD-1/PD-L1 inhibitors [8]. Based on work initially performed in melanomas, tumors have been classified into 4 groups based on the presence of tumor-infiltrating lymphocytes (TILs) and PD-L1 expression (Table 1) [3, 9]. Type I tumors exhibit a pattern of adaptive immune resistance and may be most likely to respond to immune checkpoint inhibitors. Conversely, Type II tumors show no discernable immune reaction and single agent checkpoint blockade is unlikely to be successful. Alternative approaches that include methods to recruit effector immune populations to the tumor (e.g. vaccines), possibly in combination with immune checkpoint inhibitors, are predicted to be necessary. Type III tumors exhibit intrinsic expression of PD-L1, possibly through oncogenic stimulation, with no immune reactivity. This highlights that tumor expression of PD-L1 alone cannot be used as an indicator of potential benefit of PD-1/L1 inhibition as without effector immune cells in the tumor, single agent immune checkpoint inhibition is unlikely to be beneficial. Similar to type II tumors, approaches to stimulate immune trafficking to the tumor will be necessary. Finally Type IV tumors display a pattern of tolerance to immune infiltration that is not dependent on PD-L1 expression. Thus, other suppressive signals are likely present and inhibition of other checkpoint receptors may be beneficial. Although this stratification system is based on studies in melanoma and presents several caveats (ref. [9]), it provides a framework for understanding the tumor microenvironment and rationale for the benefit of immune checkpoint inhibitors in ovarian cancer.

### Prognostic significance of ovarian cancer tumor microenvironment

Evidence of the importance of the local tumor immune microenvironment in ovarian cancer emerged in 2003 when Zhang et al. showed that infiltration of treatment naïve tumors with T-cells was associated with a significantly improved median progression free (22.4 vs 5.8 months, $p < 0.001$) and overall survival (50.3 vs 18.0 months, $p < 0.001$) compared to tumors with no T-cells present [10]. However, we have since learned that not only is presence of T cells important, but that the type of T-cell present influences outcomes. The proportion of $T_{regs}$ in the tumor negatively impacts clinical outcomes and was a predictor of increased risk of death in a multi-variate analysis [11, 12]. Multiple studies have since confirmed that the ratio of immune suppressive to effector immune infiltrates within ovarian tumors is associated with clinical outcome [13–17]. Immune responses to ovarian cancer appear to vary by histologic subtype with high-grade serous cancers most likely associated with a prognostically favorable tumor-infiltrating lymphocyte response [18, 19]. Classification of different histologic subtypes of ovarian cancers based on TIL and PD-L1 revealed that type I patterns were more common in high-grade serous cancers while type IV patterns predominated in other histologic subtypes (Table 2) [18].

### Expression of PD-L1 on ovarian cancer cells

Hamanishi and colleagues first reported that high expression of PD-L1 on ovarian cancer cells was associated with poorer outcomes [20]. The 5-year survival rate for patients with high- versus low-expressing PD-L1 tumors was $52.6 \pm 7.7\%$ versus $80.2 \pm 8.9\%$, $p = 0.016$, respectively. PD-L2 expression was also associated with poorer

**Table 1** Classification of tumors based on presence of tumor infiltrating lymphocytes (TIL) and PD-L1 expression (based on Teng et al. [9])

| Type I: Adaptive immune resistance TIL+ PD-L1+ | Type II: Immunological ignorance TIL- PD-L1- |
|---|---|
| Type III: Intrinsic induction TIL- PD-L1+ | Type IV: Tolerance TIL+ PD-L1- |

**Table 2** Classification of ovarian cancers by type of immune microenvironment (based on Webb et al. [18])

| Histologic subtype | N | % Total for histologic subtype | | | |
| | | Type I | Type II | Type III | Type IV |
|---|---|---|---|---|---|
| High-grade serous | 112 | 57.4 | 5.1 | 0 | 37.4 |
| Low-grade serous | 11 | 0 | 9.1 | 0 | 90.9 |
| Mucinous | 30 | 26.7 | 16.7 | 0 | 56.7 |
| Endometrioid | 125 | 22.4 | 14.4 | 1.6 | 61.6 |
| Clear cell | 129 | 16.2 | 30.2 | 0 | 53.5 |

outcomes but was not statistically significant. High expression of PD-L1 on ovarian cancer cells was associated with reduced infiltration of cytotoxic T lymphocytes into tumors suggesting that PD-L1 expression promotes an immunosuppressive microenvironment by inhibiting T-cell infiltration [20]. Both PD-L1 expression and TIL were independent prognostic factors, though PD-L1 expression was inversely correlated with survival. In pre-clinical models, PD-L1 expression can be induced by interferon-gamma (often produced by TILs) and administration of chemotherapy, suggesting a balance that maintains an immune suppressive environment [21, 22]. PD-1/L1 blockade causes regression of ovarian tumors in a syngeneic ovarian cancer mouse model further validating the importance of this regulatory pathway [23].

PD-L1 expression is not limited to tumor cells and has been reported on immune cells including antigen-presenting cells, T-cells, and B-cells. A recent study showed that PD-L1 expression is predominantly expressed by macrophages in ovarian cancer rather than on the ovarian cancer cells themselves; in this context, macrophage associated PD-L1 expression was a marker of favorable prognosis [18]. The differences between this study and the one above may be due to the differences in the antibodies used, but also reflect the developing understanding of PD-L1 expression and its prognostic role in ovarian cancer. PD-L1

expression may be a marker of a tumor poised to respond to immune stimulatory effects of chemotherapy or perhaps because PD-L1 may suppress the activity of immune-suppressive immune cells (i.e. $T_{regs}$), PD-L1 expression on immune cells could tip the balance towards a more favorable immune microenvironment [24]. Thus evaluating PD-L1 expression on tumor cells in isolation is not sufficient to predict immune response and efficacy of immune checkpoint blockade in ovarian cancer.

### Trials of immune checkpoint inhibitors in ovarian cancer

Several antibodies directed against PD-1, PD-L1, and CTLA-4 have been developed and are being tested clinically in patients with ovarian cancer. Table 3 reflects the latest data from studies that have reported outcomes. Table 4 shows ongoing ovarian cancer trials with immune checkpoint inhibitors as monotherapy or combined with other agents. The schema for ongoing or planned phase 3 studies are shown in Fig. 2.

### Nivolumab

Nivolumab is a fully humanized IgG4 monoclonal antibody targeting the PD-1 receptor and is FDA approved for the treatment of melanoma, NSCLC, renal cell carcinoma, and Hodgkin's lymphoma. A study of nivolumab in recurrent ovarian cancer was the first to be published

**Table 3** Studies of immune checkpoint inhibitors in ovarian cancer with reported results

| Immunotherapy agent(s) | Trial number | Disease status | Phase | N | Results (N; duration) | G3/4 adverse events | Reference |
|---|---|---|---|---|---|---|---|
| Ipilimumab | | recurrent EOC, previously treated with GVAX vaccine | I | 9 | PR (1; 35+ mos.) SD (3; 1 for 6+ mos.) | diarrhea | Hodi et al. [50] |
| BMS-936559 (anti-PD-L1) | NCT00729664 | recurrent EOC | I | 17 | 6% PR (1; 1.3+ mos.) 18% SD (3; 6+ mos.) | infusion-related reaction, adrenal insufficiency | Brahmer et al. [80] |
| Nivolumab | | platinum resistant EOC | II | 20 | 10% CR (2; 11+ mos.) 5% PR (1; 11+ mos.) 30% SD (6; 1 for 11+ mos.) | lymphocytopenia, hypoalbuminemia, elevated ALT, rash, fever, anemia | Hamanishi et al. [25] |
| Pembrolizumab | NCT02054806 | recurrent EOC, PD-L1 positive | Ib | 26 | 4% CR (1; 6+ mos.) 8% PR (2; 6+ mos.) 23% SD (8; 2 for 6+ mos.) | transaminitis | Varga et al. [26] |
| Ipilimumab | NCT01611558 | recurrent EOC | II | 40 | 10% BRR (4; NA) | NA | clinicaltrials.gov [27] |
| Avelumab | NCT01772004 | recurrent EOC | Ib | 124 | 10% PR (12; 4 for 6+ mos.) 44% SD (55; NA) | rash, edema, elevated amylase/lipase, arthritis, colitis, hyperglycemia/DM | Disis et al. [28] |
| Durvalumab + Olaparib | NCT02484404[a] | recurrent EOC | I/II | 10 | PR (1; 11+ mos.) SD (7; 4+ mos.) | Lymphopenia, anemia | Lee et al. [29] |
| Durvalumab + Cediranib | | | | 4 | PR (1; 7 mos.) SD (2; 1 for 6 mos.) | Lymphopenia, anemia, nausea, diarrhea, hypertension, PE, pulmonary hypertension, fatigue, headache | |

*Abbreviations: N* number of ovarian cancer patients treated, *EOC* epithelial ovarian cancer, *CR* complete response, *PR* partial response, *SD* stable disease, *ALT* alanine aminotransferase, *BRR* best response rate (CR/PR status not provided), *mos.* months, *NA* not available, *DM* diabetes mellitus; *PE,* pulmonary embolism
[a]As of data cut-off date: May 10, 2016

**Table 4** Ongoing studies of immune checkpoint inhibitors in ovarian cancer

| Phase | Trial number | Trial | Disease status | Immunotherapy agent(s) | Concurrent therapy |
|---|---|---|---|---|---|
| 3 | NCT02580058 | A Study Of Avelumab Alone Or In Combination With Pegylated Liposomal Doxorubicin Versus Pegylated Liposomal Doxorubicin Alone In Patients With Platinum Resistant/Refractory Ovarian Cancer (JAVELIN Ovarian 200) | recurrent platinum resistant | Avelumab | Liposomal Doxorubicin |
| 3 | NCT02718417 | Avelumab in Previously Untreated Patients With Epithelial Ovarian Cancer (JAVELIN OVARIAN 100) | primary | Avelumab | Carboplatin Paclitaxel |
| 3 | ENGOT-ov29-GCIG | A randomized, double-blinded, phase III study of atezolizumab versus placebo in patients with late relapse of epithelial ovarian, fallopian tube, or peritoneal cancer treated by platinum-based chemotherapy and bevacizumab | recurrent platinum sensitive | Atezolizumab | Carboplatin-based chemotherapy Bevacizumab |
| 2 | NCT02440425 | Dose Dense Paclitaxel With Pembrolizumab (MK-3475) in Platinum Resistant Ovarian Cancer | recurrent platinum resistant | Pembrolizumab | Dose Dense Paclitaxel |
| 2 | NCT02498600 | Nivolumab With or Without Ipilimumab in Treating Patients With Persistent or Recurrent Epithelial Ovarian, Primary Peritoneal, or Fallopian Tube Cancer | recurrent platinum sensitive/resistant | Nivolumab +/- Ipilimumab | |
| 2 | NCT02520154 | Pembrolizumab in Combination With Chemotherapy in Frontline Ovarian Cancer | primary | Pembrolizumab | Carboplatin Paclitaxel |
| 2 | NCT02659384 | Anti-programmed Cell Death-1 Ligand 1 (aPDL-1) Antibody Atezolizumab, Bevacizumab and Acetylsalicylic Acid in Recurrent Platinum Resistant Ovarian Cancer | recurrent platinum resistant | Atezolizumab | Bevacizumab Acetylsalicylic Acid |
| 2 | NCT02674061 | Efficacy and Safety Study of Pembrolizumab (MK-3475) in Women With Advanced Recurrent Ovarian Cancer (MK-3475-100/KEYNOTE-100) | recurrent platinum sensitive/resistant | Pembrolizumab | |
| 2 | NCT02764333 | TPIV200/huFR-1 (A Multi-Epitope Anti-Folate Receptor Vaccine) Plus Anti-PD-L1 MEDI4736 (Durvalumab) in Patients With Platinum Resistant Ovarian Cancer | recurrent platinum resistant | Durvalumab | TPIV200/huFR-1 (anti-folate receptor vaccine) |
| 2 | NCT02766582 | Phase II: Pembrolizumab/Carboplatin/Taxol in Epithelial Ovary Cancer | suboptimally cytoreduced primary | Pembrolizumab | Carboplatin Paclitaxel |
| 1/2 | NCT02431559 | A Phase 1/2 Study of Motolimod (VTX-2337) and MEDI4736 in Subjects With Recurrent, Platinum-Resistant Ovarian Cancer for Whom Pegylated Liposomal Doxorubicin (PLD) is Indicated | recurrent platinum resistant | Durvalumab | Motolimod Pegylated Liposomal Doxorubicin |
| 1/2 | NCT02484404 | Phase 1 and 2 Study of MEDI4736 in Combination With Olaparib or Cediranib for Advanced Solid Tumors and Recurrent Ovarian Cancer | recurrent platinum sensitive/resistant | Durvalumab | Olaparib or Cediranib |
| 1/2 | NCT02485990 | Study of Tremelimumab Alone or Combined With Olaparib for Patients With Persistent EOC (Epithelial Ovarian, Fallopian Tube or Primary Peritoneal Carcinoma) | recurrent or persistent | Tremelimumab | Olaparib |
| 1/2 | NCT02571725 | PARP-inhibition and CTLA-4 Blockade in BRCA-deficient Ovarian Cancer | BRCA-deficient recurrent platinum sensitive/resistant | Tremelimumab | Olaparib |
| 1/2 | NCT02657889 | Study of Niraparib in Combination With Pembrolizumab (MK-3475) in Patients With Triple-negative Breast Cancer or Ovarian Cancer (KEYNOTE-162) | recurrent platinum resistant | Pembrolizumab | Niraparib |
| 1/2 | NCT02726997 | Matched Paired Pharmacodynamics and Feasibility Study of Durvalumab in Combination With Chemotherapy in Frontline Ovarian Cancer | primary | Durvalumab | Carboplatin Paclitaxel |
| 1 | NCT02737787 | A Study of WT1 Vaccine and Nivolumab For Recurrent Ovarian Cancer | ≥2nd remission | Nivolumab | WT1 vaccine |
| 0 | NCT02728830 | A Study of Pembrolizumab on the Tumoral Immunoprofile of Gynecologic Cancers | primary | Pembrolizumab | |

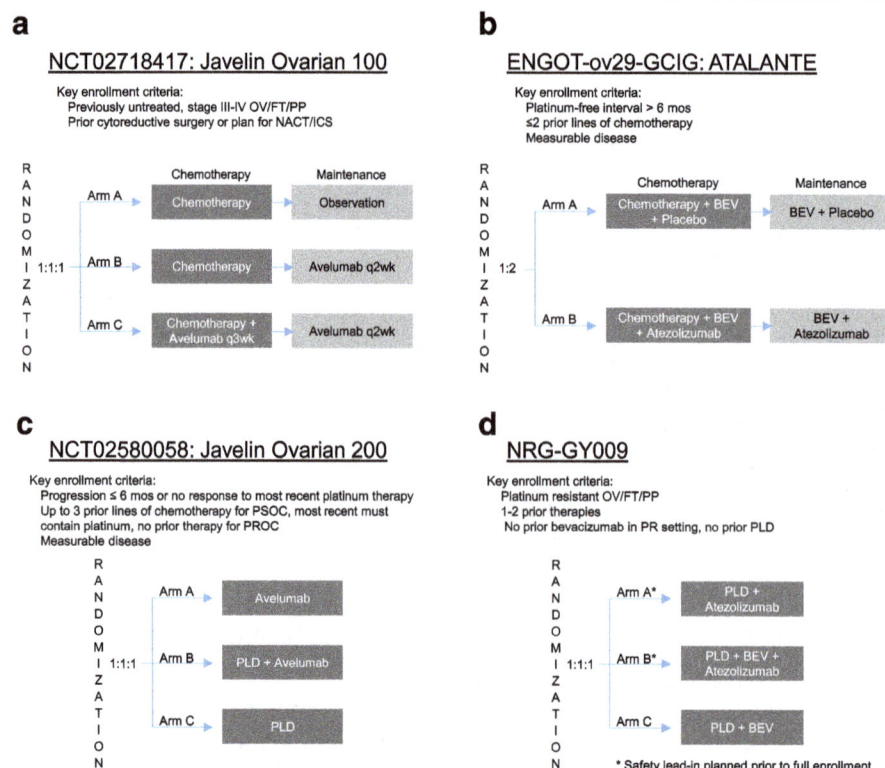

**Fig. 2** Ongoing or planned phase 3 trials in ovarian cancer with immune checkpoint inhibitors. **a** NCT02718417: Javelin Ovarian 100. **b** ENGOT-ov29-GCIG: ATALANTE. **c** NCT02580058: Javelin Ovarian 200. **d** NRG-GY009

for this patient population [25]. In this study 20 patients with platinum-resistant ovarian cancer were treated in 2 cohorts either with 1 or 3 mg/kg nivolumab every 2 weeks until progression or up to 48 weeks. Best overall response was the primary endpoint. Grade 3 or 4 adverse events occurred in 8 patients (20%) and two experienced severe adverse events (grade 3 disorientation, gait disorder, fever in 1 patient and grade 3 fever, deep venous thrombosis in the other). The best overall response was 15%. Four patients experienced prolonged disease control (2 patients in each dose cohort) with 2 patients in the 3 mg/kg cohort experiencing a durable complete response (CR). While response rates were similar to what has been seen with chemotherapy in platinum resistant disease, the durable responses are atypical in this disease and a cause for enthusiasm particularly in a very heavily pre-treated population. PD-L1 expression did not significantly correlate with objective response. Fourteen of 16 patients with PD-L1 high expression did not show a response while 1 of 4 patients with low expression was a responder.

### Pembrolizumab

Pembrolizumab is an anti-PD-1 humanized IgG4 monoclonal antibody FDA-approved for the treatment of melanoma and NSCLC. A non-randomized, multicohort phase Ib study (KEYNOTE-028, NCT02054806) was conducted of single-agent pembrolizumab in ovarian cancer patients [26]. Eligibility requirements included expression of PD-L1 in 1% of tumor nests or PD-L1 expression in stroma. Pembrolizumab 10 mg/kg was given every 2 weeks until progression, intolerable adverse effects or for up to 2 years. Twenty-six patients were treated. Objective response rate was 11.5% with 1 CR, 2 partial responses (PR), and 23% stable disease (SD). Durable responses were noted and the median time to response was 8 weeks.

### Ipilimumab

Ipilimumab is a recombinant, IgG1 human monoclonal antibody targeting CTLA-4 that is FDA-approved for the treatment of melanoma. In a phase II study of ipilimumab monotherapy in recurrent platinum-sensitive ovarian cancer (NCT01611558), 40 patients were treated with 10 mg/kg ipilimumab every 3 weeks x 4 doses (induction phase) followed by 10 mg/kg every 12 weeks until progression or unacceptable toxicity [27]. Of the 40 who started the study, 38 (95%) did not complete the induction phase because of disease progression (14, 35%), drug toxicity (17, 42.5%), death (1, 2.5%), or other/unreported (6, 15%). Twenty patients (50%) experienced drug-related adverse events of grade 3 or higher. The objective response rate (ORR) was 10.3% [95% confidence interval (CI) 2.9 to 34.2%] by RECIST criteria. Of note, the 10 mg/kg dose is higher than the FDA approved dose for the treatment of unresectable or metastatic melanoma (3 mg/kg) but is equivalent to the dose used for the adjuvant treatment of melanoma.

### Avelumab

Avelumab is a fully humanized monoclonal anti-PD-L1 IgG1 antibody that does not block PD-1 interaction with PD-L2. In a Phase Ib (NCT01772004, Javelin solid tumor study) [28], 124 patients with refractory or recurrent ovarian cancer (progression within 6 months, or after $2^{nd}/3^{rd}$ line treatment) were treated with 10 mg/kg every 2 weeks until progression or unacceptable toxicity. The median duration of treatment was 12 weeks. Grade 3/4 adverse events occurred in 6.4% of patients and 8.1% of patients discontinued treatment secondary to an adverse event. Twelve patients experienced a partial response for an ORR of 9.7%. Disease control rate (DCR, defined as ORR + SD) was 54%. ORR was 12.3% in PD-L1+ tumors and 5.9% in PD-L1- tumors (based on > =1% threshold). Differences in median PFS and OS were not statistically significant based on PD-L1 expression. There are currently two Phase 3 trials of avelumab for ovarian cancer; one for front-line therapy in combination with carboplatin and paclitaxel (Javelin ovarian 100) and the other for recurrent platinum-resistant disease (Javelin ovarian 200) (Fig. 2).

### Durvalumab

Durvalumab is an Fc optimized IgG1 monoclonal antibody directed against PD-L1, recently given breakthrough therapy designation by the FDA for PD-L1 positive urothelial bladder cancer. In an ongoing phase I/II study of durvalumab (NCT02484404) in combination with either the PARP inhibitor, olaparib, or the VEGFR inhibitor, cediranib, there was 1 PR in 9 evaluable ovarian cancer patients lasting >6 months with the combination of durvalumab and olaparib and 1 PR in 5 evaluable ovarian cancer patients treated with durvalumab and cediranib [29].

### Other immune checkpoint inhibitors

Atezolizumab is an Fc-engineered, humanized, non-glycosylated IgG1 kappa monoclonal antibody targeting PD-L1 that is FDA-approved for the treatment of bladder/urothelial carcinomas. Tremelilumab is a fully humanized antibody against CTLA-4. To date no studies have reported outcomes for patients with ovarian cancer treated with atezolizumab or tremelilumab.

Although cross trial comparisons are not feasible given the early stage of development and different trial eligibility parameters, it is remarkable that all of the studies so far have similar ORR (10–15%). This is markedly lower than was seen in early trials of PD-1 inhibitors for

Hodgkin's lymphoma where >65% of patients had a response to treatment and 17–21% achieved a complete response [30, 31], but more consistent with response rates in previously treated patients with melanoma (28%), NSCLC (18%), and renal cell carcinoma (27%) [32]. The phase Ib avelumab study suggests that ovarian cancer patients who have been treated with fewer prior courses of chemotherapy may have a greater benefit from these agents, thus chemotherapy may induce T-cell exhaustion or have other irreversible immunosuppressive effects [33].

Combining the nivolumab and avelumab studies cited above, it is notable that 4 of the 5 patients who experienced durable responses had tumors with clear cell histology [25, 28]. Histology of responding patients on other studies has not been reported. These observations run counter to the prediction that ovarian cancers with clear cell histology would be less likely to respond to PD-1 inhibitors based on low PD-1 expression and low TIL infiltration (Table 2). However, they are particularly intriguing given the characteristic chemorefractory nature of ovarian clear cell carcinomas (OCCC) [34, 35]. Because OCCC are genomically remarkably similar to RCC, it has been postulated that therapies effective for RCC may be similarly effective for OCCC [36]. Nivolumab was recently approved for the treatment of advanced RCC based on the phase III CheckMate 025 trial in which nivolumab showed an ORR of 25% and a 5 month OS benefit over everolimus (ORR 5%) [37]. Whether immune checkpoint inhibitors will result in such dramatic benefits in OCCC remains to be determined in larger cohorts.

## Opportunities to improve outcomes with immune checkpoint inhibitors
### Identification of predictive biomarkers

A critical need in this field is the development of biomarkers that can predict response to therapy, provide early indication of efficacy, and warn of the development of adverse effects. The most promising have focused on prediction of response to PD-1/L1 therapy. Indications in melanoma trials that tumor PD-L1 expression, density of TILs, and proportion of T cells expressing PD-1 or PD-L1 was associated with response led to the categorization schema outline above in an attempt to identify subsets of melanoma patients who would be most likely to respond to treatment (Table 1) [3, 9]. Further validation is still necessary to determine whether this categorization predicts better outcomes. Individually none of these factors is a reliable predictor of response.

### PD-L1 expression and TILs

Several studies of anti-PD-1/L1 therapeutic antibodies in multiple tumor types, including melanoma and NSCLC, have suggested that PD-L1 expression is associated with a greater likelihood of benefit [8, 32, 38–40]. These studies typically categorized tumors as PD-L1 positive if at least 5% of tumor cells showed cell-surface PD-L1 staining. While initial studies suggested that PD-L1 negative tumors did not show response [32, 38], subsequent studies in multiple tumor types have shown objective responses in up to 20% of PD-L1 negative tumors [39, 41, 42]. In comparison, the phase 2 nivolumab study in ovarian cancer patients showed that only 2 of 16 patients with high PD-L1 expression showed a response, while 1 of 4 patients with low expression responded [25]. Similarly, the avelumab study showed that even with a staining cut-off level of ≥1% of tumor cells in ovarian cancer, 1 of 17 patients with a PD-L1 negative tumor showed an objective response [28]. Thus, it is unclear whether PD-L1 can be used reliably as a predictive biomarker for anti-PD-1/L1 directed therapy. By contrast, PD-L1 expression status does not appear to influence response to anti-CTLA-4 therapy. In a study of previously untreated melanoma, median PFS (mPFS) in response to ipilimumab was unaffected by PD-L1 status (PD-L1 positive 3.9 months, 95% CI 2.8 to 4.2 months versus PD-L1 negative 2.8 months, 95% CI 2.8 to 3.1 months) while response to nivolumab was influenced by PD-L1 status (14.0 months, 95% CI 9.1 to not reached versus 5.3 months, 95% CI 2.8 to 7.1 in PD-L1 positive versus PD-L1 negative tumors, respectively) [43].

Other attempts at identifying predictive biomarkers have focused on T-cell infiltration. In melanoma, T-cell density, particularly at the invasive tumor border, has been associated with response to anti-PD-1 therapy, however tumors with low T cell density have also shown response [44]. However, a separate study evaluating factors associated with response to anti-PD-1 therapy in multiple solid tumors treated on a phase I clinical trial showed that the presence of TILs did not correlate with clinical outcomes [8]. Response to anti-CTLA-4 therapy has been associated with a more inflamed tumor microenvironment and potential markers include increased expression of the activation marker, inducible T-cell co-stimulator (ICOS), on peripheral blood CD4+ cells and tumor-infiltrating lymphocytes, and an increase in Teff:-Treg cell ratio in tumor tissues [45–50]. However no validated predictive biomarkers for CTLA-4 therapy are yet available.

Several factors may account for the difficulty in using receptor expression and T-cell populations as predictive biomarkers. PD-L1 expression and T-cell infiltration are dynamic processes so evaluation of tissue archived at the time of surgery may not reflect the level of expression at the time of recurrence or planned treatment. Small tumor specimens may miss focal expression of PD-L1 or T-cells localized only at the leading edge of the tumor. Scoring of immunohistochemistry for PD-L1 and TILs has not yet been standardized. Additionally, there are challenges associated with the use of different antibodies, fixation and staining techniques, and the subjective interpretation of staining thresholds. Added to this complexity is defining the importance of the subset of cells (immune versus tumor) upon which PD-L1 is expressed. At this point, there is no indication that PD-L1 expression or TIL by IHC should be used as an absolute selection criterion for therapy.

### Mutational load

Genetic alterations within a tumor (including mutations, DNA rearrangements, deletions, and insertions) have the potential to generate neo-antigens which are associated with clinical response to immune checkpoint therapies. Tumors with higher mutational loads, such as melanoma, NSCLC, and bladder cancer, have shown the greatest response rates to anti-PD-1/PD-L1 therapy, while cancers with relatively low mutation rates (pancreatic and prostate cancers) have shown low response to these therapies [51]. In melanoma, mutational load was associated with the degree of clinical benefit to CTLA-4 blockade and pembrolizumab [52–54]. However, there are patients with low mutational burden who have responded and those with high mutational burden that have not and no specific cut-off point could be determined under which patients would not derive benefit [54].

Mismatched repair (MMR) deficiency, defined by defects in one or more of 6 genes involved in the DNA mismatch repair complex, results in 10–100 fold increases in tumor mutational burden compared to MMR-competent tumors. MSI tumors express high levels of multiple immune checkpoint molecules including PD-1, PD-L1, CTLA-4 and lymphocyte activation gene 3 (LAG3) [55]. Le et al. showed that MSI-high status in colorectal cancer and mismatch-repair deficient non-colorectal cancers was able to predict clinical response to pembrolizumab in a phase 2 trial [56, 57]. There was an ORR of 48% across tumor histologies with 12 month OS and PFS rates of 79 and 54%, respectively. Germline MMR gene inactivation only occurs in ~2% of ovarian cancers, however somatic loss of expression can occur in up to 29% of ovarian cancers [58]. Whether microsatellite instability status (MSI) status may be a predictive biomarker to identify genetic subsets of ovarian tumors with an improved likelihood of response to immune checkpoint inhibition remains to be determined.

In non-MMR deficient ovarian cancers, the predominant genetic abnormality is copy number alteration and mutation rate is generally low [59]. Despite relatively low mutation burdens compared to other cancers, increased neo-antigen presentation may result from other genetic alterations. Patients with BRCA-associated tumors may be more likely to have a higher burden of genetic alterations (copy number alterations, deletions, amplifications) given the role of BRCA in homologous recombination DNA repair [60]. BRCA1-associated ovarian cancers have also been associated with increased intra-tumoral T-cell infiltration [61]. Thus it has been suggested that these patients may derive greater benefit from immune checkpoint inhibitors. Contrary to this hypothesis, no responses were seen in patients with a BRCA mutation in the avelumab phase Ib study (ORR 16% in BRCA-wildtype tumors), DCR was 11.1% in BRCA-mutation carriers versus 48.0% in BRCA-wildtype [28]. Thus at this time, there is no reason to suggest that immunotherapy trials should be limited to this patient population, beyond the stated objective of the study.

### Functional assays

Other approaches to developing predictive biomarkers include assessing functional capacity of the immune cells within the tumor microenvironment. These approaches include intracellular cytokine staining to measure interferon-gamma signaling and T-cell polyfunctionality, measurement of local inhibitory cytokine production (IL-10, TGF-beta), measurement of T-cell activation or proliferation potential, and T-cell clonality/repertoire [62–69]. However, as of yet, none of these approaches has been validated to be predictive of response to therapy.

### Combinatorial therapy to improve therapeutic outcomes

Improved therapeutic efficacy has been demonstrated with the combination of anti-PD-1 and anti-CTLA-4 inhibitors. In previously untreated melanoma patients, median PFS was 11.5 months (95% CI 8.9–16.7 months) with nivolumab and ipilimumab compared with 2.9 months (95% CI 2.8–3.4) with ipilimumab and 6.9 months (95% CI 4.3 to 9.5) with nivolumab alone [43]. Interestingly, in patients whose tumors did not express PD-1, median PFS was improved in patients receiving both drugs compared to those who received nivolumab alone; there was no difference in median PFS between these two treatment groups in patients with PD-1 expressing tumors. The frequency of treatment related toxicities was also increased with combination therapy; 55% of patients experienced grade 3/4 events in the nivolumab and ipilimumab group, 16.3% in the nivolumab group, and 27.3% in the ipilimumab group. In mouse models of ovarian cancer, 1/3 to 1/2 of TILs coexpressed PD-1 and CTLA-4 [70]. This subpopulation exhibited poor effector functions with diminished capacity to secrete effector cytokines and proliferate. Dual blockade of PD-1 and CTLA-4 increased T-cell activity and tumor regression. This treatment strategy is currently being evaluated for recurrent ovarian cancer in the NRG Oncology study GY003 (NCT02498600).

Similarly, combining immune checkpoint inhibitors with other anti-neoplastic treatments to enhance therapeutic outcomes is an active area of investigation (see Table 4 for trials for ovarian cancer). Chemotherapy, radiotherapy, tyrosine kinase inhibitors, and epigenetic modulators may be synergistic adjuncts to immunotherapy through their ability to increase tumor immunogenicity [71–74]. A particular area of interest for ovarian cancer is the combination of immune checkpoint inhibitors with anti-angiogenic agents and/or PARP inhibitors. Both anti-angiogenic agents and PARP inhibitors influence the ovarian cancer immune microenvironment in in vivo models and combination therapy is supported by preclinical studies [75–78]. Clinical trials of combination therapy are ongoing, so far phase I results of durvalumab/cediranib and durvalumab/olaparib (NCT02484404) show the combinations are feasible. It will be necessary to develop individualized approaches to determine which treatment strategy is most likely to be effective for individual patients.

## Management considerations with immune checkpoint inhibitors

### Immune-related toxicities

Related to their mechanism of action of impairing T-cell inhibition, immune checkpoint inhibitors can cause a loss of self-tolerance and thus the development of immune-related adverse effects (irAEs). While the frequency of irAEs with these agents is common (~60% with anti-CTLA-4 therapy and 40% with anti-PD-1/L1 therapy), in general serious toxicity [grade 3–5 using the Common Terminology Criteria for Adverse Events (CTCAE)] is more likely with anti-CTLA-4 therapy (>40%) than with anti-PD-1/L1 therapy (~5%) [32, 79, 80]. While the immune side effects could involve any organ system, the most common irAEs with both anti-CTLA-4 and anti-PD-1/L1 therapy are dermatologic (rash, pruritis), gastrointestinal (diarrhea), rheumatologic (arthralgia, arthritis, myalgia, myositis), endocrine disorders (thyroiditis, hypothyroidism, hypophysitis), and infusion-related reactions. Serious gastrointestinal toxicities, such as immune-mediated colitis and hepatitis, are more likely with anti-CTLA-4 therapy. Involvement of the following organ systems is much less common, especially with anti-PD-1/L1 pathways inhibitors, but have been observed including: pulmonary (pneumonitis, sarcoidosis), hematologic (hemolytic anemia, aplastic anemia, neutropenia), ocular (uveitis, conjunctivitis), cardiac (myocarditis, pericarditis), neurologic (myasthenia gravis, Guillan Barre, Bell's palsy, posterior reversible leukoencephalopathy, and aseptic meningitis). While irAEs associated with these therapies are generally reversible, without prompt management they can evolve into life-threatening conditions. Early recognition of the development of these events is critical to prevention of the progression to severe adverse effects. Vigilance, both on the part of the patient and the treating physician, is necessary to identify subtle developing signs of irAEs and specialty consultation may be necessary when irAEs are suspected but not definitive. Immune-related AEs can develop at any time during treatment and even after discontinuation of therapy. However, the onset of irAEs follows a characteristic pattern of development. For the CTLA-4 inhibitor, ipilimumab, most irAEs develop during the initial induction period (usually 4 doses given every 3 weeks). Dermatologic reactions more commonly occur early during treatment, frequently during the first few weeks, while diarrhea and colitis develop later. Endocrine disorders may be late effects, frequently developing between 7 and 20 weeks after initiation of treatment and sometimes being identified after discontinuation of treatment [81]. Combining CTLA-4 inhibitor and PD-1 inhibitors, while significantly increasing response also results in substantially more irAEs.

Spain et al. recently provided a substantive review of the management of irAEs [82]. Briefly, management is dependent on the severity of the event, usually graded using CTCAE. All references to grade in this article will be using CTCAE version 4.0 [83]. Typically grade 1 symptoms can be monitored and may not require interruption of therapy. For Grade 2 symptoms, the immune checkpoint inhibitor therapy should be withheld until symptoms improve and treatment with an immunomodulatory medication may be considered. Immune-related AEs with a higher risk of resulting in serious organ dysfunction (such as colitis, hepatitis, pneumonitis, nephritis, neurologic symptoms) likely warrant initiation of corticosteroid treatment early (Grade 2) rather than waiting for symptoms to worsen. When the severity of the irAE warrants the reversal of inflammation (≥ Grade 3), corticosteroids are the first immunomodulatory medication to be administered. Careful and timely monitoring of response to steroid therapy is required to identify steroid-refractory cases. In these situations, the use of more potent immunomodulatory agents may be necessary such as the anti-TNF-alpha antibody infliximab, the anti-metabolite mycophenylate mofetil, anti-thymocyte globulin, and/or calcineurin inhibitors (i.e. tacrolimus and cyclosporine). Consultation with, and if indicated hospitalization at, a center familiar with steroid-refractory immune checkpoint inhibitor irAEs is advised.

### Steroid use during treatment

Because of the effect of steroids on inhibiting T-cell activation, patients receiving supraphysiologic doses of corticosteroids have generally been excluded from trials of immune checkpoint inhibitors. In the most comprehensive retrospective review on the subject, Horvat et al. evaluated the effect of initiation of immunomodulatory agents for ipilimumab irAEs in melanoma patients [84]. Of the 298 patients, 85% experienced an irAE of any grade, 35% required corticosteroid treatment, and 10% required anti-TNFalpha therapy. Overall survival and time to treatment failure (median 5.7 months) was not affected by the occurrence of irAEs or the use of systemic corticosteroids. Continued anti-tumor activity has been observed in patients treated with high-dose steroids for irAEs [85]. However, data on the effects of steroid use on immune checkpoint inhibitor efficacy are still limited. Thus, it is recommended to avoid prophylactic steroids and limit therapeutic steroids as needed.

### Measurement of response: specific immune related criteria

One of the challenges faced in assessing the therapeutic value of these agents is determining the most appropriate measurement of efficacy. While response rates to immune checkpoint inhibitors as single agents is relatively low, the impressive duration in responding patients suggests that overall survival may be a better measure of efficacy. In fact, there have been patients who achieve long-term survival benefit without evidence of clinical response [53]. In addition, early studies noted that some patients had responses after initial apparent progression of disease, while others showed a mixed response or new lesions despite an overall decrease in tumor burden. Since these response patterns were not adequately captured by RECIST1.1, new immune-related response criteria (irRC) were developed to specifically accommodate the response patterns seen after treatment with immune checkpoint inhibitors [86]. Unlike in RECIST1.1, new lesions do not automatically signal progression and apparent progressive disease must be confirmed 4 weeks after initial assessment to qualify for true progression. In melanoma patients treated with either ipilimumab or pembrolizumab, 'pseudoprogression' occurred in ~ 7% of patients and has been attributed to peritumoral lymphocyte infiltration or delayed immune activity [87–89]. RECIST1.1 was noted to underestimate the benefit of pembrolizumab in this population by up to 15% [88]. However, because this phenomenon occurs relatively infrequently, many studies continue to use RECIST1.1. In order to adequately assess efficacy across studies, it will be necessary to harmonize response assessments across studies and identify more refined radiographic or biologic markers of early efficacy. In addition, the development of other immune-specific clinical trial endpoints may be necessary to account for prolonged duration of response after initial progression [90].

Rates of pseudoprogression in ovarian cancer have not been reported, but trials to date suggest it occurs less frequently than in melanoma [25, 26, 28]. Thus, in contrast to the management of melanoma, progression by

RECIST1.1 is likely true tumor progression. While treatment beyond progression is sometimes considered in melanoma patients until true progression is confirmed, further treatment after progression in ovarian cancer patients may carry additional risks as peritoneal implants could progress to cause bowel obstruction.

## Conclusions

The advent of immune checkpoint inhibitors has stimulated increased enthusiasm for immune-oncology. In ovarian cancer, while there is compelling data that the immune microenvironment influences outcomes, early results of clinical trials of immune checkpoint inhibitors suggest limited tumor response. Strategies to improve treatment outcomes and minimize immune-related toxicities are necessary and will likely require individualized approaches. There are multiple areas in which the cancer-immune system interaction can fail to result in adequate anti-tumor activity. To better understand these areas, the development of biomarkers to determine those therapies active in an individual tumors, so called 'personalized immunotherapy', are critical. Some have suggested the use of the "cancer immunogram" to describe individual tumor:-immune system interactions [91]. Biomarker guided clinical trials will be necessary to tailor these approaches to ovarian cancer patients. We anticipate that tumor genomic profiling will need to be integrated with immune profiling to provide a more comprehensive understanding of an individual patient's tumor leading to improved treatment selection and sequencing.

## Abbreviations
APC: Antigen presenting cell; CI: Confidence interval; CTCAE: Common Terminology Criteria for Adverse Events; CTLA-4: Cytotoxic T lymphocyte-associated protein 4; DC: Dendritic cell; Ig: Immunoglobulin; IL-10: Interleukin 10; irAE: Immune-related adverse event; irRC: Immune-related response criteria; LAG3: Lymphocyte activation gene 3; MDSC: Myeloid derived suppressor cell; MHC: Major histocompatibility complex; MMR: Mismatched repair; mPFS: Median PFS; MSI: Microsatellite instability; NSCLC: Non-small cell lung cancer; OCCC: Ovarian clear cell carcinoma; ORR: Objective response rate; OS: Overall survival; PD-1: Programmed cell death protein 1; PD-L1: PD-1 ligand 1; PD-L2: PD-1 ligand 2; PFS: Progression free survival; RCC: Renal cell carcinoma; RECIST: Response evaluation criteria in solid tumors; $T_{eff}$: Effector T cells; TGFbeta: Transforming growth factor beta; TIL: Tumor-infiltrating lymphocytes; TNFalpha: Tumor necrosis factor alpha; $T_{regs}$: Regulatory T cells

## Acknowledgements
The authors are grateful to Drs. Brittany Davidson, Alexandra Snyder Charen, and Kent Weinhold for their editorial expertise and review of this manuscript.

## Funding
This work was supported in part by the NIH Building Interdisciplinary Research Careers in Women's Health Program (K12 to S.L.G., Grant# 5K12HD043446-14) and the Ovarian Cancer Research Fund (2013 Liz Tilberis Grant, #258779 to S.L.G.).

## Authors' contributions
All authors were involved in the conception, design, drafting, revision, and approved the final manuscript.

## Competing interests
S.L.G. has received research funding from Bristol-Myers Squibb, Gradalis, Merck, PharmaMar, and Tetralogic, and has participated on advisory boards for Genentech and Pfizer. A.A.S. has received research funding from Amgen, Astellas Pharma, Astex Pharmaceuticals, AstraZeneca, Boehringer Ingelheim, Bristol-Myers Squibb, Eisai, Endocyte, Exelixis, Genentech, Incyte, Morphotek, Prima BioMed, and Tesaro and has participated on advisory boards for AstraZeneca, Clovis, Genentech/Roche, and Janssen.

## Author details
[1]Department of Medicine, Division of Medical Oncology, Duke Cancer Institute, 200 Trent Drive, Durham, NC 27710, USA. [2]Department of Obstetrics and Gynecology, Division of Gynecologic Oncology, Duke Cancer Institute, 200 Trent Drive, Durham, NC 27710, USA. [3]Department of Obstetrics and Gynecology, Division of Gynecologic Oncology, University of Arizona College of Medicine, 2222 E. Highland Ave., Suite 400, Phoenix, AZ 85016, USA.

## References
1. Siegel RL, Miller KD, Jemal A. Cancer statistics, 2016. CA Cancer J Clin. 2016; 66(1):7–30.
2. Chen DS, Mellman I. Oncology meets immunology: the cancer-immunity cycle. Immunity. 2013;39(1):1–10.
3. Taube JM, Anders RA, Young GD, Xu H, Sharma R, McMiller TL, Chen S, Klein AP, Pardoll DM, Topalian SL, et al. Colocalization of inflammatory response with B7-h1 expression in human melanocytic lesions supports an adaptive resistance mechanism of immune escape. Sci Transl Med. 2012;4(127):127ra137.
4. Green MR, Monti S, Rodig SJ, Juszczynski P, Currie T, O'Donnell E, Chapuy B, Takeyama K, Neuberg D, Golub TR, et al. Integrative analysis reveals selective 9p24.1 amplification, increased PD-1 ligand expression, and further induction via JAK2 in nodular sclerosing Hodgkin lymphoma and primary mediastinal large B-cell lymphoma. Blood. 2010;116(17):3268–77.
5. Atefi M, Avramis E, Lassen A, Wong DJ, Robert L, Foulad D, Cerniglia M, Titz B, Chodon T, Graeber TG, et al. Effects of MAPK and PI3K pathways on PD-L1 expression in melanoma. Clin Cancer Res. 2014;20(13):3446–57.
6. Parsa AT, Waldron JS, Panner A, Crane CA, Parney IF, Barry JJ, Cachola KE, Murray JC, Tihan T, Jensen MC, et al. Loss of tumor suppressor PTEN function increases B7-H1 expression and immunoresistance in glioma. Nat Med. 2007;13(1):84–8.
7. Fife BT, Bluestone JA. Control of peripheral T-cell tolerance and autoimmunity via the CTLA-4 and PD-1 pathways. Immunol Rev. 2008;224:166–82.
8. Taube JM, Klein A, Brahmer JR, Xu H, Pan X, Kim JH, Chen L, Pardoll DM, Topalian SL, Anders RA. Association of PD-1, PD-1 ligands, and other features of the tumor immune microenvironment with response to anti-PD-1 therapy. Clin Cancer Res. 2014;20(19):5064–74.
9. Teng MW, Ngiow SF, Ribas A, Smyth MJ. Classifying Cancers Based on T-cell Infiltration and PD-L1. Cancer Res. 2015;75(11):2139–45.
10. Zhang L, Conejo-Garcia JR, Katsaros D, Gimotty PA, Massobrio M, Regnani G, Makrigiannakis A, Gray H, Schlienger K, Liebman MN, et al. Intratumoral T cells, recurrence, and survival in epithelial ovarian cancer. N Engl J Med. 2003;348(3):203–13.
11. Sato E, Olson SH, Ahn J, Bundy B, Nishikawa H, Qian F, Jungbluth AA, Frosina D, Gnjatic S, Ambrosone C, et al. Intraepithelial CD8+ tumor-infiltrating lymphocytes and a high CD8+/regulatory T cell ratio are associated with favorable prognosis in ovarian cancer. Proc Natl Acad Sci U S A. 2005;102(51):18538–43.
12. Curiel TJ, Coukos G, Zou L, Alvarez X, Cheng P, Mottram P, Evdemon-Hogan M, Conejo-Garcia JR, Zhang L, Burow M, et al. Specific recruitment of regulatory T cells in ovarian carcinoma fosters immune privilege and predicts reduced survival. Nat Med. 2004;10(9):942–9.
13. Vermeij R, de Bock GH, Leffers N, Ten Hoor KA, Schulze U, Hollema H, van der Burg SH, van der Zee AG, Daemen T, Nijman HW. Tumor-infiltrating

cytotoxic T lymphocytes as independent prognostic factor in epithelial ovarian cancer with wilms tumor protein 1 overexpression. J Immunother. 2011;34(6):516–23.

14. Zhang Z, Huang J, Zhang C, Yang H, Qiu H, Li J, Liu Y, Qin L, Wang L, Hao S, et al. Infiltration of dendritic cells and T lymphocytes predicts favorable outcome in epithelial ovarian cancer. Cancer Gene Ther. 2015;22(4):198–206.

15. Bachmayr-Heyda A, Aust S, Heinze G, Polterauer S, Grimm C, Braicu EI, Sehouli J, Lambrechts S, Vergote I, Mahner S, et al. Prognostic impact of tumor infiltrating CD8+ T cells in association with cell proliferation in ovarian cancer patients–a study of the OVCAD consortium. BMC Cancer. 2013;13:422.

16. Webb JR, Milne K, Nelson BH. PD-1 and CD103 Are Widely Coexpressed on Prognostically Favorable Intraepithelial CD8 T Cells in Human Ovarian Cancer. Cancer Immunol Res. 2015;3(8):926–35.

17. Eisenthal A, Polyvkin N, Bramante-Schreiber L, Misonznik F, Hassner A, Lifschitz-Mercer B. Expression of dendritic cells in ovarian tumors correlates with clinical outcome in patients with ovarian cancer. Hum Pathol. 2001; 32(8):803–7.

18. Webb JR, Milne K, Kroeger DR, Nelson BH. PD-L1 expression is associated with tumor-infiltrating T cells and favorable prognosis in high-grade serous ovarian cancer. Gynecol Oncol. 2016;141(2):293–302.

19. Milne K, Kobel M, Kalloger SE, Barnes RO, Gao D, Gilks CB, Watson PH, Nelson BH. Systematic analysis of immune infiltrates in high-grade serous ovarian cancer reveals CD20, FoxP3 and TIA-1 as positive prognostic factors. PLoS One. 2009;4(7):e6412.

20. Hamanishi J, Mandai M, Iwasaki M, Okazaki T, Tanaka Y, Yamaguchi K, Higuchi T, Yagi H, Takakura K, Minato N, et al. Programmed cell death 1 ligand 1 and tumor-infiltrating CD8+ T lymphocytes are prognostic factors of human ovarian cancer. Proc Natl Acad Sci U S A. 2007;104(9):3360–5.

21. Peng J, Hamanishi J, Matsumura N, Abiko K, Murat K, Baba T, Yamaguchi K, Horikawa N, Hosoe Y, Murphy SK, et al. Chemotherapy Induces Programmed Cell Death-Ligand 1 Overexpression via the Nuclear Factor-kappaB to Foster an Immunosuppressive Tumor Microenvironment in Ovarian Cancer. Cancer Res. 2015;75(23):5034–45.

22. Abiko K, Matsumura N, Hamanishi J, Horikawa N, Murakami R, Yamaguchi K, Yoshioka Y, Baba T, Konishi I, Mandai M. IFN-gamma from lymphocytes induces PD-L1 expression and promotes progression of ovarian cancer. Br J Cancer. 2015;112(9):1501–9.

23. Duraiswamy J, Freeman GJ, Coukos G. Therapeutic PD-1 pathway blockade augments with other modalities of immunotherapy T-cell function to prevent immune decline in ovarian cancer. Cancer Res. 2013;73(23):6900–12.

24. deLeeuw RJ, Kroeger DR, Kost SE, Chang PP, Webb JR, Nelson BH. CD25 identifies a subset of CD4(+)FoxP3(-) TIL that are exhausted yet prognostically favorable in human ovarian cancer. Cancer Immunol Res. 2015;3(3):245–53.

25. Hamanishi J, Mandai M, Ikeda T, Minami M, Kawaguchi A, Murayama T, Kanai M, Mori Y, Matsumoto S, Chikuma S, et al. Safety and Antitumor Activity of Anti-PD-1 Antibody, Nivolumab, in Patients With Platinum-Resistant Ovarian Cancer. J Clin Oncol. 2015;33(34):4015–22.

26. Varga A, Piha-Paul SA, Ott PA, Mehnert JM, Berton-Rigaud D, Johnson EA, Cheng JD, Yuan S, Rubin EH, Matei DE. Antitumor activity and safety of pembrolizumab in patients (pts) with PD-L1 positive advanced ovarian cancer: Interim results from a phase Ib study. J Clin Oncol. 2015;33((suppl; abstr 5510)).

27. NCT01611558: Phase II Study of Ipilimumab Monotherapy in Recurrent Platinum-sensitive Ovarian Cancer - Study Results. https://clinicaltrials.gov/ct2/show/results/NCT01611558. Accessed 24 May 2016.

28. Disis ML, Patel MR, Pant S, Hamilton EP, Lockhart AC, Kelly K, Beck JT, Gordon MS, Weiss GJ, Taylor MH et al. Avelumab (MSB0010718C; anti-PD-L1) in patients with recurrent/refractory ovarian cancer from the JAVELIN Solid Tumor phase Ib trial: Safety and clinical activity. J Clin Oncol. 2016:34(suppl; abstr5533).

29. Lee J, Zimmer AD, Lipkowitz S, Annunziata CM, Ho TW, Chiou VL, Minasian LM, Houston ND, Ekwede I, Kohn EC. Phase I study of the PD-L1 inhibitor, durvalumab (MEDI4736; D) in combination with a PARP inhibitor, olaparib (O) or a VEGFR inhibitor, cediranib (C) in women's cancers (NCT02484404). J Clin Oncol. 2016:34(suppl; abstr 3015).

30. Ansell SM, Lesokhin AM, Borrello I, Halwani A, Scott EC, Gutierrez M, Schuster SJ, Millenson MM, Cattry D, Freeman GJ, et al. PD-1 blockade with nivolumab in relapsed or refractory Hodgkin's lymphoma. N Engl J Med. 2015;372(4):311–9.

31. Ansell SM. Where Do programmed death-1 inhibitors Fit in the management of malignant lymphoma? J Oncol Pract. 2016;12(2):101–6.

32. Topalian SL, Hodi FS, Brahmer JR, Gettinger SN, Smith DC, McDermott DF, Powderly JD, Carvajal RD, Sosman JA, Atkins MB, et al. Safety, activity, and immune correlates of anti-PD-1 antibody in cancer. N Engl J Med. 2012; 366(26):2443–54.

33. Disis ML, Patel MR, Pant S, Infante JR, Lockhart AC, Kelly K, Beck JT, Gordon MS, Weiss GJ, Ejadi S et al. Avelumab (MSB0010718C), an anti-PD-L1 antibody, in patients with previously treated, recurrent or refractory ovarian cancer: A phase Ib, open-label expansion trial. J Clin Oncol. 2015:33((suppl; abstr 5509)).

34. Crotzer DR, Sun CC, Coleman RL, Wolf JK, Levenback CF, Gershenson DM. Lack of effective systemic therapy for recurrent clear cell carcinoma of the ovary. Gynecol Oncol. 2007;105(2):404–8.

35. Takano M, Goto T, Kato M, Sasaki N, Miyamoto M, Furuya K. Short response duration even in responders to chemotherapy using conventional cytotoxic agents in recurrent or refractory clear cell carcinomas of the ovary. Int J Clin Oncol. 2013;18(3):556–7.

36. Cobb LP, Gaillard S, Wang Y, Shih I-M, Secord AA. Adenocarcinoma of Mullerian origin: review of pathogenesis, molecular biology, and emerging treatment paradigms. Gynecol Oncol Res Pract. 2015:2(1).

37. Motzer RJ, Escudier B, McDermott DF, George S, Hammers HJ, Srinivas S, Tykodi SS, Sosman JA, Procopio G, Plimack ER, et al. Nivolumab versus Everolimus in Advanced Renal-Cell Carcinoma. N Engl J Med. 2015;373(19):1803–13.

38. Brahmer JR, Drake CG, Wollner I, Powderly JD, Picus J, Sharfman WH, Stankevich E, Pons A, Salay TM, McMiller TL, et al. Phase I study of single-agent anti-programmed death-1 (MDX-1106) in refractory solid tumors: safety, clinical activity, pharmacodynamics, and immunologic correlates. J Clin Oncol. 2010;28(19):3167–75.

39. Weber JS, D'Angelo SP, Minor D, Hodi FS, Gutzmer R, Neyns B, Hoeller C, Khushalani NI, Miller Jr WH, Lao CD, et al. Nivolumab versus chemotherapy in patients with advanced melanoma who progressed after anti-CTLA-4 treatment (CheckMate 037): a randomised, controlled, open-label, phase 3 trial. Lancet Oncol. 2015;16(4):375–84.

40. Robert C, Long GV, Brady B, Dutriaux C, Maio M, Mortier L, Hassel JC, Rutkowski P, McNeil C, Kalinka-Warzocha E, et al. Nivolumab in previously untreated melanoma without BRAF mutation. N Engl J Med. 2015;372(4): 320–30.

41. Herbst RS, Soria JC, Kowanetz M, Fine GD, Hamid O, Gordon MS, Sosman JA, McDermott DF, Powderly JD, Gettinger SN, et al. Predictive correlates of response to the anti-PD-L1 antibody MPDL3280A in cancer patients. Nature. 2014;515(7528):563–7.

42. Sunshine J, Taube JM. PD-1/PD-L1 inhibitors. Curr Opin Pharmacol. 2015;23:32–8.

43. Larkin J, Chiarion-Sileni V, Gonzalez R, Grob JJ, Cowey CL, Lao CD, Schadendorf D, Dummer R, Smylie M, Rutkowski P, et al. Combined Nivolumab and Ipilimumab or Monotherapy in Untreated Melanoma. N Engl J Med. 2015;373(1):23–34.

44. Tumeh PC, Harview CL, Yearley JH, Shintaku IP, Taylor EJ, Robert L, Chmielowski B, Spasic M, Henry G, Ciobanu V, et al. PD-1 blockade induces responses by inhibiting adaptive immune resistance. Nature. 2014;515(7528):568–71.

45. Ji RR, Chasalow SD, Wang L, Hamid O, Schmidt H, Cogswell J, Alaparthy S, Berman D, Jure-Kunkel M, Siemers NO, et al. An immune-active tumor microenvironment favors clinical response to ipilimumab. Cancer Immunol Immunother. 2012;61(7):1019–31.

46. Ng Tang D, Shen Y, Sun J, Wen S, Wolchok JD, Yuan J, Allison JP, Sharma P. Increased frequency of ICOS+ CD4 T cells as a pharmacodynamic biomarker for anti-CTLA-4 therapy. Cancer Immunol Res. 2013;1(4):229–34.

47. Chen H, Liakou CI, Kamat A, Pettaway C, Ward JF, Tang DN, Sun J, Jungbluth AA, Troncoso P, Logothetis C, et al. Anti-CTLA-4 therapy results in higher CD4 + ICOShi T cell frequency and IFN-gamma levels in both nonmalignant and malignant prostate tissues. Proc Natl Acad Sci U S A. 2009;106(8):2729–34.

48. Liakou CI, Kamat A, Tang DN, Chen H, Sun J, Troncoso P, Logothetis C, Sharma P. CTLA-4 blockade increases IFNgamma-producing CD4 + ICOShi cells to shift the ratio of effector to regulatory T cells in cancer patients. Proc Natl Acad Sci U S A. 2008;105(39):14987–92.

49. Vonderheide RH, LoRusso PM, Khalil M, Gartner EM, Khaira D, Soulieres D, Dorazio P, Trosko JA, Ruter J, Mariani GL, et al. Tremelimumab in combination with exemestane in patients with advanced breast cancer and treatment-

associated modulation of inducible costimulator expression on patient T cells. Clin Cancer Res. 2010;16(13):3485–94.

50. Hodi FS, Butler M, Oble DA, Seiden MV, Haluska FG, Kruse A, Macrae S, Nelson M, Canning C, Lowy I, et al. Immunologic and clinical effects of antibody blockade of cytotoxic T lymphocyte-associated antigen 4 in previously vaccinated cancer patients. Proc Natl Acad Sci U S A. 2008; 105(8):3005–10.

51. Topalian SL, Taube JM, Anders RA, Pardoll DM. Mechanism-driven biomarkers to guide immune checkpoint blockade in cancer therapy. Nat Rev Cancer. 2016;16(5):275–87.

52. Snyder A, Makarov V, Merghoub T, Yuan J, Zaretsky JM, Desrichard A, Walsh LA, Postow MA, Wong P, Ho TS, et al. Genetic basis for clinical response to CTLA-4 blockade in melanoma. N Engl J Med. 2014;371(23):2189–99.

53. Van Allen EM, Miao D, Schilling B, Shukla SA, Blank C, Zimmer L, Sucker A, Hillen U, Foppen MH, Goldinger SM, et al. Genomic correlates of response to CTLA-4 blockade in metastatic melanoma. Science. 2015; 350(6257):207–11.

54. Rizvi NA, Hellmann MD, Snyder A, Kvistborg P, Makarov V, Havel JJ, Lee W, Yuan J, Wong P, Ho TS, et al. Cancer immunology. Mutational landscape determines sensitivity to PD-1 blockade in non-small cell lung cancer. Science. 2015;348(6230):124–8.

55. Llosa NJ, Cruise M, Tam A, Wicks EC, Hechenbleikner EM, Taube JM, Blosser RL, Fan H, Wang H, Luber BS, et al. The vigorous immune microenvironment of microsatellite instable colon cancer is balanced by multiple counter-inhibitory checkpoints. Cancer Discov. 2015;5(1):43–51.

56. Le DT, Uram JN, Wang H, Bartlett BR, Kemberling H, Eyring AD, Skora AD, Luber BS, Azad NS, Laheru D, et al. PD-1 Blockade in Tumors with Mismatch-Repair Deficiency. N Engl J Med. 2015;372(26):2509–20.

57. Diaz LA, Uram JN, Wang H, Bartlett B, Kemberling H, Eyring A, Azad NS, Dauses T, Laheru D, Lee JJ et al. Programmed death-1 blockade in mismatch repair deficient cancer independent of tumor histology. J Clin Oncol. 2016:34(suppl; abstr 3003).

58. Xiao X, Melton DW, Gourley C. Mismatch repair deficiency in ovarian cancer – molecular characteristics and clinical implications. Gynecol Oncol. 2014; 132(2):506–12.

59. Integrated genomic analyses of ovarian carcinoma. Nature. 2011:474(7353): 609-15.

60. Patch AM, Christie EL, Etemadmoghadam D, Garsed DW, George J, Fereday S, Nones K, Cowin P, Alsop K, Bailey PJ, et al. Whole-genome characterization of chemoresistant ovarian cancer. Nature. 2015; 521(7553):489–94.

61. George J, Alsop K, Etemadmoghadam D, Hondow H, Mikeska T, Dobrovic A, deFazio A, Australian Ovarian Cancer Study G, Smyth GK, Levine DA, et al. Nonequivalent gene expression and copy number alterations in high-grade serous ovarian cancers with BRCA1 and BRCA2 mutations. Clin Cancer Res. 2013;19(13):3474–84.

62. Daud AI, Loo K, Pauli ML, Sanchez-Rodriguez R, Sandoval PM, Taravati K, Tsai K, Nosrati A, Nardo L, Alvarado MD, et al. Tumor immune profiling predicts response to anti-PD-1 therapy in human melanoma. J Clin Invest. 2016; 126(9):3447–52.

63. Robert L, Tsoi J, Wang X, Emerson R, Homet B, Chodon T, Mok S, Huang RR, Cochran AJ, Comin-Anduix B, et al. CTLA4 blockade broadens the peripheral T-cell receptor repertoire. Clin Cancer Res. 2014;20(9):2424–32.

64. Robert L, Harview C, Emerson R, Wang X, Mok S, Homet B, Comin-Anduix B, Koya RC, Robins H, Tumeh PC, et al. Distinct immunological mechanisms of CTLA-4 and PD-1 blockade revealed by analyzing TCR usage in blood lymphocytes. Oncoimmunology. 2014;3:e29244.

65. Maker AV, Attia P, Rosenberg SA. Analysis of the Cellular Mechanism of Antitumor Responses and Autoimmunity in Patients Treated with CTLA-4 Blockade. J Immunol. 2005;175(11):7746–54.

66. Zaretsky JM, Blum SM, Faja LR, Emerson RO, Ribas A. TCR use and cytokine response in PD-1 blockade. J Clin Oncol. 2015:33((suppl; abstr 3027)).

67. Goldinger SM, Courtier A, Jaberg-Bentele NF, Schindler S, Manuel M, Plantier N, Treillard B, Noel M, Nguyen Kim TDL, Raaijmakers MIG et al. The peripheral blood TCR repertoire to facilitate patient stratification for immune checkpoint blockade inhibition in metastatic melanoma. J Clin Oncol. 2016:34((suppl; abstr 3026)).

68. Yuan J, Gnjatic S, Li H, Powel S, Gallardo HF, Ritter E, Ku GY, Jungbluth AA, Segal NH, Rasalan TS, et al. CTLA-4 blockade enhances polyfunctional NY-ESO-1 specific T cell responses in metastatic melanoma patients with clinical benefit. Proc Natl Acad Sci U S A. 2008;105(51):20410–5.

69. Lizotte PH, Ivanova EV, Awad MM, Jones RE, Keogh L, Liu H, Dries R, Almonte C, Herter-Sprie GS, Santos A, et al. Multiparametric profiling of non-small-cell lung cancers reveals distinct immunophenotypes. JCI Insight. 2016;1(14):e89014.

70. Duraiswamy J, Kaluza KM, Freeman GJ, Coukos G. Dual blockade of PD-1 and CTLA-4 combined with tumor vaccine effectively restores T-cell rejection function in tumors. Cancer Res. 2013;73(12):3591–603.

71. Chen G, Emens LA. Chemoimmunotherapy: reengineering tumor immunity. Cancer Immunol Immunother. 2013;62(2):203–16.

72. Salama AK, Postow MA, Salama JK. Irradiation and immunotherapy: From concept to the clinic. Cancer. 2016;122(11):1659–71.

73. Topalian SL, Drake CG, Pardoll DM. Immune checkpoint blockade: a common denominator approach to cancer therapy. Cancer Cell. 2015; 27(4):450–61.

74. Atkins MB, Larkin J. Immunotherapy combined or sequenced with targeted therapy in the treatment of solid tumors: current perspectives. J Natl Cancer Inst. 2016;108(6):djv414.

75. Huang J, Wang L, Cong Z, Amoozgar Z, Kiner E, Xing D, Orsulic S, Matulonis U, Goldberg MS. The PARP1 inhibitor BMN 673 exhibits immunoregulatory effects in a Brca1(-/-) murine model of ovarian cancer. Biochem Biophys Res Commun. 2015;463(4):551–6.

76. Rivera LB, Bergers G. Intertwined regulation of angiogenesis and immunity by myeloid cells. Trends Immunol. 2015;36(4):240–9.

77. Higuchi T, Flies DB, Marjon NA, Mantia-Smaldone G, Ronner L, Gimotty PA, Adams SF. CTLA-4 Blockade Synergizes Therapeutically with PARP Inhibition in BRCA1-Deficient Ovarian Cancer. Cancer Immunol Res. 2015;3(11):1257–68.

78. Ziogas AC, Gavalas NG, Tsiatas M, Tsitsilonis O, Politi E, Terpos E, Rodolakis A, Vlahos G, Thomakos N, Haidopoulos D, et al. VEGF directly suppresses activation of T cells from ovarian cancer patients and healthy individuals via VEGF receptor Type 2. Int J Cancer. 2012;130(4):857–64.

79. Hodi FS, O'Day SJ, McDermott DF, Weber RW, Sosman JA, Haanen JB, Gonzalez R, Robert C, Schadendorf D, Hassel JC, et al. Improved survival with ipilimumab in patients with metastatic melanoma. N Engl J Med. 2010; 363(8):711–23.

80. Brahmer JR, Tykodi SS, Chow LQ, Hwu WJ, Topalian SL, Hwu P, Drake CG, Camacho LH, Kauh J, Odunsi K, et al. Safety and activity of anti-PD-L1 antibody in patients with advanced cancer. N Engl J Med. 2012; 366(26):2455–65.

81. Weber JS, Dummer R, de Pril V, Lebbe C, Hodi FS, Investigators MDX. Patterns of onset and resolution of immune-related adverse events of special interest with ipilimumab: detailed safety analysis from a phase 3 trial in patients with advanced melanoma. Cancer. 2013;119(9):1675–82.

82. Spain L, Diem S, Larkin J. Management of toxicities of immune checkpoint inhibitors. Cancer Treat Rev. 2016;44:51–60.

83. Common Terminology Criteria for Adverse Events (CTCAE) Version 4.0. http://evs.nci.nih.gov/ftp1/CTCAE/CTCAE_4.03_2010-06-14_QuickReference_ 8.5x11.pdf. Accessed 20 June 2016.

84. Horvat TZ, Adel NG, Dang TO, Momtaz P, Postow MA, Callahan MK, Carvajal RD, Dickson MA, D'Angelo SP, Woo KM, et al. Immune-related adverse events, need for systemic immunosuppression, and effects on survival and time to treatment failure in patients with melanoma treated with ipilimumab at memorial Sloan Kettering cancer center. J Clin Oncol. 2015;33(28):3193–8.

85. Harmankaya K, Erasim C, Koelblinger C, Ibrahim R, Hoos A, Pehamberger H, Binder M. Continuous systemic corticosteroids do not affect the ongoing regression of metastatic melanoma for more than two years following ipilimumab therapy. Med Oncol. 2011;28(4):1140–4.

86. Wolchok JD, Hoos A, O'Day S, Weber JS, Hamid O, Lebbe C, Maio M, Binder M, Bohnsack O, Nichol G, et al. Guidelines for the evaluation of immune therapy activity in solid tumors: immune-related response criteria. Clin Cancer Res. 2009;15(23):7412–20.

87. pO'Day SJ, Maio M, Chiarion-Sileni V, Gajewski TF, Pehamberger H, Bondarenko IN, Queirolo P, Lundgren L, Mikhailov S, Roman L, et al. Efficacy and safety of ipilimumab monotherapy in patients with pretreated advanced melanoma: a multicenter single-arm phase II study. Ann Oncol. 2010; 21(8):1712–7.

88. Hodi FS, Hwu WJ, Kefford R, Weber JS, Daud A, Hamid O, Patnaik A, Ribas A, Robert C, Gangadhar TC, et al. Evaluation of Immune-Related Response Criteria and RECIST v1.1 in Patients With Advanced Melanoma Treated With Pembrolizumab. J Clin Oncol. 2016;34(13):1510–7.

# Characteristics and outcomes for patients with advanced vaginal or vulvar cancer referred to a phase I clinical trials program: the MD Anderson cancer center experience

Siqing Fu[1*], Naiyi Shi[1], Jennifer Wheler[1], Aung Naing[1], Filip Janku[1], Sarina Piha-Paul[1], Jing Gong[1], David Hong[1], Apostolia Tsimberidou[1], Ralph Zinner[1], Vivek Subbiah[1], Ming-Mo Hou[1], Pedro Ramirez[2], Lois Ramondetta[2], Karen Lu[2] and Funda Meric-Bernstam[1]

## Abstract

**Background:** Early-stage vaginal and vulvar cancer can be cured. But outcomes of patients with metastatic disease are poor. Thus, new therapeutic strategies are urgently required.

**Methods:** In this retrospective study, we analyzed the clinical outcomes of consecutive patients with metastatic vaginal or vulvar cancer who were referred to a phase I trial clinic between January 2006 and December 2013. Demographic and clinical data were obtained from patients' electronic medical records.

**Results:** Patients with metastatic vaginal ($n = 16$) and vulvar ($n = 20$) cancer who were referred for phase I trial therapy had median overall survival durations of 6.2 and 4.6 months, respectively. Among those who underwent therapy ($n = 27$), one experienced a partial response and three experienced stable disease for at least 6 months. Patients with a body mass index ≥30 had a significantly longer median overall survival duration than did those with a body mass index <30 (13.2 months versus 4.4 months, $p = 0.04$). Preliminary data revealed differences in molecular profiling between patients with advanced vaginal cancer and those with advanced vaginal cancer.

**Conclusions:** Metastatic vaginal and vulvar cancers remain to be difficult-to-treat diseases with poor clinical outcomes. The currently available phase I trial agents provided little meaningful clinical benefits. Understanding these tumors' molecular mechanisms may allow us to develop more effective therapeutic strategies than are currently available regimens.

**Keywords:** Vaginal cancer, Vulvar cancer, Phase I trial, Body mass index, Molecular analysis

## Background

Vaginal and vulvar cancers comprise approximately 8 % of all malignant neoplasms of the female genital tract: approximately 3,000 vaginal cancers and 4,500 vulvar cancers are diagnosed annually in the United States [1]. Most of these tumors are squamous cell carcinomas, but melanoma, sarcoma, adenocarcinoma, and other histological types also occur [2–6]. All vaginal and vulvar cancers are associated with similar risk factors: cigarette smoking, human papillomavirus infection, and a history of other gynecological malignancies [7, 8]. Early-stage vaginal and vulvar cancer can be cured, but if the disease is not amenable to radical local excision or curative chemoradiation therapy [9–11], patients with recurrent or metastatic vaginal or vulvar cancers have a poor prognosis [12, 13]. Palliative systemic therapy results in limited clinical benefit [14].

The overall poor prognosis of these patients warrants the development of novel therapeutic regimens [15]. Therefore, we conducted a retrospective chart review to identify the demographic characteristics and major

* Correspondence: siqingfu@mdanderson.org
[1]Department of Investigational Cancer Therapeutics, Unit 0455, The University of Texas MD Anderson Cancer Center, 1515 Holcombe Boulevard, Houston, TX 77030, USA
Full list of author information is available at the end of the article

clinical outcomes, such as mutational status, clinical response, and survival duration, of patients with metastatic vaginal or vulvar cancer who were referred to a designated phase I trial clinic. These data may lead to the development of new drugs for the treatment of patients with these diseases.

## Methods

### Patient selection

We included all consecutive patients with metastatic or recurrent vaginal or vulvar carcinoma who were referred to the Department of Investigational Cancer Therapeutics (a phase I clinical trials program) at The University of Texas MD Anderson Cancer Center between January 1, 2006, and December 31, 2013 in this retrospective chart review. Follow-up was defined as the time of the initial phase I clinic visit until death or the last date of the study, censored on August 8, 2014. This study was conducted in accordance with MD Anderson's institutional review board guidelines.

### Data collection

During the data collection phase, two members of the research team worked independently: one reviewed patients' electronic medical records, and the other audited and checked the accuracy of the collected data. Any data discrepancy was resolved by a consensus after group discussion. The collected clinical information included race, treatment history (e.g., surgery, radiation therapy, and chemotherapy), date of birth, Eastern Cooperative Oncology Group performance status at the initial phase I clinic visit, mutation profile of the tumor specimen, phase I clinical trial therapies, and clinical outcomes (progression-free survival [PFS], overall survival [OS], and objective responses, including complete remission [CR], partial response [PR], and stable disease for 6 months or longer [SD ≥6 months]).

Clinical objective responses were evaluated using Response Evaluation Criteria in Solid Tumors software version 1.0 or 1.1, per individual study protocols [16, 17]. The PFS duration was defined as the interval from the date of initial treatment to the first objective documentation of disease progression, the time of death, or the last date of contact (August 8, 2014), at which time the patients' data were censored. OS duration was estimated from the date of the initial phase I clinical trial therapy to death or the last date of contact. The enrollment of eligible patients into specific phase I trials was dependent on trial availability at the time of presentation and the preference of the treating physician, according to good clinical practice. If a phase I agent was unsuccessful, another was used as long as the patient was eligible and willing to participate.

**Table 1** Baseline patient demographics ($n = 36$)

| Characteristics | Vaginal cancer ($n = 16$) | Vulvar cancer ($n = 20$) |
|---|---|---|
| Median age, years (range) | 60 (30 to 85) | 55 (33 to 78) |
| Race, n (%) | | |
| White | 13 (81 %) | 19 (95 %) |
| Black | 1 (6 %) | 0 |
| Hispanic | 2 (13 %) | 0 |
| Asian | 0 | 1 (5 %) |
| Body Mass Index, n (%) | | |
| Underweight (<18.5) | 0 | 1 (5 %) |
| Normal Weight (18.5 to 25) | 10 (62 %) | 13 (65 %) |
| Overweight (>25) | 6 (38 %) | 6 (30 %) |
| The Eastern Cooperative Oncology Group Performance Status, n (%) | | |
| 0 | 4 (25 %) | 0 |
| 1 | 9 (56 %) | 18 (90 %) |
| 2 | 3 (19 %) | 2 (10 %) |
| Prior Chemotherapy | | |
| Yes, n (%) | 14 (88 %) | 16 (80 %) |
| Median number (range) | 2 (0 to 4) | 1 (0 to 6) |
| Prior Radiation Therapy | | |
| Yes, n (%) | 15 (94 %) | 17 (85 %) |
| Pathological Diagnosis, n (%) | | |
| Squamous Cell Carcinoma | 7 (44 %) | 17 (85 %) |
| Adenocarcinoma | 4 (25 %) | 0 |
| Melanoma | 3 (19 %) | 3 (15 %) |
| Carcinosarcoma | 1 (6 %) | 0 |
| High-grade neuroendocrine carcinoma | 1 (6 %) | 0 |
| Phase I Trial Enrollment, n (%) | 11 (69 %) | 16 (80 %) |

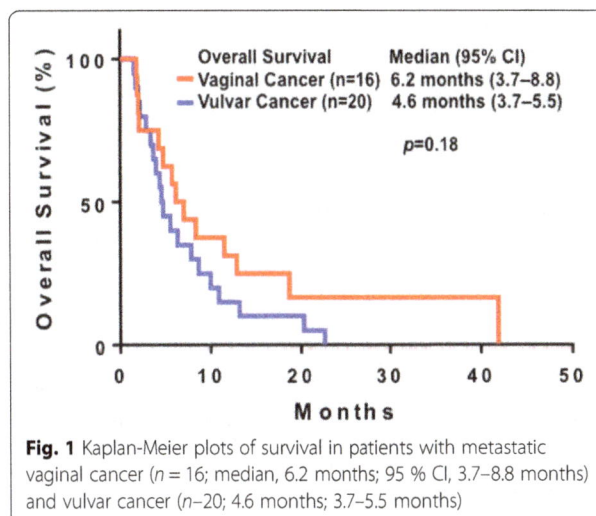

**Fig. 1** Kaplan-Meier plots of survival in patients with metastatic vaginal cancer ($n = 16$; median, 6.2 months; 95 % CI, 3.7–8.8 months) and vulvar cancer ($n$–20; 4.6 months; 3.7–5.5 months)

**Table 2** Major characteristics and clinical outcomes in patients receiving a phase I trial therapy ($n = 27$)

| Age | Pathology | Prior therapy | OS | BMI | MDACC score | Phase I trials | PFS | CMS46 or Foundation Med |
|---|---|---|---|---|---|---|---|---|
| Vaginal cancer | | | | | | | | |
| 45 | A | 2 | 41.9 | 33.2 | 1 | Bevacizumab and Temsirolimus | 1.0 | ND |
| 81 | S | 0 | 5.8 | 21.9 | 0 | Gemcitabine and Dasatinib | 0.9 | ND |
| 61 | M | 4 | 2.0 | 23.0 | 3 | PI3K Inhibitor and Paclitaxel | 0.9 | ND |
| 59 | A | 3 | 4.8 | 37.8 | 2 | Bevacizumab and Temsirolimus plus Carboplatin | PFS1 = 1.4 | ND |
| | | | | | | CHK1 Inhibitor | PFS2 = 1.5 | |
| | | | | | | Erlotinib and Pralatrexate | PFS3 = 2.2 | |
| 53 | S | 2 | 12.9 | 18.6 | 0 | Aurora Kinase Inhibitor | 4.9 | ND |
| 57 | S | 1 | 1.8 | 22.9 | 2 | Trientine and Carboplatin | 0.7 | PIK3CA (E545K) |
| 57 | S | 0 | 28+ | 21.3 | 1 | Everolimus and Pazopanib | PFS1 = 18.2 | PIK3CA (E545K), PTPRD (S1845fs*2) and STK11 loss |
| | | | | | | PI3K Inhibitor | PFS2 = 1.9 | |
| 72 | M | 1 | 4.3 | 21.0 | 1 | Ipilimumab and Imatinib | 2.3 | PTEN loss, C17orf39, KDR, KIT and MYST3 amplification |
| 58 | S | 1 | 15+ | 19.5 | 1 | Erlotinib and Pralatrexate | 14.6+ | ERBB2 (S310F), ERBB4 (D609N), FBXW7 (R479Q), RB1 (E539*), ARID2 (Q1194*) and amplification of EPHBI, PIK3CA and SOX2 |
| 67 | A | 2 | 8.4 | 31.3 | 1 | Anastrozole and Everolimus | 2.6 | PTEN (210-1G > A), KRAS (G12V), CTNNB1 (D32N), MPL (P106L), and amplification of MCL1, MYC and NFKB1A |
| 52 | S | 1 | 7.1 | 24.0 | 0 | Erlotinib and Valproic Acid | 2.8 | ND |
| Vulvar cancer | | | | | | | | |
| 37 | S | 1 | 3.7 | 21.2 | 2 | PI3K inhibitor plus Caboplatin and Paclitaxel | PFS1 = 1.4 | PIK3CA: mutation not detected |
| | | | | | | Erlotinib and Valporic acid | PFS2 = 0.6 | |
| 58 | S | 1 | 13.2 | 30.5 | 1 | Erlotinib and Valporic acid | PFS1 = 3.9 | BRAF, KRAS and PIK3CA: no mutation detected |
| | | | | | | Bevacizumab and Cetuximab plus Erlotinib | PFS2 = 7.2 | |
| 74 | S | 1 | 6.4 | 23.7 | 1 | Microtube Inhibitor | 3.1 | ND |
| 60 | M | 6 | 4.4 | 22.3 | 2 | PI3K Inhibitor | 2.0 | Single Gene: c-KIT (L576P) |
| 42 | S | 1 | 2.0 | 23.7 | 1 | Bevacizumab and Trastuzumab plus Lapatinib | 0.7 | ND |
| 42 | S | 0 | 1.5 | 19.9 | 2 | Src Inhibitor | 0.5 | ND |
| 78 | S | 0 | 20.3 | 35.5 | 1 | Erlotinib and Valporic Acid | 6.1 | ND |
| 37 | S | 1 | 1.7 | 18.7 | 2 | Camptothecin | 0.8 | ND |
| 55 | S | 3 | 4.8 | 15.8 | 1 | Histone Deacetylase Inhibitor | 0.5 | ND |
| 41 | S | 0 | 2.2 | 18.8 | 2 | Sirolimus and Docetaxel | 1.7 | ND |
| 54 | S | 1 | 2.9 | 26.6 | 1 | Lapatinib and Sirolimus | 1.5 | Single Gene: BRAF (V600E) |
| 60 | M | 2 | 4.6 | 22.9 | 3 | Multikinase Inhibitor | 2.9 | ND |
| 69 | S | 1 | 22.6 | 30.9 | 2 | Carboplatin and Trientine | 0.9 | A 46-gene panel: no mutation detected |
| 33 | S | 1 | 10.0 | 24.8 | 2 | Lenalidomide and Temsirolimus | 1.9 | ND |
| 73 | S | 1 | 5.6 | 22.4 | 2 | Crizotinib and Pazopanib | 1.6 | KRAS (R102T), TET2 (W1198*), TP53 (R248Q), and CDK2NA/B loss |
| 55 | M | 1 | 3.4 | 24.2 | 2 | Translation Initiation Inhibition | 1.0 | ND |

*OS* overall survival, *BMI* body mass index, *MDACC score* the sum of five variables (low serum albumin, high serum lactate dehydrogenase, *ECOG performance status of 1 or higher* more than two metastatic sites, and gastrointestinal tumor type), *PFS* progression-free survival (1, 2, or 3 indicates the first, second, or third line of phase I trial), * deletion , *A* adenocarcinoma, *S* squamous cell carcinoma, *M* melanoma, *ND* not done

## Statistical analyses

Categorical data were described using contingency tables. Continuously scaled measures were summarized with descriptive statistical measures (i.e., the median and the range), whereas PFS and OS rates were estimated using the Kaplan-Meier method. Patients who were still alive at the time of data analysis were censored at that time. Fisher's exact test was used to assess the association between categorical variables. Statistical inferences were based on two-sided tests at a significance level of $p < 0.05$. Statistical analyses were carried out using SPSS Statistics software version 22 (IBM, Inc., Armonk, NY).

## Results

### Study population

This study included 36 consecutive patients with metastatic vaginal ($n = 16$) or vulvar ($n = 20$) cancer who were evaluated in the phase I clinic at MD Anderson. The majority of these patients were white ($n = 32$ [89 %]); presented with squamous cell carcinoma ($n = 24$ [67 %]); had adequate functional status, with an Eastern Cooperative Oncology Group performance status of 0 or 1 ($n = 31$ [86 %]); and had undergone systemic chemotherapy ($n = 30$ [83 %]) or radiation therapy ($n = 32$ [89 %]). The patients' baseline characteristics are listed in Table 1. All patients had undergone systemic chemotherapy or chemoradiation therapy for locally advanced or metastatic disease before they were referred. Most patients ($n = 27$ [75 %]) were enrolled in a phase I trial.

### Major clinical outcomes

The 36 patients had a median OS duration of 5.6 months (95 % CI, 3.7–7.5 months). A similar duration was observed in patients with vaginal cancer (6.2 months; 3.7–8.8 months) and vulvar cancer (4.6 months; 3.7–5.5 months ($p = 0.18$), as shown in Fig. 1.

The baseline demographics, major clinical outcomes, and molecular aberrations of the 27 patients who underwent phase I trial therapy, are listed in Table 2, associated with a median OS duration of 5.6 months (95 % CI, 3.1–8.1 months). There was no difference in the median OS duration between patients with vaginal cancer (7.1 months; 3.2–11 months) and vulvar cancer (4.4 months; 2.6–6.2 months; $p = 0.1$), as shown in Fig. 2. In this cohort of patients who underwent phase I trial therapy, six (22 %) were classified as obese (BMI ≥30), one (4 %) overweight (BMI 25–30), 19 (70 %) normal (BMI 18.5–25), and one (4 %) underweight (BMI <18.5). Obese patients had a median OS duration of 13.2 months (95 % CI, 0–27.5 months), which was significantly longer than that of those who were not obese (4.4 months; 3.1–5.7; $p = 0.04$), as shown in Fig. 3.

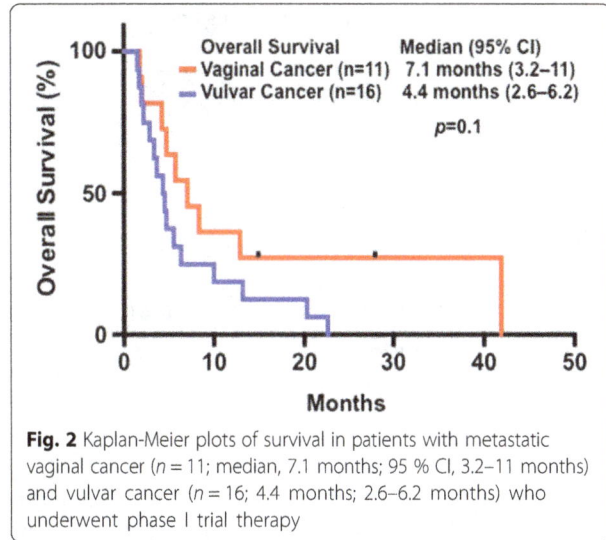

**Fig. 2** Kaplan-Meier plots of survival in patients with metastatic vaginal cancer ($n = 11$; median, 7.1 months; 95 % CI, 3.2–11 months) and vulvar cancer ($n = 16$; 4.4 months; 2.6–6.2 months) who underwent phase I trial therapy

### Exploratory molecular analysis

Molecular marker studies were performed of available tumor specimens in a Clinical Laboratory Improvement Amendments-certified molecular diagnostic laboratory. Table 3 lists the limited molecular aberrations per tumor type. In patients with metastatic vaginal cancer, the PI3K/AKT/mTOR pathway was activated, which was supported by the finding of frequent PIK3CA mutations and PTEN loss or mutation. A loss of STK11 and FBXW7 mutations was also observed in these patients. Furthermore, treatment with everolimus and pazopanib led to a partial response for 18.2 months in one patient with metastatic squamous cell carcinoma that harbored PIK3CA (E545K), PTPRD (S1845fs*2), and STK11 losses.

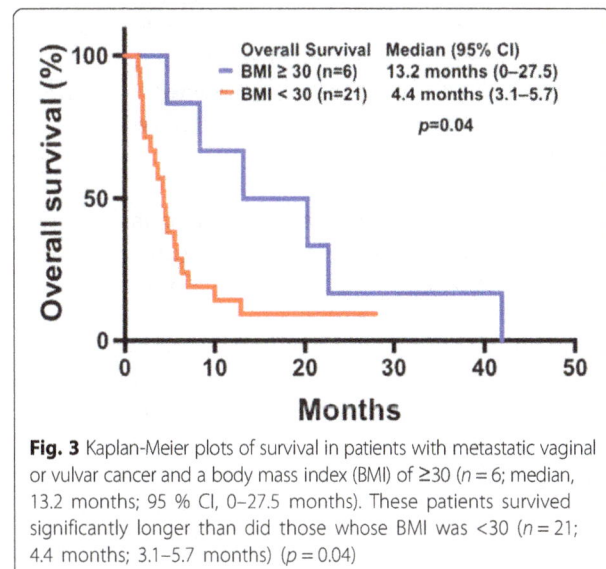

**Fig. 3** Kaplan-Meier plots of survival in patients with metastatic vaginal or vulvar cancer and a body mass index (BMI) of ≥30 ($n = 6$; median, 13.2 months; 95 % CI, 0–27.5 months). These patients survived significantly longer than did those whose BMI was <30 ($n = 21$; 4.4 months; 3.1–5.7 months) ($p = 0.04$)

**Table 3** Summary of molecular aberrations per tumor type

|  | Vaginal cancer, n (%) | Vulvar cancer, n (%) |
|---|---|---|
| PIK3CA | 33 % (n = 9) | 0 % (n = 8) |
| PTEN | 67 % (n = 6) | 0 % (n = 4) |
| KRAS | 10 % (n = 10) | 13 % (n = 8) |
| NRAS | 10 % (n = 10) | 0 % (n = 4) |
| EGFR | 0 % (n = 9) | 0 % (n = 6) |
| BRAF | 0 % (n = 9) | 14 % (n = 7) |
| C-MET | 0 % (n = 7) | 0 % (n = 3) |
| TP53 | 0 % (n = 6) | 33 % (n = 3) |
| C-KIT | 0 % (n = 8) | 20 % (n = 3) |

Treatment with erlotinib and pralatrexate resulted in stable disease for approximately 15 months in a patient with metastatic squamous cell carcinoma that harbored ERBB2 (S310F), ERBB4 (D609N), FBXW7 (R479Q), RB1 (E539*), and ARID2 (Q1194*) and amplification of EPHBI, PIK3CA, and SOX2. In patients with metastatic vulvar cancer, we found no common intracellular transduction pathway mutations; rather, mutations were found in *TP53, c-KIT, BRAF,* and *KRAS.* One patient with metastatic KRAS wild-type squamous cell carcinoma experienced stable disease for about 11 months after being treated with epithelial growth factor inhibition-based phase I trial regimens, while another patient had stable disease for 6 months after being treated with erlotinib and valproic acid.

## Discussion

Patients with metastatic or recurrent vaginal or vulvar cancer have limited therapeutic treatment options [18–20]. In this study, we found that these patients did not experience a meaningful clinical benefit from novel phase I therapeutics: there were low rates of objective responses and a median OS duration of only 5.6 months. Further evaluation is warranted to determine the effects of novel cancer therapeutics, molecular profiling, and targeted therapy on patient outcomes in the phase I setting.

There were several notable observations in our study. In general, patients with metastatic vaginal squamous cell carcinoma had a median OS duration of 7.1 months compared with 4.4 months in those with metastatic vulvar squamous cell carcinoma. Both cohorts of patients had poor clinical outcomes and low antitumor activity in response to currently available phase I agents. These patients had significantly shorter OS durations than did other patients with other metastatic or recurrent solid tumors [21–23]. Second, patients with metastatic vaginal cancer had a higher prevalence of PI3K/AKT/mTOR pathway activation, while patients with metastatic vulvar

cancer had no common transduction pathway mutations. Therefore, early molecular profiling is urgently required to further explore therapeutic options for these patients. Third, since the association between obesity and survival in patients with metastatic gynecological malignancies remains equivocal, we determined the relationship between BMI and major clinical outcomes. Patients with BMIs of ≥30 had a significantly longer median OS duration (13.2 months) than did those with BMIs <30 (4.4 months), suggesting that further studies are warranted of the effects of excess body weight on tumor biology. Elucidating the molecular mechanisms of vaginal and vulvar cancer may result in the development of more effective therapeutic strategies [24, 25].

A limited sample size was available for subgroup analyses, which confounded our ability to validate statistical significance in the category assessment. Nevertheless, the findings of this retrospective study should be considered preliminary evidence for generating hypotheses that will require further validation in larger prospective studies.

## Conclusion

In conclusion, metastatic vaginal and vulvar cancers are difficult-to-treat diseases with poor clinical outcomes. The currently available phase I trial agents provided little meaningful clinical benefits. Preliminary data revealed differences in molecular profiling between patients with advanced vaginal cancer and those with advanced vaginal cancer. Therefore, we advocate the earlier use of molecular profiling to obtain a better understanding of their tumorigenesis and development. Biomarker-driven therapies based on complex molecular profiles may be an initial step to develop effective therapeutic regimens treating these malignancies.

**Competing interests**
The authors declare that they have no competing interests.

**Authors' contributions**
SF contributed to study conception and design. SF, NS, and JG acquired the data and drafted the manuscript, and all other co-authors critically revised the manuscript. SF, JW, AN, FJ, SPP, DH, AT, RZ, VS, PR, LR, and KL observed the patients and collected the data. All authors have approved the final version of the manuscript.

**Acknowledgements**
The authors thank Ellen Chiu in the Department of Investigational Cancer Therapeutics at MD Anderson for conducting database searches and Ann M Sutton in the Department of Scientific Publications at MD Anderson for editing the manuscript.

**Author details**
[1]Department of Investigational Cancer Therapeutics, Unit 0455, The University of Texas MD Anderson Cancer Center, 1515 Holcombe Boulevard, Houston, TX 77030, USA. [2]Department of Gynecologic Oncology, The University of Texas MD Anderson Cancer Center, Houston, TX, USA.

Characteristics and outcomes for patients with advanced vaginal or vulvar cancer referred to a phase I clinical...

139

## References

1. Siegel R, Ma J, Zou Z, Jemal A. Cancer statistics, 2014. CA Cancer J Clin. 2014;64(1):9–29.

2. Woelber L, Mahner S, Voelker K, Eulenburg CZ, Gieseking F, Choschzick M, et al. Clinicopathological prognostic factors and patterns of recurrence in vulvar cancer. Anticancer Res. 2009;29(2):545–52.

3. Zweizig S, Korets S, Cain JM. Key concepts in management of vulvar cancer. Best Pract Res Clin Obstet Gynaecol. 2014.

4. Beller U, Benedet JL, Creasman WT, Ngan HY, Quinn MA, Maisonneuve P, et al. Carcinoma of the vagina. FIGO 26th annual report on the results of treatment in gynecological cancer. Int J Gynaecol Obstet. 2006;95 Suppl 1:S29–42.

5. Beller U, Quinn MA, Benedet JL, Creasman WT, Ngan HY, Maisonneuve P, et al. Carcinoma of the vulva. FIGO 26th annual report on the results of treatment in gynecological cancer. Int J Gynaecol Obstet. 2006;95 Suppl 1:S7–27.

6. Sznurkowski JJ, Milczek T, Emerich J. Prognostic factors and a value of 2009 FIGO staging system in vulvar cancer. Arch Gynecol Obstet. 2013;287(6):1211–8.

7. Sinno AK, Saraiya M, Thompson TD, Hernandez BY, Goodman MT, Steinau M, et al. Human papillomavirus genotype prevalence in invasive vaginal cancer from a registry-based population. Obstet Gynecol. 2014;123(4):817–21.

8. Ioffe YJ, Massad LS. Clinical behavior of HPV-negative and HPV-positive vulvar cancers. Gynecol Oncol. 2013;131(1):247.

9. Sardain H, Lavoue V, Laviolle B, Henno S, Foucher F, Leveque J. Prognostic factors for curative pelvic exenterations in patients with recurrent uterine cervical or vaginal cancer. Int J Gynecol Cancer. 2014;24(9):1679–85.

10. Micheletti L, Preti M. Surgery of the vulva in vulvar cancer. Best Pract Res Clin Obstet Gynaecol. 2014.

11. Miyamoto DT, Viswanathan AN. Concurrent chemoradiation for vaginal cancer. PLoS One. 2013;8(6):e65048.

12. Witteveen PO, van der Velden J, Vergote I, Guerra C, Scarabeli C, Coens C, et al. Phase II study on paclitaxel in patients with recurrent, metastatic or locally advanced vulvar cancer not amenable to surgery or radiotherapy: a study of the EORTC-GCG (European Organisation for Research and Treatment of Cancer–Gynaecological Cancer Group). Ann Oncol. 2009;20(9):1511–6.

13. Salom EM, Penalver M. Recurrent vulvar cancer. Curr Treat Options in Oncol. 2002;3(2):143–53.

14. Woelber L, Trillsch F, Kock L, Grimm D, Petersen C, Choschzick M, et al. Management of patients with vulvar cancer: a perspective review according to tumour stage. Ther Adv Med Oncol. 2013;5(3):183–92.

15. Deppe G, Mert I, Winer IS. Management of squamous cell vulvar cancer: a review. J Obstet Gynaecol Res. 2014;40(5):1217–25.

16. Therasse P, Arbuck SG, Eisenhauer EA, Wanders J, Kaplan RS, Rubinstein L, et al. New guidelines to evaluate the response to treatment in solid tumors. European organization for research and treatment of cancer, national cancer institute of the United States, national cancer institute of Canada. J Natl Cancer Inst. 2000;92(3):205–16.

17. Eisenhauer EA, Therasse P, Bogaerts J, Schwartz LH, Sargent D, Ford R, et al. New response evaluation criteria in solid tumours: revised RECIST guideline (version 1.1). Eur J Cancer. 2009;45(2):228–47.

18. Hacker NF, Eifel PJ, van der Velden J. Cancer of the vulva. Int J Gynaecol Obstet. 2012;119 Suppl 2:S90–6.

19. Stehman FB, Look KY. Carcinoma of the vulva. Obstet Gynecol. 2006;107(3):719–33.

20. Hacker NF, Eifel PJ, van der Velden J. Cancer of the vagina. Int J Gynaecol Obstet. 2012;119 Suppl 2:S97–9.

21. Wheler J, Tsimberidou AM, Hong D, Naing A, Falchook G, Piha-Paul S, et al. Survival of 1,181 patients in a phase I clinic: the MD Anderson Clinical Center for targeted therapy experience. Clin Cancer Res Off J Am Assoc Cancer Res. 2012;18(10):2922–9.

22. Hou MM, Liu X, Wheler J, Naing A, Hong D, Bodurka D, et al. Outcomes of patients with metastatic cervical cancer in a phase I clinical trials program. Anticancer Res. 2014;34(5):2349–55.

23. Hou MM, Liu X, Wheler J, Naing A, Hong D, Coleman RL, et al. Targeted PI3K/AKT/mTOR therapy for metastatic carcinomas of the cervix: a phase I clinical experience. Oncotarget. 2014.

24. Modesitt S, Walker J. Obesity crisis in cancer care: gynecologic cancer prevention, treatment, and survivorship in obese women in the United States. Gynecol Oncol. 2014;133(1):1–3.

25. von Gruenigen VE, Tian C, Frasure H, Waggoner S, Keys H, Barakat RR. Treatment effects, disease recurrence, and survival in obese women with early endometrial carcinoma : a Gynecologic Oncology Group study. Cancer. 2006;107(12):2786–91.

# Transversus abdominis plane block with liposomal bupivacaine compared to oral opioids alone for acute postoperative pain after laparoscopic hysterectomy for early endometrial cancer: a cost-effectiveness analysis

Brandon-Luke L. Seagle[1][*], Emily S. Miller[1], Anna E. Strohl[1], Anna Hoekstra[2] and Shohreh Shahabi[1]

**Abstract**

**Background:** To determine the cost-effectiveness of transversus abdominis plane block with liposomal bupivacaine (TAP) compared to oral opioids alone for acute postoperative pain after laparoscopic hysterectomy for early endometrial cancer.

**Methods:** A cost-effectiveness analysis using a decision tree structure with a 30.5 day time-horizon was used to calculate incremental cost-effectiveness ratio (ICER) values per quality-adjusted life-year (QALY). Base-case costs, probabilities, and QALY values were identified from recently published all-payer national database studies, 2017 Medicare fee-schedules, randomized trials, institutional case series, or assumed, when published values were not available. One-way, two-way and multiple probabilistic sensitivity analyses were performed.

**Results:** The TAP strategy dominated the oral opioid-only strategy, with decreased costs and increased effectiveness. Specifically, the TAP strategy saved $235.90 under the base-case assumptions. Threshold analyses demonstrated that if the relative same-day discharge probability was ≥ 12% higher in the TAP group, then TAP was cost-saving over oral opioids-alone. Similarly, TAP was cost-saving whenever the costs saved by same-day discharge compared to admission were ≥ $1115.22. Cost-effectiveness of the TAP strategy was highly robust of a variety of sensitivity analyses.

**Conclusions:** TAP with liposomal bupivacaine was robustly cost-effective at conventional willingness-to-pay thresholds. Further, TAP was cost-saving compared to opioids-only when the same-day discharge rate among TAP users was greater than among opioid-only users.

**Keywords:** Endometrial cancer, Pain, Analgesia, Bupivacaine, Transversus abdominis plane block

* Correspondence: brandon.seagle@northwestern.edu
[1]Department of Obstetrics and Gynecology, Prentice Women's Hospital, Northwestern University, Feinberg School of Medicine, 250 E Superior Street, Suite 05-2168, Chicago, IL 60611, USA
Full list of author information is available at the end of the article

## Background

Enhanced recovery protocols have become the standard-of-care for gynecologic oncology surgery [1, 2]. These comprehensive protocols result in shorter lengths of stay, fewer complications, earlier return of bowel function, and increased patient satisfaction [1, 2]. Optimal analgesia for acute postoperative pain requires a multi-class medication strategy with the goal of opioid minimization [1, 2]. Epidural and patient-controlled analgesia (PCA) have lost favor in many practices given immediate initiation of oral intake and the concurrent goals of early ambulation and opioid minimization in the early postoperative period. Much of the experience supporting a potential benefit of either incisional or regional injection of long-acting local analgesics such as liposomal bupivacaine was not published at the time of development of the ERAS® Society guidelines [1, 2].

Recently, the Mayo clinic reported a series of gynecologic oncology patients who received surgeon-injected regular or liposomal bupivacaine at the laparotomy incision [3]. Women who received liposomal bupivacaine used less rescue intravenous or PCA opioids [3]. There was no difference in total pharmacy costs despite the higher cost of liposomal bupivacaine [3]. Women who received liposomal bupivacaine also had decreased nausea and ileus [3]. Because the innervation of the anterior abdominal wall anatomically travels from lateral to medial, and laparoscopy requires placement of laterally-located port sites, injection of liposomal bupivacaine by bilateral transversus abdominis plane (TAP) block may be particularly useful for women undergoing laparoscopic or robotic hysterectomy.

Anesthesiologists at one of the author's hospitals routinely give TAP blocks with liposomal bupivacaine preoperatively to women undergoing laparoscopic or robotic surgery. This quality-improvement practice facilitated an 86% rate of same-day discharge (SDD) among women undergoing surgical staging for gynecologic malignancies in the last two-years. High SDD rates were also reported by a trial of women undergoing robotic hysterectomy and randomized to TAP with regular versus liposomal bupivacaine [4]. 60.7% (17/28) of women who received liposomal bupivacaine had same-day discharge [4]. Women who received liposomal bupivacaine had decreased pain scores throughout their first 72-h after surgery, significantly decreased opioid use, and less nausea and vomiting [4]. We believe that presumptions about higher costs and, in some systems, pharmacy formulary decisions against liposomal bupivacaine, have limited access to TAP blocks with liposomal bupivacaine. To address this concern, we performed a cost-effectiveness analysis of TAP with liposomal bupivacaine versus routine oral opioid-only analgesia for women undergoing laparoscopic hysterectomy for early endometrial cancer.

## Methods

### Decision tree

A decision tree was built to evaluate the cost-effectiveness of TAP block with liposomal bupivacaine versus routine oral opioid-only postoperative analgesia among women undergoing laparoscopic hysterectomy for early endometrial cancer (Additional files 1, 2 and 3: Figures S1–S3). The model was built from a healthcare system perspective, meaning that costs to the healthcare system but not greater societal costs were included. Incremental cost-effectiveness ratio (ICER) values were calculated in terms of costs per quality-adjusted life-year (QALY). An ICER value of < 50,000/QALY was considered cost-effective.

The decision node of the model was split by TAP with liposomal bupivacaine versus no TAP. In both arms of the decision tree women had a chance of SDD or admission, a chance of readmission or no readmission within 30 days, and a chance of opioid use or no opioid use. Downstream of opioid use, there was a complication subtree including costs and probabilities related to narcotic-use for aspiration and ileus. In the TAP arm, possibilities of a TAP procedure complication or liposomal bupivacaine adverse event were additionally modeled. Any patient who experienced either a TAP procedure complication or bupivacaine adverse event was assumed to be admitted. Probabilities reflecting the chances of overall 30-day mortality and of a composite complication (most commonly urinary tract infection) for women undergoing laparoscopic hysterectomy were included as chance events throughout both arms. Additional probabilities of death were modeled specifically for a bupivacaine adverse event, aspiration, or bowel perforation, which was assumed to be a very rare complication only in the postoperative ileus population. Finally, among women who used opioids, the 30-day mortality rate was increased by the prescription opioid fatal overdose risk of the population. At the end of model, each patient was either alive without complications, alive with complications, alive after perforation, alive after perforation and additional complications, or deceased. Model building and implementation, statistical analyses and figure creation were performed with TreeAge Pro 2016 (TreeAge Software Inc., Williamstown, MA).

The model operates under several additional noteworthy assumptions. First is the assumption that SDD is typically higher among women who have a TAP block than women who receive only oral opioids. This assumption is based on our experience and also the published SDD rates, decreased pain scores, better 72-h pain control, and decreased postoperative nausea and vomiting associated with use of liposomal bupivacaine for acute postoperative pain reported by previous studies

[3, 4]. Since the major discharge criteria for SDD are adequate pain control and ability to tolerate oral analgesics and anti-emetics, if needed, this assumption is reasonable. Differences in opioid use were modeled as use or non-use rather than by quantity of use, given limitations of the existing literature. Further, since the serious narcotic-associated complications are uncommon, alternative modeling of these parameters would not change the statistical inferences resulting from this cost-effectiveness analysis. Complications were allowed even among women who were not readmitted, so as to not bias the model toward TAP block with its associated higher SDD probability, since readmission has been observed to be less common among women who had SDD. The analysis reasonably assumes no systematic differences in surgical procedures or oncologic outcomes among women who receive TAP versus opioid-only analgesia. The model used a short time-horizon of only 30.5 days as outcome differences related to strategy for postoperative pain management are assumed to be none by or before 30 days after surgery. Finally, the model assumes that anesthesiology personal are readily available to place TAP blocks, and that TAP blocks are placed in pre-operative holding before women enter the operating room, which is our routine practice. Therefore, there are no systematic differences in operating room time, or time under general anesthesia, among women who do versus do not receive TAP blocks.

## Costs

Cost data are shown in Table 1. Drug prices were the average wholesale prices, updated monthly, as referenced on UpToDate® drug information pages. Liposomal

**Table 1** Cost estimates

| Cost | Base-case ($) | Range ($) | Reference |
|---|---|---|---|
| 30 day mortality | 5000 | 2000–10,000 | Assumed |
| Aspiration | 30 | 0–100 | UpToDate |
| Liposomal bupivacaine | 204 | 50–350 | UpToDate |
| Liposomal bupivacaine adverse event | 209.76 | 100–300 | CMS |
| Composite complication | 18.72 | 10–30 | UpToDate |
| Postoperative ileus | 8296 | 1000–15,000 | 8 |
| Oral opioids | 16.23 | 10–25 | UpToDate |
| Nonfatal bowel perforation | 138,000 | 20,000–200,000 | 9 |
| Readmission | 10,000 | 5000–15,000 | 10 |
| Laparoscopic hysterectomy | 6679 | 5197–8673 | 6 |
| Cost reduction for same-day discharge | 2400 | 1000–4000 | 7 |
| TAP procedure | 83.12 | 75–100 | CMS |
| TAP complication | 315.70 | 200–450 | CMS |

Abbreviations: *CMS* Centers for Medicare & Medicaid Services

bupivacaine administration was modeled as typical TAP block use of a single vial of Exparel®, base-case cost of $204. The wholesale acquisition cost has been reported to be as low as $14.25 per vial [5]. Northwestern Memorial Hospital's pharmacy has a hospital cost of $315 per vial. Prophylactic treatment for uncomplicated aspiration was presumed to be ampicillin-clavulanate 875–125 mg orally twice daily for 3 days. The online 2017 physician fee schedule facility limiting charges from the Centers for Medicare & Medicaid Services were used for reimbursement costs based on CPT codes. TAP procedure cost was per CPT code 64488 for bilateral injection. Cost of a serious bupivacaine adverse event was considered the cost of a cardiopulmonary resuscitation using CPT code 92950. Total cost for surgical admission, including costs of complications, were considered the observed costs for laparoscopic hysterectomy from Wright et al. using the nationally-representative all-payer Premier database [6]. Costs for same-day surgery were modeled as the costs from Wright et al. minus $2400, the average cost per inpatient day in the United States among nonprofit hospitals [7]. This assumes that admitted patients are typically discharge home on postoperative day 1, although some patients stay longer [7]. Costs of additional complications were considered the cost to treat a urinary tract infection, the most common complication after laparoscopic hysterectomy, with trimethoprim-sulphamethoxazole double-strength orally twice daily for 3 days. Costs of postoperative ileus were from Asgeirsson et al. [8]. Costs of routine opioid prescription were considered oxycodone 5 mg × 30 tablates. Costs of nonfatal bowel perforation were from Cohn et al. [9]. General readmission costs were used similarly as by Seagle et al. [10]. Cost of a serious TAP block complication was considered the cost of a computed tomography scan of the abdomen and pelvis (CPT 74177) to diagnose the complication [11].

## Effectiveness

Effectiveness was framed in terms of QALY values. Alive states were given baseline QALY values of 0.85. This calculation accounted for 70% of women with clinically early endometrial cancer being surgically staged as stage I and therefore without evidence of disease after surgery. These women have a high expectation of cure. In contrast, 30% were considered to be alive with cancer or with pathologic high-risk factors requiring adjuvant therapy, and were assigned a QALY of 0.5 [12]. Having experienced a complication is assumed to further decrease the QALY value by 30% of baseline, except for having survived a bowel perforation, assumed to decrease the QALY by 80% of baseline during the 30 day study period. A randomized trial in laparoscopic hysterectomy reported a 10% increase in patient satisfaction scores comparing TAP with liposomal bupivacaine to TAP with regular bupivacaine [4]. While QALY values and patient satisfaction are not the same, we sought to incorporate this finding by assigning surviving women who underwent TAP with liposomal bupivacaine, compared to oral opioids-only, an additional 0.1 QALY value. Finally, all QALY values were adjusted to 30.5 day values by multiplication by 30.5/365.

## Probabilities

Probabilities were assigned as listed in Table 2. Composite complication probabilities for surgery were considered to occur with a 9.0% probability for the base-case and varied from 5.0–12.0% based on Wright et al. (laparoscopic hysterectomy for benign disease from the Premier database) and Scalici et al. (laparoscopic staging for endometrial cancer from the ACS-NSQIP database) [6, 13]. Probability of dying from bowel perforation was considered 25% from Cohn et al. [9]. The 30-day mortality probability for laparoscopic endometrial cancer surgery was 0.14% from Gildea et al. [14]. For women using opioids, the 30-day mortality probability was increased

**Table 2** Probability estimates

| Probability | Base value (%) | Range (%) | Reference |
|---|---|---|---|
| 30 day mortality | 0.14 | 0.02–1.0 | 14 |
| Fatal opioid overdose | 0.001 | 0–0.002 | 15 |
| Postoperative ileus without opioids | 0.17 | 0–0.34 | 16 |
| Postoperative ileus with opioids | 1.43 | 0.43–2.43 | 16 |
| Aspiration with ileus | 5 | 0–10 | Assumed |
| Aspiration without ileus | 1 | 0–2 | Assumed |
| Death by aspiration | 1 | 0–2 | Assumed |
| Bowel perforation with ileus | 0.1 | 0–0.2 | Assumed |
| Death from bowel perforation | 25 | 10–40 | 9 |
| Composite complication | 9 | 5–12 | 6, 13 |
| Opioid use without TAP block | 95 | 90–100 | Assumed |
| Fractional opioid difference with TAP | 50 | 100–30 | 4 |
| Same-day discharge (SDD), TAP | 90 | 80–99 | 4 |
| Fractional SDD difference, no TAP | 78 | 90–50 | 19, 21 |
| Readmission after SDD, TAP | 2.5 | 1–5 | 19 |
| Readmission after SDD, no TAP | 2.5 | 1–5 | 19 |
| Readmission after admission, TAP | 4.0 | 1–5 | 19 |
| Readmission after admission, no TAP | 4.0 | 1–5 | 19 |
| TAP procedure complication | 0.1 | 0–0.2 | 11 |
| Bupivacaine adverse event | 1.5 | 0–3 | 11 |
| Death by bupivacaine adverse events | 0.1 | 0–0.2 | Assumed |

by 100/10,000,000, the population probability of prescription opioid fatal overdose [15]. Probabilities of postoperative ileus with or without opioid use among patients who had abdominal surgery were from Goettesch et al. [16]. Probabilities of an aspiration event without or with ileus were assumed to be 1 and 5% due to lack of literature references for these values. There are no estimates in the English language literature for some less common risks, which were therefore assumed (Table 2). For instance, there were no cases of local anesthetic complications reported with use in TAP block, per a published literature review [11]. There are also no case reports of death from a TAP block procedure complication [11]. However, we estimated a low-risk of serious liposomal bupivacaine adverse event based on tachycardia or bradycardia probabilities [17]. Bowel perforation as a very rare complication of postoperative ileus or obstruction was modeled based on case reports and series with an assumed base-case probability of 1/1000 cases of ileus [18]. Probability of readmission within 30 days was 2.5% for women who had SDD and 4.0% for admitted patients based on an ACS-NSQIP study [19]. Probability of SDD among women who got TAP with liposomal bupivacaine was estimated at 90% for the base-case model. The base-case probability of SDD was considered to be 0.78 × the SDD probability of women who underwent TAP, based on SDD proportions without TAP blocks reported as high as 70–75% in series where SDD was prioritized [20, 21]. These high SDD rates, however, are far from typical, with national surveillance database estimates being about 8–9% [19]. Finally, use of postoperative opioids among women given a TAP block is modeled as 50% of the probability of opioid use in the opioid-only group [4].

## Sensitivity analyses

One-way sensitivity analyses were performed and reported as tornado diagrams to evaluate how potential variation in each model parameter impacts the calculated ICER value estimates. Cost and probability estimates were varied across the ranges shown in Tables 1 and 2 for one-way sensitivity analyses and for probabilistic sensitivity analyses, using triangle distributions. A two-way sensitivity analysis was performed on the SDD probability in the TAP group and the proportional difference in SDD among the oral opioid group to better describe the results in terms of these important parameters. The probabilistic sensitivity analysis (1000 parameter re-samplings) was used to generate 95% confidence intervals for the base-case model ICER value estimate. Additionally, cost-effectiveness acceptability curves were plotted. Finally, the probabilistic sensitivity analyses were repeated with difference specifications of the base-case estimates, as indicated with Results, to test how our statistical inferences may vary under different major assumptions of the model.

## Results

### Base-case analysis

The TAP block strategy dominated the oral opioid-only strategy, with negative ICER values indicating decreased costs and increased effectiveness associated with TAP block use (Table 3). Specifically, the TAP block strategy was cost-saving of $235.90 under the base-case assumptions. Due to the short time-horizon of the analysis, the absolute QALY difference is low. If the increased QALY associated with patient satisfaction was assumed to be 0 rather than 0.1 in the base-case, TAP block was still cost-saving, as it had decreased cost at the same effectiveness.

### One-way sensitivity analyses

Tornado plots for one-way sensitivity analyses for all cost and probability estimates are shown in Figs. 1 and 2. For costs, ICER values were most sensitive to costs saved by SDD and costs of bupivacaine (Fig. 1). For probabilities, ICER values were most sensitive to the proportional difference in SDD in the no TAP group (Fig. 2). However, when this difference was 1.0, meaning that both strategies had an equal 90% SDD rate, the ICER for TAP was still cost-effective compared to a conventional willingness-to-pay of $50,000/QALY (Fig. 2).

Threshold analyses for when TAP block would no longer be cost-saving demonstrated that if the SDD probability was ≥12% higher (relative difference, not absolute difference) in the TAP group than the oral opioid group, then TAP was cost-saving over oral opioids-alone. Similarly, TAP was cost-saving when the costs saved by SDD were ≥ $1115.22 compared to admission, which would be true even in states with the lowest daily hospitalization costs [7].

### Two-way sensitivity analysis

A two-way sensitivity analysis for the probability of SDD in the TAP group (range 50%–99%) versus the proportional difference in SDD in the oral opioid group (range 0.50–1.00), with willingness-to-pay set to $0/QALY to indicate the cost-saving strategy, showed that even at a low 50% SDD probability in the TAP group, TAP was cost-saving compared to oral opioids-only so long as the

absolute SDD probability was ≤ 40% in the oral opioid-only group (Fig. 3).

### Probabilistic sensitivity analyses

In the initial probabilistic sensitivity analysis, TAP was cost-effective compared to a conventional willingness-to-pay of $50,000/QALY in 99.5% of simulations, and cost-saving with ICER < $0/QALY in 89.3% of simulations. Cost acceptability curves for each strategy are shown in Fig. 4.

Additional probabilistic sensitivity analyses were performed under different major assumptions of the model and demonstrated highly robust results. First, if the oral opioid group was allowed to have an equal probability of SDD as the TAP group in sensitivity analyses, then TAP was cost-saving in 80.5% of simulations. Second, if the base-case probabilities of SDD were assumed to be 90% in both the TAP and oral opioid groups, with the opioid group allowed to have equal probability of SDD as the TAP group in sensitivity analyses, TAP was still cost-saving in 65.4% of simulations and cost-effective in 96.7% of simulations. Third, if the cost of liposomal bupivacaine was changed to the price of $315 (Northwestern Memorial Hospital's cost to purchase) with range of $200–400 per vial, TAP was cost saving in 76.9% of simulations and cost-effective in 98.8% of simulations. Fourth, if the probabilities of readmission were assumed to be equally low at 2.5% (range 1–5%) in both groups, TAP remained cost-saving in 89% of simulations. Finally, if the QALY increase associated with TAP use was removed from the model, TAP remained cost-saving in 90.2%.

## Discussion

Compared to the routine practice of prescribing oral opioids after laparoscopic hysterectomy, TAP block with liposomal bupivacaine is robustly cost-effective and in most scenarios is also cost-saving. This finding is robust to many alternative specifications of base-case parameters, and to changing their likeliest values used for probabilistic sensitivity analyses. Therefore, even if the major model assumptions are not agreed upon by all readers or representative of some practices (for instance, those with lower SDD rates), the main results are robust to alternatives in model assumptions. The cost-effectiveness of the TAP strategy was most sensitive to the difference in SDD probability between women who received TAP versus oral opioids-only. The two-way sensitivity analysis

**Table 3** Cost effectiveness of TAP with liposomal bupivacaine compared to oral opioids

| Regimen | Cost ($) | Incremental cost ($) | 30 day QALY | Incremental | ICER ($/QALY) | 95% CI ($/QALY) |
|---|---|---|---|---|---|---|
| TAP | 5193.30 | −235.90 | 0.08 | 0.01 | −28,274.70 | −10,177.86, |
| No TAP | 5429.20 | | 0.07 | | | −112,226.67 |

Abbreviations: *TAP* transverses abdominis plane block, *QALY* quality-adjusted life-year, *ICER* incremental cost effectiveness ratio, *CI* confidence interval

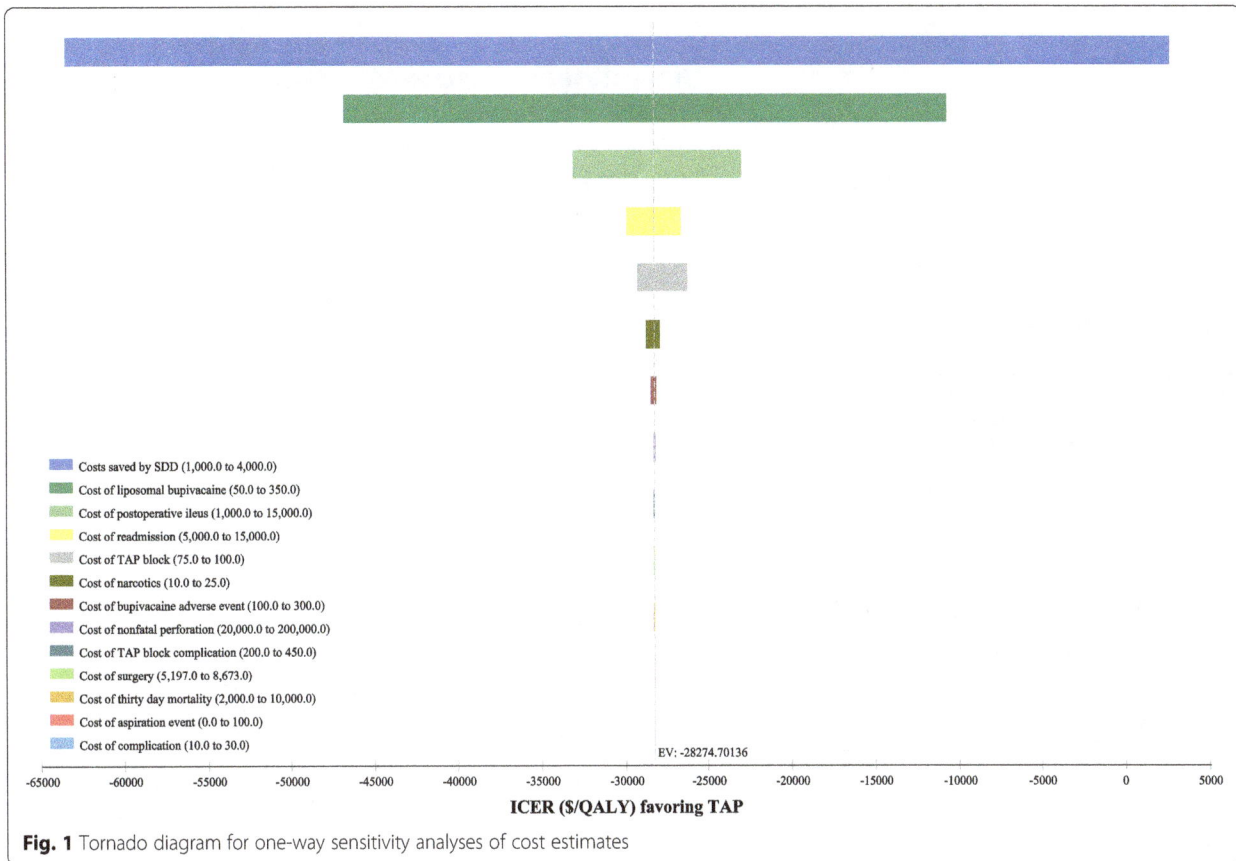

**Fig. 1** Tornado diagram for one-way sensitivity analyses of cost estimates

showed that TAP was cost-saving even at a low SDD probability of 50% among TAP users, with a 20% decreased relative SDD probability among oral opioid-only users, giving them an also low SDD probability of 40%.

Nationally, the SDD rate after laparoscopic surgical staging remains low at 8–9%, despite an only 2.5% readmission probability after SDD [19]. Some institutions have reported high (70–75%) SDD rates without use of TAP blocks [20, 21]. The randomized trial of TAP with regular versus liposomal bupivacaine had > 60% SDD in the liposomal bupivacaine arm [4]. In our experience, high SDD rates are routinely achieved using TAP with liposomal bupivacaine. The cost-effectiveness analysis here confirms that TAP block with the more expensive but longer-acting liposomal formulation of bupivacaine is typically cost-saving.

Achieving routine SDD for women undergoing laparoscopic or robotically-assisted laparoscopic surgical staging for early endometrial cancer offers an opportunity for healthcare system cost-savings, with improved postoperative recovery and patient satisfaction. Implementing routine SDD requires system and practice-wide commitments, beginning with preoperative patient counselling to expect outpatient surgery. Operative times for surgical procedures need to be consistently efficient, which can be more difficult to achieve in training

environments with rotating surgical teams. Multidisciplinary support for SDD, with collaboration from operating room and recovery room anesthesiologists and nurses, is critical to ensure the success of SDD protocols. In fact, much of the success of a SDD program likely depends on anesthesiology and nursing practices.

In addition to limitations related to the base-case model assumptions, limitations of this study include that not all possible specific complications were modeled. For instance, postoperative pneumonia and venous thromboembolism were not specifically considered. However, these complications would presumably occur more often among women who were admitted to the hospital, favoring the TAP block strategy. Furthermore, cost estimates used for the surgical admission were total inpatient cost estimates including costs related to the full-spectrum of complications experienced, based on a nationally-representative all-payer database analysis, and therefore include costs of other additional complications. Also, because major complications are uncommon, consistent with the one-way sensitivity analysis results, the results are not sensitive to major complication costs. Therefore, disagreement about assumptions of modeling uncommon major complications, leading to alternative modeling of complications, would not meaningfully change the result that the TAP strategy is robustly cost-

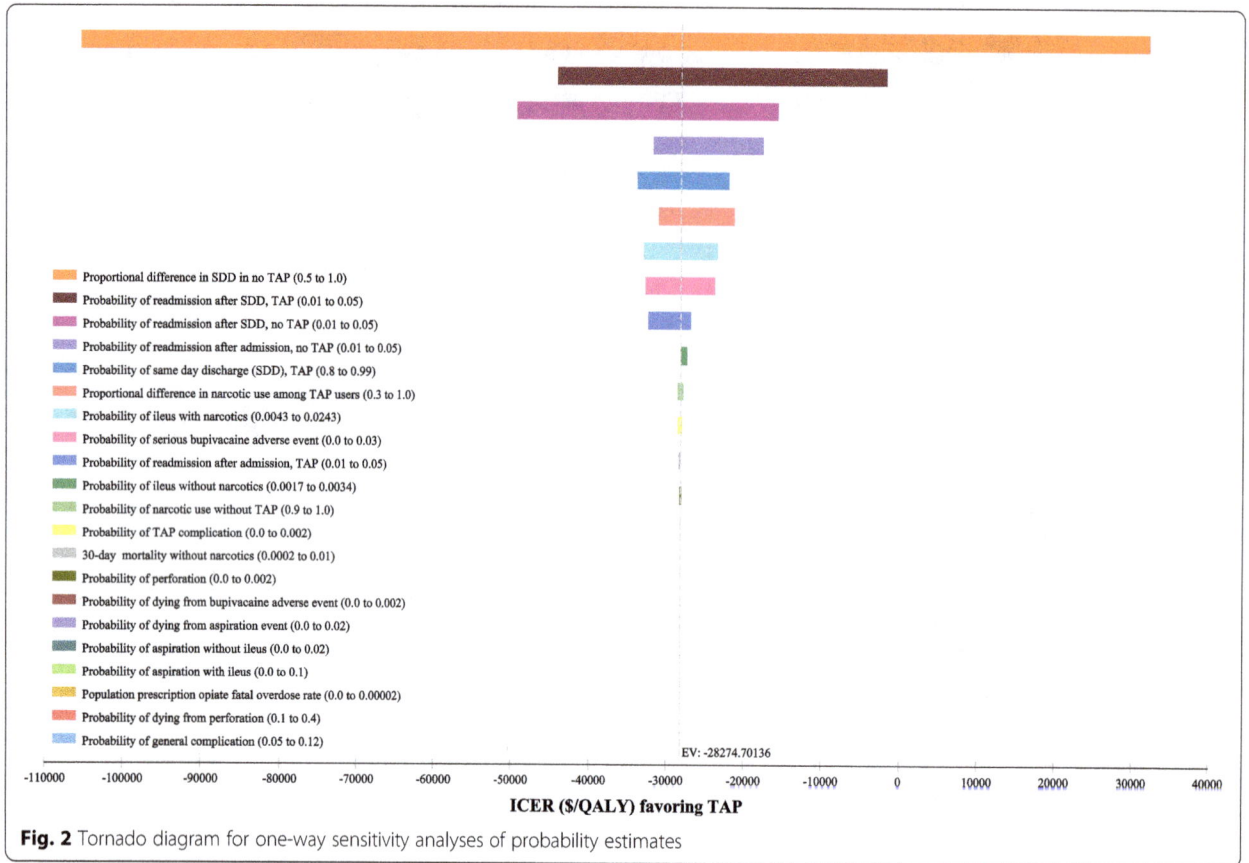

**Fig. 2** Tornado diagram for one-way sensitivity analyses of probability estimates

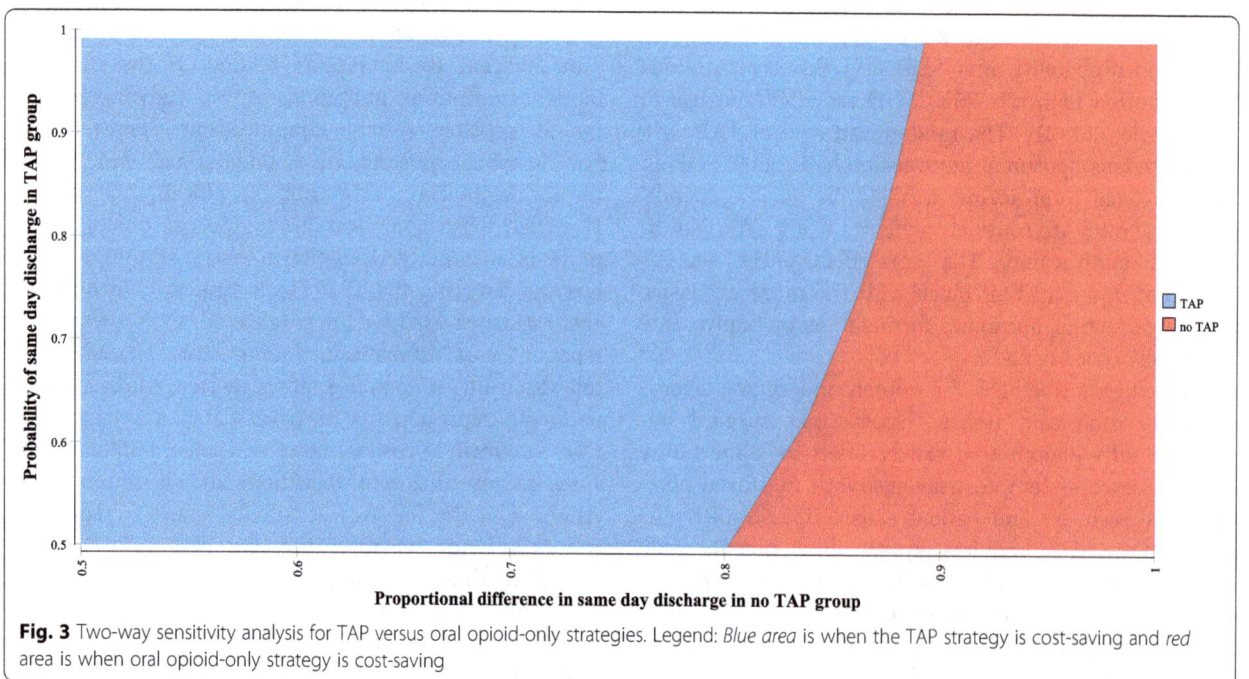

**Fig. 3** Two-way sensitivity analysis for TAP versus oral opioid-only strategies. Legend: *Blue area* is when the TAP strategy is cost-saving and *red* area is when oral opioid-only strategy is cost-saving

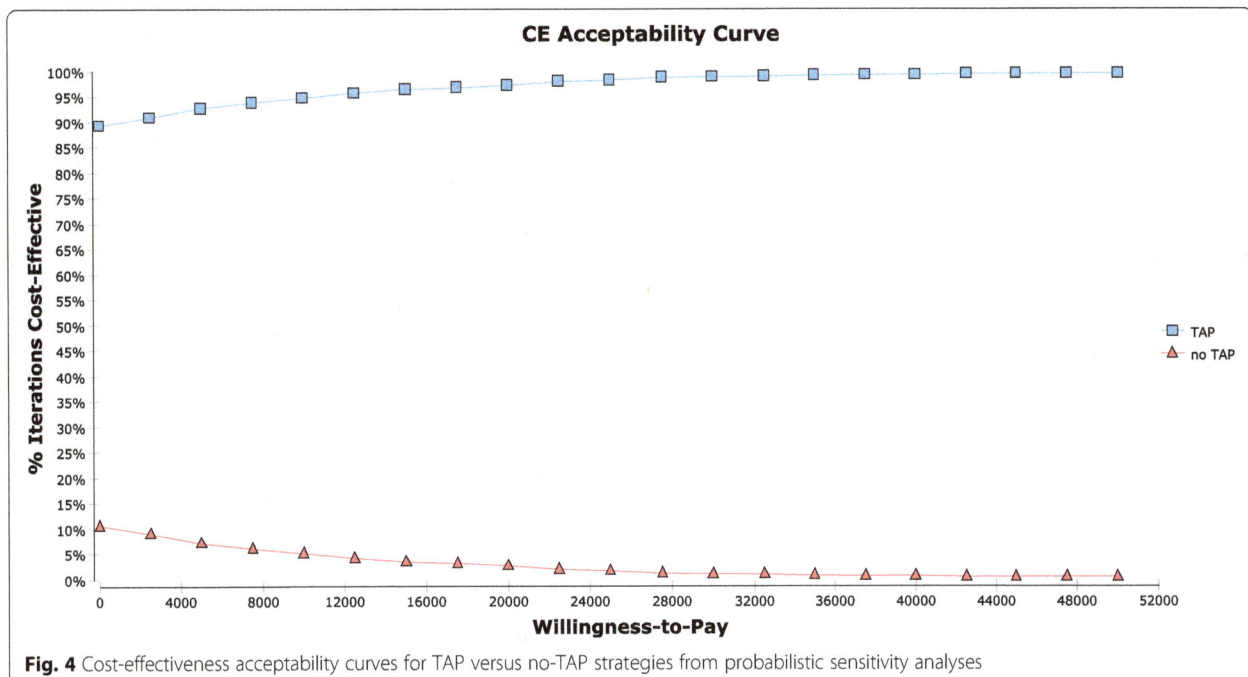

**Fig. 4** Cost-effectiveness acceptability curves for TAP versus no-TAP strategies from probabilistic sensitivity analyses

effective and often cost-saving. Surgical procedure costs used pertained to women undergoing hysterectomy for benign disease rather than for cancer. If higher surgical admission costs specifically for cancer or for robotic hysterectomy were used, the results would be very similar because the difference in SDD probabilities and cost-saving associated with SDD would be the same. These SDD parameters are the most important factors for determining the relative cost-effectiveness and the cost-savings of the TAP strategy. As for the potential concerns about assumptions of effectiveness estimates (QALY values) used here, it should be noted that no case report of death resulting from a TAP block with a local analgesic has been reported, and therefore the probability of death due to the TAP strategy that was assumed could arguably be removed from the model. This would allow us to transform the analysis to a cost-minimization, without consideration of effectiveness estimates or alternative time-horizons. A cost-minimization would show the TAP strategy to be most often cost-saving, consistent with the cost-effectiveness analysis results. Finally, use of non-opioid analgesic agents was assumed to be similar among the model arms in this decision analysis and was therefore not modeled. Given modern enhanced recovery protocols, it is likely that any institution using TAP blocks routinely also uses multi-modal oral analgesia strategies as part of good practice.

## Conclusions

TAP with liposomal bupivacaine is robustly cost-effective and most often cost-saving. This finding should

be considered by hospital administrators and pharmacists when making their pharmacy formulary decisions. Anesthesiologists and surgeons with concerns about seemingly increased costs related to use of liposomal bupivacaine should be reassured that so long as SDD is routine for women with laparoscopic/robotic surgery, then the TAP strategy is cost-saving. Furthermore, cost-savings associated with use of liposomal bupivacaine may not hinge entirely on superior SDD probabilities among women who receive TAP. For instance, in our probabilistic sensitivity analysis that assumed high and equal 90% SDD probabilities in both the TAP and oral opioid-only groups, TAP remained cost-saving in 65% of simulations. Use of bilateral TAP blocks with liposomal bupivacaine as an analgesic strategy to facilitate SDD is most often cost-saving, and nearly always cost-effective compared to conventional willingness-to-pay thresholds.

**Abbreviations**

ICER: Incremental cost-effectiveness ratio; PCA: Patient-controlled analgesia; QALY: Quality-adjusted life-year; SDD: Same-day discharge; TAP: Transversus abdominis plane block

**Acknowledgements**

None.

**Funding**

BLS is supported by funds of the Division of Gynecologic Oncology at Northwestern and the Jean Donovan Estate. Funding sources had no role in the design of the study, collection of data, analysis, interpretation of the data, or writing of the manuscript.

## Authors' contributions

BLS: concept, data analysis and interpretation, wrote manuscript; ESM: discussed and reviewed analysis, edited manuscript; AES: edited manuscript; AH & SS: concept, edited manuscript. All authors read and approved the final manuscript.

## Competing interests

The authors declare that they have no competing interests.

## Author details

[1]Department of Obstetrics and Gynecology, Prentice Women's Hospital, Northwestern University, Feinberg School of Medicine, 250 E Superior Street, Suite 05-2168, Chicago, IL 60611, USA. [2]West Michigan Cancer Center and Western Michigan University, Homer Stryker School of Medicine, Kalamazoo, MI, USA.

## References

1.  Nelson G, Altman AD, Nick A, Meyer LA, Ramirez PT, Achtari C, et al. Guidelines for pre- and intra-operative care in gynecologic/oncology surgery: enhanced recovery after surgery (ERAS®) society recommendations – part I. Gynecol Oncol. 2016;140:313–22.

2.  Nelson G, Altman AD, Nick A, Meyer LA, Ramirez PT, Achtari C, et al. Guidelines for postoperative care in gynecologic/oncology surgery: enhanced recovery after surgery (ERAS®) society recommendations – part II. Gynecol Oncol. 2016;140:323–32.

3.  Kalogera E, Bakkum-Gamez JN, Weaver AL, Moriarty JP, Borah BJ, Langstraat CL, et al. Abdominal incision injection of liposomal bupivacaine and opioid use after laparotomy for gynecologic malignancies. Obstet Gynecol. 2016; 128:1009–17.

4.  Hutchins J, Delaney D, Vogel RI, Ghebre RG, Downs LS Jr, Carson L, et al. Ultrasound guided subcostal transversus abdominis plane (TAP) infiltration with liposomal bupivacaine for patients undergoing robotic assisted hysterectomy: a prospective randomized controlled study. Gynecol Oncol. 2015;138:609–13.

5.  Lambrechts M, O'Brien MJ, Savoie FH, You Z. Liposomal extended-release bupivacaine for postsurgical analgesia. Patient Prefer Adherence. 2013;7: 885–90.

6.  Wright JD, Ananth CV, Lewin SN, Burke WM, Lu YS, Neugut AI, et al. Robotically assisted vs laparoscopic hysterectomy among women with benign gynecologic disease. JAMA. 2013;309:689–98.

7.  Kaiser State Health Facts. Available at: http://kff.org/health-costs/state-indicator/expenses-per-inpatient-day-by -ownership. Accessed 6 Mar 2017.

8.  Asgeirsson T, El-Badawi K, Mahmood A, Barletta J, Luchtefeld M, Senagore AJ. Postoperative ileus: it costs more than you expect. J Am Coll Surg. 2010; 210:228–31.

9.  Cohn DE, Kim KH, Resnick KE, O'Malley DM, Straughn JM Jr. At what cost does a potential survival advantage of bevacizumab make sense for the primary treatment of ovarian cancer? A cost-effectiveness analysis. J Clin Oncol. 2011;29:1247–51.

10. Seagle BL, Shahabi S. Cost-effectiveness analysis of dose-dense versus standard intravenous chemotherapy for ovarian cancer: an economic analysis of results from the gynecologic oncology group protocol 262 randomized controlled trial. Gynecol Oncol. 2017;145:9–14.

11. Young MJ, Gorlin AW, Modest VE, Quiraishi SA. Clinical implications of the transversus abdominis plane block in adults. Anesthesiol Res Pract. 2012; 2012:731645.

12. Kang R, Goodney PP, Wong SL. Importance of cost-effectiveness and value in cancer care and healthcare policy. J Surg Oncol. 2016;114:275–80.

13. Scalici J, Laughlin BB, Finan MA, Wang B, Rocconi RP. The trend towards minimally invasive surgery (MIS) for endometrial cancer: an ACS-NSQIP evaluation of surgical outcomes. Gynecol Oncol. 2015;136:512–5.

14. Gildea C, Nordin A, Hirschowitz L, Poole J. Thirty-day postoperative mortality for endometrial carcinoma in England: a population-based study. BJOG. 2016;123:1853–61.

15. Paulozzi LJ, Budnitz DS, Xi Y. Increasing deaths from opioid analgesics in the United States. Pharmacoepidemiol Drug Saf. 2006;15:618–27.

16. Goettsch WG, Sukel MP, van der Peet DL, van Riemsdijk MM, Herings RM. In-hospital use of opioids increases rate of coded postoperative paralytic ileus. Pharmacoepidemiol Drug Saf. 2007;16:668–74.

17. Uskova A, O'Connor JE. Liposomal bupivacaine for regional anesthesia. Curr Opin Anaesthesiol. 2015;28:593–7.

18. Tenofsky PL, Beamer RL, Smith RS. Ogilvie syndrome as a postoperative complication. Arch Surg. 2000;135:682–7.

19. Lee J, Aphinyanaphongs Y, Curtin J, Chern JY, Frey MK, Boyd LR. The safety of same-day discharge after laparoscopic hysterectomy for endometrial cancer. Gynecol Oncol. 2016;142:508–13.

20. Rettenmaier MA, Mendivil AA, Brown JV III, Abaid LN, Micha JP, Goldstein BH. Same-day discharge in clinical stage I endometrial cancer patients treated with total laparoscopic hysterectomy, bilaterally salpingo-oophorectomy, and bilateral pelvic lymphadenectomy. Oncology. 2012;82:321–6.

21. Melamed A, Katz Eriksen JL, Hinchcliff EM, Worley MJ Jr, Berkowitz NS, Muto MG, et al. Same-day discharge after laparoscopic hysterectomy for endometrial cancer. Ann Surg Oncol. 2016;23:178–85.

# 18

# Response to pembrolizumab in a heavily treated patient with metastatic ovarian carcinosarcoma

Graziela Zibetti Dal Molin[1], Carina Meira Abrahão[2], Robert L. Coleman[3] and Fernando Cotait Maluf[4*]

## Abstract

**Background:** Ovarian carcinosarcoma is a rare malignancy associated with a high rate of cancer-related mortality even at early stages. Guidelines for systemic treatment have been difficult to establish because the disease is commonly excluded from prospective clinical trials. Ovarian carcinosarcoma is usually managed as high-grade epithelial ovarian cancer despite major histologic differences. Owing to the rarity and poor prognosis of ovarian carcinosarcoma, salvage treatments and their efficacy have been poorly described.

**Case presentation:** A patient heavily treated for ovarian carcinosarcoma showed an objective response to an immune checkpoint inhibitor, pembrolizumab. Pembrolizumab in this patient appeared to provide tumor control in multifocal metastatic sites.

**Conclusions:** Pembrolizumab should be evaluated in prospective trials for the treatment of ovarian carcinosarcoma and further work is needed to identify patients most likely to respond to this type of intervention.

**Keywords:** Immunotherapy, Pembrolizumab, Immune checkpoint inhibitors, Ovarian carcinosarcoma, Anti-PD1 antibody

## Background

Ovarian carcinosarcoma (OCS), also known as malignant mixed mesodermal tumor or malignant mixed müllerian tumor, is a rare and highly aggressive malignancy that contains both sarcomatous and carcinomatous elements [1]. OCS accounts for 1–4% of all primary ovarian carcinomas [2]. According to an analysis of the Surveillance, Epidemiology and End Results data, the rate of OCS is 0.19 per 100,000 women [3]. Despite the rarity of OCS, it is associated with a high rate of cancer-related mortality even at early stages [4]. OCS typically occurs in postmenopausal women at a median age of 65 years and is staged according to FIGO criteria for epithelial ovarian cancer (EOC) [5]. More than 70% of patients present with advanced stage (stage III-IV) disease at the time of diagnosis [4]. The most common symptoms resemble those observed with EOC, including pelvic and/or abdominal pain, early satiety, bloating, and abdominal

* Correspondence: fernandocotaitmaluf@gmail.com
[4]Hospital BP Mirante, Martiniano de Carvalho Street, 965, São Paulo 01323-90, Brazil
Full list of author information is available at the end of the article

distention [6]. OCS often presents as a large tumor with massive areas of hemorrhage and necrosis. The morphological features and biology of the tumor seem identical regardless of its site of origin in the female genital tract [7].

Several clinical prognostic factors associated with poor outcome have been described, including age, advanced stage at presentation, and suboptimal surgical resection [6]. Other reports indicate that the use of adjuvant chemotherapy may have a clinical benefit, although the limited number of patients in these retrospective studies does not allow definitive conclusions in this regard [8].

The epithelial component of OCS seems to drive the prognosis and survival characteristics and is usually the dominant histologic characteristic in metastatic sites. OCS has a pattern of spread similar to EOC, with early dissemination to the serosa and peritoneum of the pelvic and abdominal cavity [2]. Despite the lack of specific data, OCS is usually treated as a high-grade EOC despite major differences in histologic characteristics, molecular features, response to systemic therapy, and outcome [8]. Median overall survival was also shown to be significantly decreased in women with OCS (24 months) compared with those with EOC (41 months) [9]. Owing to the rarity of OCS and the poor prognosis, salvage treatments and their efficacy have been poorly described. We describe a patient heavily treated for OCS that had an objective response to an immune checkpoint inhibitor, pembrolizumab.

## Case presentation

A 62-year-old woman, who was negative for the BRCA1/2 germline mutation, presented to our institution with abdominal pain in October 2011. She was referred from another institution, where she had undergone a primary suboptimal cytoreduction. Pathologic analysis revealed a carcinosarcoma with a high-grade serous adenocarcinoma component associated with high-grade endometrial sarcoma in the right ovary and fallopian tube, with angiolymphatic embolization. There were also peritoneal implants in the upper abdomen and pelvis. The uterus, left fallopian tube and ovary, and lymph nodes had no evidence of disease; however, peritoneal cytologic analysis was positive for malignancy. Immunohistochemistry of the right ovary demonstrated that the tumor was positive for estrogen and progesterone receptor but HER2/neu-negative.

From April through June 2012, the patient received adjuvant carboplatin (AUC 6) and paclitaxel (175 mg/m$^2$) every 3 weeks for four cycles. In July 2012, she underwent an interval cytoreduction (optimal) followed by treatment with intraperitoneal cisplatin (75 mg/m$^2$) and intravenous (135 mg/m$^2$) and intraperitoneal paclitaxel (60 mg/m$^2$) for six additional cycles. After the end of chemotherapy, she received tamoxifen as maintenance treatment for 4 months. She was observed off treatment for 6 months. In May 2013, retroperitoneal adenopathy was discovered following a serial rise in CA125, which prompted radiographic assessment. She

received carboplatin (AUC 5), pegylated liposomal doxorubicin (30 mg/m$^2$), and bevacizumab (10 mg/kg) for four cycles and had a partial response. Paclitaxel was not used again owing to residual neuropathy. In light of localized recurrence and response, she underwent a tertiary debulking procedure with complete macroscopic gross resection. Unfortunately, 6 months later a positron emission tomography/computed tomography study (PET-CT) revealed disease progression in a right retropectoral lymph node, as well as in paraesophageal lymph nodes. She then received cisplatin (35 mg/m$^2$), gemcitabine (800 mg/m$^2$), and bevacizumab (10 mg/kg), but had disease progression.

From April 2014 through December 2015, the patient received various treatments for platinum-resistant disease: pemetrexed, nab-paclitaxel, megestrol, capecitabine, and vinorelbine. The metastatic sites were predominantly lymphatic and peritoneal. Despite the extensive pretreatment, she remained largely asymptomatic and had a good performance status. However, owing to disease progression, in January 2016 she initiated treatment with pembrolizumab (200 mg every 3 weeks). Unfortunately, there was not enough material to test the status of microsatellite instability, mutational load, or PD-L1 expression in the tumor. Also, the tumor was not analyzed for druggable mutations due to lack of insurance coverage. After the third cycle, she developed thyroiditis grade 1 but no other adverse events. After the fourth cycle, PET/CT showed objective partial response in the left external iliac lymph nodes (Fig. 1), as well as in the right-posterior pectoral lymph node conglomerate (Fig. 2). Another major site of metastatic disease was the right retropulmonary lymph nodes. With the goal of increasing local control and potentially causing an abscopal effect, she underwent radiotherapy (24 Gy in three fractions of 8 Gy). She then received an additional four cycles of pembrolizumab.

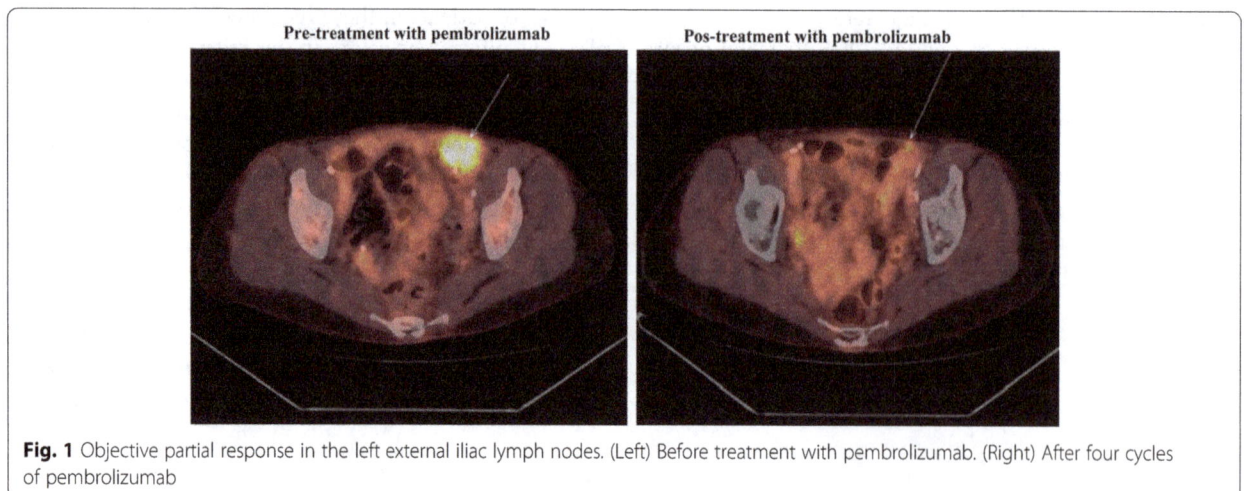

**Fig. 1** Objective partial response in the left external iliac lymph nodes. (Left) Before treatment with pembrolizumab. (Right) After four cycles of pembrolizumab

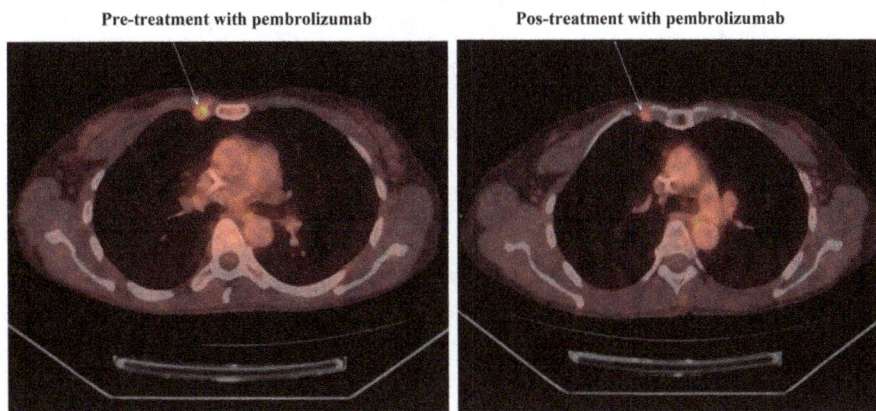

Pre-treatment with pembrolizumab            Pos-treatment with pembrolizumab

**Fig. 2** Objective partial response in the right-posterior pectoral lymph node conglomerate. (Left) Before treatment with pembrolizumab. (Right) After four cycles of pembrolizumab

Unfortunately, disease progression was discovered in the liver shortly thereafter. She received olaparib (400 mg twice per day) for 2 months but without response, and she died in October 2016.

## Discussion and conclusions

In the past few decades, overall survival has not improved for women with OCS; the median overall survival is less than 2 years. Currently, there is no clear evidence to establish consensus guidelines for systemic management of OCS [10].

Published data evaluating the benefit of chemotherapy are scarce, and treatment recommendations are generally based on a few nonrandomized prospective studies and some retrospective analyses. Adding to this difficulty is the common exclusion of patients with OCS from prospective therapeutic clinical trials. Active agents given to patients with OCS include carboplatin, cisplatin, ifosfamide, paclitaxel, doxorubicin, and dacarbazine [1, 10]. Common treatment combinations include platinum plus paclitaxel and platinum plus ifosfamide, although the benefit of multiagent chemotherapy over single-agent chemotherapy is unclear. The overall response rate (ORR) to platinum-based chemotherapy for patients with OCS varies between 25 and 70%, whereas median overall survival ranges from 8 to 16 months [11]. There is little evidence regarding the effectiveness of second-line therapies. In a study of single-agent ifosfamide, an ORR of 17.9% in patients with recurrent disease was recorded [12]. Owing to the high rate of recurrence, even for those with early-stage disease, adjuvant systemic therapy is generally considered, although there is no clear consensus on the standard first-line therapy in the adjuvant and metastatic setting [10].

Several studies have verified the role of molecular signaling pathways in the treatment of OCS. OCS most frequently contains high-grade serous components, which often contain a *TP53* mutation, and the precursor lesions may originate from normal-appearing fallopian tube epithelium that contains a *TP53* signature [13]. Given the poor response of OCS to standard available therapies, researchers have sought insight from molecular characterizations such as next-generation whole-exome sequencing [14]. Unsurprisingly, given the high rate of serous adenomatous components in OCS, the most common alteration is in *TP53* [13]. Other alterations described include mutations in *H2A* and *H2B*, deletions of *TP53* and *MBD3*, and amplification of chromosome segments containing *PIK3CA*, *TERT*, and *MYC*. However, few of these mutations are directly druggable [14].

Nevertheless, some EOCs have been known to induce a strong immune response characterized by high tumor T-cell infiltrates. As such, immune checkpoint inhibitors and combinations with chemotherapy, anti-angiogenesis agents, poly (ADP-ribose) polymerase (PARP) inhibitors, and other immune active compounds are under active investigation. Immunologic effector cells may be blocked by inhibitory regulatory pathways controlled by specific molecules often called immune checkpoints. These checkpoints serve to control or turn off the immune response when it is no longer needed to prevent tissue injury and auto-immunity [15]. Immune responses to ovarian cancer appear to vary by histologic subtype; high-grade serous cancers are most likely to be associated with a prognostically favorable tumor-infiltrating lymphocyte response. Classification of various histologic subtypes of ovarian cancers on the basis of tumor-infiltrating lymphocytes and PD-L1 expression revealed that

**Table 1** Clinical trial results for PD-1 and PD-L1 inhibitors in ovarian cancer

| Result | Agent | | | | |
|---|---|---|---|---|---|
| | Nivolumab [19] | Pembrolizumab [17] | Avelumab [20] | Atezolizumab [23] | Durvalumab [24] |
| No. of patients | 20 | 26 | 124 | 12 | 15 |
| Prior therapies | ≥4 in 55% of cases | ≥5 in 38.5% of cases | ≥3 in 65.3% of cases | ≥6 in 58% of cases | median 4 |
| PD-L1+ prevalence | 80% (IC 66%) | 100% (> 1% TC) | 77% (IC 66%) | 83% (> 1% TC) | 73% (> 5% TC) |
| Overall response rate | 15% | 11.5% | 9.7% | 25% | Not reported |
| Median progression-free survival | 3.5 months | Not reached | 2.6 months | 2.9 months | Not reported |
| Median overall survival | 20 months | Not reached | 10.8 months | 17.4 months | Not reported |

*IC* immune cells, *TC* tumor cells

type I patterns were more common in high-grade serous cancers and type IV patterns predominated in other histologic subtypes [16].

A phase Ib trial evaluated the safety and antitumor activity of pembrolizumab, an anti-PD-1 antibody, in patients with PD-L1-positive advanced solid tumors. One of the 26 patients with advanced EOC obtained a complete response and two patients experienced a partial response. The ORR was 11.5%, and the most common adverse events reported were fatigue, anemia, and decreased appetite [17]. Pembrolizumab has been studied in various scenarios in EOC: neoadjuvant setting, maintenance treatment, and recurrent or metastatic disease [18].

Another anti-PD-1 antibody, nivolumab, has also been studied in ovarian cancer. In a phase II trial, nivolumab was administered in patients with platinum-resistant EOC. Two complete responses were observed, as well as one partial response. The ORR was 15%, and the disease control rate was 45% [19]. Avelumab, a fully-humanized anti-PD-L1 IgG1 antibody, was studied in a phase I trial in patients with recurrent or refractory EOC. The ORR was 9.7% and the disease control rate was 54% [20]. A summary of the results of single-agent trials of PD-1/PD-L1 inhibitors is presented in Table 1. Ongoing studies are also evaluating the role of an anti-CTLA-4 antibody. Independent from the prognostic significance of PD-L1 expression, PD-L1/PD-1 receptor B7/CTLA-4 interactions are important immune escape mechanisms, allowing tumor progression [18].

To the best of our knowledge, this case report represents the first data on the use of pembrolizumab in OCS. The objective response in our patient suggests that OCS, like EOC, is an immunogenic malignancy. Interestingly, our patient was heavily pretreated with multiple locoregional and systemic therapies. It is unknown whether radiotherapy may have contributed to the objective response according to the suggested abscopal effect [21]. The biologic phenomenon underlying this effect is not completely understood, but it may be mediated by immunologic mechanisms [22].

In conclusion, pembrolizumab in this patient appeared to provide some tumor control in multifocal metastatic sites, despite the effects being short-lived. OCS should be evaluated in prospective trials and further work is needed to identify patients most likely to respond to this type of intervention.

**Abbreviations**
EOC: Epithelial ovarian cancer; OCS: Ovarian carcinosarcoma; ORR: Overall response rate

**Acknowledgments**
We would like to thank the Department of Scientific Publications of MD Anderson Cancer Center.

**Funding**
RLC is supported by CPRIT RP120214, the Ann Rife Cox Chair in Gynecology, Judy Reis/Albert Pisani, and the MD Anderson ovarian cancer research fund. All other authors have no funding to declare. No funding was received to publish this manuscript.

**Authors' contributions**
GZDM and CMA contributed to write the manuscript. GZDM, CMR, RLC and FCT edited the manuscript. All authors read and approved the final manuscript.

**Consent for publication**
We obtained consent to publish from the legal parent to report individual patient data.

**Competing interests**
RLC has clinical research funding from Merck, AstraZeneca/Medimmune, Genentech/Roche, Novartis, Clovis Oncology, Abbvie, and Janssen pharmaceuticals. All other authors have no competing interests to declare.

**Author details**
[1]Department of Gynecologic Oncology and Reproductive Medicine, The University of Texas MD Anderson Cancer Center, Houston, TX, USA. [2]Hospital BP Mirante, São Paulo, Brazil. [3]Department of Gynecologic Oncology and

Reproductive Medicine, The University of Texas MD Anderson Cancer Center, Houston, TX, USA. [4]Hospital BP Mirante, Martiniano de Carvalho Street, 965, São Paulo 01323-90, Brazil.

## References

1. del Carmen MG, Birrer M, Schorge JO. Carcinosarcoma of the ovary: a review of the literature. Gynecol Oncol. 2012;125(1):271–7.
2. Paulsson G, Anderson S, Sorbe B. A population-based series of ovarian carcinosarcomas with long-term follow-up. Anticancer Res. 2013;33:1003–8.
3. Howlader N, Noone AM, Krapcho M, Neyman N, Aminon R, Altekruse SF, et al., editors. SEER cancer statistics review, 1975–2009. Bethesda: National Cancer Institute; 2012.
4. Kyoung-Chul C, Jae-Joon K, Dae-Yeon K, Jong-Hyeok K, Yong-Man K, Joo-Hyun N, et al. Optimal debulking surgery followed by paclitaxel/platinum chemotherapy is very effective in treating ovarian carcinosarcomas: a single center experience. Gynecol Ostet Invest. 2011;72:208–14.
5. FIGO Committee on Gynecologic Oncology. FIGO staging for carcinoma of the vulva, cervix, and corpus uteri. Int J Gynaecol Obstet. 2014;125:97–8.
6. Brown E, Stewart M, Rye T, Al-Nafussi A, Williams AR, Bradburn M, et al. Carcinosarcoma of the ovary: 19 years of prospective data from a single center. Cancer. 2004;100(10):2148–53.
7. D'Angelo E, Prat J. Pathology of mixed Müllerian tumours. Best Pract Res Clin Obstet Gynaecol. 2011;25:705–18.
8. Rauh-Hain JA, Growdon WB, Rodriguez N, et al. Carcinosarcoma of the ovary: a case-control study. Gynecol Oncol. 2011;121:477–81.
9. Dictor M. Malignant mixed mesodermal tumor of the ovary: a report of 22 cases. Obstet Gynecol. 1985;65:720–4.
10. Berton-Rigaud D, Devouassoux-Shisheboran M, Ledermann JA, Leitao MM, Powell MA, Poveda A, et al. Gynecologic Cancer intergroup (GCIG) consensus review for uterine and ovarian carcinosarcoma. Int J Gynecol Cancer. 2014;24:S55–60.
11. Cicin I, Saip P, Eralp Y, Selam M, Topuz S, Ozluk Y, et al. Ovarian carcinosarcomas: clinicopathological prognostic factors and evaluation of chemotherapy regimens containing platinum. Gynecol Oncol. 2008; 108(1):136–40.
12. Shylasree TS, Bryant A, Athavale R. Chemotherapy and/or radiotherapy in combination with surgery for ovarian carcinosarcoma. Cochrane Database Syst Rev. 2013;28(2):CD006246.
13. Ardighieri L. Identical TP53 mutations in pelvic carcinosarcomas and associated serous tubal intraepithelial carcinomas provide evidence of their clonal relationship. Virchows Arch. 2016;469:61–9.
14. Zhao S, Bellone S, Lopez S, Thakral D, Schwab C, English DP, et al. Mutational landscape of uterine and ovarian carcinosarcoma implicates histone genes in epithelial-mesenchymal transition. Proc Natl Acad Sci U S A. 2016;113(43):12238–43.
15. Sharon E, Streicher H, Goncalves P, Chen HX. Immune checkpoint inhibitors in clinical trials. Chin J Cancer. 2014;33(9):434–44.
16. Webb JR, Milne K, Kroeger DR, Nelson BH. PD-L1 expression is associated with tumor-infiltrating T cells and favorable prognosis in high-grade serous ovarian cancer. Gynecol Oncol. 2016;141(2):293–302.
17. Varga A, Piha-Paul SA, Ott PA, Mehnert JM, Berton-Rigaud D, Johnson EA, et al. Antitumor activity and safety of pembrolizumab in patients (pts) with PD-L1 positive advanced ovarian cancer: interim results from a phase Ib study. J Clin Oncol. 2015;33(suppl 5510):5510.
18. Mittica G, Genta S, Aglietta M, Valabrega G. Immune checkpoint inhibitors: a new opportunity in the treatment of ovarian cancer? Int J Mol Sci. 2016; 17(7):1169.
19. Hamanishi J, Mandai M, Ikeda T, Minami M, Kawaguchi A, Murayama T, et al. Safety and antitumor activity of anti-PD-1 antibody, nivolumab, in patients with platinum resistant ovarian cancer. J Clin Oncol. 2015;33: 4015–22.
20. Disis ML, Patel MR, Pant S, Hamilton EP, Lockhart AC, Kelly K, et al. Avelumab (MSB0010718C; anti-PD-L1) in patients with recurrent/refractory ovarian cancer from the JAVELIN Solid Tumor phase Ib trial: safety and clinical activity. J Clin Oncol. 2016;34(suppl 5533):5533.
21. Mole RH. Whole body irradiation: radiobiology or medicine? Br J Radiol. 1953;26:234–41.
22. Drake C. Radiation-induced immune modulation. In: DeWeese TL, Laiho M, editors. Molecular determinants of radiation response. New York: Springer; 2011. p. 251–63.
23. Infante JR, Braiteh F, Emens LA, Balmanoukian AS, Oaknin A, Wang Y, et al. Safety, clinical activity and biomarkers of atezolizumab in advanced ovarian cancer. Ann Oncol. 2016;27(suppl 6):abstract 871P.
24. Lee J-M, Cimino-Mathews A, Peer CJ, Zimmer A, Lipkowitz S, Annunziata CM, et al. Safety and clinical activity of the programmed death-ligand 1 inhibitor durvalumab in combination with Poly(ADP-Ribose) polymerase inhibitor olaparib or vascular endothelial growth factor receptor 1–3 inhibitor cediranib in women's cancer: a dose escalation, phase I study. J Clin Oncol. 2016;34(suppl):abstract 3015.

# 19

# Preparation in the business and practice of medicine: perspectives from recent gynecologic oncology graduates and program directors

Matthew Schlumbrecht[1]*[iD], John Siemon[2], Guillermo Morales[1], Marilyn Huang[1] and Brian Slomovitz[1]

## Abstract

**Background:** Preparation in the business of medicine is reported to be poor across a number of specialties. No data exist about such preparation in gynecologic oncology training programs. Our objectives were to evaluate current time dedicated to these initiatives, report recent graduate perceptions about personal preparedness, and assess areas where improvements in training can occur.

**Methods:** Two separate surveys were created and distributed, one to 183 Society of Gynecologic Oncology candidate members and the other to 48 gynecologic oncology fellowship program directors. Candidate member surveys included questions about perceived preparedness for independent research, teaching, job-hunting, insurance, and billing. Program director surveys assessed current and desired time dedicated to the topics asked concurrently on the candidate survey. Statistical analysis was performed using Chi-squared (or Fisher's exact test if appropriate) and logistic regression.

**Results:** Survey response rates of candidate members and program directors were 28% and 40%, respectively. Candidate members wanted increased training in all measures except retrospective protocol writing. Female candidates wanted more training on writing letters of intent (LOI) ($p = 0.01$) and billing ($p < 0.01$). Compared to their current schedules, program directors desired more time to teach how to write an investigator initiated trial ($p = 0.01$). 94% of program directors reported having career goal discussions with their fellows, while only 72% of candidate members reported that this occurred ($p = 0.05$).

**Conclusion:** Recent graduates want more preparation in the non-clinical aspects of their careers. Reconciling program director and fellow desires and increasing communication between the two may serve to achieve the educational goals of each.

**Keywords:** Fellowship education, Program directors, Survey, Gynecologic oncology

## Background

Gynecologic oncology training programs have evolved much over the last ten years, and the volume of information that fellows are required to master has significantly increased. As it is has been reported that matriculating fellows are often ill-equipped for the rigors of a gynecologic oncology fellowship [1], there are increasing pressures on training programs to ensure adequate surgical experiences

while providing thorough didactic teaching in a short amount of time. Education in the non-clinical aspects of medicine, including skills to be a successful academician, experience with trial development, and exposure to different types of practice environments, may be lacking in lieu of basic science and clinical programs. At a time when recent fellowship graduates report dissatisfaction with their fellowship didactic lectures [2], it is important to understand the areas where they perceive weaknesses, and address these concerns in order to work towards further optimization of training programs. Our objective was to evaluate the perceptions of recent fellowship graduates in

* Correspondence: mschlumbrecht@miami.edu
[1]Division of Gynecologic Oncology, Sylvester Comprehensive Cancer Center, University of Miami, 1121 NW 14th St, Suite 345C, Miami, FL 33136, USA
Full list of author information is available at the end of the article

regards to their preparation for the non-clinical responsibilities of medicine, to evaluate current fellowship program education for such non-clinical responsibilities, and to determine if fellowship program directors are themselves satisfied with their own content curricula.

## Methods

Approval was obtained from the University of Miami Institutional Review Board. Two separate de novo surveys were created (Additional files 1 and 2). The first survey was for recent gynecologic oncology fellowship graduates who had not yet passed the oral certification exam in gynecologic oncology. These individuals are candidates for membership in the Society of Gynecologic Oncology (SGO), and were identified by a query of the SGO member database. The candidate survey contained questions about demographics, education history, and current practice setting. Additional questions about perceived preparation for a number of issues in post-training practice were posed in yes/no format, and addressed comfort with grant writing, protocol writing, effective teaching, billing and coding, malpractice insurance and medical-legal issues, financial planning, and disability; follow-up questions about these topics asked whether or not they would have preferred more training on each. Candidate members were also asked about how they obtained their first jobs, including faculty mentorship during the process, use of a headhunter, and contract review.

The second survey was developed for current gynecologic oncology fellowship program directors. As the subspecialty of gynecologic oncology is currently undergoing a transition in oversight from the American Board of Obstetrics and Gynecology (ABOG) to the Accreditation Council for Graduate Medical Education (ACGME), program directors were identified by a query of both organizations. Associate program directors were not included. Length of the program was ascertained. The survey then inquired about current number of didactic hours dedicated to each of the following topics over the length of fellowship training: protocol writing, drafting a grant proposal/letter of intent, being an effective teacher, billing/coding, medical-legal concerns, financial planning, disability, and the Affordable Care Act. Program directors were then asked how many hours they would *prefer* to spend on each of these topics.

The surveys for both program directors and candidate members were released via email in January, 2017, with a link to the questionnaire. The survey link was active for six weeks, and three separate email invitations to participate were sent. A statement of implied informed consent was included in the survey instructions. Responses were collected anonymously and stored in a RedCap database.

Statistical analyses were completed using STATA IC (StataCorp, College Station, TX). All data was used, even if the surveys were not completed in toto. Summary statistics were generated to describe the cohort. Chi-square testing (or Fisher's exact when appropriate) was used to analyze proportional associations between groups. Logistic regression was used to estimate associations between binary variables. All tests were two-sided, and $p$-values <0.05 were considered statistically significant.

## Results

Of the 183 candidate members contacted, fifty-one (28%) completed the survey. Demographic characteristics are shown in Table 1. Seventy one percent (71%) of the respondents were female, and the median age was 36 years (range 32–44). The majority had completed their fellowships after 2013, with 75% attending three-year programs. Nearly 57% of participants were in university-based practices, while 33% reported being employed in community/academic hybrid programs, and 10% in community based programs.

Ninety-two percent of respondents felt comfortable writing a retrospective protocol and 74% felt comfortable drafting a letter of intent, but only 26% reported comfort writing a grant proposal. Even fewer (14%) felt comfortable writing an investigator initiated therapeutic trial. There were no differences in reported

**Table 1** Demographics of candidate member respondents ($n = 51$)

| | N (%) |
|---|---|
| **Gender** | |
| Male | 14 (27.5) |
| Female | 36 (70.6) |
| Other | 1 (1.9) |
| **Current Age** | |
| Less than 35 years | 15 (29.4) |
| 35–39 years | 29 (56.9) |
| 40–44 years | 7 (13.7) |
| **Year of Fellowship Graduation** | |
| 2008–2010 | 3 (5.8) |
| 2011–2014 | 14 (27.5) |
| 2014–2016 | 34 (66.7) |
| **Length of Fellowship Program** | |
| 3 years | 38 (74.5) |
| 4 years | 13 (25.5) |
| **Current Practice Setting** | |
| Community based | 5 (9.8) |
| University based | 26 (56.9) |
| Community/Academic hybrid | 17 (33.3) |

comfort levels by gender, age, time since fellowship, or length of fellowship.

Figure 1 shows candidate-reported exposure to educational opportunities and career development during their training. Twenty percent or fewer of respondents had attended a protocol writing workshop (20%) or billing and coding courses (2%), and reported little education in documentation and coding (14%), ICD-10 transition (14%), the Affordable Care Act (10%), malpractice insurance (20%), and disability insurance (12%).

Figure 2 shows areas in which candidate members reported whether or not they received adequate education on non-clinical topics during fellowship. The greatest proportions of candidate members wanted additional education in billing, coding, and documentation (94%) and the Affordable Care Act (82%). Topics about which additional education was least desired included retrospective protocol writing (48%), how to be an effective teacher (64%), and writing letters of intent (64%). Despite this, working in an academic practice was highly associated with the desire for more training in writing a letter of intent (OR 3.45 [95% CI 1.03–11.55], $p$ = 0.04). Academic candidate members were also more likely to want additional training in drafting IIT, though this did not reach statistical significance (OR 2.97 [95% CI 0.80–10.90, $p$ = 0.10). Age, length of fellowship, and time since completion of fellowship were not associated with reported interest in more education about any topic queried. Compared with males, a greater proportion of females wanted more teaching on billing and coding (79% vs. 100%, $x^2$ = 10.37, $p$ = 0.005) and writing letters of intent (36% vs. 74%, $x^2$ = 6.40, $p$ = 0.01). Males were

less likely to want more training on disability insurance (OR 0.28 [95% CI 0.07–1.09], $p$ = 0.059) and grant writing (OR 0.30 [95% CI 0.08–1.10], $p$ = 0.07), though these did not reach statistical significance. Formal education in certain subject areas was negatively associated with a desire for further training on those subjects, including how to be an effective teacher (OR 0.11 [95% CI 0.03–0.45], $p$ = 0.002), the Affordable Care Act (0.03 [95% CI 0.002–0.34], $p$ = 0.004), and disability insurance (OR 0.22 [95% CI 0.06–0.87], $p$ = 0.03). Of those who did not receive any teaching on the Affordable Care Act, 89% reported wanting more training.

Of the 48 fellowship program directors contacted, 19 completed the survey for a response rate of 40%. Sixty-five percent of the respondents directed three-year programs, while 35% directed four-year programs. The current didactic time for each program dedicated to the non-clinical practice of medicine is reported in Table 2. There were no associations between the length of the program and the amount of didactic time spent on any one topic. Program directors did indicate, however, that they would prefer more didactic time be spent on how to write an investigator-initiated trial compared to the current time allotted in their programs ($x^2$ = 6.11, $p$ = 0.01).

Table 3 shows candidate member and fellowship director responses to mentorship and job-hunting questions. Compared with fellowship directors, fewer candidate members reported that career goals were discussed (72% vs. 94%, $x^2$ = 3.89, $p$ = 0.05) and that they received encouragement from their program directors to review employment agreements with a

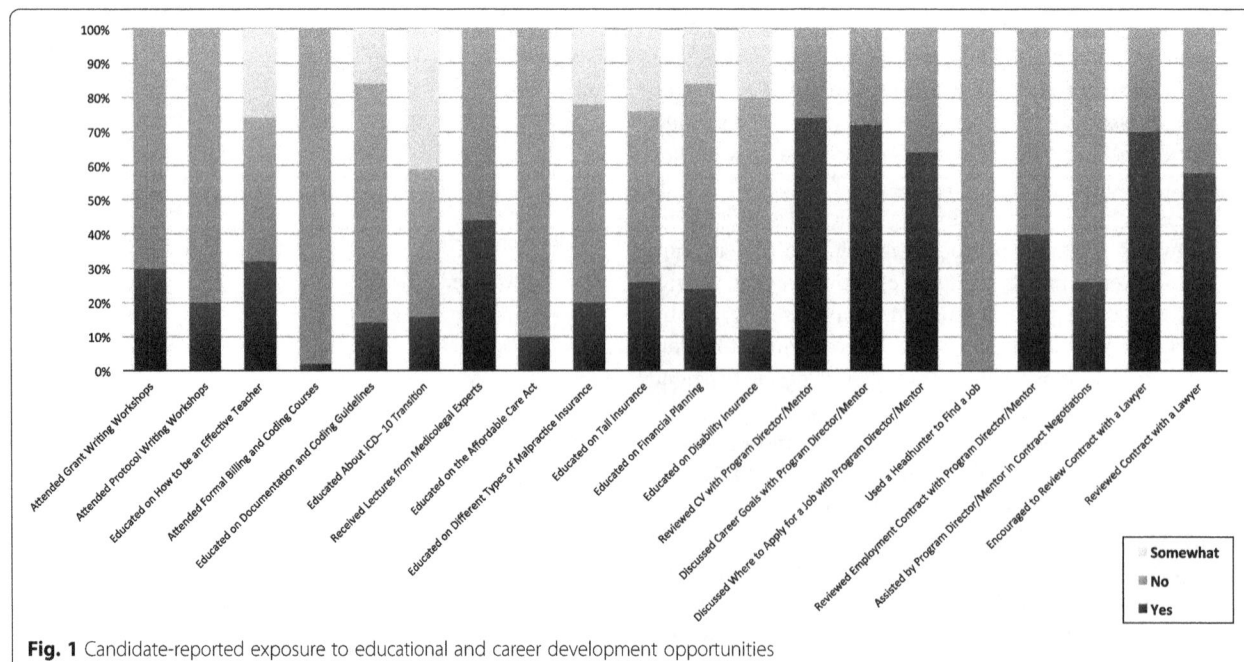

**Fig. 1** Candidate-reported exposure to educational and career development opportunities

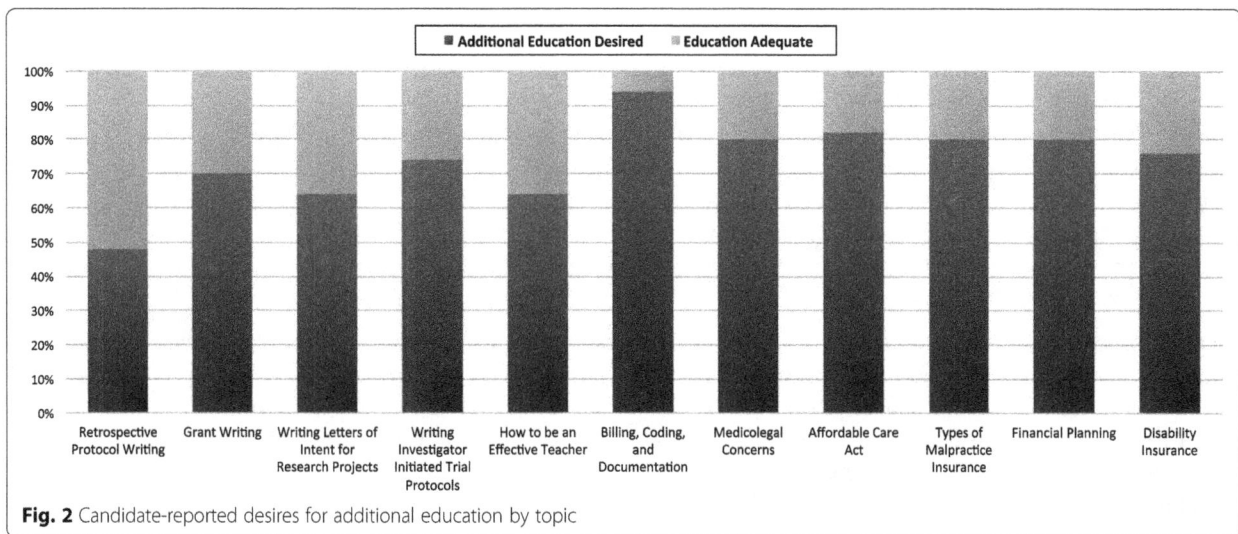

**Fig. 2** Candidate-reported desires for additional education by topic

lawyer (70% vs. 94%, $\chi^2$ = 4.39, p = 0.05). Notably, those who were encouraged to review their contracts with a lawyer were more likely to actually do so compared with those who did not (OR 6.87 [95% CI 1.77–26.76], $p$ = 0.005).

## Discussion

With increasing pressure on fellowship programs to train competent gynecologic oncologists in an era of rapidly advancing surgical and chemotherapeutic evolution, it is important to also recognize the concerns of trainees about adequate preparation for the practical aspects of being independent physicians. Our study shows that while recent fellowship graduates indicate a high level of comfort with some aspects of both the academic and business components of post-training employment, there remains a significant disparity in the perceived preparation for many of these important facets of practice.

The findings reported here are not unique to gynecologic oncology. In fact, other surgical specialties have reported a recognition of the importance of training in the business of medicine and a lack of trainee knowledge in this arena. Fakhry et al. [3] published the results of a survey of surgical residents and attending physicians, which included self-assessments of perceived knowledge and expertise in billing, coding, documentation, and insurance reimbursement. While 92% of residents reported that expertise in documentation and coding would make a difference in their practices, only 54% of residents accurately answered questions about billing correctly. Nearly 90% of both residents and faculty, however, thought further education on the topic was a crucial part of residency training. Similarly, a survey of general

**Table 2** Program director report of current didactic time versus desired didactic time per topic (n = number of programs) over the entire length of fellowship

| Educational Topic | Current Time 0–2 h (n) | Current Time ≥ 3 h (n) | Desired Time 0–2 h (n) | Desired Time ≥ 3 h (n) | $\chi^2$ p-value |
|---|---|---|---|---|---|
| Retrospective protocol writing | 11 | 8 | 7 | 11 | 0.25 |
| Writing letter of intent | 12 | 7 | 7 | 11 | 0.14 |
| Writing grant proposal | 11 | 8 | 6 | 12 | 0.13 |
| Writing investigator initiated trial | 13 | 6 | 5 | 13 | 0.01 |
| Being an effective teacher | 10 | 9 | 5 | 13 | 0.12 |
| Billing, coding, and documentation | 12 | 7 | 7 | 11 | 0.14 |
| Medical-legal concerns | 12 | 7 | 9 | 9 | 0.42 |
| Affordable Care Act | 17 | 2 | 14 | 4 | 0.34 |
| Types of malpractice insurance | 17 | 2 | 13 | 5 | 0.18 |
| Financial planning | 17 | 2 | 13 | 5 | 0.18 |
| Disability insurance | 18 | 1 | 14 | 4 | 0.13 |

**Table 3** Comparison of affirmative candidate member and program director experience of mentorship and job preparation

| Item | Trainee | Program Director | $X^2$ p-value |
|---|---|---|---|
| Faculty mentor or program director review CV | 74% | 72% | 0.88 |
| Faculty mentor or program director discuss career goals | 72% | 94% | 0.05 |
| Program director recommends where to apply for job | 64% | 78% | 0.38 |
| Faculty mentor or program director assist in contract negotiation | 26% | 50% | 0.06 |
| Fellows encouraged to review contracts with a lawyer | 70% | 94% | 0.05 |

surgery program directors found that 87% agreed trainees should receive education in practice management [4]. Despite this, 34% of programs offered no training in the business of medicine, and 70% indicated that their residents were inadequately trained.

There are limited data on the importance of education in the more traditionally academic components of employment, such as preparation for protocol development and teaching. A survey of maternal fetal medicine fellows demonstrated that the percentage of respondents who felt they had adequate training to apply for grants was 20% [5], which is not dissimilar from the 26% reported here. However, assessments of other key components of an academic practice such as teaching and protocol development are lacking in the post-graduate medical literature. Multiple studies have highlighted the importance of mentorship, which likely serves as a surrogate for roles in university-based medicine. In both gynecologic oncology and maternal fetal medicine fellowship, having a close research mentor has been associated with completion of the thesis, fellowship satisfaction, and productivity [5, 6]. Having a faculty advisor or mentor has also been associated with a fellow's desire to enter academic practice. In our study, the similarity in responses to questions between program directors and fellows regarding mentorship may suggest a close relationship between trainee and educator, though response bias cannot be ruled out as a factor in these findings. However, the discrepancy between the two groups regarding a discussion of career goals is striking. Faculty advisors and program directors may, therefore, need to be more explicit or transparent about their intentions for career counseling with trainees.

The amount of time dedicated to certain topics varies by program, and it is apparent that program directors have different opinions about the need for time spent to achieve competency. This is true of surgical training programs, as well, and is apparent in the diverse approach to education in the practice of non-clinical medicine. A number of strategies have been proposed to increase competency with contract negotiation, coding compliance, and financial planning. Jones, et al. [7] reported on a 10-lecture curriculum in managed care and coding compliance given over two years to surgical residents. Its efficacy was impressive; surgical coding

compliance increased nearly 50% over a 12-month period. Other approaches have included weekend retreats and mock trial presentations, all of which demonstrated significant improvement in measured knowledge categories and high participant satisfaction [8, 9].

There are several weaknesses to this study. The survey that was released was developed de novo, and is not validated, so its reproducibility may be in question. The response rates of 28% and 40% for candidate members and fellowship directors, respectively, are low, but are in line with other studies requiring physician response to survey invitations. There is also a likely component of bias, as more than two-thirds of candidate respondents had less than three years of experience, and about 90% of had a university appointment or were in a community/academic hybrid practice. Relative overrepresentation of this population may skew perceptions on the need for additional academic-based professional training, but demonstrates that there are clearly concerns regarding tools for success as an academic gynecologic oncologist. Additionally, candidates were not queried about advanced training in research, business, or administration, which may have influenced their responses. Despite these limitations, this is the first study within the gynecologic oncology subspecialty to evaluate perceived preparation for measures outside of the usually studied surgical and medical oncology realm, and as such provides new insight into areas in which changes in didactic programs may be made. Larger investigations across multiple subspecialties, both on the residency and fellowship level, may assist in clarifying perceived additional educational need, with consideration being given to including such training as a core measure for trainee professionalism.

At our institution, we have initiated a more comprehensive program of didactics based on the current findings, now including lectures from risk management, billing and coding, and the institutional review board. Our approach, however, may not be universally applicable to all gynecologic oncology programs. In fact, since preparation in the business and academic practice of medicine is not a component of any core competency for training, creativity in curricula development should be encouraged. It is clear, though, that new graduates from gynecologic oncology fellowships feel inadequately prepared for some of the responsibilities they will have post-training. It remains incumbent on those entrusted to educate them to continuously strive to improve their programs and maintain open communication with the fellows so that a truly collaborative teaching environment can be developed.

## Conclusion

Recent gynecologic oncology fellowship graduates want more training in the non-clinical, academic and business practice of medicine. Modifying curricula to more effectively prepare graduates for professional lives should be considered. Improved dialogue between trainer and trainee will be a crucial component of such a curricular evolution.

### Abbreviations

ABOG: American Board of Obstetrics and Gynecology; ACGME: Accreditation Council for Graduate Medical Education; LOI: Letters of Intent; SGO: Society of Gynecologic Oncology

### Acknowledgements

The authors would like to acknowledge the support and feedback from the Division of Gynecologic Oncology at the Sylvester Comprehensive Cancer Center, University of Miami.

### Funding

Funding in part provided by Sylvester Comprehensive Cancer Center.

### Authors' contributions

MS conceived the study, drafted the protocol, designed the questionnaires, performed the data analysis, and was primarily responsible for writing the manuscript. JS collected data, assisted in data analysis, created figures and tables, and assisted in writing the manuscript. GM participated in data collection and analysis. MH participated in study design and writing the manuscript. BS participated in conception of the study and writing the manuscript. All authors read and approved the final manuscript.

### Author information

Dr. Schlumbrecht is an Associate Professor of Clinical Obstetrics and Gynecology in the Division of Gynecologic Oncology at Sylvester Comprehensive Cancer Center at the University of Miami. He serves as the Associate Director for the Gynecologic Oncology Fellowship Program and the Co-Director of Cancer Control and Prevention for Gynecologic Oncology.

### Consent for publication

Not applicable.

### Competing interests

The authors declare that they have no competing interests.

### Author details

[1]Division of Gynecologic Oncology, Sylvester Comprehensive Cancer Center, University of Miami, 1121 NW 14th St, Suite 345C, Miami, FL 33136, USA. [2]Department of Obstetrics and Gynecology, University of Miami, Miami, USA.

### References

1. Doo D, et al. Preparedness of Ob/Gyn residents for fellowship training in gynecologic oncology. Gynecol Oncol Rep. 2015;12:55–60.
2. Scribner DJ, Baldwin J, Mannel R. Gynecologic oncologists' perceptions of fellowship training. J Reprod Med. 2005;50(1):29–34.
3. Fakhry S, et al. Surgical residents' knowledge of documentation and coding for professional services: an opportunity for focused educational offering. Am J Surg. 2007;194:236–67.
4. Lusco V, Martinez S, Polk H. Program directors in surgery agree that residents should be formally trained in business and practice management. Am J Surg. 2005;189:11–3.
5. Sciscione A, Colmorgen G, D'Alton M. Factors affecting fellowship satisfaction, thesis completion, and career direction among maternal-fetal medicine fellows. Obstet Gynecol. 1998;91(6):1023–6.
6. Ramondetta L, et al. Mentorship and productivity among gynecologic oncology fellows. J Cancer Educ. 2003;18(1):15–9.
7. Jones K, et al. Practice management education during surgical residency. Am J Surg. 2008;196:878–82.
8. Holak E, Kaslow O, Pagel P. Facilitating the transition to practice: a weekend retreat curriculum for business-of-medicine education of United States anesthesiology residents. J Anesth. 2010;24:807–10.
9. Drukteinis D, et al. Preparing emergency physicians for malpractice litigation: a joint emergency medicine residency-law school mock trial competition. J Emerg Med. 2014;46(1):95–103.

# 20

# PARP inhibitors as potential therapeutic agents for various cancers: focus on niraparib and its first global approval for maintenance therapy of gynecologic cancers

Mekonnen Sisay[1]* [iD] and Dumessa Edessa[2]

**Abstract**

Poly (ADP-ribose) polymerases (PARPs) are an important family of nucleoproteins highly implicated in DNA damage repair. Among the PARP families, the most studied are PARP1, PARP2 and PARP 3. PARP1 is found to be the most abundant nuclear enzyme under the PARP series. These enzymes are primarily involved in base excision repair as one of the major single strand break (SSB) repair mechanisms. Being double stranded, DNA engages itself in reparation of a sub-lethal SSB with the aid of PARP. Moreover, by having a sister chromatid, DNA can also repair double strand breaks with either error-free homologous recombination or error-prone non-homologous end-joining. For effective homologous recombination repair, DNA requires functional heterozygous *breast cancer genes* (BRCA) which encode BRCA1/2. Currently, the development of PARP inhibitors has been one of the promising breakthroughs for cancer chemotherapy. In March 2017, the United States Food and Drug Administration (FDA) approved niraparib for maintenance therapy of recurrent gynecologic cancers (epithelial ovarian, primary peritoneal and fallopian tube carcinomas) which are sensitive to previous platinum based chemotherapy irrespective of *BRCA* mutation and homologous recombination deficiency status. It is the third drug in this class to receive FDA approval, following olaparib and rucaparib and is the first global approval for maintenance therapy of the aforementioned cancers. Niraparib preferentially blocks both PARP1 and PARP2 enzymes. The daily tolerated dose of niraparib is 300 mg, above which dose limiting grade 3 and 4 toxicities were observed. In combination with humanized antibody, pembrolizumab, it is also under investigation for those patients who have triple negative breast cancer. By and large, there are several clinical trials that are underway investigating clinical efficacy and safety, as well as other pharmacokinetic and pharmacodynamic profiles of this drug for various malignancies.

**Keywords:** PARP, PARP inhibitors, DNA repair, Cancer, Malignant tumors, Maintenance therapy, Niraparib, Mk-4827, Zejula, Companion diagnostic*

* Correspondence: mekonnensisay27@yahoo.com
[1]Department of Pharmacology and Toxicology, School of Pharmacy, College of Health and Medical Sciences, Haramaya University, P.O.Box 235, Harar, Ethiopia
Full list of author information is available at the end of the article

## Introduction

### General principles of DNA repair

The human genome is constantly under stress due to insults from both endogenous (free radicals or reactive oxygen species derived from metabolic processes) and exogenous (irradiation, chemicals, clinical drugs, and viruses, among others) sources. This results in routine DNA damage that may in turn lead to a serious genetic instability and cell death if it is left unrepaired. Being double stranded and having a sister chromatid, DNA repairs itself prior to cell division in any one of the following repair mechanisms (Fig. 1) [1–3].

Direct reversal is highly efficient, applicable when there is a single lesion, and is essentially error-free. The lesion may be tolerated or bypassed if it does not have a significant risk on the ongoing DNA replication and the genetic stability in general. Coming to the single strand break (SSB) repair, since the damage involves one strand of replicating DNA, it can be repaired by undergoing either excision of damaged site (base or nucleotide) or correcting the mismatch bases complementary to the anti-sense (template) strand [2, 4, 5].When a SSB is left unrepaired due to genetic and/or epigenetic factors, it will progress to double strand break (DSB) during DNA replication. By having homologous chromosomes, DNA has a back up to undergo DSB repair either by error-free homologous recombination (HR) or error-prone non-homologous end-joining (NHEJ). If the DSB is left unrepaired, it leads to a breakdown of the chromosome into smaller fragments, genomic instability, cell cycle arrest and apoptosis [1, 4, 6, 7]. The more faithful process of HR repair of DSBs involves localization of BRCA-1 and BRCA-2 proteins encoded from *breast cancer gene* to sites of DNA damage, resection of the DSB, and gap-filling DNA synthesis using the homologous sister chromatid as a template [8]. Before the DNA enters the repair process, cellular response depends upon the magnitude of the damage, resulting in induction of cell-cycle checkpoint pathways and DNA repair mechanisms. G2/M check point is a critical point where DNA must be repaired before the cell enters cell division/mitosis. If the damage is extensive and irreparable, induction of cell death occurs [3, 7].

### The role of poly (ADP-ribose) polymerases (PARPs) in DNA repair

PARPs are a member of nuclear protein enzymes highly implicated in DNA damage repair. During SSB, PARP detects the damaged site and undergoes post translational modification of targeted proteins by the process known as ADP-ribosylation. This process creates a conducive environment for recruiting several DNA repair proteins including topoisomerases, DNA ligase III, DNA polymerase β, and scaffolding proteins such as X-ray cross complementing protein 1 (XRCC1), among others. The ribosylation process also leads in relaxation of tightened chromatins and histones and results in unwinding of DNA to make it accessible for repair processes. What is more, PARP facilitates HR by recruiting factors such as ataxia telangiectasia-mutated kinase (ATM), mitotic recombination 11 (Mre11), and Nijmegen breakage syndrome 1 (Nbs1) to sites of DSBs (Fig. 2) [9–11]. When PARP activity is compromised, these SSBs cannot be repaired and progress to DSBs at DNA replication forks. In a normal cell, there is a cellular

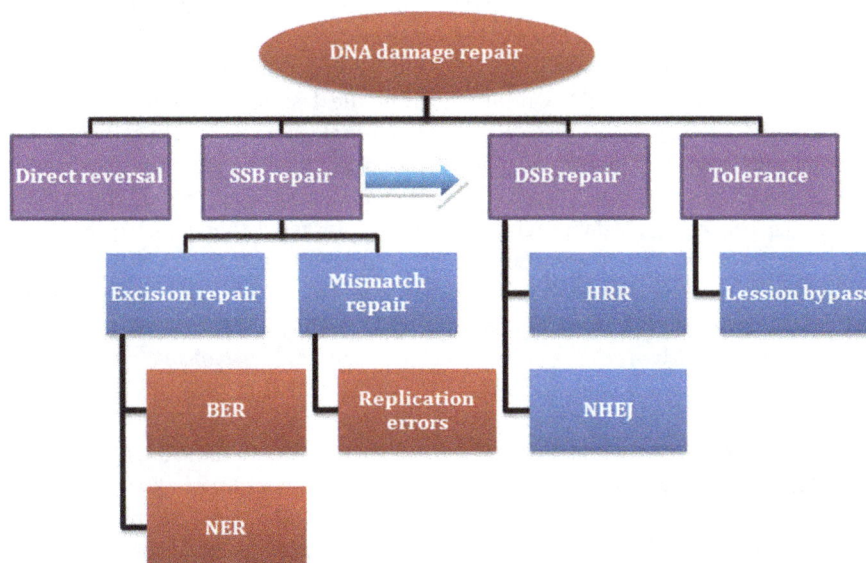

**Fig. 1** Illustrated diagram describing DNA repair pathways. (Note: BER, base excision repair; DSB, double strand break; HRR, homologous recombination repair; NER, nucleoside excision repair; NHEJ, non-homologous end-joining; SSB, single strand break)

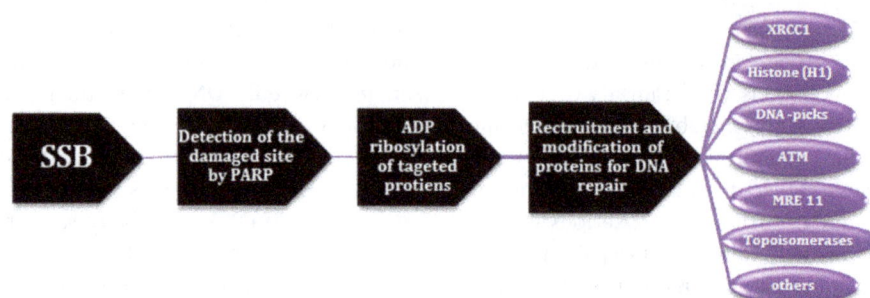

**Fig. 2** DNA repair processes with the aids of poly (ADP-ribose) polymerase. (Notes: XRCC1, X-ray cross complementing protein 1; ATM, ataxia telangiectasia-mutated kinase; MRE11, mitotic recombination 11. Others include: - Nijmegen breakage syndrome 1 (Nbs1), DNA ligase III, and DNA polymerase β)

backup by which DSBs are repaired with the aid of HR, a mechanism different from base excision repair (BER) and hence, even in the absence of PARP activity and loss of BER, DNA repair can be effectively taken place by this pathway. However, cells can have a double-hit whereby both BER and HR are compromised. These cells rely on error-prone NHEJ for damage repair, which results in DNA instability and chromosomal aberrations, eventually resulting in apoptosis. The dual-insult of HR and BER defects results in "synthetic lethality" justifying the potent and lethal synergy between these two otherwise non-lethal event when they occur alone [1, 11]. Therefore, this review aims to address the role of common PARP inhibitors on cancer chemotherapy with special focus on niraparib and its first global approval for maintenance therapy of gynecologic cancers.

## Methods

A total of 945 articles were retrieved from various legitimate data bases and indexing services (Directory of open access journals, PubMed, PubMed Central, MEDLINE, Scopus and ProQuest), as well as other supplemental sources and search engines (CrosRef, WorldCat, and Google Scholar) with the aid of key terms: "PARP", "PARP inhibitors", "DNA repair", "cancer", "malignant tumors", "Niraparib", "MK-4827", "Zejula", "maintenance therapy" and "companion diagnostic*". Boolean operators (AND, OR, NOT) were appropriately used for increasing the chance of obtaining relevant literature for this topic. Moreover, truncation was also applied to expand the literature searches and increase the number of related articles for inclusion. Following database searches and in-depth screening of each article by authors, majority of articles were removed from this study including duplicate articles from various databases and search engines; unrelated titles and abstracts; abstracts without full texts and full texts with insufficient information for data extraction. Finally, 68 references were included for the study from which, 22 articles were critically reviewed to summarize the current therapeutic profile of niraparib. Coming to the data extraction process, general background information concerning the role of PARP in DNA repair, cancer therapeutics

and earlier inhibitors of this enzyme (s) were highlighted. Coming to the drug of interest, niraparib, data regarding the chemistry, pharmacology, primary outcomes of preclinical studies as well as completed clinical trials were extracted from respective individual studies. Furthermore, important data about ongoing clinical trials were also retrieved upon visiting https://clinicaltrials.gov/ web site. Data were collected from June to August, 2017.

## Review

### The role of PARP inhibitors in cancer chemotherapy

Ovarian cancer is the 5th leading cause of cancer-related deaths in women in the United States. It is estimated that in 2017, more than 22,440 women will be diagnosed with ovarian cancer leading to more than 14,080 deaths. However, cancer chemotherapy has shown little improvement over time [12, 13]. So far, recurrent ovarian cancer has been dichotomized into two categories based on the sensitivity of platinum based therapy as 'platinum sensitive' and 'platinum resistant'. This classification considers the number of months within which the patient can be freed from platinum based therapy from the last time of infusion to recorded recurrence. From molecular perspective, there is no clear cut demarcation to divide cancers based on sensitivity to platinum chemotherapy. With advancement in science and technology, targeted therapies like PARP inhibitors have led to a more holistic approach to the treatment of disease recurrence [14–16]. It is estimated that approximately 50% of high-grade serous ovarian cancer (HGSOC) show alterations in the *Fanconi anemia–BRCA* pathway [17]. Mutations in this pathway, including genes involved in HR repair such as RAD51C/D, and BRIP1 have been associated with homologous recombination deficiency (HRD) and hereditary ovarian cancer [18]. Epigenetic mechanisms can also contribute to the development of HRD. For example, silencing of BRCA1 in HGSOC has been shown to occur via epigenetic changes such as hypermethylation of BRCA1 promoter [17]. PARP inhibitors have been developed in the recurrence and maintenance treatment settings in epithelial ovarian cancer. As they inhibit SSB repair, inducing synthetic lethality in cells with underlying HRD as seen in BRCA1/2 mutant tumors (Fig. 3). Marked responses have been observed in ovarian cancers with BRCA1/2 mutation, even if up to 50% of HGSOC having HRD may also be better treated compared to cancers with HRD negative (HR proficient) genotypes [19, 20].

Among the newly diagnosed ovarian cancers, around 25% of them carry BRCA1/2 mutations from which majority (18%) are germline mutations whereas the remaining (7%) cancers are associated with somatic mutations [21]. In the absence of either germline or somatic mutations of BRCA1/2, HRD can occur in a variety of mechanisms as studied in several serious malignancies. The HR defects that occur due to aberration in genes other than BRCA exhibit closely resembling phenotypic characteristics secondary to PARP inhibitors and the condition is referred to as 'BRCA-ness. This has been clearly demonstrated in either genetic mutations of ATM, RAD51C/D, check point kinases 2 (CHK2), phosphatase and tensin homolog (PTEN) or epigenetic silencing of BRCA1/2 promoter as having difficulty of effectively repairing DSBs by HR [22–25].

## Overview of common PARP inhibitors that got FDA approval

Beginning from the first efficacious in vitro study of PARP inhibitors, several agents have been studied in ovarian cancer [26, 27]. The best studied include olaparib, veliparib, talazoparib, rucaparib and niraparib (Table 1). Each PARP inhibitor possesses subtly different targets of PARP isoenzymes [28, 29]. PARP-1 is the most abundant and founding member of poly ADP-ribosylating proteins (a family of around 17 proteins) known as the ADP-ribosyltransferase diphtheria toxin-like proteins [16, 30]. In addition to the canonical targets of niraparib, PARP1 and PARP2, subsequent functional validation suggested that inhibition of deoxycytidine kinase by it could have detrimental effects when combined with nucleoside analogs used for the treatment of various diseases [31].

## Olaparib

The PARP inhibitor olaparib (Lynparza®) was the first to be approved in advanced ovarian cancer therapy for those with gBRCA1/2 mutations. Following phase I safety and efficacy studies, a multicenter phase II study demonstrated response to olaparib in patients with gBRCA1/2 mutations in recurrent ovarian cancer and breast cancer with at least 3 prior chemotherapy regimens. A subgroup analysis of patients with advanced ovarian cancer patients revealed an overall response rate (ORR) of 34% [32, 33]. These findings led to the fast track approval of olaparib capsules in the USA in December, 2014 as fourth line therapy. The approval of olaparib for advanced ovarian cancer patients with BRCA 1/2 mutation and who are intensively pretreated with chemotherapy becomes a major therapeutic breakthrough for this lethal and difficult to treat disease. Even if it is the first agent in its class to get fast track approval by FDA, rucaparib and niraparib received recent approval in slightly different settings. Several PARP inhibitors are also under clinical development either alone or in combination with other treatment modalities including radiation therapies, cytotoxic agents and antiangiogenic agents [6] (Table 1). On August 17, 2017, FDA granted regular approval to olaparib tablets (Lynparza, AstraZeneca) for the maintenance treatment settings of adult patients with recurrent gynecologic cancers, who are in a complete or partial response to platinum-based chemotherapy [34]. The recent approval of olaparib in the maintenance setting was based on two randomized, placebo-controlled, double-blind, multicenter trials in patients with recurrent gynecologic cancers who were in response to platinum-based therapy.

Study 19 (NCT00753545), a phase II trial engaged 265 patients with platinum sensitive HGSOC regardless of BRCA status (1:1) to receive olaparib capsules 400 mg orally twice daily or placebo. Study 19 demonstrated a statistically significant improvement in investigator-assessed progression-free survival (PFS) in patients treated with olaparib compared to

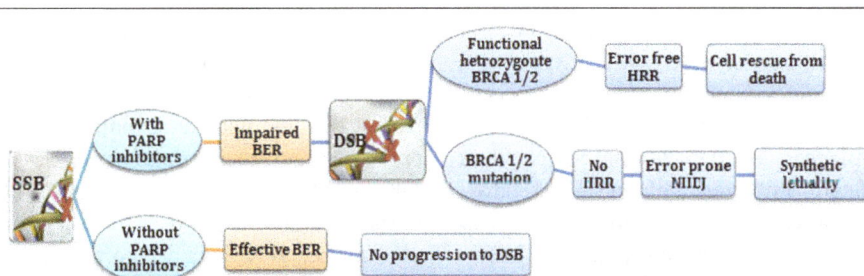

**Fig. 3** The influence of PARP inhibitors and BRCA mutation status in DNA repair and apoptosis of cancer cell. (Note: SSB, single strand break; BER, base excision repair; DSB, double strand break; HRR, homologous recombination repair; NHEJ, Non-homologous end-joining)

**Table 1** Overview of common FDA approved and investigational PARP inhibitors and their treatment profile

| Name of the drug | Approval by FDA | Clinical conditions for which the drug are approved or under investigation | Route | Targeted PARP enzyme(s) (Affinity) | $IC_{50}$ | Line of previous chemotherapy | References |
|---|---|---|---|---|---|---|---|
| Veliparib (ABT-888) | Under investigation (its efficacy and safety have not been established yet) | FDA grants orphan drug designation for advanced squamous non-small cell lung cancer (Phase III) | PO | PARP 1and PARP2 | 5.2 nM/2.9 nM (PARP1/2) | _____ | [63] |
| Fluzoparib (SHR3162) | Under investigation (phase I) in combination with apatinib | Recurrent ovarian cancer TNBC | PO | PARP 1 and PARP 2 | _____ | Two lines of platinum-based therapy (gynecologic cancers) and only one line of standard chemotherapy (TNBC) | [64] |
| Talazoparib (BMN 673) | Investigational drug | Under development for advanced breast cancer patients with gBRCA mutations | PO | PARP 1/2 >>>>PARP3 | 1.2 nM/0.9 nM (PARP1/2) | _____ | [65] |
| Olaparib (Lynparza®) | December 2014 (First FDA approval) | Patients with germline BRCA1/2-mutated advanced recurrent ovarian cancer | PO | PARP 1 > PARP2>> PARP3 | 5 nM/1 nM (PARP1/2) | ≥ 3 prior lines of chemotherapy | [9, 32, 33]. |
| | Approved again on Aug 17, 2017 | For the maintenance treatment of adult patients with recurrent gynecologic cancers | PO | _____ | _____ | ≥ 2 lines of therapy | [34] |
| Rucaparib (Rubraca®) | December 2016 (Second approval) | Treatment of ovarian cancer patients with somatic and/or germline BRCA mutations | PO | PARP 1>>>>> PARP2/3 | 1.4 nM (PARP1) | One line earlier than olaparib (patients who have received ≥2 prior lines of chemotherapy) | [37, 38, 60] |
| | Sought FDA approval for second time on October 10, 2017 | For maintenance treatment settings | PO | _____ | _____ | ≥ 3 lines of therapy | [40] |
| Niraparib (Zejula™) | March 2017 (Third Approval) | Maintenance therapy of adult patients with recurrent gynecologic cancers irrespective of the status of BRCA mutations and/or HRD status | PO | PARP1 and PARP2 | 3.2 nM/4 nM (PARP1/2) | - CR or PR to previous (at least two) platinum-based chemotherapy. | [42, 56] |

Abbreviations: *IC* intracellular concentrations, *BRCA* breast cancer genem, *PO* per oral, *PARP* Poly(ADP-ribose) polymerase, *CR* complete response, *PR* partial response, *FDA* Food and Drug Administration, *HRD* homologous recombination deficiency, *TNBC* triple negative breast cancer

placebo (Hazard Ratio (HR') = 0.35; 95% CI: 0.25, 0.49; $p < 0.0001$). The estimated median PFS was 8.4 months and 4.8 months in the olaparib and placebo arms, respectively. Clinical outcomes between placebo- and olaparib-treated patients with somatic BRCA1/2 mutations were similar to those with germline BRCA1/2 mutations, indicating that patients with somatic BRCA1/2 mutations benefit from treatment with olaparib in maintenance setting [35]. SOLO-2/ENGOT-Ov21 (NCT01874353), a phase III clinical trial, randomized 295 patients with recurrent germline BRCA-mutated gynecologic cancers (2:1) to receive olaparib tablets 300 mg orally twice daily or placebo. SOLO-2 demonstrated a statistically significant improvement in investigator-assessed PFS in patients randomized to olaparib compared with those who received placebo (HR' = 0.30; 95% CI: 0.22, 0.41; $p < 0.0001$). The estimated median PFS was 19.1 and 5.5 months in the olaparib and placebo arms, respectively [36].

**Rucaparib**

Coming to rucaparib (Rubraca®), it is a potent inhibitor of PARP1, PARP2 and PARP 3 with the greatest affinity towards PARP1. Both phase I and II clinical trials demonstrated that it has a promising efficacy in ovarian cancers with both BRCA mutation (including germline and somatic subtypes) and tumors with HRD positive. In December, 2016, US FDA approved rucaparib for the treatment of advanced ovarian cancer patients with general BRCA1/2 mutation and who took at least 2 lines of previous platinum based therapy. The accelerated approval was based upon ORR (54%) [37]. In ARIEL2 part 1, patients with recurrent, platinum-sensitive, high-grade ovarian carcinomas were classified into one of three predefined HRD subgroups on the basis of tumor mutational analysis: *BRCA* mutant (deleterious germline or somatic), *BRCA* wild-type and loss of heterozygosity (LOH) high (LOH high group), or *BRCA* wild-type and LOH low (LOH low group). Median PFS after rucaparib treatment was 12·8 months (95% CI 9·0–14·7) in the

*BRCA* mutant subgroup, 5·7 months (5·3–7·6) in the LOH high subgroup, and 5·2 months (3·6–5·5) in the LOH low subgroup. PFS was significantly longer in the *BRCA* mutant (HR' = 0·27, 95% CI 0·16–0·44, $p < 0.0001$) and LOH high (0·62, 0·42–0·90, $p = 0.011$) subgroups compared with the LOH low subgroup. Part 2 of the ARIEL2 trial is ongoing, and it will prospectively evaluate rucaparib responsiveness in patient sub-groups defined by LOH scores [38].

ARIEL3 (NCT01968213), a randomised, double-blind, placebo-controlled, phase 3 trial, demonstrated improved PFS by investigator review for rucaparib compared with placebo in all three primary efficacy analyses: BRCA mutation (16.6 months vs. 5.4 months; HR': 0.23, $P < 0.001$); HRD-positive (13.6 months vs. 5.4 months; HR': 0.32, $P < 0.001$); overall intent-to-treat populations (10.8 months vs. 5.4 months; HR': 0.36, $P < 0.001$) [39]. On October 10, 2017, FDA approval was sought for maintenance therapy of rucaparib in ovarian cancer following promising findings from ARIEL3 clinical trial (Table 1) [40].

### Niraparib

Among the PARP inhibitor series, niraparib (Zejula) is the third drug in this class, to receive FDA approval for cancer chemotherapy. However, the previous PARP inhibitors, olaparib and rucaparib have been approved for simple treatment rather than maintenance for those patients who are responsive to previous chemotherapy. Niraparib has become the first drug that got global approval for maintenance therapy of patients with recurrent gynecologic cancers regardless of their BRCA mutation and HRD status [41, 42] (Table 1). Hereafter, this review focuses on summarizing the chemistry, pharmacology, preclinical studies, completed and ongoing clinical trials as well as toxicological concerns of niraparib.

### Chemistry, pharmacology and preclinical data of niraparib

Niraparib (Zejula, MK-4827; (2-[4-[(3S)-piperidin-3-yl], phenyl]indazole-7-carboxamide) is a potent and selective inhibitor of PARP-1 and PARP-2 enzymes. Its molecular formula is $C_{19}H_{20}N_4O$ and has a molar mass of 320.396 g/mol (Fig. 4) [43].

Niraparib is administered orally on once daily basis and can be taken without consideration to meals since food

does not significantly affect the absorption and/or the metabolism of niraparib [44]. It is readily absorbed from the oral route and its bioavailability is approximately 73% in humans as per the phase III clinical trials revealed. There is no significant difference in pharmacokinetic parameters between the feeding and fasting states. For example, the mean ratios of maximum plasma concentration ($C_{max}$) and area under the curve ($AUC_{0-\infty}$) in the fed to fasted state were 0.83 and 1.08, respectively. In both cases, niraparib possesses long terminal half-life ($t_{1/2}$) of greater than 2 days (57 and 59 h for feeding and fasting states, respectively). This is consistent with once daily dosing of niraparib for cancer chemotherapy [45]. Coming to the metabolic profile of niraparib, it had been shown that niraparib is moderately metabolized in humans primarily via hydrolytic (phase I) and conjugative (Phase II) pathways in the liver. The hepatic phase I metabolism is via carboxylesterase-catalyzed amide hydrolysis, leading to the formation of inactive metabolite (carboxylic acid derivative) which in turn undergoes a phase II conjugation reaction called glucuronidation for ease of biliary and renal excretion [46]. Unlike rucaparib and olaparib, studies indicated that cytochrome P-450 enzymes (CYP) including CYP 1A2 play a negligible role in the metabolism of niraparib in humans [46–48]. Moreover, from the total administered dose, 31.6% and 40.0% are recovered in feces and urine, respectively, whereas 29.9% of the dose is excreted unchanged in the urine and feces [46].

In preclinical trial of rodent's model, it was also indicated that almost similar concentration-time profile of niraparib was obtained from both brain and plasma samples, and the mean brain-to-plasma concentration ratios following a single oral dose ranged from 0.85–0.99 of the brain $T_{max}$ (Table 2) [49]. Moreover, different preclinical and clinical studies indicated that niraparib induces chemo- and radio-sentiziation and hence facilitates cell death in cancer cells. Combinational therapy of niraparib with topoisomerase inhibitors such as irinotecan chemosensitize cancer cells as observed both in in-vivo and in vitro studies. In several breast and lung cancer models, niraparib enhances the therapeutic effects of radiation therapy independent of the tumor suppressor P-53 function (Table 3). Having impaired the BER function by niraparib, exposure of radiation converts the sub-lethal SSBs into lethal DSBs leading to synthetic lethality of cancer cells [50–52].

The activity of niraparib in sporadic prostate cancer provides a strong clinical evidence for developing PARP inhibitor based therapies for metastatic castration resistant prostate cancer (CRPC). Erythroblast transformation-specific (ETS) gene rearrangement and loss of PTEN are among the common genetic alterations in prostate cancer and have been linked to increased sensitivity to PARP inhibitors in preclinical models [4]. Moreover, compared to other PARP inhibitors, niraparib was found to be effective as a monotherapeutic agent in several cell

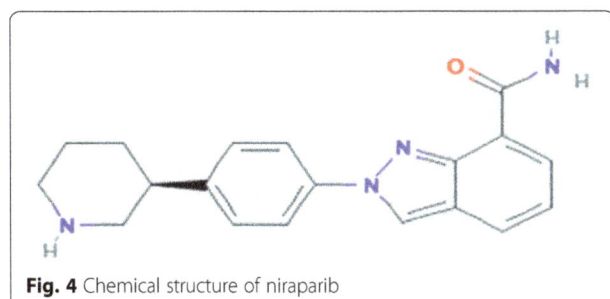

**Fig. 4** Chemical structure of niraparib

**Table 2** Overview of the pharmacokinetic profile of niraparib in preclinical and clinical studies

| Description of study population | Methods | Results | References |
|---|---|---|---|
| Patients with ovarian cancer | Two-way crossover design ((feeding versus fasting)<br>- each subject received 2 separate 300-mg doses of niraparib, 1 each in a fasting and a fed state<br>- investigating pharmacokinetic parameters based on feeding state | - The mean ratios of $C_{max}$ and $AUC_{0\text{-inf}}$ in the fed (test) versus fasted state (reference) were 0.83 and 1.08, respectively<br>- The mean $t_{1/2}$ of feeding and fasting states are 57 and 59 h, respectively<br>- Median $T_{max}$ in the feeding condition is almost 2 times to that of fasting state | [45] |
| Rodents with BRCA2-mutant (Capan-1) and MDA-MB-436 (BRCA-1 mutant) human pancreatic cancer xenograft model | Randomized cohorts of Balb/c nude mice bearing either subcutaneous Capan-1 tumors, or intracranial Capan-1-luc tumors<br>- Dosing of niraparib (15, 30, or 45 mg/kg QD)<br>- Up to 50 days<br>- Investigating the brain and plasma levels of niraparib | - Similar Concentration-time profiles of niraparib in the brain and plasma<br>- Mean brain-to-plasma concentration ratios for niraparib following a single oral dose to rats were 0.85–0.99 of the brain Tmax<br>- Brain Ctrough levels (24 h) were 2–4 times greater than observed in plasma, indicating niraparib is able to penetrate the brain in rodents<br>- Have therapeutic benefit in an IC BRCA-mutant human xenograft model | [49] |

Abbreviations: *QD* every day, *BRCA* breast cancer, *IC* intracranial

lines tested in pediatric diffuse intrinsic pontine glioma and pediatric high-grade astrocytoma [53].

### Evidences from clinical trials of niraparib

Niraparib is approved for the maintenance therapy of adult patients with recurrent gynecologic cancers that are in a complete or partial response to previous platinum-based chemotherapy. In Europe, it is under review by European Medicine Agency for maintenance therapy of recurrent ovarian cancer patients who are sensitive to earlier platinum chemotherapy [42].

In a phase 1 dose-escalation study, 100 patients with advanced solid tumors were enrolled in two parts. In part A, cohorts of three to six patients, enriched for

**Table 3** Preclinical studies of niraparib on different cancer models

| Study characteristics | Methods | Primary outcomes observed | References |
|---|---|---|---|
| Panel of 25 TNBC PDX models in mice | Gapped sequential design (cyclophosphamide followed by niraparib after 14 days)<br>✓ investigating the antitumor efficacy of niraparib alone or in combination with alkylating agent, cyclophosphamide (standard chemotherapy of TNBC) | - Cyclophosphamide showed partial to complete tumor regression<br>- For niraparib, significant antitumor response occurs with BRCA mutations or a high HRD score<br>- Potentiation with inhibition of tumor relapse after discontinuing cyclophosphamide (in niraparib sensitive tumor sub types)<br>- In niraparib responder cells, superior efficacy compared to sequential therapy of cyclophosphamide alone | [66] |
| Panel of 17 BBC PDXmodels in mice | - Experimental design in which groups were treated with niraparib (50 mg/kg/day) and vehicle control separately<br>- 13 of BBC were TNBC cells<br>- Treatment continued for 28 days<br>- Tumor volume and body weight measurements | - No sign of body weight reduction relative to the vehicle control<br>- Niraparib exhibited robust efficacy in five of the 17 models. All five responsive models were TNBC<br>- Niraparib is generally effective in subset of TNBC patients | [67] |
| Four neuroblastoma cell lines (in vitro) and a murine xenograft model of metastatic neuroblastoma (in vivo) | - Clonogenic survival assays<br>- ELISA (PARP assay)<br>  o Poly ADP<br>- Immunohistochemistry<br>  ✓ Measurement of cleaved caspase-3, γ-H2AX, and Ki67 | - Reduced clonogenicity<br>- Additive effects with radiation<br>- Significantly prolonged survival in combined modalities<br>- ↑cleaved caspase-3 and γ-H2AX | [68] |
| Tumor cell lines derived from lung, breast, and prostate cancers (MDA-MB-231, LnCaP, MDA-MB-436, CCD-16, and MCF-10A cells) plus normal cell lines | - Clonogenic survival analyses | - µM conc of niraparib radiosensitized tumor cell lines independently of their p53 status but not cell lines derived from normal tissues<br>- It also sensitized tumor cells to $H_2O_2$ | [50] |

Abbreviations: *TNBC* triple negative breast cancer, *ADP* adenosine diphosphate, *ELISA* enzyme linked immunosorbet assay, *HRD* homologous recombination deficiency, *PDX* patient derived xenograft, *BBC* basal breast cancer, ↑ increased

*BRCA1* and *BRCA2* mutation carriers, received niraparib daily at ten escalating doses from 30 mg to 400 mg in a 21-day cycle to establish the maximum tolerated dose. In part B, further investigation was conducted to determine the maximum tolerated dose in patients with sporadic platinum-resistant high-grade serous ovarian cancer and sporadic prostate cancer. Considering various side effects associated with dose escalation, 300 mg/day was established as the maximum tolerated dose (Table 4). Niraparib was found to inhibit tumor growth in models with loss of BRCA activity and loss of function mutation of tumor suppressor PTEN proteins. Sandhu et al. administered niraparib to a small cohort of patients enriched for BRCA-deficient and sporadic cancers associated with defects in HR repair. Thirty-nine patients were treated, 11 of whom had gBRCA1/2 mutations. Eight of the BRCA1/2 mutation carriers with ovarian

cancer had a partial response. What is more, antitumor activity was also found in sporadic HGSOC [54].

While only a minority of prostate cancer patients carries germline mutations, many sporadic CRPCs harbor epigenetic and genetic disruption of genes that are crucial for the HR pathway including *BRCA1, BRCA2, FANC, ATM, CHEK1/2, MRE11A* and *RAD51*. Some of these aberrations have been associated with responsiveness to PARP inhibitors and platinum, justifying a synthetic lethality between platinum or PARP inhibitors and these sporadic DNA repair gene defects [55] (Table 4).

In the multinational, randomized, double blind, phase III clinical trial (ENGOT-OV16/NOVA trial), adult patients were dichotomized in two cohorts, each containing two arms, based on the status of *gBRCA* mutation (gBRCA cohort and non-gBRCA cohort). The categorization was based on BRCAnalysis CDx$_{BRCA}$

**Table 4** Clinical trials of niraparib for cancer patient with different histological subtypes

| Description of Study participants | Phases | Methods | Observed outcomes (primary and/or secondary) | References |
|---|---|---|---|---|
| Hundred patients with advanced solid tumors in three sites ((dose escalation study) | phase I | Two cohort studies with single arm in each<br>Part A: 60 patients<br>• enriched for BRCA1 and BRCA2 mutation carriers<br>• received niraparib daily at ten escalating doses from 30 mg to 400 mg in a 21-day cycle to establish the maximum tolerated dose<br>Part B: 40 patients<br>• sporadic platinum-resistant HGSOC and sporadic prostate cancer<br>• investigating the maximum tolerated dose | - maximum tolerated dose is 300 mg/day dose liming toxic effects (Initial cycle)<br>- Grade 3 fatigue (30 mg/day) and pnemonitis (60 mg/day) were observed during first cycle<br>- Grade 4 thrombocytopenia (400 mg/day)<br>- Other common treatment related grade 1 and 2 side effects<br>- Inhibition of PARP exceeds 50% at dose greater than 80 mg/day (80 mg > ED50)<br>- Antitumor effect was observed beyond 60 mg/day | [54] |
| Patients with sporadic CRPC | Phase I | randomized clinical trial with two treatment arms (21 patients)<br>- Arm 1: niraparib 290–300 mg/day<br>- Arm 2: placebo | - Stabilization of CRPC<br>- in 43% of patients with a median duration of response of 254 days<br>- 30% of patients had a decrease of circulating tumor cells<br>- No correlation between ERG rearrangements/loss of PTEN expression and treatment response. | [55] |
| Patients with recurrent OC (553 patients) | phase III | Randomized double blind clinical trial with two category ad two arms per category<br>- Arm 1: Niraparib 300 mg once daily<br>• 138 patients<br>- Arm 2: placebo<br>• 65 patients<br>➤ Both arm 1 and 2 patients are with gBRCA mutant tumors<br>- Arm 3: Niraparib 300 mg once daily<br>• 234 patients<br>- Arm 4: Placebo<br>• 116 patients<br>➤ Both arm 3 and 4 patients are with non-gBRCA mutant (wild type) tumors irrespective of HR status | The primary outcomes were PFS<br>In gBRCA cohort<br>• (21 months vs. 5.5 months for treatment to placebo)<br>For non-gBRCA cohort with HRD positivity<br>• The PFS was found to be 12.9 and 3.8 months for niraparib and placebo arms, respectively.<br>Overall PFS in non-gBRCa cohor<br>• 9.3 months vs 3.9 months | [56] |
| 181 patients with recurrent OC, no prior use PARP inhibitors and at least 2 previous platinum therapy | Phase III | Randomized double blind clinical trial (two cohorts based on gBRCA status) | Platinum resistance rates were 42%, 53% and 49% for gBRCA, non-gBRCA and pooled cohorts, respectively | [57] |

Abbreviations: *HGSOC* high grade serious ovarian cancer, *PFS* progression free survival, *OC* ovarian cancer, *CRPC* castration resistant prostate cancer

testing (Myriad Genetics, Salt Lake City, USA). Patients were randomly assigned in 2:1 ratio to receive 300 mg niraparib or placebo in each cohort. In this study, the primary end point (outcome) measured was the PFS. To further fine tune the efficacy of niraparib on different ovarian cancer histological subtypes, the non gBRCA cohort was further classified in to HRD positive (HR deficient) and HRD negative (HR proficient) based on myChoice HRD™ test (Myriad Genetics). In this trial, the total number of patients enrolled was 553 and from those 203 were assigned to gBRCA cohort (138 to treatment arm (niraparib) and 65 to placebo) while the remaining 350 patients were assigned to non gBRCA cohort (234:116 for niraparib to placebo group). In gBRCA cohort, patient in the niraparib arm had significantly longer median PFS period (21 months) compared to placebo group (5.5 months) [HR', 0.27; 95% CI: 0.17–0.4. Coming to the non gBRCA cohort with HRD positive patients, the median PFS was found to be 12.9 months and 3.8 months for niraparib and placebo groups, respectively [HR', 0.38; (95% CI: 0.24–0.59]. The overall PFS in non-gBRCA cohort regardless of HRD status was 9.3 months vs 3.9 months [HR', 0.45; 95% CI: 0.34–0.61]. Generally, from this clinical trial, we can conclude that niraparib can be given to recurrent ovarian cancer patients regardless of gBRCA and HRD status (Table 4) [56].

The successful phase 3 niraparib ENGOT-OV16/NOVA trial also included a substantial number of patients with platinum resistant ovarian cancer. In this study, 181 patients were assigned to placebo (65 gBRCA-muts and 116 non-gBRCAmuts). The prevalence of platinum resistance estimated for the gBRCAmut, non-gBRCAmut, and pooled cohorts were 42%, 53%, and 49%, respectively (Table 4). Approximately half of the patients in the NOVA study, where niraparib treatment met its primary endpoint by prolonging PFS following a response to platinum, had developed resistance at last line of chemotherapy (Table 4) [57].

### Toxicological concerns of niraparib

In phase I dose escalation trial, common treatment-related toxic effects were anemia (48%), nausea (42%), fatigue (42%), thrombocytopenia (35%), anorexia (26%), neutropenia (24%), constipation (23%), and vomiting (20%), and were predominantly grade 1 or 2. The most common grade 3 or 4 adverse events that were reported in the niraparib group were thrombocytopenia (33.8%), anemia (25.3%), and neutropenia (19.6%), which were managed with dose modifications [54]. Niraparib is also associated with serious risks, such as hypertension, hypertensive crisis, myelodysplastic syndrome, acute myeloid leukemia, and bone marrow suppression. Women who are pregnant or breastfeeding should not

take niraparib because it may cause harm to a developing conceptus or a newborn baby [41, 56].

### Companion diagnostic tests

Companion diagnostic tests are very critical to identify cancer patients who are best treated by PARP inhibitors. Myriad's BRCA analysis CDx™ is the only FDA-approved test to determine olaparib treatment eligibility. Rucaparib's companion diagnostic test (FoundationFocus™CDx$_{BRCA}$ test that detects germline and somatic BRCA1/2 mut) is the first FDA-approved next-generation sequencing (NGS)-based test designed to identify patients likely to respond to rucaparib [58–60]. Coming to niraparib, the eligibility is determined with myChoice HRD™ test (Myriad Genetics). While BRCA analysis CDx™, as the name explains, evaluates only BRCA, myChoiceHRD™, developed by the same company, evaluates LOH beyond BRCA and can be considered an enhancement of BRCA analysis CDx™. It is an NGS-based assay that assesses BRCA1/2 sequences, and genomic scarring (HRD score), composed by LOH, telomeric allelic balance and large-scale transitions [61].

### Ongoing clinical trials

There are several clinical trials that are underway for invesigating safety, tolerability, efficacy, and other pharmacokinetic and pharmacodynamic profiles of niraparib in different treatment modalities (single and/or combination therapies) and cancers of diverse histological origin. Several phase I clinical trials are underway investigating the maximum tolerated dose of niraparib when used in combiation with different treatment modalitites: with enzalutamide in CRPC, with everolimus in ovarian cancer, as well as with temozolomide and irinotecan in case of ewing sarcoma, among others. In phase II clinical trials, the safety and efficacy of niraparib alone is on the way to be investigated. Coming to the phase III clinical trials, the primary outcome measures of niraparib alone and in comparison with physician's choice have been under evaluation for maintenance therapy of advanced ovarian cancer patients following a response to front line platinum based therapy and human epidermal growth factor receptor 2 negative (HER2-), gBRCA mut-positive breast cancer patients, respectively(Table 5) [62].

### Conclusion and future prospects

The role of PARP family enzymes in DNA repair and cancer therapeutics was well emphasized in this review article. The development of PARP inhibitors has become one of the promising breakthroughs and hot spots in the area of experimental oncology. As documented in various histological subtypes of cancer, there are several germline and/or somatic mutations, as well as epigenetic alterations compromising effective reparation of DSBs

**Table 5** Ongoing clinical trials of niraparib alone or in combination with other agents for treatment of various malignancies [62]

| ClinicalTrials.gov Identifier | Title | Conditions under study | Phase | Interventions (Experimental arms) | Primary outcome measures of niraparib | Recruitment status |
|---|---|---|---|---|---|---|
| NCT03209401 | Niraparib plus carboplatin in patients with HRD advanced solid tumor malignancies | Solid malignancies in adult patients with evidence of HRD | Phase 1 | Niraparib Carboplatin | The dose of niraparib required to combine with carboplatin | Not yet recruiting |
| NCT03076203 | Phase IB Trial of Radium-223 and niraparib in patients with CRPC (RAPARP) | Prostate carcinoma metastatic to the bone Stage IV prostate adenocarcinoma Hormone-refractory prostate cancer | Phase I | Niraparib Radium R$_a$ 223 Dichloride | To determine MTD to combine with radiation | Not yet recruiting |
| NCT02500901 | Enzalutamide and niraparib in the treatment of CRPC | Metastatic prostate pancer | Phase I | Enzalutamide Niraparib | MTD | Active, but not recruiting |
| NCT03154281 | Evaluation of the safety and tolerability of niraparib with everolimus in ovarian and breast cancer | Breast cancer Ovarian cancer | Phase I | Niraparib Everolimus | MTD | Not yet recruiting |
| NCT02044120 | ESP1/SARC025 global collaboration: a phase I study of a combination of the PARP inhibitor, niraparib and temozolomide or irinotecan in patients with previously treated, incurable Ewing sarcoma | Ewing sarcoma | Phase I | Niraparib Temozolomide Irinotecan | DLT and MTD | Recruiting |
| NCT02924766 | A safety and pharmacokinetics study of niraparib plus an androgen receptor-targeted therapy in men with metastatic CRPC (BEDIVERE) | Prostatic neoplasms | Phase I | Niraparib Apalutamide Abiraterone Acetate Prednison | Determine Recommended Phase 2 dose | Recruiting |
| NCT03207347 | A Trial of niraparib in BAP1 and Other DNA DSB repair deficient neoplasms (UF-STO-ETI-001) | Mesothelioma Uveal melanoma Renal cell carcinoma Cholangiocarcinoma | Phase II | Niraparib | ORR | Not yet recruiting |
| NCT02657889 | Study of niraparib in combination with pembrolizumab (MK-3475) in patients with TNBC or Ovarian Cancer (TOPACIO) | TNBC Ovarian cancer Stage IV breast cancer Fallopian tube cancer Peritoneal cancer | Phase I/II | Niraparib Pembrolizumab | Evaluate DLT | Recruiting |
| NCT02354131 | Niraparib versus niraparib-bevacizumab combination in women with platinum-sensitive epithelial ovarian cancer (AVANOVA) | Ovarian cancer | Phase I/II | Niraparib Bevacizumab | PFS | Recruiting |
| NCT02854436 | An efficacy and safety study of niraparib in men with metastatic CRPC and DNA-Repair anomalies (Galahad) | Prostatic neoplasms | Phase II | Niraparib | ORR | Suspended |
| NCT02354586 | A study of niraparib in patients with ovarian cancer who have received three or four previous chemotherapy regimens (QUADRA) | Ovarian cancer | Phase II | Niraparib | Evaluation of antitumor activity | Recruiting |
| NCT01905592 | A phase III trial of niraparib versus physician's choice in HER2-, germline BRCA mutation-positive breast cancer patients (BRAVO) | Breast cancer HER 2-breast cancer BRCA1/2 gene mutation | Phase III | Niraparib Physician's choice | PFS | Active, but not recruiting |
| NCT02655016 | A study of niraparib maintenance treatment in patients with advanced ovarian cancer following response on front-line platinum-based chemotherapy | Ovarian cancer | Phase III | Niraparib | PFS | Recruiting |

Abbreviations: *ORR* Objective response rate, *DLT* dose limiting toxicity, *MTD* maximum tolerated dose, *HRD* homologous recombination deficiency, *TNBC* triple negative breast cancer, *CRPC* castaration resistant prostate cancer, *HER2* human epethilial growth factor receptor 2 negative

by HR repair. This will create medically important and selective situation whereby cancer cells will be subjected to dual insult of PARP inhibitors and mutations of HR genes including BRCA1/2. Normal cells are less likely to be affected by PARP inhibitors since they have functional HR for DSB. Based on this evidence, scientists are striving to discover PARP inhibitors which have superior safety and efficacy profiles than the existing medications for cancer chemotherapy. Even if niraparib is the third drug to get FDA approval from its class, it is the first one to receive global approval for maintenance therapy of patients with recurrent gynecologic cancers regardless of BRCA and HRD status. Maintenance therapy is an important part of cancer chemotherapy for patients who have responded positively to a primary treatment. Niraparib offers patients a new treatment option that may help delay the future growth of these cancers, regardless of whether they have a specific genetic mutation. Niraparib has also several important pharmacokinetic features including negligible interaction with food; once daily dosing regimen; less likely to interact with other coadministered drugs since it is primarily metabolized by hydrolytic and conjugative pathways, and lower dosage requirement than previously approved PARP inhibitors (olaparib and rucaparib). It is also a potent inhibitor of PARP 1 and PARP 2 enzymes. Evidence from randomized phase III clinical trials indicated that niraparib can be given to any ovarian cancer patients who are responsive to previous therapy. Additional feature here is that this drug can also be given to patients irrespective of HRD status: HRD negative (HR proficient) and HRD positive (HR deficient) cells as statistically significant median PFS was observed in niraparib arms of both cohorts compared to placebo. Generally, niraparib is under investigation either alone or in combination with other treatment modalities for several cancer types. Among them, niraparib alone is under study in phase III clinical trial for maintenance treatment of patients with advanced ovarian cancer following a response on front line platinum based therapy. In combination with pembrolizumab, it is at the transition of phase I/II trials investigating the dose limiting toxicity in triple negative breast cancer patients. Moreover, the efficacy (PFS) of niraparib in comparison with physicians' choice is also under consideration in phase III (BRAVO) trial for HER2- breast cancer patients.

## Abbreviations

BER: Base Excision Repair; BRCA: Breast Cancer gene; CHK2: Check point Kinase 2; CRPC: Castration Resistant Prostate Cancer; DSB: Double Strand Break; ETS: Erythroblast Transformation-Specific gene; FDA: Food and Drug Administration; gBRCA: Germline mutation of Breast Cancer gene; HER2-: Human Epidermal growth factor Receptor 2 negative; HGSOC: High Grade Serious Ovarian Cancer; HR: Homologous Recombination; HR': Hazard Ratio; HRD: Homologous Recombination Deficiency; LOH: Loss of Heterozygosity; NHEJ: Non Homologous End Joining; PARP: Poly (ADP-Ribose) Ploymerase; PFS: Progression Free Survival; PTEN: Phosphatase and Tensin homolog; SSB: Single Strand Break; TNBC: Triple Negative Breast Cancer

## Acknowledgments

We would like to thank Haramaya University School of Pharmacy staffs who gave us invaluable intellectual feedback for the realization of this article.

## Funding

We didn't receive any specific grant for this review article.

## Authors' contributions

Both authors designed the study, collected scientific literatures, critically appraised individual articles for inclusion, wrote the review article and drafted the manuscript. MS also prepared the final manuscript for publication. Both authors read and approved the final version.

## Consent for publication

Not applicable

## Competing interests

The authors declare that they have no competing interests.

## Author details

[1]Department of Pharmacology and Toxicology, School of Pharmacy, College of Health and Medical Sciences, Haramaya University, P.O.Box 235, Harar, Ethiopia. [2]Department of Clinical Pharmacy, School of Pharmacy, College of Health and Medical Sciences, Haramaya University, P.O. Box 235, Harar, Ethiopia.

## References

1.  Liu JF, Matulonis UA. What is the place of PARP inhibitors in ovarian cancer treatment? Curr Oncol Rep. 2016;18(5):29.
2.  Rabenau K, Hofstatter E. DNA damage repair and the emerging role of poly (ADP-ribose) polymerase inhibition in cancer therapeutics. Clin Ther. 2016; 38(7):1577–88.
3.  Jackson SP, Bartek J. The DNA-damage response in human biology and disease. Nature. 2009;461(7267):1071.
4.  Zhang J. Poly (ADP-ribose) polymerase inhibitor: an evolving paradigm in the treatment of prostate cancer. Asian J Androl. 2014;16(3):401–6.
5.  Dantzer F, de la Rubia G, Ménissier-de Murcia J, Hostomsky Z, de Murcia G, Schreiber V. Base excision repair is impaired in mammalian cells lacking poly (ADP-ribose) polymerase-1. Biochemistry. 2000;39(25):7559–64.
6.  Coyne GOS, Chen A, Kummar S. Delivering on the promise: PARP inhibition as targeted anti-cancer therapy. Curr Opin Oncol. 2015;27(6):475–81.
7.  Frey MK, Pothuri B. Targeting DNA repair: poly (ADP-ribose) polymerase inhibitors. Trans Cancer Res. 2015;4(1):84–96.
8.  Gudmundsdottir K, Ashworth A. The roles of BRCA1 and BRCA2 and associated proteins in the maintenance of genomic stability. Oncogene. 2006;25(43):5864–74.
9.  Shen Y, Aoyagi-Scharber M, Wang B. Trapping poly(ADP-ribose) polymerase. J Pharmacol Exp Ther. 2015;353(3):446–57.
10. Do K, Chen AP. Molecular pathways: targeting PARP in cancer treatment. Clin Cancer Res. 2013;19(5):977–84.
11. Fortini P, Pascucci B, Parlanti E, D'errico M, Simonelli V, Dogliotti E. The base excision repair: mechanisms and its relevance for cancer susceptibility. Biochimie. 2003;85(11):1053–71.
12. American Cancer Society. Cancer facts and figures 2017. Atlanta: American Cancer Society; 2017.
13. Miller RE, Ledermann JA. The status of poly (adenosine diphosphate-ribose) polymerase (PARP) inhibitors in ovarian cancer, part 2: extending the scope beyond olaparib and BRCA1/2 mutations. Clin Adv Hematol Oncol. 2016; 14(9):704–11.
14. Alvarez RD, Matulonis UA, Herzog TJ, Coleman RL, Monk BJ, Markman M. Moving beyond the platinum sensitive/resistant paradigm for patients with recurrent ovarian cancer. Gynecol Oncol. 2016;141(3):405–9.

15. Pujade-Lauraine E, Combe P. Recurrent ovarian cancer. Ann Oncol. 2016; 27(suppl_1):i63–5.

16. Coyne GOS, Chen AP, Meehan R, Doroshow JH. PARP inhibitors in reproductive system cancers: current use and developments. Drugs. 2017;77(2):113–30.

17. Konstantinopoulos PA, Ceccaldi R, Shapiro GI, D'Andrea AD. Homologous recombination deficiency: exploiting the fundamental vulnerability of ovarian cancer. Cancer Discov. 2015;5(11):1137–54.

18. Pennington KP, Swisher EM. Hereditary ovarian cancer: beyond the usual suspects. Gynecol Oncol. 2012;124(2):347–53.

19. Kanjanapan Y, Lheureux S, Oza AM. Niraparib for the treatment of ovarian cancer. Expert Opin Pharmacother. 2017;18(6):631–40.

20. Sabatucci I, Lorusso D. Il ruolo di niraparib nel trattamento del carcinoma ovarico: attualita e prospettive. Recenti Prog Med. 2017;108(6):265–8.

21. Pennington KP, Walsh T, Harrell MI, Lee MK, Pennil CC, Rendi MH, et al. Germline and somatic mutations in homologous recombination genes predict platinum response and survival in ovarian, fallopian tube, and peritoneal carcinomas. Clin Cancer Res. 2014;20(3):764–75.

22. McCabe N, Turner NC, Lord CJ, Kluzek K, Białkowska A, Swift S, et al. Deficiency in the repair of DNA damage by homologous recombination and sensitivity to poly (ADP-ribose) polymerase inhibition. Cancer Res. 2006;66(16):8109–15.

23. Anwar M, Aslam HM, Anwar S. PARP inhibitors. Hered Cancer Clin Prac. 2015;13(1):4.

24. Konstantinopoulos P, Spentzos D, Karlan B, Taniguchi T, Fountzilas E, Francoeur N, et al. A gene expression profile of BRCAness that correlates with responsiveness to platinum and PARP inhibitors. J Clin Oncol. 2010; 28(15_suppl):5004.

25. Dedes KJ, Wetterskog D, Mendes-Pereira AM, Natrajan R, Lambros MB, Geyer FC, et al. PTEN deficiency in endometrioid endometrial adenocarcinomas predicts sensitivity to PARP inhibitors. Sci Transl Med. 2010;2(53):53ra75.

26. Bryant HE, Schultz N, Thomas HD. Specific killing of BRCA2-deficient tumours with inhibitors of poly(ADP-ribose) polymerase. Nature. 2005; 434(7035):913–7.

27. Farmer H, McCabe N, Lord CJ. Targeting the DNA repair defect in BRCA mutant cells as a therapeutic strategy. Nature. 2005;434(7035):917–21.

28. Scott C, Swisher E, Kaufmann S. Poly (ADP-ribose) polymerase inhibitors: recent advances and future development. J Clin Oncol. 2015;33(12):1397–406.

29. Thorsell AG, Ekblad T, Karlberg T, Low M, Pinto AF, Tresaugues L, et al. Structural basis for potency and promiscuity in poly(ADP-ribose) polymerase (PARP) and Tankyrase inhibitors. J Med Chem. 2017;60(4):1262–71.

30. Hassa PO, Hottiger MO. The diverse biological roles of mammalian PARPS, a small but powerful family of poly-ADP-ribose polymerases. Front Biosci:J virtual library. 2008;13(13):3046–82.

31. Knezevic CE, Wright G, Remsing Rix LL, Kim W, Kuenzi BM, Luo Y, et al. Proteome-wide profiling of clinical PARP inhibitors reveals compound-specific secondary targets. Cell Chem Biol. 2016;23(12):1490–503.

32. Kaufman B, Shapira-Frommer R, Schmutzler RK, et al. Olaparib monotherapy in patients with advanced cancer and a germline BRCA1/2 mutation. J Clin Oncol. 2015;33(3):244–50.

33. Domchek SM, Aghajanian C, Shapira-Frommer R, et al. Efficacy and safety of olaparib monotherapy in germline BRCA1/2 mutation carriers with advanced ovarian cancer and three or more lines of prior therapy. Gynecol Oncol. 2016;140(2):199–203.

34. US FDA. FDA approves olaparib tablets for maintenance treatment in ovarian cancer. Available at:- https://www.fda.gov/Drugs/InformationOnDrugs/ApprovedDrugs/ucm572143.htm. Accessed 10 Oct 2017.

35. Dougherty BA, Lai Z, Hodgson DR, Orr MCM, Hawryluk M, Sun J, et al. Biological and clinical evidence for somatic mutations in BRCA1 and BRCA2 as predictive markers for olaparib response in high-grade serous ovarian cancers in the maintenance setting. Oncotarget. 2017;8(27):43653–61.

36. Pujade-Lauraine E, Ledermann JA, Selle F, Gebski V, Penson RT, Oza AM, et al. Olaparib tablets as maintenance therapy in patients with platinum-sensitive, relapsed ovarian cancer and a BRCA1/2 mutation (SOLO2/ENGOT-Ov21): a double blind, randomised, placebo-controlled, phase 3 trial. Lancet Oncol. 18(9):1274–1284.

37. Dockery L, Gunderson C, Moore K. Rucaparib: the past, present, and future of a newly approved PARP inhibitor for ovarian cancer. OncoTargets Ther. 2017;10:3029–37.

38. Swisher EM, Lin KK, Oza AM, Scott CL, Giordano H, Sun J, et al. Rucaparib in relapsed, platinum-sensitive high-grade ovarian carcinoma (ARIEL2 Part 1): an international, multicentre, open-label, phase 2 trial. Lancet Oncol. 2017;18(1):75–87.

39. Coleman RL, Oza AM, Lorusso D, Aghajanian C, Oaknin A, Dean A, et al. Rucaparib maintenance treatment for recurrent ovarian carcinoma after response to platinum therapy (ARIEL3): a randomised, double-blind, placebo-controlled, phase 3 trial. Lancet. 2017;390(10106):1949–61.

40. Broderick JM: FDA Approval Sought for Maintenance Rucaparib in Ovarian Cancer. Available at: http://www.onclive.com/web-exclusives/fda-approval-sought-for-maintenance-rucaparib-in-ovarian-cancer. Accessed 20 Oct 2017.

41. Tarapchak P. FDA Approves Maintenance Treatment for Recurrent Epithelial Ovarian, Fallopian Tube, or Primary Peritoneal Cancers. Oncology Times 2017: http://journals.lww.com/oncology-times/blog/fdaactionsandupdates/pages/post.aspx?PostID=231.

42. Scott LJ. Niraparib: first global approval. drugs; 2017. p. 1–6.

43. National Center for Biotechnology Information. PubChem Compound Database; CID=24958200. Available at: https://pubchem.ncbi.nlm.nih.gov/compound/1038915-60-4#section=Top. Accessed 15 Oct 2017.

44. Gonzalez-Martin A, Backes FJ, Baumann KH, Chase DM, Fehr MK, Coleman RL, et al. A randomized, double-blind phase III trial of niraparib maintenance treatment in patients with HRD+ advanced ovarian cancer after response to front-line platinum-based chemotherapy. J Clin Oncol. 2016;34(15 suppl): TPS5606-TPS5606.

45. Moore KN, Zhang Z-Y, Agarwal S, Patel MR, Burris HA, Martell RE, et al. Food effect substudy of a phase 3 randomized double-blind trial of maintenance with niraparib (MK4827), a poly(ADP)ribose polymerase (PARP) inhibitor versus placebo in patients with platinum-sensitive ovarian cancer. J Clin Oncol. 2014;32(15_suppl):e16531.

46. van Andel L, Zhang Z, Lu S, Kansra V, Agarwal S, Hughes L, et al. Human mass balance study and metabolite profiling of 14C–niraparib, a novel poly(ADP-Ribose) polymerase (PARP)-1 and PARP-2 inhibitor, in patients with advanced cancer. Investig New Drugs. 2017.

47. United States Product Insert. 2017. Available from: http://www.accessdata.fda. gov/drugsatfda_docs/label/2016/209115s000lbl.pdf. Accessed 3 Aug 2017.

48. Zhang Z-Y, Kansra V, van Andel L, Tibben M, Rosing H, Lu S, et al. Characterization of absorption, metabolism, and elimination of Niraparib, an investigational poly (ADP-ribose) polymerase inhibitor, in cancer patients. Clin Ther. 2017;39(8):e7–8.

49. Mikule K, Wilcoxen K. Abstract B168: the PARP inhibitor, niraparib, crosses the blood brain barrier in rodents and is efficacious in a BRCA2-mutant intracranial tumor model. AACR; 2015.

50. Bridges KA, Toniatti C, Buser CA, Liu H, Buchholz TA, Meyn RE. Niraparib (MK-4827), a novel poly(ADP-ribose) polymerase inhibitor, radiosensitizes human lung and breast cancer cells. Oncotarget. 2014;5(13):5076–86.

51. Wang L, Mason KA, Ang KK, Buchholz T, Valdecanas D, Mathur A, et al. MK-4827, a PARP-1/−2 inhibitor, strongly enhances response of human lung and breast cancer xenografts to radiation. Investig New Drugs. 2012;30(6): 2113–20.

52. Williams SMG, Kuznicki AM, Andrade P, Dolinski BM, Elbi C, O'Hagan RC, et al. Treatment with the PARP inhibitor, niraparib, sensitizes colorectal cancer cell lines to irinotecan regardless of MSI/MSS status. Cancer Cell Int. 2015;15(1):14.

53. Chornenkyy Y, Agnihotri S, Yu M, Buczkowicz P, Rakopoulos P, Golbourn B, et al. Poly-ADP-ribose polymerase as a therapeutic target in pediatric diffuse intrinsic Pontine Glioma and pediatric high-grade Astrocytoma. Mol Cancer Ther. 2015;14(11):2560–8.

54. Sandhu SK, Schelman WR, Wilding G, Moreno V, Baird RD, Miranda S, et al. The poly(ADP-ribose) polymerase inhibitor niraparib (MK4827) in BRCA mutation carriers and patients with sporadic cancer: a phase 1 dose-escalation trial. Lancet Oncol. 2013;14(9):882–92.

55. Nappi L, Gleave ME. PARP inhibition in castration-resistant prostate cancer. Future Med. 2016;12(5). https://doi.org/10.2217/fon.2216.2211.

56. Mirza MR, Monk BJ, Herrstedt J, Oza AM, Mahner S, Redondo A, et al. Niraparib maintenance therapy in platinum-sensitive, recurrent ovarian cancer. N Engl J Med. 2016;375(22):2154–64.

57. Campo JMD, Mirza MR, Berek JS, Provencher DM, Emons G, Fabbro M, et al. The successful phase 3 niraparib ENGOT-OV16/NOVA trial included a substantial number of patients with platinum resistant ovarian cancer (OC). J Clin Oncol. 2017;35(15_suppl):5560.

58. Frampton GM, Fichtenholtz A, Otto GA, Wang K, Downing SR, He J, et al. Development and validation of a clinical cancer genomic profiling test based on massively parallel DNA sequencing. Nat Biotechnol. 2013; 31(11):1023–31.

59. Lin K, Sun J, Maloney L, Goble S, Oza A, Coleman R, et al. 2701 quantification of genomic loss of heterozygosity enables prospective selection of ovarian cancer patients who may derive benefit from the PARP inhibitor rucaparib. Eur J Cancer. 2015;51:S531–2.

60. Jenner ZB, Sood AK, Coleman RL. Evaluation of rucaparib and companion diagnostics in the PARP inhibitor landscape for recurrent ovarian cancer therapy. Future Oncol. 2016;12(12):1439–56.

61. Wilcoxen KM, Becker M, Neff C, Abkevich V, Jones JT, Hou X, et al. Use of homologous recombination deficiency (HRD) score to enrich for niraparib sensitive high grade ovarian tumors. J Clin Oncol. 2015;33

62. US National Library of Medicine. clinicaltrials.gov. Available online at: https://clinicaltrials.gov/ct2/results?cond=Cancer&term=Niraparib&cntry1= &state1=&recrs. Accessed 10 Aug 2017.

63. FDA: FDA grants orphan drug designation to veliparib for advanced NSCLC. HemOnc Today 2016.

64. US National Library of Medicine. clinicaltrials.gov. Available at: https://clinicaltrials. gov/ct2/show/NCT03075462?term=fluzoparib&rank=2. Accessed 16 Oct 2017.

65. Litton JK, Scoggins M, Whitman GJ, Barcenas CH, Moulder SL, Murthy RK, et al. A feasibility study of neoadjuvant talazoparib for early-stage breast cancer patients with a germline BRCA pathogenic variant: NCT02282345. Am Soc Clin Oncol. 2017.

66. Deas O, Cairo S, Wilcoxen K, Mikule K, Tran T-A, Timms K, et al: Preclinical evaluation of the PARP inhibitor niraparib and cytotoxic chemotherapy alone or in combination in a panel of 25 triple-negative breast cancer PDX models: relevance of BRCA mutations, HRD status and other biomarkers. AACR; 2016.

67. Wang Y, Cairo S, Nicolle D, Cristescu R, Loboda A, Nebozhyn M, et al. The PARP inhibitor niraparib demonstrates robust activity in a subset of patient-derived triple-negative breast cancer xenograft models. AACR; 2014.

68. Mueller S, Bhargava S, Molinaro AM, Yang X, Kolkowitz I, Olow A, et al. Poly (ADP-ribose) polymerase inhibitor MK-4827 together with radiation as a novel therapy for metastatic neuroblastoma. Anticancer Res. 2013;33(3):755–62.

# 21

# Clinical trial experience with CA4P anticancer therapy: focus on efficacy, cardiovascular adverse events, and hypertension management

Rachel Grisham[1]* ⓘ, Bonnie Ky[2], Krishnansu S. Tewari[3], David J. Chaplin[4] and Joan Walker[5]

## Abstract

Combretastatin A4-phosphate (CA4P) is a vascular-disrupting agent (VDA) in clinical development for the treatment of ovarian and other cancers. In contrast to antiangiogenic agents, such as bevacizumab, which suppress the development of new tumor vasculature, VDAs target established tumor vasculature. These differing but complementary mechanisms of action are currently being explored in clinical trials combining CA4P and bevacizumab. Clinical experience to date has highlighted an important need to better understand the cardiovascular adverse events of CA4P, both alone and in combination with antiangiogenic agents, which can also be associated with cardiovascular adverse events.

An acute but transient increase in blood pressure is often the most clinically relevant toxicity associated with CA4P. Increases in CA4P-related blood pressure typically occur 0.5 to 1 h after initiation of the 10-min infusion, peak by 2 h, and return to baseline 3 to 4 h after the infusion. Post-infusion increases in blood pressure are likely to recur in subsequent treatment cycles; however, the severity does not appear to increase with successive cycles. Other cardiovascular adverse events, such as transient, predominantly grade 1–2 tachycardia, bradycardia, QTc prolongation, and in rare cases myocardial ischemia, have also been observed with CA4P but at markedly lower frequencies than hypertension.

The clinical trial experience with CA4P suggests that cardiovascular assessment of patients prior to CA4P treatment and careful management of blood pressure during CA4P treatment can largely mitigate the risk of cardiovascular adverse events. Accordingly, we have developed a blood pressure management algorithm for use in the ongoing phase II/III FOCUS study of the triple combination of CA4P with physician's choice chemotherapy and bevacizumab.

**Keywords:** Bevacizumab, Blood pressure, CA4P, Cardiovascular, Combretastatin A4-phosphate, Focus, Fosbretabulin, Hypertension

## Introduction

Tumor vasculature is a long-established target of anticancer therapy [1]. Vascular-targeted anticancer therapies include two broad categories of agents with complementary mechanisms of action [2]: antiangiogenic agents (AAs), which prevent tumor neovascularization by inhibiting vascular endothelial growth factor and other pro-angiogenic factors, and vascular disrupting agents (VDAs), which destroy established tumor vasculature. The most extensive preclinical and clinical VDA data profile is associated with the tubulin-binding VDA, combretastatin A4-phosphate (CA4P) [3]. CA4P binds to tubulin, at or close to the colchicine binding site, causing disruption of the tumor endothelial cell cytoskeleton and junctions between endothelial cells. This results in endothelial cell shape change, leaky vessels, congestion within the blood vessel lumen, cessation of blood flow, and ultimately tumor necrosis [4, 5]. The preferential targeting of tubulin-binding VDAs to tumor vasculature as opposed to that of normal vasculature is

* Correspondence: grishamr@mskcc.org
[1]Memorial Sloan Kettering Cancer Center and Weil Cornell Medical College, New York, NY, USA
Full list of author information is available at the end of the article

due to the relative immaturity and instability of tumor vasculature [6].

VDAs, including CA4P, demonstrate limited single-agent antitumor activity [7, 8]. Preclinical data indicate that this limited single-agent activity is attributable to a remaining viable rim of tumor cells that are supported by oxygen and nutrients from the surrounding normal vasculature [4, 7–9]. Without additional treatment the tumor can rapidly revascularize. It has been proposed that the combined use of AAs and VDAs might circumvent this issue since AAs can inhibit this neovascularization while VDAs target the already formed, but abnormal, tumor vasculature inducing extensive cellular necrosis at the tumor core [10, 11]. This combined approach is being studied for the treatment of ovarian cancer (OC) in a phase II/III trial of physician's choice chemotherapy and bevacizumab with or without CA4P and in a phase I/II trial of CA4P plus pazopanib. Clinical experience with CA4P to date suggests that the most frequently occurring adverse events (AEs) associated with CA4P treatment are acute but transient blood pressure (BP) increases. Hypertension (HTN) is also associated with bevacizumab [12], pazopanib [13], and other AAs [14]. Thus, establishing an understanding of the cardiovascular safety profile of CA4P–antiangiogenic combination therapies is an important step in the clinical development of these therapeutic regimens. This article reviews the cardiovascular safety profile of CA4P as a single-agent and in combination regimens and reports a BP management algorithm developed by an expert panel based on these data and clinical experience.

## Review
### CA4P clinical studies: Efficacy
CA4P has been studied in phase II trials in several tumor types [15–19]. In the phase II FALCON study, 63 patients with chemotherapy-naive stage IIIb/IV non–small cell lung cancer (NSCLC) were randomized to CP and bevacizumab with or without CA4P (60 mg/m$^2$) [16]. CA4P did not confer a significant survival benefit (median OS 13.6 vs 16.2 months; HR = 1.06 [95% confidence interval [CI], 0.55–2.03]), but it was associated with a substantial increase in response rate compared with the control arm (50% vs 32%, respectively). Interestingly, post hoc analyses showed a trend toward longer survival with CA4P–CP–bevacizumab compared with CP–bevacizumab in patients with tumors >10 cm (median OS 14.2 vs 11.0 months; HR = 0.67 [95% CI, 0.26–1.70]).

A single-arm, phase II study evaluated the combination of CA4P (63 mg/m$^2$) and CP in 44 patients with OC that had recurred <6 months after platinum therapy

[17]. A confirmed response (all partial responses) was observed in 5 of 37 (13.5%) patients who were evaluable by Response Evaluation Criteria in Solid Tumors. The response rate was 34% in the 38 patients evaluable by Gynecologic Cancer InterGroup CA 125 criteria. GOG-0186I—a randomized, phase II study—evaluated CA4P (60 mg/m$^2$) in combination with bevacizumab versus bevacizumab alone in 107 patients with recurrent OC [18, 19]. Patients in the CA4P arm had a near-3-month PFS benefit (median PFS, 7.3 vs 4.8 months; HR = 0.69 [90% CI 0.47–1.00], $p = 0.05$) [18]. Notably, in the 81 patients with measurable disease, the PFS benefit was enhanced in those treated with CA4P + bevacizumab compared with those receiving bevacizumab alone (9.8 vs 6.1 months; HR = 0.60, $p = 0.027$) [19]. The PFS benefit was further enhanced in patients with tumors greater than the median size (>5.7 cm) for the study population with measurable disease at baseline (10.5 vs 4.3 months; HR = 0.554, $p = 0.071$), again demonstrating a greater benefit in patients with larger tumor size [19]. Together, the clinical data support the potential for CA4P in the management of varied cancer types, with clear signals in recurrent OC as well as ATC and NSCLC [15–19].

### CA4P clinical studies: Safety
In the studies to date, CA4P has been studied as monotherapy and in combination with other treatments, such as antiangiogenic therapy (eg, bevacizumab) and chemotherapy (eg, CP). CA4P has been generally well tolerated with the most notable AEs across studies being hematologic toxicity, tumor pain, and HTN.

#### Cardiovascular AEs
Cardiovascular AEs have been the most frequently and consistently reported AEs across CA4P studies (Table 1). By far, the most common of these has been an acute, transient increase in BP (see Table 1). Typically, in studies of single-agent CA4P or CA4P + CP, increases of approximately 10% to 15% above baseline were seen at 0.5 to 1-h post-infusion. These resolved by 3 to 4 h post-infusion [17, 20, 21] (Fig. 1).

The HTN observed in these studies was predominantly grade 1–2 [15, 17, 20–22]. In the FACT study in ATC, grade 1–2 HTN was increased with the addition of CA4P to CP (29.4% vs 0% with CP) [15]. The incidence of grade 3 HTN was similar with CP with and without CA4P (3.9% and 4.2%, respectively), and no grade 4 HTN was observed. In the single-arm, phase II study of CP and CA4P in patients with recurrent OC, grade ≤ 2 HTN was observed in 23% of patients, but no grade 3 or 4 HTN was observed [17]. Notably, there was no cumulative hypertensive effect demonstrated with consecutive treatment cycles.

**Table 1** Adverse events related to the cardiovascular system in studies of CA4P

| Study | | Phase II single-arm CA4P (63 mg/m²) + CP (n = 44) [17] | Phase II, two-arm[a] Bev (15 mg/kg) + CA4P (60 mg/m²) (n = 54) OR Bev (n = 53) [18, 24] | Phase II single-arm CA4P (60 mg/m²) (n = 51) [15] | Phase II, two-arm[a] CP + Bev (15 mg/kg) + CA4P (60 mg/m²) (n = 31) OR CP + Bev (n = 29) [16] | Phase I single-arm CA4P (doses from 18 mg/m² to 90 mg/m²) (n = 25) [21, 22][b] | Phase I single-arm CA4P (doses from 5 mg/m² to 114 mg/m²) (n = 34) [20] | Phase I single-arm CA4P (doses from 45 mg/m² to 63 mg/m²) + Bev (10 mg/kg) (n = 15) [23] |
|---|---|---|---|---|---|---|---|---|
| Tumor type | | Platinum-resistant ovarian cancer | Recurrent ovarian cancer | Anaplastic thyroid cancer | Stage IIIb/IV NSCLC | Solid tumors | Solid tumors | Solid tumors |
| Hypertension, n (%) | All-grades | 10 (23) | 32/53 (60) | 17 (33) | 17 (55) | 1 (4) | 12 (35) | 11 (73) |
| | Grade ≤ 2 | 10 (23) | NR | 15 (29) | NR | 1 (4) | 12 (35) | 11 (73) |
| | Grade 3 | 0 | 19 (35) | 2 (4) | NR | 0 | 0 | 0 |
| | Grade 4 | | | 0 | NR | 0 | 0 | 0 |
| Tachycardia, n (%) | All-grades | 15 (34) | 2 (4) | 6 (12) | 8 (26) | NR | 19 (56) | 1 (7) |
| | Grade ≤ 2 | 14 (32) | NR | 6 (12) | NR | NR | 19 (56) | 1 (7) |
| | Grade 3 | 1 (2) | NR | 0 | NR | NR | 0 | 0 |
| | Grade 4 | | NR | 0 | NR | NR | NR | 0 |
| Bradycardia, n (%) | All-grades | 1 (2) | 3 (6) | 2 (4) | 4 (13) | NR | 8 (24) | NR |
| | Grade ≤ 2 | 1 (2) | NR | 1 (2) | NR | NR | 8 (24) | NR |
| | Grade 3 | 0 | NR | 1 (2) | NR | NR | 0 | NR |
| | Grade 4 | | NR | 0 | NR | NR | NR | NR |
| Hypotension, n (%) | All grades | 2 (5) | 3 (6) | NR | NR | NR | 6 (18) | NR |
| | Grade ≤ 2 | 2 (5) | NR | NR | NR | NR | 6 (18) | NR |
| | Grade 3 | 0 | NR | NR | NR | NR | 1 (3) | NR |
| | Grade 4 | | NR | NR | NR | NR | NR | NR |
| Arrhythmia, n (%) | All grades | 2 (5) | 2 (4) | 0 | NR | 2 (8) | NR | 1 (7) |
| | Grade ≤ 2 | 1 (2) | NR | 0 | NR | 2 (8) | NR | 0 |
| | Grade 3 | 1 (2) | NR | 0 | NR | 0 | NR | 1 (7) |
| | Grade 4 | | NR | 0 | NR | 0 | NR | 0 |
| Myocardial ischemia, n (%) | All grades | 1 (2) | NR | 2 (4) | 2 (6) | 2 (8)[c] | NR | NR |
| | Grade ≤ 2 | 1 (2) | NR | 2 (4) | 0 | 1 (4) | NR | NR |
| | Grade 3 | 0 | NR | 0 | 2 (6) | 0 | NR | NR |
| | Grade 4 | | NR | 0 | 0 | 1 (4)[c] | NR | NR |
| >QTc, n (%) | All grades | 2 (5) | NR | 8 (16) | NR | 7 (28) | 0 | NR |
| | Grade ≤ 2 | 2 (5) | NR | 6 (12) | NR | 7 (28) | 0 | NR |
| | Grade 3 | 0 | NR | 2 (4) | NR | 0 | 0 | NR |

**Table 1** Adverse events related to the cardiovascular system in studies of CA4P *(Continued)*

| Study | | Phase II single-arm CA4P (63 mg/m²) + CP (n = 44) [17] | Phase II, two-arm[a] Bev (15 mg/kg) + CA4P (60 mg/m²) OR Bev (n = 54) OR (n = 53) [18, 24] | Phase II single-arm CA4P (60 mg/m²) + CP (n = 51) [15] | Phase II, two-arm[a] CP + Bev (15 mg/kg) + CA4P (60 mg/m²) (n = 31) OR CP + Bev (n = 29) [16] | Phase I single-arm CA4P (doses from 18 mg/m² to 90 mg/m²) (n = 25) [21, 22][b] | Phase I single-arm CA4P (doses from 5 mg/m² to 114 mg/m²) (n = 34) [20] | Phase I single-arm CA4P (doses from 45 mg/m² to 63 mg/m²) + Bev (10 mg/kg) (n = 15) [23] |
|---|---|---|---|---|---|---|---|---|
| | Grade 4 | NR | NR | 0 | NR | 0 | 0 | NR |
| AV block, n (%) | All grades | NR | NR | 1 (2) | NR | NR | NR | NR |
| | Grade ≤ 2 | NR | NR | 1 (2) | NR | NR | NR | NR |
| | Grade 3 | NR | NR | 0 | NR | NR | NR | NR |
| | Grade 4 | NR | NR | 0 | NR | NR | NR | NR |

[a]In two-arm studies, adverse events are shown only for the CA4P-containing arms

[b]These manuscripts describe the same patient cohort so safety data were combined

[c]Grade 4 myocardial ischemia occurred in a patient receiving 90 mg/m² of CA4P

*AV* atrioventricular, *Bev* bevacizumab, *CA4P* combretastatin A4-phosphate, *CP* carboplatin and paclitaxel, *MI* myocardial infarction, *NR* not reported, *NSCLC* non–small cell lung cancer

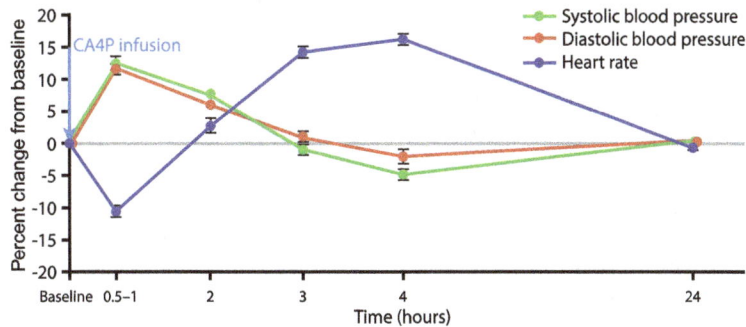

**Fig. 1** Time course of mean [20, 21] and median [17] heart rate changes from baseline, and mean [16, 20, 23] and median [17] blood pressure changes [17, 20, 23] from baseline in combretastatin A4-phosphate (CA4P) studies reporting such data. CA4P infusion occurred at time 0. Means of published data points are shown. Standard error of the mean is indicated with error bars

Bevacizumab is commonly associated with sustained HTN. In a meta-analysis of 12,656 patients treated with bevacizumab, HTN was demonstrated in 23.6% of patients, including 7.9% who had HTN categorized as grade $\geq 3$ [12]. Given the established association of HTN and bevacizumab, the incidence of HTN in patients receiving CA4P in combination with bevacizumab is of particular interest. Consistent with studies of single-agent CA4P or chemotherapy + CA4P, increases in transient BP were seen in patients receiving CA4P + bevacizumab. The time course was similar to prior studies. Increases in BP typically occurred within the first 30 min to 1 h after infusion, persisted for approximately 2 h, and returned to baseline by 4 h [16, 23]. The addition of bevacizumab to CA4P appeared to increase the magnitude of the increases in BP during the first three bevacizumab-containing cycles but not in subsequent cycles. Systolic and diastolic BP were increased by approximately 10% in these combination-treatment cycles compared with values with CA4P alone in cycle 1 [23]. Notably, there was no grade 3 or higher HTN. The addition of bevacizumab to CA4P also appears to increase the incidence of HTN overall. In the FALCON study of CA4P in combination with CP–bevacizumab in patients with NSCLC, all-grade HTN was increased in the CP–bevacizumab–CA4P arm relative to the CP–bevacizumab arm (55% vs 45%) [16]. In the GOG-0186I trial, in which patients were randomized to bevacizumab with and without CA4P, grade $\geq 3$ HTN was increased with bevacizumab–CA4P (35% vs 20% with bevacizumab alone; relative risk, 1.77 [95% CI, 0.90–3.45]) [18]. Because of the increased incidence of HTN reported with CA4P + bevacizumab, active monitoring of BP and management in clinical trials of this combination is essential.

Other cardiovascular AEs, such as tachycardia, bradycardia, and QTc prolongation, have also been observed with CA4P [15–18]. In phase II studies to date,

tachycardia and bradycardia have been reported in 4% to 34% and 2% to 13% of patients, respectively (see Table 1) [15–17]. With the exception of one case of grade 3 tachycardia [17] and one case of grade 3 bradycardia [15], all events have been grade 1 or 2. The heart rate changes are typically characterized by a decrease in heart rate within the first hour after infusion followed by an increase between 3 and 4 h post-infusion, and a return to baseline by 24 h [17, 20–22]. The typical time course of heart rate changes following CA4P administration are shown in Fig. 1.

QTc prolongation has also been reported in CA4P studies; however, to date, a dedicated QTc study has not yet been performed. In the FACT study in ATC, all-grade and grade 3 QTc prolongation were reported for 16% and 4% of patients receiving CP–CA4P, respectively, and one patient discontinued treatment because of QTc prolongation. There were no reports of QTc prolongation in the control arm; however, since electrocardiograms were not routinely collected in the control arm, the rate of QTc prolongation in the control arm may have been under-reported [15]. QTc prolongations were also reported in two single-arm studies of CA4P, but all were grade 1 or 2 [17, 21, 22] and deemed clinically insignificant [21, 22].

To date, across eight studies, seven patients administered CA4P-containing regimens have experienced myocardial ischemia [15–17, 21, 22]. In the phase II FALCON study, two patients in the CA4P–CP–bevacizumab arm, both with a history of HTN, experienced three episodes of grade 3 myocardial ischemia, which resulted in treatment discontinuation [16]. One event occurred concurrently with a post-CA4P infusion BP increase and another occurred during the bevacizumab infusion, 24 h after the CA4P infusion. Three patients in the other phase II studies experienced myocardial ischemia, but it was asymptomatic and grade 1 in two patients [15] and grade 1–2 in the other [17]. In a single-agent CA4P dose-finding study, two patients (one treated with 60 mg/m$^2$ CA4P and one with 90 mg/m$^2$ CA4P) had myocardial ischemia (one grade 2; one grade 4) [22]. The patient treated with 60 mg/m$^2$ CA4P had a grade 2 event and subsequently was found to have coronary artery disease, which was treated with angioplasty. The patient recovered fully with no further cardiac issues during the 11 months he was followed after treatment discontinuation [21, 22]. The patient treated with 90 mg/m$^2$ of CA4P experienced grade 4 myocardial ischemia secondary to coronary artery vasospasm. An electrocardiogram was performed, and it was consistent with myocardial infarction. Cardiac catheterization showed subtotal stenosis. Serial troponin levels were normal. The patient recovered the same day with a normal electrocardiogram and left ventricular ejection fraction [21, 22].

### Hematologic toxicity

The rate of all-grade hematologic toxicity increased with the addition of CA4P to chemotherapy [15] (all-grade leukopenia CP 4% vs CP + CA4P 41%; all-grade neutropenia CP 21% vs CP + CA4P 57%) and to chemotherapy + bevacizumab [16] (all-grade leukopenia CP + bevacizumab 24% vs CP + bevacizumab + CA4P 45%; all-grade neutropenia CP + bevacizumab 18% vs CP + bevacizumab + CA4P 81%). However, in GOG-0186I, in which neither treatment arm contained chemotherapy, the rates of all-grade leukopenia (21% vs 15%) and all-grade neutropenia (13% vs 15%) were similar in the bevacizumab alone and the CA4P + bevacizumab study arms [24].

### Tumor pain

Grade 3–4 tumor pain was reported in the CA4P arm of the FACT study but not in the control arm (6% vs 0%) [15]. Grade 3–4 pain was also observed in 18% of patients with recurrent OC treated with CP and CA4P in the single-arm phase II study [17]. In most cases, tumor pain occurred within an hour after CA4P infusion and resolved with pain medication. No patient discontinued treatment due to pain. Tumor pain has also been observed in several phase I studies of CA4P [20, 21, 25]. This tumor pain was observed more frequently in patients with OC who responded to treatment (67% vs 48%), though this correlation was not statistically significant [17]. A potential relationship between tumor pain and heart rate and/or BP should not be overlooked because tumor pain may exacerbate these AEs. Active management with pain medication is recommended.

### Management of CA4P-induced BP increases: Best practice

Preclinical data demonstrate that the cardiovascular AEs associated with CA4P can be prevented by pretreatment with calcium channel blockers, suggesting that CA4P does not induce direct cardiotoxic effects [26]. Administration of CA4P to hypertensive rats resulted in a significant increase in mean arterial pressure and, in a number of animals, circulating troponin I. The calcium channel blockers diltiazem and nicardipine completely eliminated the hypertensive effects and pretreatment with diltiazem prevented increases in serum troponin in these animals [26]. Similarly, administration of the tubulin-binding VDA ZD6126 has been shown to elevate BP in rats, increase circulating troponin, and induce left ventricular myocardial fiber necrosis [27]. These effects were all blocked when animals were pretreated with a calcium channel blocker in combination with a beta blocker to prevent HTN [27].

Preclinical and clinical data suggest that CA4P-induced BP increases are a compensatory response to an increase in peripheral resistance [28, 29]. In a preclinical study in rats, which measured blood flow using a radiolabel and quantitative autoradiography, arterial BP was increased at 1 and 6 h after CA4P administration, and by 6 h, mean tumor blood flow was reduced by more than 100-fold [28]. Blood flow was also reduced in other tissues, most notably, the spleen (seven-fold decrease). In a clinical study using positron emission tomography to evaluate 13 patients treated with a radiolabel and CA4P, mean tumor perfusion was reduced (−49%), beginning 30 min after administration of CA4P [29]. Decreases were also observed in spleen perfusion (−35%) and kidney perfusion (−6%).

Because of their transient nature, the underlying pathophysiology of the BP increases associated with CA4P appear to differ from that of the sustained BP increases observed with bevacizumab therapy [30]. This supports different management strategies for HTN associated with CA4P and bevacizumab. The clinical trial experience with CA4P lends support to careful patient selection prior to CA4P therapy along with cardiovascular assessment and careful management of BP during and after CA4P infusion.

To optimize the cardiovascular risk profile of CA4P therapy, an expert panel was convened to develop a BP management algorithm for use in the phase II/III FOCUS study [31] (Fig. 2). The panel agreed that different treatment strategies should be used for patients with baseline HTN (defined for this study as systolic BP >130 mmHg) and those without. For those with baseline HTN, the panel recommended that their current antihypertensive medication be optimized. Carvedilol was recommended as an initial agent for BP control because it acts at both alpha- and beta-adrenergic receptors, is fairly well tolerated, and combines well with other antihypertensive agents. Moreover, a beta blocker strategy would be beneficial

**Pre-CA4P Infusion**

This is a guideline only, medical judgement can and should be used by each investigator when managing individual patients

**Managing Patients with Pre-existing Hypertension/High BP**
- BP should be well controlled prior to entering the study
- Patients initiating bevacizumab will be at risk for chronic increases in BP from their baseline levels

Baseline SBP >130 mmHg

- Optimize original anti-hypertensive agent (if on one) OR
- Add carvedilol 20 mg PO QD

- If SBP remains elevated, add carvedilol 20 mg PO QD (if not added already) OR
- Increase carvedilol to 40 mg PO QD

**Managing Patients at "High Risk" of BP Increase**
- If patient has had a CA4P post-infusion BP increase on a prior cycle OR
- SBP >130 mmHg 30 minutes prior to CA4P infusion PLUS a CV risk factor (i.e., prior anthracycline-based therapies, diabetes, dyslipidemia, previously uncontrolled hypertension [BP >140/90], previous MI, previous stents, previous CABG)

- Prophylactically treat 30 to 60 minutes prior to CA4P infusion with either:
  – Labetalol 100 mg x1 – may re-dose with 100 mg after 30 minutes up to a maximum of 300 mg
  – Diltiazem 30 mg x1 – may re-dose with 30 mg after 30 minutes up to a maximum of 120 mg

**Post-CA4P Infusion\***

This is a guideline only, medical judgement can and should be used by each investigator when managing individual patients

**Managing Acute Post-infusion CA4P BP Increases**
Note: CA4P-induced BP increases generally resolve within 4-6 hours post infusion

Post-infusion SBP increases to >140 mmHg

Repeat BP within 5-10 minutes prior to treatment to confirm reading

Consider treatment with:
- Diltiazem 30 mg x1 OR
- Labetalol 100 mg x1

Consider re-treatment at one hour, if SBP remains >140 mmHg

Retreat with:
- Diltiazem 30 mg x1 OR
- Labetalol 100 mg x1

If patient has symptoms of hypertensive emergency (e.g., chest pain, SOB, blurred vision, severe HA), then IV anti-hypertensives are required – transfer to ER for management (e.g., nitroglycerin or nitroprusside)

\*Monitor BP at 15, 30, 60, 90, and 120 minutes post-infusion

**Fig. 2** Combretastatin A4-phosphate (CA4P) blood pressure management algorithm. BP = blood pressure; CV = cardiovascular; ER = emergency room; HA = headache; PO = orally; QD = daily; SBP = systolic blood pressure; SOB = shortness of breath

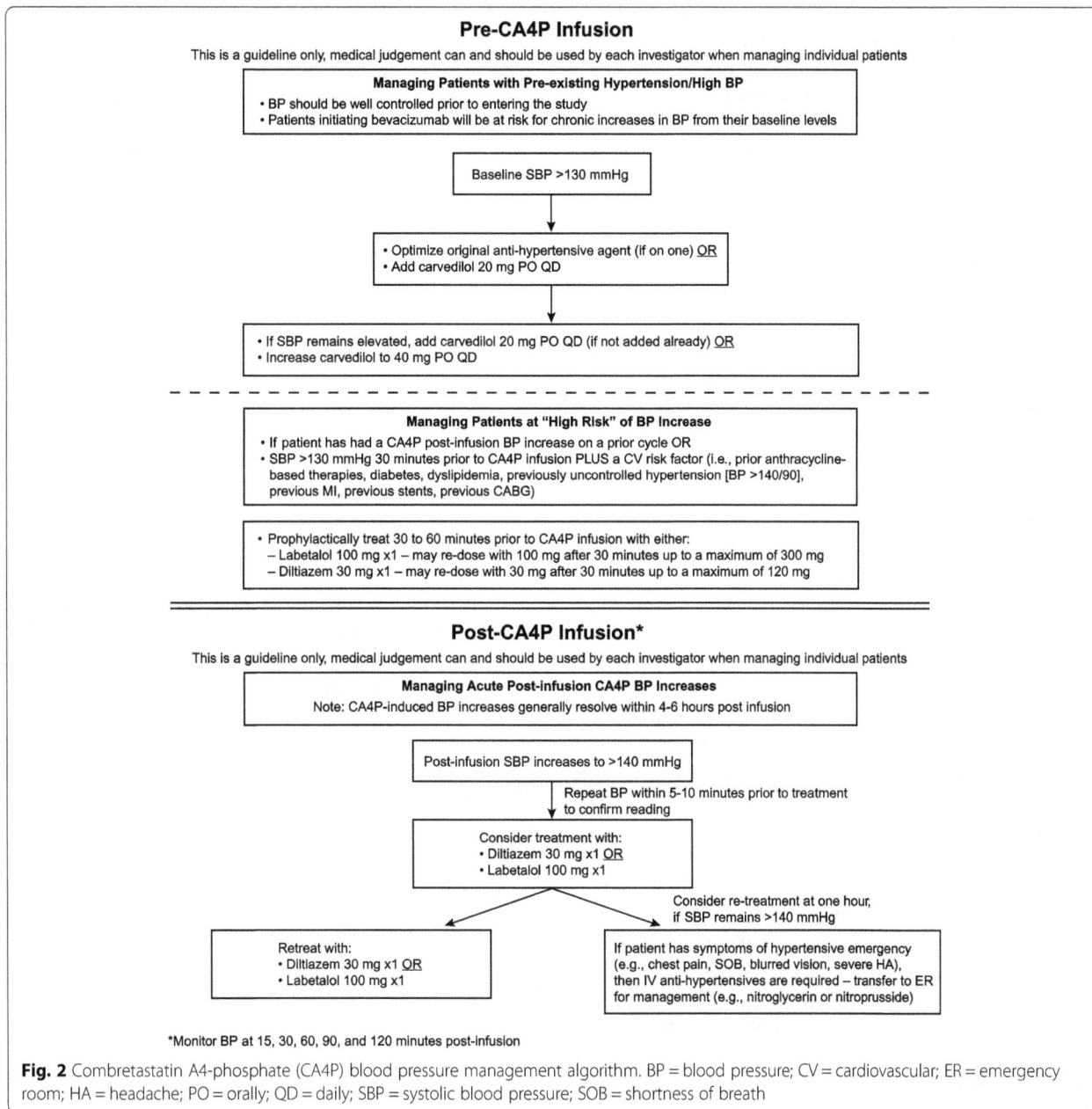

in the setting of myocardial ischemia, and there is a longstanding literature suggesting a cardioprotective and beneficial cardiac remodeling effect with carvedilol [32, 33]. The most common side effect associated with carvedilol is dizziness [34, 35]. Of note, carvedilol carries an FDA black-box warning against abrupt cessation of treatment in patients with coronary artery disease as this can exacerbate angina or result in myocardial infarction or ventricular arrythmia. Therefore, it is critical that cessation of therapy is strictly monitored and carried out in accordance with the prescribing information [34, 35].

For patients without baseline HTN, the panel recommended that an evaluation of cardiovascular risk factors be performed before therapy is started. Cardiovascular risk factors should include prior anthracyclines, diabetes, dyslipidemia, prior uncontrolled HTN, previous myocardial infarction, previous stents, or previous coronary artery bypass grafting. Consideration of patients as "high risk" is recommended if patients had a previous CA4P-induced BP increase or if they have systolic BP >130 mmHg 30 min prior to CA4P infusion plus a cardiovascular risk factor as defined above.

The panel recommended that BP be monitored frequently after infusion at intervals of 15, 30, 60, 90, and 120 min. Should systolic BP reach 140 mmHg, treatment with diltiazem or labetalol with continuous monitoring was advised. If systolic BP remains at or above 140 mmHg at 1 h, retreatment with diltiazem or labetalol is advised or, if patients experience symptoms of hypertensive emergency, patients should be transferred to emergency room care.

The recommended antihypertensive agents were chosen for several reasons. As discussed earlier, CA4P-induced BP increases typically begin 0.5 to 1 h post-infusion and resolve by 3 to 4 h post-infusion [17, 20–22]. Thus, to avoid hypotension, it is important that the antihypertensive agents used to manage these BP increases have a quick onset of action and are short-acting. Additionally, agents that could result in reflex tachycardia should be avoided, given the risk of CA4P-associated tachycardia.

The alpha- and beta-adrenergic receptor blocker, labetalol, and the calcium channel blocker diltiazem have pharmacokinetic profiles that mesh well with the time course of CA4P-induced BP increases. The onset of the antihypertensive effect of oral labetalol is between 30 and 120 min, the maximum effects are observed within 1 to 3 h after administration and the plasma half-life is 6 to 8 h [36]. The onset of action for immediate release diltiazem is between 30 and 60 min, peak plasma levels are observed 2 to 3 h after administration and the plasma half-life is 3.5 h [37].

Because patients with cancer are typically being treated with multiple medications, the potential for drug–drug interactions and additional side-effects are another key consideration when developing an antihypertensive strategy. Labetalol has a relatively low-risk of drug–drug interaction [36]; however, diltiazem is metabolized by CYP34A so care should be taken when prescribing it to patients taking other drugs that interact with CYP34A [37]. Side-effects of labetalol include, dizziness, nausea, and fatigue [36] and side effects of dilitiazem include edema, headaches, nausea, and dizziness [37]. Labetalol may have an added advantage in that some data suggest that tumor cells express beta 1-, beta 2- and beta 3-adrenergic receptors and that these receptors can mediate tumor cell proliferation and facilitate metastasis [38, 39]. Some retrospective studies suggest that blockade of these receptors is associated with improved outcomes in patients with cancer [40–42]. However, other studies have not found such an association [43, 44].

## Conclusions

VDAs, including CA4P, disrupt the existing tumor vasculature within the interior of tumors, a region that is often resistant to standard therapies, such as chemotherapy and radiation, and may have particular benefit in patients with bulky disease. CA4P has a contrasting and complementary activity compared with AAs, such as bevacizumab, and the combination of these agents is supported both by a mechanistic rationale and promising clinical data. While CA4P and bevacizumab are associated with toxicity profiles dominated by BP effects, the agents appear to be able to be used safely in combination with appropriate patient selection and active monitoring and treatment. While bevacizumab primarily causes sustained HTN that requires modulation of a daily antihypertensive regimen, the BP surges seen with CA4P most commonly resolve within hours after drug administration and are best treated either with pretreatment in selected high-risk patients or with immediate administration of antihypertensive therapy at the time of the first BP increase. Frequent BP monitoring is essential immediately after CA4P administration to mitigate associated complications. It is anticipated that the ongoing FOCUS phase II/III trial of physician's choice chemotherapy, bevacizumab, and CA4P in patients with platinum-resistant OC, which employs a proactive BP management strategy, will provide key data on the efficacy and safety of triple combination therapy [31].

**Abbreviations**
AA: Antiangiogenic agent; AE: Adverse event; ATC: Anaplastic thyroid cancer; BP: Blood pressure; CA4P: Combretastatin A4-phosphate;; CI: Confidence interval; CP: Carboplatin–Paclitaxel; CV: Cardiovascular; ER: Emergency room; HA: Headache; HR: Hazard ratio; HTN: Hypertension; NSCLC: Non–small cell lung cancer; OC: Ovarian cancer; OS: Overall survival; PFS: Progression-free survival; PO: Orally; QD: Daily; SBP: Systolic blood pressure; SOB: Shortness of breath; VDA: Vascular-disrupting agent

**Acknowledgements**
Writing assistance was provided by Twist Medical and funded by Mateon Therapeutics.

**Funding**
Writing assistance was funded by Mateon Therapeutics.

**Authors' contributions**
All authors contributed to the writing of this manuscript and approved the submitted manuscript.

**Consent for publication**
Not applicable

**Competing interests**
RG receives grant funding from Cycle for Survival and the Ovarian Cancer Research Fund Alliance. She has also served as a consultant for Mateon Therapeutics.
BK has served as a consultant for Mateon Therapeutics.

KT has served on speakers' bureaus for Astra Zeneca, Clovis, Merck, Roche, and Vermillion. He has served on advisory boards for Caris, Clovis, Genentech, and Mateon Therapeutics. He serves on the scientific steering committee for Mateon Therapeutics.

DC is an employee of Mateon Therapeutics.

JW has served as a consultant for Mateon Therapeutics.

## Author details

[1]Memorial Sloan Kettering Cancer Center and Weil Cornell Medical College, New York, NY, USA. [2]Perelman School of Medicine, University of Pennsylvania, Philadelphia, PA, USA. [3]Division of Gynecologic Oncology, University of California Irvine, Orange, CA, USA. [4]Mateon Therapeutics, South San Francisco, CA, USA. [5]The Stephenson Cancer Center, University of Oklahoma, Oklahoma City, OK, USA.

## References

1. Folkman J. Tumor angiogenesis: therapeutic implications. N Engl J Med. 1971;285:1182–6.

2. Siemann DW, Bibby MC, Dark GG, Dicker AP, Eskens FA, Horsman MR, et al. Differentiation and definition of vascular-targeted therapies. Clin Cancer Res. 2005;11:416–20.

3. Chase DM, Chaplin DJ, Monk BJ. The development and use of vascular targeted therapy in ovarian cancer. Gynecol Oncol. 2017;145:393–406.

4. Tozer GM, Kanthou C, Baguley BC. Disrupting tumour blood vessels. Nat Rev Cancer. 2005;5:423–35.

5. Siemann DW. The unique characteristics of tumor vasculature and preclinical evidence for its selective disruption by tumor-vascular disrupting agents. Cancer Treat Rev. 2011;37:63–74.

6. Siemann DW, Chaplin DJ, Horsman MR. Vascular-targeting therapies for treatment of malignant disease. Cancer. 2004;100:2491–9.

7. Chaplin DJ, Pettit GR, Hill SA. Anti-vascular approaches to solid tumour therapy: evaluation of combretastatin A4 phosphate. Anticancer Res. 1999; 19:189–95.

8. Horsman MR, Siemann DW. Pathophysiologic effects of vascular-targeting agents and the implications for combination with conventional therapies. Cancer Res. 2006;66:11520–39.

9. Salmon BA, Siemann DW. Characterizing the tumor response to treatment with combretastatin A4 phosphate. Int J Radiat Oncol Biol Phys. 2007;68:211–7.

10. Siemann DW, Shi W. Dual targeting of tumor vasculature: combining Avastin and vascular disrupting agents (CA4P or OXi4503). Anticancer Res. 2008;28:2027–31.

11. Kendrew J, Odedra R, Logié A, Taylor PJ, Pearsall S, Ogilvie DJ, et al. Anti-tumour and anti-vascular effects of cediranib (AZD2171) alone and in combination with other anti-tumour therapies. Cancer Chemother Pharmacol. 2013;71:1021–32.

12. Ranpura V, Pulipati B, Chu D, Zhu X, Wu S. Increased risk of high-grade hypertension with bevacizumab in cancer patients: a meta-analysis. Am J Hypertens. 2010;23:460–8.

13. Qi WX, Lin F, Sun YJ, Tang LN, He AN, Yao Y, et al. Incidence and risk of hypertension with pazopanib in patients with cancer: a meta-analysis. Cancer Chemother Pharmacol. 2013;71:431–9.

14. Faruque LI, Lin M, Battistella M, Wiebe N, Reiman T, Hemmelgarn B, et al. Systematic review of the risk of adverse outcomes associated with vascular endothelial growth factor inhibitors for the treatment of cancer. PLoS One. 2014;9:e101145.

15. Sosa JA, Elisei R, Jarzab B, Balkisson J, Lu SP, Bal C, et al. Randomized safety and efficacy study of fosbretabulin with paclitaxel/carboplatin against anaplastic thyroid carcinoma. Thyroid. 2014;24:232–40.

16. Garon EB, Neidhart JD, Gabrail NY, de Oliveira MR, Balkisson J, Kabbinavar F. A randomized phase II trial of the tumor vascular disrupting agent CA4P (fosbretabulin tromethamine) with carboplatin, paclitaxel, and bevacizumab in advanced nonsquamous non-small-cell lung cancer. Onco Targets Ther. 2016;9:7275–83.

17. Zweifel M, Jayson GC, Reed NS, Osborne R, Hassan B, Ledermann J, et al. Phase II trial of combretastatin A4 phosphate, carboplatin, and paclitaxel in patients with platinum-resistant ovarian cancer. Ann Oncol. 2011;22:2036–41.

18. Monk BJ, Sill MW, Walker JL, et al. Randomized phase II evaluation of bevacizumab versus bevacizumab plus CA4P in recurrent ovarian, tubal, or peritoneal carcinoma: an NRG oncology/gynecologic oncology group study. J Clin Oncol. 2016;34:2279–86.

19. Tewari KS, Abrouk N, Coleman R, Aghajanian C, Couchenour R, Nelson J, et al. Improved progression-free survival among women with measurable recurrent ovarian carcinoma treated with ca4p plus bevacizumab: a post-hoc analysis of GOG-0186l. Int J Gynecol Cancer. 2016;26(Suppl 3):651–2.

20. Rustin GJ, Galbraith SM, Anderson H, Stratford M, Folkes LK, Sena L, et al. Phase I clinical trial of weekly combretastatin A4 phosphate: clinical and pharmacokinetic results. J Clin Oncol. 2003;21:2815–22.

21. Cooney MM, Radivoyevitch T, Dowlati A, Overmoyer B, Levitan N, Robertson K, et al. Cardiovascular safety profile of combretastatin a4 phosphate in a single-dose phase I study in patients with advanced cancer. Clin Cancer Res. 2004;10: 96–100.

22. Dowlati A, Robertson K, Cooney M, Petros WP, Stratford M, Jesberger J, et al. A phase I pharmacokinetic and translational study of the novel vascular targeting agent combretastatin a-4 phosphate on a single-dose intravenous schedule in patients with advanced cancer. Cancer Res. 2002;62:3408–16.

23. Nathan P, Zweifel M, Padhani AR, Koh DM, Ng M, Collins DJ, et al. Phase I trial of combretastatin A4 phosphate (CA4P) in combination with bevacizumab in patients with advanced cancer. Clin Cancer Res. 2012;18:3428–39.

24. Clinicaltrials.gov. https://clinicaltrials.gov/ct2/show/results/ NCT01305213?term=GOG-0186l&rank=1&sect=X40156#othr accessed: 29 Aug 2017.

25. Stevenson JP, Rosen M, Sun W, Gallagher M, Haller DG, Vaughn D, et al. Phase I trial of the antivascular agent combretastatin A4 phosphate on a 5-day schedule to patients with cancer: magnetic resonance imaging evidence for altered tumor blood flow. J Clin Oncol. 2003;21:4428–38.

26. Ke Q, Samad MA, Bae S, Chaplin DJ, Kang PM. Exaggerated hypertensive response to combretastatin A-4 phosphate in hypertensive rats: effective pharmacological inhibition by diltiazem. Vasc Pharmacol. 2015;74:73–9.

27. Gould S, Westwood FR, Curwen JO, Ashton SE, Roberts DW, Lovick SC, et al. Effect of pretreatment with atenolol and nifedipine on ZD6126-induced cardiac toxicity in rats. J Natl Cancer Inst. 2007;99:1724–8.

28. Tozer GM, Prise VE, Wilson J, Locke RJ, Vojnovic B, Stratford MR, et al. Combretastatin A-4 phosphate as a tumor vascular-targeting agent: early effects in tumors and normal tissues. Cancer Res. 1999;59:1626–34.

29. Anderson HL, Yap JT, Miller MP, Robbins A, Jones T, Price PM. Assessment of pharmacodynamic vascular response in a phase I trial of combretastatin A4 phosphate. J Clin Oncol. 2003;21:2823–30.

30. Syrigos KN, Karapanagiotou E, Boura P, Manegold C, Harrington K. Bevacizumab-induced hypertension: pathogenesis and management. BioDrugs. 2011;25:159–69.

31. Monk BJ, Herzog T, Alvarez R, et al. FOCUS study: physician's choice chemotherapy (PCC) plus bevacizumab and CA4P versus PCC plus bevacizumab and placebo in platinum-resistant ovarian cancer. Int J Gynecol Cancer. 2016;26(Suppl 3):878–9.

32. Williams RE. Early initiation of beta blockade in heart failure: issues and evidence. J Clin Hypertens (Greenwich). 2005;7:520–8.

33. Stafylas PC, Sarafidis PA. Carvedilol in hypertension treatment. Vasc Health Risk Manag. 2008;4:23–30.

34. Coreg [package insert]. Research Triangle Park, NC: GlaxoSmithKline, plc; 2015.

35. Coreg CR [package insert]. Research Triangle Park, NC: GlaxoSmithKline; 2015.

36. Trandate [package insert]. San Diego: Prometheus Laboratories, Inc.; 2010.

37. Cardizem [package insert]. Bridgewater: Valeant Pharmaceuticals North America LLC; 2014.

38. Powe DG, Voss MJ, Habashy HO, Zanker KS, Green AR, Ellis IO, et al. Alpha- and beta-adrenergic receptor (AR) protein expression is associated with poor clinical outcome in breast cancer: an immunohistochemical study. Breast Cancer Res Treat. 2011;130:457–63.

39. Montoya A, Amaya CN, Belmont A, Diab N, Trevino R, Villanueva G, et al. Use of non-selective β-blockers is associated with decreased tumor proliferative indices in early stage breast cancer. Oncotarget. 2017;8: 6446–60.

40. Barron TI, Connolly RM, Sharp L, Bennett K, Visvanathan K. Beta blockers and breast cancer mortality: a population-based study. J Clin Oncol. 2011;29: 2635–44.

41. Grytli HH, Fagerland MW, Fosså SD, Taskén KA. Association between use of β-blockers and prostate cancer-specific survival: a cohort study of 3561 prostate cancer patients with high-risk or metastatic disease. Eur Urol. 2014; 65:635–41.

42. Watkins JL, Thaker PH, Nick AM, Ramondetta LM, Kumar S, Urbauer DL, et al. Clinical impact of selective and nonselective beta-blockers on survival in patients with ovarian cancer. Cancer. 2015;121:3444–51.

43. Shah SM, Carey IM, Owen CG, Harris T, Dewilde S, Cook DG. Does β-adrenoceptor blocker therapy improve cancer survival? Findings from a population-based retrospective cohort study. Br J Clin Pharmacol. 2011;72:157–61.

44. Cardwell CR, Coleman HG, Murray LJ, O'Sullivan JM, Powe DG. Beta-blocker usage and prostate cancer survival: a nested case-control study in the UK clinical practice research Datalink cohort. Cancer Epidemiol. 2014;38:279–85.

# 22

# Bringing new medicines to women with epithelial ovarian cancer: what is the unmet medical need?

Thomas J. Herzog[1*] and Bradley J. Monk[2]

**Abstract**

**Background:** Therapy for advanced epithelial ovarian cancer (OC) includes first line platinum/taxane-containing chemotherapy and re-treatment with platinum-containing regimens for disease recurrence in patients likely to respond again. Single-agent, non-platinum, cytotoxic agents are commonly used to treat patients resistant to platinum retreatment, but these agents are associated with dose-limiting toxicities and response rates below 20%.

**Main body:** Recent advances have led to novel targeted treatments for recurrent OC that offer opportunities to improve response rates and prolong progression-free intervals. However, they also add complexity to the process of selecting treatment for individual patients at different stages of the disease process. Advanced and recurrent OC is rarely cured. Multiple lines of platinum combinations, and nonplatinum chemotherapeutics eventually fail to achieve clinical benefit, thus other active and tolerable systemic therapies are needed. Consequently, the US Food and Drug Administration has created a mechanism for "accelerated approval" of new medicines in situations of high unmet medical need.

**Conclusion:** We review the clinical implications of recent key clinical studies in these settings and outline the path forward for study design and approval of novel therapeutics to treat recurrent OC.

**Keywords:** BRCA1/2, Ovarian cancer, PARP, Platinum-refractory

## Introduction

More than 70% of women with epithelial ovarian cancer (OC), which typically also includes fallopian tube and primary peritoneal cancers, have advanced disease at the time of first diagnosis. Although many patients with advanced disease achieve complete remission after surgical cytoreduction and platinum- and taxane-based chemotherapy, up to 80% eventually experience recurrence [1]. Two major goals of recent and ongoing clinical studies in OC have been to achieve a more durable disease-free interval after induction therapy and better response rates for regimens administered beyond first line therapy. We provide a succinct overview of recent studies addressing these two goals and outline the unmet need for additional treatment options.

* Correspondence: herzogtj@ucmail.uc.edu
[1]University of Cincinnati Cancer Institute, University of Cincinnati, Medical Sciences Bldg, Suite 2005H, ML0662, 231 Albert Sabin Way, Cincinnati, OH 45267-0662, USA
Full list of author information is available at the end of the article

## Review

### What is the role of maintenance therapy as part of first line therapy?

Platinum-containing induction chemotherapy remains a standard first-line treatment for women with advanced OC. However, there has been vigorous debate regarding the role of maintenance chemotherapy in patients with advanced OC who achieve an objective response during induction chemotherapy [1, 2]. In the 1990s, studies of extended platinum chemotherapy (8–12 cycles) found no evidence for improved progression-free survival (PFS) or overall survival (OS) versus 5–6 cycles (reviewed in Markman 2015) [2]. Furthermore, extended platinum regimens were associated with increased toxicity versus standard regimens.

In the early 2000s, a true maintenance study assessed paclitaxel maintenance therapy in women who had achieved an objective complete response to induction platinum-paclitaxel [3]. Patients were randomized to either 12 or 3 additional cycles of single-agent paclitaxel.

The study was terminated early because patients in the 12-cycle arm had significantly longer PFS than patients in the 3-cycle arm. At mature follow-up, PFS was 22 versus 14 months ($P = 0.006$), but there was no significant effect on OS (53 versus 48 months; $P = 0.34$) [4]. The lack of a significant effect on OS may have several explanations, including exposure to subsequent active treatment regimens [2]. Patients in the 12-cycle arm experienced higher rates of peripheral neuropathy. Another study of single-agent paclitaxel (6 cycles) after complete or pathologic response to platinum-paclitaxel induction demonstrated no improvement in PFS or OS, and increased rates of peripheral neuropathy in the paclitaxel arm [5]. Recently, those findings were confirmed by another phase 3 study (GOG-212), which also demonstrated no OS benefit for patients who received maintenance paclitaxel [6].

Two studies (GOG-218 and ICON7) have explored use of the anti-angiogenesis agent bevacizumab to extend the disease-free interval after first line chemotherapy [7, 8]. In both studies, bevacizumab was added to standard chemotherapy (5 or 6 cycles of carboplatin-paclitaxel), and bevacizumab monotherapy was continued (for 12–22 cycles) after cessation of chemotherapy. Initially, both studies reported improved PFS when extended bevacizumab treatment was added to chemotherapy [7, 8]. However, long-term follow-up of the ICON7 study found no significant improvement in PFS or OS in the overall study population, although there was evidence of benefit in high-risk patients [9]. The GOG-218 study had three treatment arms, all of which received 6 cycles of carboplatin-paclitaxel [7]. One arm received bevacizumab concurrent with chemotherapy, a second arm received bevacizumab concurrently and during an extended period (up to cycle 22), and the third arm received only chemotherapy. A placebo was administered as appropriate control in this double-blind study. Patients in the extended-bevacizumab arm had the longest PFS (14.1 months), which was significantly longer than the chemotherapy-alone arm (10.3 months; hazard ratio [HR]: 0.717; 95% confidence interval [CI]: 0.625–0.824; $P < 0.001$). The PFS in the concurrent-bevacizumab arm was 11.2 months [7]. In both studies, bevacizumab was associated with increased risk of adverse events, especially gastrointestinal events [10], and neither study found a benefit in terms of OS for the overall study population. Exposure to bevacizumab or other active regimens after the study may have confounded any OS effect; nonetheless, the role of bevacizumab in front-line therapy for advanced OC—either concurrently with chemotherapy or for an extended duration—continues to be controversial. SOLO-1 is an ongoing study of olaparib maintenance monotherapy after first line platinum-based chemotherapy. Also, the randomized,

phase 3 PAOLA-1 study (NCT02477644) is comparing olaparib and bevacizumab versus placebo and bevacizumab as maintenance therapy in patients with advanced OC following first line treatment with platinum chemotherapy and bevacizumab [11]. Olaparib and other Poly (ADP-ribose) polymerase (PARP) inhibitors are discussed in more detail below.

**Recurrent ovarian cancer**

Selection of treatment for recurrence of advanced epithelial OC is generally guided by the progression-free interval [12] (Fig. 1). When the time to progression is >6 months after cessation of initial platinum-containing chemotherapy, the disease is considered to be platinum-sensitive. In these patients, treatment using a combination platinum-containing chemotherapy (typically including a taxane, pegylated liposomal doxorubicin [PLD], gemcitabine, or bevacizumab in carefully selected patients) is considered a preferred treatment option [13]. Response rates to second line, combination platinum-containing chemotherapy in patients with platinum-sensitive tumors are approximately 50%–65% [14–16]. Combination therapy demonstrated advantages over single-agent platinum regimens in terms of both PFS and OS [17]. When progression after first line therapy occurs less than 6 months after cessation of chemotherapy, the disease is considered to be platinum-resistant; recommended second line therapies in these patients include mostly single-agent, nonplatinum-containing chemotherapy regimens, with the possible addition of bevacizumab or pazopanib in carefully selected patients [13]. When progression occurs during chemotherapy or within 1 month of cessation, the disease is considered platinum-refractory [12].

Until recent years, there were essentially no treatment options other than repeated courses of chemotherapy in patients with 2 or more prior lines of chemotherapy. Furthermore, nearly all patients eventually become resistant to platinum-containing regimens [12]. Thus, the concept of platinum sensitivity becomes less important beyond 2 or 3 lines of chemotherapy, and its relevance to treatment selection in such patients is not well understood. The limited available evidence indicates that responsiveness to platinum-containing regimens declines dramatically after 2 prior lines, even in patients who were initially platinum-sensitive. In one study of 63 patients who received at least 3 lines of chemotherapy, only 11.9% had a clinical response to third line chemotherapy, although 52% had responded to second line [18]. Nonplatinum-containing regimens—such as PLD, paclitaxel, gemcitabine, or topotecan—have similar response profiles (range 10%–15%), PFS (3–4 months), and OS (~12 months) when used as late-line therapies [12]. A retrospective analysis of 3 large European clinical

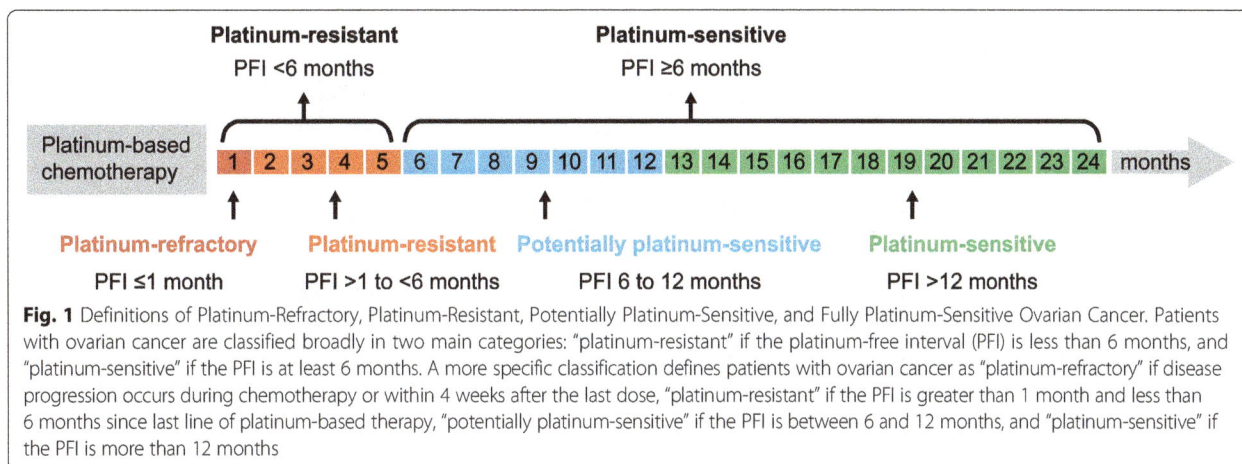

**Fig. 1** Definitions of Platinum-Refractory, Platinum-Resistant, Potentially Platinum-Sensitive, and Fully Platinum-Sensitive Ovarian Cancer. Patients with ovarian cancer are classified broadly in two main categories: "platinum-resistant" if the platinum-free interval (PFI) is less than 6 months, and "platinum-sensitive" if the PFI is at least 6 months. A more specific classification defines patients with ovarian cancer as "platinum-refractory" if disease progression occurs during chemotherapy or within 4 weeks after the last dose, "platinum-resistant" if the PFI is greater than 1 month and less than 6 months since last line of platinum-based therapy, "potentially platinum-sensitive" if the PFI is between 6 and 12 months, and "platinum-sensitive" if the PFI is more than 12 months

studies of chemotherapy in patients with OC ($N$ = 1620) found that the benefits of chemotherapy in terms of increased PFS or OS declined with successive recurrences (Fig. 2) [19]. Although chemotherapy for a fourth recurrence was still associated with a small benefit in terms of OS, the authors concluded that this benefit was mostly due to patients with platinum-sensitive disease, and that chemotherapy beyond three recurrences was not beneficial in patients with platinum-resistant disease. This conclusion, however, may need to be revisited as more data accumulate from studies of patient subgroups, and from new and emerging treatment strategies for patients with multiple recurrences.

Because of reduced potential for benefit after 2 prior lines of chemotherapy, and severe effects on quality of life (QOL), some patients forego chemotherapy after 2 prior lines, although many patients prefer to continue receiving additional lines of chemotherapy even if it confers diminishing benefits [20]. Undoubtedly, many patients withstand the side effects from subsequent lines of chemotherapy but obtain limited benefit. Furthermore, repeated chemotherapy regimens may expose patients to cumulative toxicities associated with many of these regimens [1, 19].

Recently, molecularly targeted inhibitors of vascular endothelial growth factor (VEGF; ie, bevacizumab) and PARP (ie, olaparib, rucaparib, and niraparib) have emerged as treatment options in patients with advanced epithelial OC after multiple prior lines of chemotherapy (Table 1) [21–32]. Both bevacizumab and PARP inhibitors require careful patient selection, the criteria for which are still evolving.

### Which patients are candidates for bevacizumab in recurrent OC

Bevacizumab, in combination with paclitaxel, PLD, or topotecan is approved for the treatment of patients with platinum-resistant recurrent epithelial OC who received no

more than 2 prior lines of chemotherapy [21, 22, 25, 33]. In the AURELIA study, patients with platinum-resistant OC and 2 or fewer prior lines of chemotherapy had response rates of 27.3% in the bevacizumab plus chemotherapy arm versus 11.8% in the chemotherapy-alone arm ($P$ = 0.001). Note that this study excluded patients who were platinum-refractory (progression during previous platinum-containing therapy) [25].

In patients with platinum-sensitive, recurrent OC, the OCEANS study found significantly increased objective response rate (ORR; 78% versus 57%; $P$ < 0.001) and PFS (12.4 versus 8.4 months; $P$ < 0.001) when bevacizumab was added to gemcitabine plus carboplatin, but there was no improvement in OS [26, 27]. Another randomized phase 3 study (GOG-213) found a statistically significant improvement in response rate (78% versus 59% in a subset of patients with evaluable data from imaging; $P$ < 0.001) and PFS (13.8 versus 10.4 months; $P$ < 0.001) when bevacizumab was added to paclitaxel plus carboplatin [28]. In the primary analysis of this study, OS was better in the group that received bevacizumab (42.2 versus 37.7 months), although this incremental improvement narrowly missed achieving statistical significance ($P$ = 0.056). However, when miscalculations of the prior platinum-free interval were corrected, the difference in OS achieved statistical significance ($P$ = 0.045) [28].

Single-agent bevacizumab has also shown activity (clinical response rate 16%–21%) in patients with 1 to 3 prior lines of chemotherapy, most of whom were platinum-resistant [21, 22]. Other small studies have reported responses to single-agent bevacizumab as a later line of therapy in patients with recurrent, platinum-resistant OC, with response rates ranging from 13% to 16% [21, 23, 24].

Thus, there is evidence to support the use of bevacizumab in multiple settings, including in combination with chemotherapy (typically PLD, weekly paclitaxel, or topotecan) in platinum-resistant patients with no more than 2

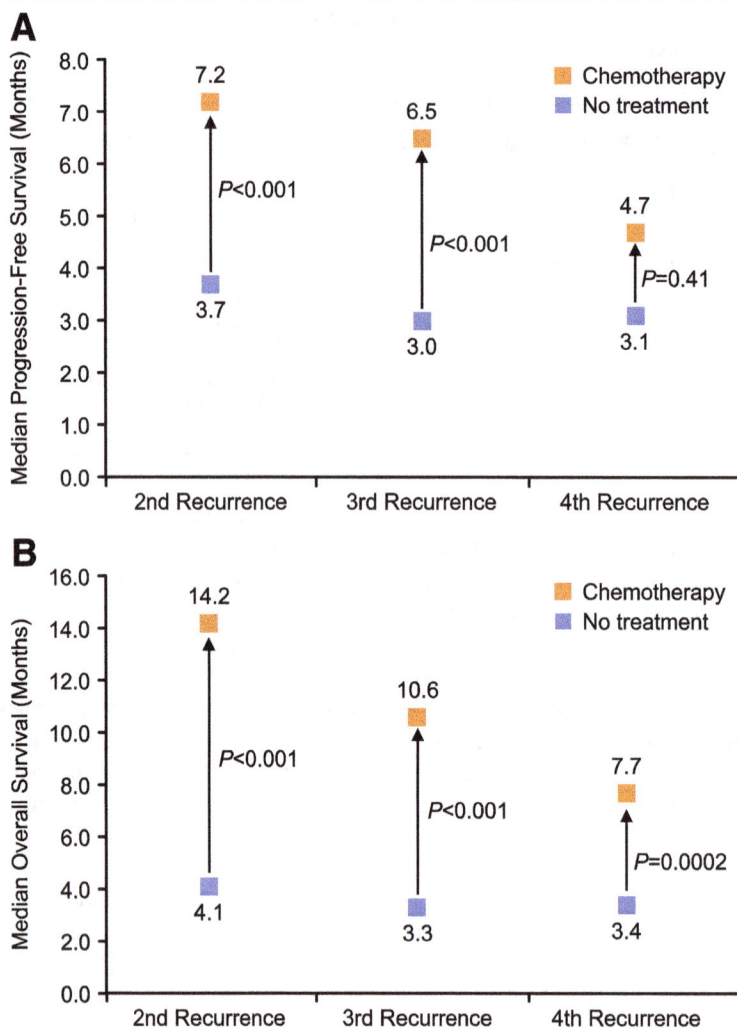

**Fig. 2** Median Progression-Free Survival (**a**) and Overall Survival (**b**) Associated with Successive Lines of Chemotherapy (Versus no Treatment) in a Retrospective Analysis of Three Randomized Trials in Patients with Advanced Ovarian Cancer [19]. Data from Hanker et al. *Ann Oncol.* 2012;23:2605–12. Hanker et al. performed a retrospective, pooled analysis of three randomized, phase 3 studies of primary taxane-platinum-based chemotherapy. The analysis included 1620 patients for whom complete data were available. Responsiveness to platinum-containing regimens declined dramatically after 2 prior *lines*, even in patients who were initially platinum-sensitive [19]

prior lines of chemotherapy. But bevacizumab may also provide benefit in platinum-sensitive patients in combination with carboplatin-gemcitabine or carboplatin-paclitaxel. The United States Food and Drug Administration (US FDA)-approved indications for bevacizumab in OC are summarized in Table 2 [33]. Perhaps just as important to the selection of patients for bevacizumab is the strict exclusion of patients who are at increased risk of bowel perforation. Restrictive exclusion criteria used in clinical studies are commonly followed [21, 25]. These criteria exclude any patient with a history of bowel obstruction (including subocclusive disease) related to underlying disease, history of abdominal fistula, gastrointestinal perforation, intra-abdominal abscess, evidence of rectosigmoidal involvement by pelvic exam, bowel involvement on computed tomography, or clinical symptoms of bowel

obstruction [25]. The role of bevacizumab after previous exposure requires further study; thus, some clinicians will withhold repeat courses until further data are reported.

### What is the role of PARP inhibitors for treatment of recurrent OC?

Recent clinical studies have evaluated the potential roles of PARP inhibitors for treatment of patients with advanced OC in two distinct settings: 1) when disease has recurred or progressed after 2–3 or more prior lines of platinum-containing chemotherapy, and 2) when the disease is in a state of response after completion of a recent course of platinum-containing chemotherapy (maintenance therapy). Some of these studies enrolled only patients with known deleterious *BRCA* mutations (germline or somatic).

**Table 1** Clinical activity of targeted therapies for treatment of recurrent ovarian cancer in heavily pretreated patients

| | Phase | Patients with OC, n | Previous therapies | ORR, n (%) | CR, n (%) | Median DoR, mo | Median PFS, mo | OS, mo |
|---|---|---|---|---|---|---|---|---|
| Bevacizumab Monotherapy | | | | | | | | |
| Cannistra 2007 [21] | 2 | 44 | 2–3 | 7 (16) | 0 | 4.2 | 4.4 | 10.7 |
| Burger 2007 [22] | 2 | 62 | 1–2 | 13 (21) | 2 (3) | 10.3 | 4.7 | 16.9 |
| Monk 2006 [23] | | 32 | 5 (range: 2–10) | 5 (16) | 1 (3) | NR | 5.5 | 6.9 |
| Pietzner 2011 [24] | | 15 | 5.4 (range: 1–7) | 2 (13) | 0 | NR | NR | 15.0 |
| Bevacizumab-Chemotherapy Combination | | | | | | | | |
| AURELIA [25] | 3 | 361 | ≤2 | 27.3% | NR | NR | 6.7 | 16.6 |
| OCEANS [26, 27] | 2 | 484 | ≤1 | 190/242 (78.5) | 42 (17) | 10.4 | 12.4 | 33.6 |
| GOG-213 [28] | 3 | 674 | ≥3 | 196/249 (78) | 79/249 (32) | NR | 13.8 | 42.2 |
| Olaparib Monotherapy | | | | | | | | |
| Kaufman 2015 [29] | 2 | 193 | 4.3 ± 2.2 (SD) | 60 (31) | 6 (3) | 7.5 | 7 | 16.6 |
| ≥ 3 Prior lines [30][a] | | 137[a] | ≥3 | 46 (34) | 2 (2) | 7.9 | 6.7 | NR |
| Gelmon 2011 [31] | 2 | 65 | 3 (range: 1–10) | 18 (29) | 0 | NR | 7.3 | NR |
| Rucaparib Monotherapy | | | | | | | | |
| Swisher 2017 [32] | 2 | | | | | | | |
| BRCA mutant | | 40 | 1–2 | 32 (80) | NR | 9.2 | 12.8 | NR |
| BRCA wild-type | | | | | | | | |
| LOH high | | 82 | 1–2 | 24 (29) | NR | 10.8 | 5.7 | NR |
| LOH low | | 70 | 1–2 | 7 (10) | | 5.6 | 5.2 | |

CR complete response, DoR duration of response, LOH loss-of-heterozygosity score, mo months, NR not reported, OC ovarian cancer, ORR objective/overall response rate, OS overall survival, PFS progression-free survival, SD standard deviation
[a]Subset of patients in Kaufman/Domchek who had measurable disease at baseline and ≥3 prior lines of chemotherapy

### Which patients with recurrent ovarian cancer are candidates for a PARP inhibitor?

In late 2014, olaparib received accelerated approval by the US FDA as monotherapy for patients with advanced OC harboring deleterious or suspected deleterious germline BRCA (gBRCA) mutations and who were previously treated with 3 or more lines of chemotherapy. Approval was primarily based on data from a single-arm study of patients with advanced OC and gBRCA1/2 mutations [29, 30], most of whom had received multiple prior lines of chemotherapy (mean 4.3). Among 137 patients who had measurable disease at baseline and who had received 3 or more prior lines of chemotherapy, the ORR was 34% and the median duration of response was 7.9 months (Table 1) [30]. Although patients with platinum-sensitive disease had the highest ORR (18/39; 46%), the response rate observed in patients with platinum-resistant disease (24/81; 30%) suggests that platinum resistance does not preclude responsiveness to olaparib as late-line therapy in patients with OC and a BRCA mutation. In contrast, the ORR was 14% (2/14) among patients with platinum-refractory disease [30].

In late 2016, another PARP inhibitor, rucaparib (Table 2), was approved for treatment of patients with advanced OC associated with deleterious BRCA mutation (germline or somatic) and who had progressed after 2 or more prior

lines of chemotherapy. The accelerated approval was based upon ORR (54%) [34] and median duration of response (9.2 months) in patients with a BRCA mutation from the single-arm, phase 2 study (ARIEL2 Part 1) that enrolled women with high-grade, relapsed, platinum-sensitive OC [32]. The ARIEL2 study results are shown in Table 1 [32].

One of the goals of the ARIEL2 study was to explore biomarkers of response to PARP inhibition. Thus, the study also included patients who had wild-type BRCA, but tumor samples were analyzed for genetic loss of heterozygosity (LOH) as a potential surrogate marker of homologous recombination deficiency (HRD). Although patients with wild-type BRCA but high LOH scores had lower rates of ORR and shorter PFS than patients with BRCA mutation, both cohorts (those with BRCA mutation and those with wild-type BRCA but high LOH scores, indicating presence of HRD) had ORR and PFS that were significantly better than patients with wild-type BRCA and low LOH scores ($P < 0.02$) [32]. These results demonstrated that PARP inhibitors appear active in a broader set of patients than only those harboring deleterious BRCA mutations. Part 2 of the ARIEL2 trial is ongoing, and it will prospectively evaluate rucaparib responsiveness in patient subgroups defined by LOH scores.

**Table 2** US FDA-approved targeted therapies for ovarian cancer

|  | Drug class | Ovarian cancer indication | Black box warnings | Warnings and precautions |
|---|---|---|---|---|
| Bevacizumab [33] | VEGF inhibitor; anti-angiogenesis | Platinum-resistant recurrent disease • In combination with paclitaxel, PLD, or topotecan with no more than 2 prior lines of chemotherapy Platinum-sensitive recurrent disease • In combination with carboplatin and paclitaxel, or carboplatin and gemcitabine; followed by single-agent bevacizumab | • Gastrointestinal perforations • Surgery and wound healing complications • Hemorrhage | • Perforation or fistula • Arterial and venous thromboembolic events • Hypertension • Posterior reversible encephalopathy syndrome • Proteinuria • Infusion reactions • Embryo-fetal toxicity • Ovarian failure |
| Niraparib [36] | PARP inhibitor | Maintenance treatment of recurrent disease in complete or partial response to platinum-based chemotherapy | None | • Myelodysplastic syndrome/acute myeloid leukemia • Bone marrow suppression • Cardiovascular effects (blood pressure and heart rate) • Embryo-fetal toxicity |
| Olaparib [35] | PARP inhibitor | Maintenance treatment of recurrent disease in complete or partial response to platinum-based chemotherapy Treatment of deleterious or suspected deleterious germline BRCA-mutated disease with ≥3 prior lines of chemotherapy; requires FDA-approved companion diagnostic test | None | • Myelodysplastic syndrome/acute myeloid leukemia • Pneumonitis • Embryo-fetal toxicity |
| Rucaparib [34] | PARP inhibitor | Monotherapy in patients with deleterious BRCA mutations treated with two or more prior chemotherapies; requires companion diagnostic test | None | • Myelodysplastic syndrome/acute myeloid leukemia • Embryo-fetal toxicity |

PARP poly (ADP-ribose) polymerase, PLD pegylated liposomal doxorubicin, VEGF vascular endothelial growth factor

PARP inhibitors are also associated with side effects, although not usually as severe as those observed with chemotherapy. However, a small percentage (1% or less) in both olaparib [35] and rucaparib [34] studies developed myelodysplastic syndrome/acute myeloid leukemia. Patients should be monitored for hematologic toxicities at baseline and during treatment.

**Is there a role for PARP inhibitors in maintenance therapy?**
Both olaparib [35] and niraparib [36] (Table 2), have been approved as maintenance therapies in patients who are in a complete or partial response to platinum-based chemotherapy [37–39]. Some have questioned use of the term "maintenance therapy" in this setting, on the basis that many patients had only a partial response to chemotherapy rather than a complete response. Nevertheless, this term has been adopted by regulatory agencies, and it will continue to be used in this context.

The maintenance therapy studies of PARP inhibitors enrolled patients with OC who were in response (partial or complete) after their most recent platinum-containing regimen and who had responded for at least 6 months after the preceding platinum-containing regimen. In the phase 2 olaparib study (Study 19), patients in the olaparib arm had significantly longer PFS than those in the placebo arm (8.4 versus 4.8 months; $P < 0.001$) [37]. Further analysis according to BRCA

status revealed that patients with a deleterious BRCA mutation (germline or somatic) had the greatest benefit from olaparib versus placebo (PFS 11.2 versus 4.3 months; $P < 0.001$), but even patients with wild-type BRCA benefited from olaparib maintenance therapy (PFS 7.4 versus 5.5 months; $P = 0.007$) [40]. While no significant difference in OS was found for the general population, patients with BRCA mutation-positive, platinum-sensitive, recurrent OC benefited from longer survival when treated with olaparib [41]. The recently reported SOLO-2 study was a confirmatory phase 3 trial to determine the efficacy of olaparib tablets as maintenance monotherapy in patients with platinum-sensitive, relapsed OC and germline BRCA-mutation [39]. In this study, olaparib maintenance therapy was associated with marked improvements in PFS versus placebo (Table 3). Health-related QOL also was evaluated in the SOLO-2 study. Patients maintained their QOL while on olaparib maintenance therapy, exhibiting no significant negative effect on health-related QOL versus placebo. Patients receiving olaparib (versus placebo) experienced a significant improvement in multiple assessments of patient-centered benefits [42].

The phase 3 niraparib study (NOVA) enrolled 2 cohorts of patients according to the presence or absence of a gBRCA mutation [38]. In the gBRCA cohort, niraparib treatment was also associated with markedly longer PFS

**Table 3** Phase 3 studies of PARP inhibitors for maintenance therapy in patients with platinum-sensitive ovarian cancer

| | Prior lines of chemotherapy | Inclusion biomarkers | Median PFS, months | | HR for PFS (95% CI) | P value |
|---|---|---|---|---|---|---|
| | | | Active therapy | Placebo | | |
| **Niraparib Monotherapy** | | | | | | |
| NOVA [38] | ≥2 | None Patients stratified according to gBRCA status and HRD score | gBRCA: 21.0 | 5.5 | 0.27 (0.17–0.41) | <0.001 |
| | | | Non-gBRCA: 9.3 | 3.9 | 0.45 (0.34–0.61) | <0.001 |
| | | | HRD-positive: 12.9 | 3.8 | 0.38 (0.24–0.59) | <0.001 |
| | | | HRD-negative: 6.9 | 3.8 | 0.58 (0.36–0.92) | 0.02 |
| **Olaparib Monotherapy** | | | | | | |
| SOLO-2 [39] | ≥2 | BRCA1/2 mutation | 30.2 | 5.5 | 0.25 (0.18–0.35) | <0.001 |
| **Rucaparib Monotherapy** | | | | | | |
| ARIEL3 [45, 46] | ≥3[a] | None | BRCA mutation: 16.6 | 5.4 | 0.23 | <0.001 |
| | | | HRD-positive: 13.6 | 5.4 | 0.32 | <0.001 |
| | | | ITT population: 10.8 | 5.4 | 0.36 | <0.001 |

CI confidence interval, gBRCA germline BRCA mutation, HR hazard ratio, HRD homologous recombination deficiency, ITT intent-to treat, PARP poly (ADP-ribose) polymerase, PFS progression-free survival

[a]Received ≥2 prior platinum-based treatment regimens including platinum based regimen and no more than 1 non-platinum chemotherapy regimen

than placebo (Table 3). Patients in the non-gBRCA cohort also had significant benefits from niraparib therapy. Interestingly, even patients who did not have a gBRCA mutation, and who did not exhibit HRD, experienced a longer PFS with niraparib versus placebo [38]. In a subgroup analysis, niraparib provided significant benefit in patients with recurrent OC who achieved a partial response following platinum therapy [43]. In addition, 49% of the total patient population was found to have developed platinum resistance to previous chemotherapy, yet the study met its primary endpoint of prolonged PFS following response to most recent platinum therapy [44]. Results for OS have not yet been reported from either the SOLO-2 or NOVA studies.

With appropriate caution regarding toxicities, PARP inhibitors are emerging as a potential maintenance therapy in patients with OC who have responded to at least 2 prior lines of platinum-containing chemotherapy and are in response (complete or partial) to the most recent course. Although BRCA mutations and deficiency in homologous recombination repair appear to be relative markers predictive of response to PARP inhibitors, lack of these markers does not preclude a response. This concept is especially notable in the NOVA trial, which led to recent approval of niraparib irrespective of biomarker status. Thus, neither BRCA status nor HRD score are requisites for use of niraparib. The ongoing ARIEL3 study (NCT01968213) is exploring the use of rucaparib as maintenance therapy, with enrollment criteria similar to those in the olaparib and niraparib maintenance therapy studies, but without restrictions related to BRCA status. As reported in June 2017, the phase 3 ARIEL3 study demonstrated improved PFS (Table 3) by investigator review for rucaparib compared with placebo in all three primary efficacy analyses: BRCA mutation

(16.6 months vs 5.4 months; HR: 0.23, $P < 0.001$); HRD-positive (13.6 months vs 5.4 months; HR: 0.32, $P < 0.001$); overall intent-to-treat populations (10.8 months vs 5.4 months; HR: 0.36, $P < 0.001$) [45, 46].

## What percentage of patients with advanced ovarian cancer have BRCA mutations?

In population-based studies of unselected patients with OC, 5%–18% of cases were found to be associated with gBRCA mutations [47]. Limited available data suggest that another 5%–10% arise from somatic BRCA mutations [48]. Thus, at initial diagnosis the percentage of patients with OC whose cancer is BRCA-related is modest. However, patients with BRCA-related OC have better long-term survival than non-carriers [49, 50], which may in part be related to better responsiveness to platinum-based chemotherapy [50, 51]. Thus, patient groups who have undergone multiple lines of chemotherapy may become enriched for BRCA mutation carriers.

## What are the prospects for the unmet needs of patients requiring third line therapy and beyond?

Several studies are investigating treatment options for patients who have platinum-resistant disease or who have progressed after multiple lines of treatment, including the third line setting and beyond (Table 4). With regard to PARP inhibitors, the phase 3 SOLO-3 study is measuring PFS for olaparib versus single-agent investigator's choice nonplatinum-based chemotherapy in patients with platinum-sensitive high-grade serous OC or high-grade endometrioid cancer who progressed at least 6 months after last platinum treatment, and have received 2 or more platinum-based lines of therapy (NCT02282020) [52]. To determine the most sensitive and specific assays to assess HRD and more accurately

**Table 4** Ongoing phase 2 and 3 studies investigating late-line therapies in ovarian cancer

| Agent | NCT #<br>Study name | Phase | Est. N | Setting | Expected completion |
|---|---|---|---|---|---|
| PARP Inhibitors | | | | | |
| Niraparib | NCT02354586<br>QUADRA | 2 | 400 | Recurrent, ≥4th- 5th-line | October 2017 |
| Olaparib | NCT02282020<br>SOLO-3 | 3 | 411 | Recurrent, ≥3rd-line | December 2017 |
| Olaparib | NCT02889900<br>CONCERTO | 2 | 100 | Recurrent, ≥3rd-line | November 2018 |
| Rucaparib | NCT01891344<br>ARIEL2 | 2 | 480 | Recurrent, ≥4th-line | March 2017 |
| Rucaparib | NCT01968213<br>ARIEL3 | 3 | 540 | Recurrent, ≥3rd-line | March 2017 |
| Mirvetuximab soravtansine (an antibody-drug conjugate targeting the folate-alpha receptor) | | | | | |
| | NCT02631876<br>FORWARD1 | 3 | 333 | Platinum-resistant; 1–3 prior lines of chemotherapy | February 2019 |
| NUC-1031 (gemcitabine prodrug[a]) | | | | | |
| | NCT03146663 | 2 | 64 | Platinum-resistant; ≥3 prior lines of chemotherapy | June 2020 |
| Trabectedin (novel alkylating chemotherapy agent) | | | | | |
| | NCT01846611<br>ORCHYD | 3 | 670 | Platinum-sensitive; 3rd line; known BRCA1/2 mutation | December 2019 |
| Ipilimumab (immune checkpoint inhibitor) | | | | | |
| | NCT01611558 | 2 | 49 | Platinum-sensitive; ≤4 prior lines of chemotherapy | July 2019 |
| Birinapant (SMAC mimetic and IAP inhibitor) | | | | | |
| | NCT02756130 | 2 | 34 | In combination with carboplatin in newly diagnosed or recurrent disease | June 2020 |
| Volasertib (Plk1 inhibitor) | | | | | |
| | | | | In development; no ongoing phase 2 or phase 3 studies | |

IAP inhibitor of apoptosis protein, Plk1 polo-like kinase 1, SMAC second mitochondrial-derived activator of caspases
[a]Prodrug is a compound that is metabolized into a pharmacologically active drug after administration

predict patients who may respond to treatment with olaparib, the phase 2 LIGHT study (NCT02983799) is evaluating the efficacy and safety of olaparib in patients with platinum-sensitive, relapsed OC who have received ≥2 prior lines of platinum-based chemotherapy. Patients will be stratified by use of different HRD genetic tests [53].

The combination of olaparib with cediranib, an antiangiogenic VEGF receptor inhibitor, is of interest. The phase 2 NCI-2012-02938 study (NCT01116648) in women with recurrent platinum-sensitive OC reported significantly longer median PFS for those treated with combination therapy versus olaparib alone (16.5 vs 8.2 months, HR: 0.50, $P$ = 0.007). This effect was greatest for patients without known gBRCA mutations: median PFS was 23.7 versus 5.7 months (HR: 0.32, $P$ = 0.002) and median OS was 37.8 versus 23.0 months (HR: 0.48, $P$ = 0.074) with combination therapy versus olaparib alone, respectively. These results suggest that the combination of a PARP inhibitor and an antiangiogenic may

result in increased activity in these patients [54]. Ongoing studies for this combination include: the phase 3 NRG-GY004 study (NCT02446600) in platinum-sensitive OC compared to olaparib alone or platinum-based chemotherapy [55]; the single arm phase 2 CONCERTO study (NCT02889900) in women with platinum-resistant relapsed disease without a gBRCA mutation [56]; and the phase 2/3 NRG-GY005 study (NCT02502266) in patients with platinum-resistant disease who have received no more than 3 prior treatment regimens [57].

The phase 2 QUADRA study (NCT02354586) is evaluating the antitumor activity of niraparib in patients with advanced, relapsed, high-grade serous epithelial ovarian, fallopian tube, or primary peritoneal cancer who received 3 or more prior chemotherapy regimens [58]. In platinum-resistant disease, ongoing studies are investigating the use of the antibody-drug conjugate mirvetuximab soravtansine and the gemcitabine prodrug NUC-103. Other agents are also being investigated in phase 2 studies, including the

Bringing new medicines to women with epithelial ovarian cancer: what is the unmet medical...

191

alkylating agent trabectedin, an antibody-drug conjugate targeting the folic acid receptor (mirvetuximab soravtensine), the immune checkpoint inhibitors ipilimumab, durvalumab, and tremelimumab, and the targeted agents birinapant and volasertib (Table 4). AZD1775, an inhibitor of the WEE1 tyrosine kinase, is also is being explored in platinum-resistant OC (NCT02272790) [59]. Numerous other agents are being studied as earlier lines of therapy for advanced OC, including the folic acid receptor antibody farletuzumab and several inhibitors of histone deactylase (HDAC). The HDAC inhibitors most clinically advanced for treatment of OC are entinostat (NCT02915523), vorinostat (NCT00132067), and ricolinostat (NCT02661815). Finally, several vaccines are being studied as potential treatments for advanced OC [60, 61]. Selected examples include dendritic cell vaccines, patient-specific autologous tumor cell vaccines, and vaccines targeting various antigens enriched in tumor cells, such as folate receptor alpha, HER2, brachyury, insulin-like growth factor binding protein-2, survivin, and carcinoembryonic antigen. These emerging therapies are of interest owing to the very limited treatment options for women who have failed 2 or more lines of chemotherapy, including platinum-based agents, and who have received or were ineligible to receive bevacizumab or a PARP inhibitor.

Another important aspect of addressing the unmet need for treatments in advanced OC is the regulatory pathway for accelerated approval in the United States [62, 63]. The Accelerated Approval Program allows earlier approval of drugs that treat serious conditions and fill an unmet need. In this program, oncology drugs can be approved based on a surrogate endpoint (such as objective response rate rather than survival), when those drugs fill an unmet need, have acceptable toxicity, and satisfy criteria for chemistry, manufacturing, and controls. Typically, approval is provisional and a confirmatory phase 3 trial is expected to be undertaken. This program has been beneficial for patients with OC, which has lagged behind other cancers with regard to treatment options.

A good example of how accelerated approval has aided the OC community is PLD, which was granted accelerated approval in 1999. Under accelerated approval, which was based on three phase 2 studies, PLD was indicated for the treatment of metastatic OC in patients with disease that was refractory to both paclitaxel- and platinum-based chemotherapy. According to the terms of the accelerated approval, a randomized, phase 3 clinical study was then completed to formally demonstrate the drug's clinical benefit in patients with relapsed OC [64, 65]. On the basis of that trial, full approval of PLD was granted in 2005. More recently, the PARP inhibitor olaparib was granted accelerated approval in 2014 and the phase 3 SOLO-2 trial was submitted as a confirmatory study; the ongoing SOLO-3 trial may serve as a second confirmatory study. Rucaparib was also granted accelerated approval in 2016, with ARIEL3 and ARIEL4 serving as confirmatory studies. Given the continuing unmet need for therapies in many patients with OC, it is encouraging that the accelerated approval program exists to usher in new treatment options in a manner that allows access that ensures an appropriate level of patient safety.

Despite new therapeutic strategies approved in recent years and promising strategies and agents on the horizon, there continue to be unmet needs for patients with advanced OC. Addressing those needs will require a reexamination and possibly a redesign of the drug discovery and development process. The cancer drug development process is facing many challenges, including inefficient clinical study designs, relative paucity of new drug targets but a proliferation of "me-too" drugs, and the dilution of the patient population available for enrollment into clinical studies. That dilution has many contributing causes, including the progress toward personalized medicine in which few patients may qualify for a given treatment, as well as the proliferation of clinical studies needed to test the large numbers of drugs with similar or identical mechanisms of action. Novel study designs including master protocols for umbrella, basket, and platform studies are being used to address this need [66]. Furthermore, many emerging therapies require biomarker tests, which must be developed and approved, and which are often expensive and provide low yields. These problems extend well beyond the OC arena, and their solutions call for a concerted and creative effort on the part of the scientific, pharmaceutical, and regulatory communities.

## Conclusions

Platinum-based chemotherapy is recommended as first line therapy in women with advanced epithelial OC. Bevacizumab may have roles in selected patients with recurrent disease in combination with 5 approved chemotherapy backbones. For those patients who achieve an objective response to retreatment with platinum-based chemotherapy, a recent phase 3 study showed that niraparib can extend PFS when used as maintenance monotherapy. The recently reported phase 3 SOLO-2 study confirmed the efficacy of olaparib tablets as maintenance monotherapy in patients with platinum-sensitive, relapsed OC with a gBRCA mutation. Currently, there are limited treatment options for women with recurrent OC who have failed two or more lines of chemotherapy and have received or were ineligible to receive bevacizumab or a PARP inhibitor [39]. The US FDA's accelerated approval of olaparib and rucaparib for the treatment of recurrent disease offers exciting new treatment options. Accelerated FDA approval poses an opportunity for additional new medicines to become rapidly available to address unmet needs.

## Abbreviations

CI: Confidence interval; CR: Complete response; DoR: Duration of response; gBRCA: germline BRCA; HR: Hazard ratio; HRD: Homologous recombination deficiency; ITT: Intent-to-treat; LOH: Loss of heterozygosity; NR: Not reported; OC: Ovarian cancer; ORR: Objective response rate; OS: Overall survival; PARP: Poly(ADP-ribose) polymerase; PFI: Platinum-free interval; PFS: Progression-free survival; PLD: Pegylated liposomal doxorubicin; QOL: Quality of life; SD: Standard deviation; VEGF: Vascular endothelial growth factor

## Acknowledgments

The authors express thanks to Ken Scholz, PhD, Greg Tardie, PhD, Joan Hudson, and The Lockwood Group, Stamford, CT, for medical writing and editorial support, which was in accordance with Good Publication Practice (GPP3) guidelines.

## Funding

Funding for medical writing and editorial support was provided by AstraZeneca LP.

## Authors' contributions

Both authors were involved in drafting the article or revising it critically for important intellectual content, and both authors approved the final version to be submitted for publication. Development of the manuscript adhered to both authorship guidelines for Good Publication Practice and International Society for Medical Publication Professionals.

## Consent for publication

Not applicable.

## Competing interests

Dr. Monk discloses that he has received honoraria for speaker bureaus from Roche/Genentech, AstraZeneca, Janssen/Johnson & Johnson, Myriad, Clovis, and TESARO. Additionally, Dr. Monk has been a consultant for Roche/Genentech, Merck, TESARO, AstraZeneca, Gradalis, Advaxis, Cerulean, Amgen, Vermillion, ImmunoGen, Pfizer, Bayer, NuCana, Insys, GlaxoSmithKline, Verastem, Mateon (formally OxiGENE), Clovis, Precision Oncology, Perthera, Biodesix, and ImmunoGen. Dr. Herzog discloses that he has been a consultant for Roche, Johnson &Johnson, AstraZeneca, TESARO, Clovis, and Caris within past 1 year.

## Author details

[1]University of Cincinnati Cancer Institute, University of Cincinnati, Medical Sciences Bldg, Suite 2005H, ML0662, 231 Albert Sabin Way, Cincinnati, OH 45267-0662, USA. [2]Arizona Oncology (US Oncology Network), University of Arizona College of Medicine and Creighton University School of Medicine at Dignity Health St. Joseph's Hospital and Medical Center, Phoenix, AZ 85013, USA.

## References

1. Korkmaz T, Seber S, Basaran G. Review of the current role of targeted therapies as maintenance therapies in first and second line treatment of epithelial ovarian cancer; in the light of completed trials. Crit Rev Oncol Hematol. 2016;98:180–8.
2. Markman M. Maintenance chemotherapy in the management of epithelial ovarian cancer. Cancer Metastasis Rev. 2015;34(1):11–7.
3. Markman M, Liu PY, Wilczynski S, Monk B, Copeland LJ, Alvarez RD, et al. Phase III randomized trial of 12 versus 3 months of maintenance paclitaxel

in patients with advanced ovarian cancer after complete response to platinum and paclitaxel-based chemotherapy: a southwest oncology group and gynecologic oncology group trial. J Clin Oncol. 2003;21(13):2460–5.
4. Markman M, Liu PY, Moon J, Monk BJ, Copeland L, Wilczynski S, et al. Impact on survival of 12 versus 3 monthly cycles of paclitaxel (175 mg/m2) administered to patients with advanced ovarian cancer who attained a complete response to primary platinum-paclitaxel: follow-up of a southwest oncology group and gynecologic oncology group phase 3 trial. Gynecol Oncol. 2009;114(2):195–8.
5. Pecorelli S, Favalli G, Gadducci A, Katsaros D, Panici PB, Carpi A, et al. Phase III trial of observation versus six courses of paclitaxel in patients with advanced epithelial ovarian cancer in complete response after six courses of paclitaxel/platinum-based chemotherapy: final results of the After-6 protocol 1. J Clin Oncol. 2009;27(28):4642–8.
6. Copeland LJ, Brady MF, Burger RA, Rodgers WH, Huang H, Cella D, et al. A phase III trial of maintenance therapy in women with advanced ovarian/fallopian tube/peritoneal cancer (O/PC/FT ) after a complete clinical response (CCR) to first-line therapy: an NRG oncology study [late-breaking abstract]. National Harbor, Maryland: SGO Annual Meeting on Women's Cancer; 2017.
7. Burger RA, Brady MF, Bookman MA, Fleming GF, Monk BJ, Huang H, et al. Incorporation of bevacizumab in the primary treatment of ovarian cancer. N Engl J Med. 2011;365(26):2473–83.
8. Perren TJ, Swart AM, Pfisterer J, Ledermann JA, Pujade-Lauraine E, Kristensen G, et al. A phase 3 trial of bevacizumab in ovarian cancer. N Engl J Med. 2011;365(26):2484–96.
9. Oza AM, Cook AD, Pfisterer J, Embleton A, Ledermann JA, Pujade-Lauraine E, et al. Standard chemotherapy with or without bevacizumab for women with newly diagnosed ovarian cancer (ICON7): overall survival results of a phase 3 randomised trial. Lancet Oncol. 2015;16(8):928–36.
10. Burger RA, Brady MF, Bookman MA, Monk BJ, Walker JL, Homesley HD, et al. Risk factors for GI adverse events in a phase III randomized trial of bevacizumab in first-line therapy of advanced ovarian cancer: a gynecologic oncology group study. J Clin Oncol. 2014;32(12):1210–7.
11. Ray-Coquard IL, Harter P, Martin AG, Cropet C, Pignata S, Fujiwara K, et al. PAOLA-1: An ENGOT/GCIG phase III trial of olaparib versus placebo combined with bevacizumab as maintenance treatment in patients with advanced ovarian cancer following first-line platinum-based chemotherapy plus bevacizumab [abstract and poster presented at 2017 ASCO Annual Meeting]. J Clin Oncol. 2017;35(suppl):abstr TPS5605.
12. Pujade-Lauraine E, Combe P. Recurrent ovarian cancer. Ann Oncol. 2016; 27(Suppl 1):i63–5.
13. National Comprehensive Cancer Network. NCCN Clinical Practice Guidelines in Oncology. Ovarian Cancer Including Fallopian Tube Cancer and Primary Peritoneal Cancer. Version 1.2016. https://www.tri-kobe.org/nccn/guideline/gynecological/english/ovarian.pdf. Accessed 15 March 2017.
14. Alberts DS, Liu PY, Wilczynski SP, Clouser MC, Lopez AM, Michelin DP, et al. Randomized trial of pegylated liposomal doxorubicin (PLD) plus carboplatin versus carboplatin in platinum-sensitive (PS) patients with recurrent epithelial ovarian or peritoneal carcinoma after failure of initial platinum-based chemotherapy (southwest oncology group protocol S0200). Gynecol Oncol. 2008;108(1):90–4.
15. Parmar MK, Ledermann JA, Colombo N, du Bois A, Delaloye JF, Kristensen GB, et al. Paclitaxel plus platinum-based chemotherapy versus conventional platinum-based chemotherapy in women with relapsed ovarian cancer: the ICON4/AGO-OVAR-2.2 Trial. Lancet. 2003;361(9375):2099–106.
16. Pfisterer J, Plante M, Vergote I, du Bois A, Hirte H, Lacave AJ, et al. Gemcitabine plus carboplatin compared with carboplatin in patients with platinum-sensitive recurrent ovarian cancer: an intergroup trial of the AGO-OVAR, the NCIC CTG, and the EORTC GCG. J Clin Oncol. 2006;24(29):4699–707.
17. Raja FA, Counsell N, Colombo N, Pfisterer J, du Bois A, Parmar MK, et al. Platinum versus platinum-combination chemotherapy in platinum-sensitive recurrent ovarian cancer: a meta-analysis using individual patient data. Ann Oncol. 2013;24(12):3028–34.
18. Bruchim I, Jarchowsky-Dolberg O, Fishman A. Advanced (>second) line chemotherapy in the treatment of patients with recurrent epithelial ovarian cancer. Eur J Obstet Gynecol Reprod Biol. 2013;166(1):94–8.
19. Hanker LC, Loibl S, Burchardi N, Pfisterer J, Meier W, Pujade-Lauraine E, et al. The impact of second to sixth line therapy on survival of relapsed ovarian cancer after primary taxane/platinum-based therapy. Ann Oncol. 2012; 23(10):2605–12.

20. Penson RT, Dignan F, Seiden MV, Lee H, Gallagher CJ, Matulonis UA, et al. Attitudes to chemotherapy in patients with ovarian cancer. Gynecol Oncol. 2004;94(2):427–35.

21. Cannistra SA, Matulonis UA, Penson RT, Hambleton J, Dupont J, Mackey H, et al. Phase II study of bevacizumab in patients with platinum-resistant ovarian cancer or peritoneal serous cancer. J Clin Oncol. 2007;25(33):5180–6.

22. Burger RA, Sill MW, Monk BJ, Greer BE, Sorosky JI. Phase II trial of bevacizumab in persistent or recurrent epithelial ovarian cancer or primary peritoneal cancer: a gynecologic oncology group study. J Clin Oncol. 2007; 25(33):5165–71.

23. Monk BJ, Han E, Josephs-Cowan CA, Pugmire G, Burger RA. Salvage bevacizumab (rhuMAB VEGF)-based therapy after multiple prior cytotoxic regimens in advanced refractory epithelial ovarian cancer. Gynecol Oncol. 2006;102(2):140–4.

24. Pietzner K, Richter R, Chekerov R, Erol E, Oskay-Ozcelik G, Lichtenegger W, et al. Bevacizumab in heavily pre-treated and platinum resistant ovarian cancer: a retrospective study of the north-eastern German Society of Gynaecologic Oncology (NOGGO) ovarian cancer study group. Anticancer Res. 2011;31(8):2679–82.

25. Pujade-Lauraine E, Hilpert F, Weber B, Reuss A, Poveda A, Kristensen G, et al. Bevacizumab combined with chemotherapy for platinum-resistant recurrent ovarian cancer: the AURELIA open-label randomized phase III trial. J Clin Oncol. 2014;32(13):1302–8.

26. Aghajanian C, Blank SV, Goff BA, Judson PL, Teneriello MG, Husain A, et al. OCEANS: a randomized, double-blind, placebo-controlled phase III trial of chemotherapy with or without bevacizumab in patients with platinum-sensitive recurrent epithelial ovarian, primary peritoneal, or fallopian tube cancer. J Clin Oncol. 2012;30(17):2039–45.

27. Aghajanian C, Goff B, Nycum LR, Wang YV, Husain A, Blank SV. Final overall survival and safety analysis of OCEANS, a phase 3 trial of chemotherapy with or without bevacizumab in patients with platinum-sensitive recurrent ovarian cancer. Gynecol Oncol. 2015;139(1):10–6.

28. Coleman RL, Brady MF, Herzog TJ, Sabbatini P, Armstrong DK, Walker JL, et al. Bevacizumab and paclitaxel–carboplatin chemotherapy and secondary cytoreduction in recurrent, platinum-sensitive ovarian cancer (NRG oncology/gynecologic oncology group study GOG-0213): a multicentre, open-label, randomised, phase 3 trial. Lancet Oncol. 2017;18(6):779–91.

29. Kaufman B, Shapira-Frommer R, Schmutzler RK, Audeh MW, Friedlander M, Balmana J, et al. Olaparib monotherapy in patients with advanced cancer and a germline BRCA1/2 mutation. J Clin Oncol. 2015;33(3):244–50.

30. Domchek SM, Aghajanian C, Shapira-Frommer R, Schmutzler RK, Audeh MW, Friedlander M, et al. Efficacy and safety of olaparib monotherapy in germline BRCA1/2 mutation carriers with advanced ovarian cancer and three or more lines of prior therapy. Gynecol Oncol. 2016;140(2):199–203.

31. Gelmon KA, Tischkowitz M, Mackay H, Swenerton K, Robidoux A, Tonkin K, et al. Olaparib in patients with recurrent high-grade serous or poorly differentiated ovarian carcinoma or triple-negative breast cancer: a phase 2, multicentre, open-label, non-randomised study. Lancet Oncol. 2011;12(9): 852–61.

32. Swisher EM, Lin KK, Oza AM, Scott CL, Giordano H, Sun J, et al. Rucaparib in relapsed, platinum-sensitive high-grade ovarian carcinoma (ARIEL2 part 1): an international, multicentre, open-label, phase 2 trial. Lancet Oncol. 2017; 18(1):75–87.

33. Avastin (bevacizumab) [prescribing information]. South San Francisco: Genentech, Inc.; 2016.

34. Clovis Oncology Inc. Rubraca (rucaparib) tablets [prescribing information]. Boulder, CO: Clovis Oncology, Inc.; 2016.

35. AstraZeneca Pharmaceuticals LP. Lynparza (olaparib) capsules [prescribing information]. AstraZeneca Pharmaceuticals LP: Wilmington, DE; 2017.

36. Tesaro Inc. Zejula (niraparib) capsules [prescribing information]. Waltham, MA: Tesaro, Inc.; 2017.

37. Ledermann J, Harter P, Gourley C, Friedlander M, Vergote I, Rustin G, et al. Olaparib maintenance therapy in platinum-sensitive relapsed ovarian cancer. N Engl J Med. 2012;366(15):1302–92.

38. Mirza MR, Monk BJ, Herrstedt J, Oza AM, Mahner S, Redondo A, et al. Niraparib maintenance therapy in platinum-sensitive, recurrent ovarian cancer. N Engl J Med. 2016;375(22):2154–64.

39. Pujade-Lauraine E, Ledermann JA, Penson RT, Oza AM, Korach J, Huzarski T, et al. Treatment with olaparib monotherapy in the maintenance setting significantly improves progression-free survival in patients with platinum-sensitive relapsed ovarian cancer: results from the phase III SOLO-2 study

40. Ledermann J, Harter P, Gourley C, Friedlander M, Vergote I, Rustin G, et al. Olaparib maintenance therapy in patients with platinum-sensitive relapsed serous ovarian cancer: a preplanned retrospective analysis of outcomes by BRCA status in a randomised phase 2 trial. Lancet Oncol. 2014;15(8):852–61.

41. Ledermann JA, Harter P, Gourley C, Friedlander M, Vergote I, Rustin G, et al. Overall survival in patients with platinum-sensitive recurrent serous ovarian cancer receiving olaparib maintenance monotherapy: an updated analysis from a randomised, placebo-controlled, double-blind, phase 2 trial. Lancet Oncol. 2016;17(11):1579–89.

42. Friedlander M, Gebski V, Gibbs E, Bloomfield R, Hilpert F, Wenzel LB, et al. Health-related quality of life (HRQOL) and patient-centered outcomes with maintenance olaparib compared with placebo following chemotherapy in patients with germline (g) BRCA-mutated (m) platinum-sensitive relapsed serous ovarian cancer (PSR SOC): SOLO-2 phase III trial [abstract presented at 2017 ASCO Annual Meeting]. J Clin Oncol. 2017;35(suppl):abstr 5507.

43. Mirza MR, Monk BJ, Gil-Martin M, Gilbert L, Canzler U, Follana P, et al. Efficacy of niraparib on progression-free survival (PFS) in patients (pts) with recurrent ovarian cancer (OC) with partial response (PR) to the last platinum-based chemotherapy [abstract and poster presented at 2017 ASCO Annual Meeting]. J Clin Oncol. 2017;35(suppl):abstr 5517.

44. Del Campo JM, Mirza MR, Berek JS, Provencher DM, Emons G, Fabbro M, et al. The successful phase 3 niraparib ENGOT-OV16/NOVA trial included a substantial number of patients with platinum resistant ovarian cancer (OC) [abstract and poster presented at 2017 ASCO Annual Meeting]. J Clin Oncol. 2017;35(suppl):abstr 5560.

45. Clovis Oncology Inc. Rucaparib significantly improved progression-free survival in all ovarian cancer patient populations studied in phase 3 ARIEL3 maintenance treatment trial (press release June 19, 2017). http://phx. corporate-ir.net/phoenix.zhtml?c=247187&p=irol-newsArticle&ID=2281511. Accessed 20 June 2017.

46. Clovis Oncology Inc. A study of rucaparib as switch maintenance following platinum-based chemotherapy in patients with platinum-sensitive, high-grade serous or endometrioid epithelial ovarian, primary peritoneal or fallopian tube cancer (ARIEL3). https://clinicaltrials.gov/ct2/show/NCT01968213?term= NCT01968213&rank=1 Accessed: 20 June 2017.

47. Ramus SJ, Gayther SA. The contribution of BRCA1 and BRCA2 to ovarian cancer. Mol Oncol. 2009;3(2):138–50.

48. Hennessy BT, Timms KM, Carey MS, Gutin A, Meyer LA, Flake DD 2nd, et al. Somatic mutations in BRCA1 and BRCA2 could expand the number of patients that benefit from poly (ADP ribose) polymerase inhibitors in ovarian cancer. J Clin Oncol. 2010;28(22):3570–6.

49. Chetrit A, Hirsh-Yechezkel G, Ben-David Y, Lubin F, Friedman E, Sadetzki S. Effect of BRCA1/2 mutations on long-term survival of patients with invasive ovarian cancer: the national Israeli study of ovarian cancer. J Clin Oncol. 2008;26(1):20–5.

50. Alsop K, Fereday S, Meldrum C. deFazio a, Emmanuel C, George J, et al. BRCA mutation frequency and patterns of treatment response in BRCA mutation-positive women with ovarian cancer: a report from the Australian ovarian cancer study group. J Clin Oncol. 2012;30(21):2654–63.

51. Pothuri B. BRCA1- and BRCA2-related mutations: therapeutic implications in ovarian cancer. Ann Oncol. 2013;24(Suppl 8):viii22-viii7.

52. AstraZeneca Pharmaceuticals LP. Olaparib treatment in relapsed germline breast cancer susceptibility gene (BRCA) mutated ovarian cancer patients who have progressed at least 6 months after last platinum treatment and have received at least 2 prior platinum treatments (SOLO-3). https:// clinicaltrials.gov/ct2/show/NCT02282020?term=NCT02282020&rank=1 Accessed 12 May 2017.

53. Cadoo KA, Aghajanian C, Fraser C, Milner A, Kolvenbag G. A phase 2 study to assess olaparib by homologous recombination deficiency status in patients with platinum-sensitive, relapsed, ovarian, fallopian tube, or primary peritoneal cancer [abstract and poster presented at 2017 ASCO Annual Meeting]. J Clin Oncol. 2017;35(suppl):abstr TPS5606.

54. Liu JF, Barry WT, Birrer MJ, Lee JM, Buckanovich RJ, Fleming GF, et al. Overall survival and updated progression-free survival results from a randomized phase 2 trial comparing the combination of olaparib and cediranib against olaparib alone in recurrent platinum-sensitive ovarian cancer [abstract and poster presented at 2017 ASCO Annual Meeting]. J Clin Oncol. 2017; 35(suppl):abstr 5535.

(abstract and presentation slides). National Harbor, Maryland: SGO Annual Meeting on Women's Cancer; 2017.

55. AstraZeneca Pharmaceuticals LP. Olaparib or cediranib maleate and olaparib compared with standard platinum-based chemotherapy in treating patients with recurrent platinum-sensitive ovarian, fallopian tube, or primary peritoneal cancer. https://clinicaltrials.gov/ct2/show/NCT02446600?term=NCT02446600&rank=1 Accessed 15 June 2017.

56. AstraZeneca Pharmaceuticals LP. Efficacy and safety study of cediranib in combination with olaparib in patients with recurrent platinum-resistant ovarian cancer (CONCERTO). https://clinicaltrials.gov/ct2/show/NCT02889900?term=NCT02889900&rank=1 Accessed 15 June 2017.

57. National Cancer Institute. Cediranib maleate and olaparib or standard chemotherapy in treating patients with recurrent platinum-resistant or -refractory ovarian, fallopian tube, or primary peritoneal cancer. https://clinicaltrials.gov/ct2/show/NCT02502266?term=NCT02502266&rank=1 Accessed 15 June 2017.

58. Tesaro Inc. A study of niraparib in patients with ovarian cancer who have received three or four previous chemotherapy regimens (QUADRA). https://clinicaltrials.gov/ct2/show/NCT02354586?term=NCT02354586&rank=1 Accessed 12 May 2017.

59. AstraZeneca Pharmaceuticals LP. AZD1775 plus chemotherapy in patients with platinum-resistant ovarian, fallopian tube, or primary peritoneal cancer. https://clinicaltrials.gov/ct2/show/NCT02272790?term=NCT02272790&rank=1 Accessed: 15 June 2017.

60. Leffers N, Daemen T, Boezen HM, Melief KJ, Nijman HW. Vaccine-based clinical trials in ovarian cancer. Expert Rev Vaccines. 2011;10(6):775–84.

61. Liao JB, Disis ML. Therapeutic vaccines for ovarian cancer. Gynecol Oncol. 2013;130(3):667–73.

62. United States Food and Drug Administration. Accelerated Approval Program 2016. https://www.fda.gov/drugs/resourcesforyou/healthprofessionals/ucm313768.htm Accessed: 12 May 2017.

63. United States Food and Drug Administration. Guidance for Industry: Expedited Programs for Serious Conditions – Drugs and Biologics. May 2014 Procedural. https://wwwfdagov/downloads/drugs/guidancecomplianceregulatoryinformation/guidances/ucm358301pdf Accessed: 12 May 2017.

64. Gordon AN, Fleagle JT, Guthrie D, Parkin DE, Gore ME, Lacave AJ. Recurrent epithelial ovarian carcinoma: a randomized phase III study of pegylated liposomal doxorubicin versus topotecan. J Clin Oncol. 2001;19(14):3312–22.

65. Gordon AN, Tonda M, Sun S, Rackoff W. Doxil study investigators. Long-term survival advantage for women treated with pegylated liposomal doxorubicin compared with topotecan in a phase 3 randomized study of recurrent and refractory epithelial ovarian cancer. Gynecol Oncol. 2004;95(1):1–8.

66. Woodcock J, LaVange LM. Master protocols to study multiple therapies, multiple diseases, or both. N Engl J Med. 2017;377(1):62–70.

# 23

# A small molecule inhibitor of the perinucleolar compartment, ML246, attenuates growth and spread of ovarian cancer

Margaux J. Kanis[1], Wenan Qiang[2,3], Mario Pineda[1], Kruti P. Maniar[3] and J. Julie Kim[2,4]* (iD)

## Abstract

**Background:** Ovarian cancer remains a major health problem for women as it is often diagnosed at a late stage with metastatic disease. There are limited therapeutic agents and survival rates remain poor. The perinucleolar compartment (PNC) has been shown to be associated with malignancy and is considered a surrogate phenotypic marker for metastatic cancer cells. A small molecule, ML246, was derived from a screen against PNCs. In this study, the effect of ML246 on ovarian cancer growth and spread was investigated.

**Methods:** SKOV3 or OVCAR3 cells were treated with ML246 in vitro and PNC was visualized with immunofluorescent staining. Cell invasion was assessed using Matrigel-coated transwell systems. SKOV3 cells were xenografted orthotopically under the ovarian bursa of immunocompromised mice. Additionally, a patient derived ovarian cancer cell line was grafted subcutaneously. Mice were treated with ML246 and tumor growth and spread was assessed.

**Results:** PNCs were prevalent in the ovarian cancer cell lines OVCAR3 and SKOV3 with higher prevalence in OVCAR3 cells. Treatment with ML246 significantly reduced PNC prevalence in OVCAR3 and SKOV3 cells. Moreover, the invasive activity of both cell lines was significantly inhibited in vitro. Orthotopic implantation of SKOV3 cells resulted in growth of the tumor on the ovary as well as spread of tumor tissues outside of the primary site on organs into the abdominal cavity. Treatment with ML246 decreased the incidence of tumors outside of the ovary. In addition, a patient-derived xenograft (PDX) line was grafted subcutaneously to monitor tumor growth. ML246 significantly attenuated growth of tumors over a 5-week treatment period.

**Conclusions:** PNC's are present in ovarian cancer cells and treatment with ML246 decreases invasion in vitro and tumor growth and spread in vivo. Additional studies are warranted to determine the efficacy of ML246 as an inhibitor of metastatic disease in ovarian cancer and to determine its precise mechanism of action.

**Keywords:** Perinucleolar compartment, Ovarian cancer, ML246, Metarrestin

* Correspondence: j-kim4@northwestern.edu
[2]Division of Reproductive Science in Medicine, Department of Obstetrics and Gynecology, Northwestern University Feinberg School of Medicine, Chicago, IL, USA
[4]Robert H. Lurie Comprehensive Cancer Center, Northwestern University, 303 E. Superior Street, 4-117, Chicago, IL 60611, USA
Full list of author information is available at the end of the article

## Background

Ovarian cancer is the most lethal of the gynecologic cancers with approximately 14,000 women dying annually in the United States from this disease [1]. Although most of these cancers are responsive to initial chemotherapy, relapse from remission frequently occurs, resulting in death from widespread metastatic disease. Effective therapeutics are currently lacking to successfully overcome this disease leading to the low long-term survival rates for ovarian cancer patients. Novel treatments that inhibit ovarian cancer progression are in urgent need to improve the outcomes of these patients.

Targeted therapy is changing the therapeutic landscape in oncology and agents including angiogenesis inhibitors and PARP inhibitors, alone or in combination with chemotherapies, have been shown to be promising advancements for the treatment of ovarian cancer [2]. While these agents target physiological processes such as angiogenesis and DNA repair, targeting cellular structures that form specifically in malignant cells is another approach to tackle cancer. The perinucleolar compartment (PNC) is a nuclear body, containing RNA polymerase III transcripts and polypyrimidine tract-binding protein (PTB), that is adherent to but distinct from the nucleolus [3–5]. They are observed in various metastatic solid tumors and transformed cell lines including breast, prostate, pancreatic and colorectal cancers, but absent in normal cells including embryonic stem cells [6–9]. PNC prevalence in tumors of breast and colorectal cancer were shown to be positively associated with disease severity and inversely correlated with patient survival [6, 8]. Its prevalence was high, particularly in metastatic tumors and metastatically transformed cancer cell lines, making it a potential pan-marker for metastatic progression. Although the precise function of PNCs remains unclear, studies have implicated possible roles in RNA metabolism [10–13], and thus, inhibition of PNCs could render the cancer cells unable to grow and spread by dysregulating the ribosome machinery. A compound to decrease PNC prevalence in cancer cells, ML246 (*Metarrestin*) was identified through a high throughput screen [14, 15]. Given the growth and metastatic characteristics of ovarian cancer and the urgent need to better treat this deadly disease, we investigated the effects of the novel drug, ML246 on PNC prevalence and invasive activity of ovarian cancer cells in vitro and tested its efficacy on tumor growth and spread in xenograft models.

## Methods

### Cell lines and PDX

The human ovarian cancer cell lines SKOV3 and OVCAR3 were obtained from the laboratory of Dr. Jian-Jun Wei (Northwestern University) [16]. SKOV3 was cultured in McCoy's 5A supplemented with 10% fetal bovine serum (FBS) and 1% penicillin/streptomycin and cultured in a humidified incubator (5% $CO_2$) at 37 °C. OVCAR3 cells were cultured in Dulbecco's modified Eagle's medium (DMEM) supplemented with FBS 20%. All cell lines were authenticated.

The PDX line used in this study was originally obtained from primary ovarian high grade serous carcinoma at the time of surgery at the Prentice Women's Hospital of Northwestern University, Chicago, USA. This line was propagated in NSG mice and characterized as previously described [17]. For this study, frozen PDX tumor fragments at passage 3 were repropagated in NSG mice.

### Immunofluorescence for detection of PNC

SKOV3 and OVCAR3 cells were cultured on glass cover slips for 24 h. Cells were treated for 24 h with DMSO, 0.05 µM, 1 µM or 2 µM of ML246 and then fixed with 4% paraformaldehyde in PBS for 10 min, washed, and solubilized in 0.5% Triton X-100 in PBS for 5 min. Cells were incubated with anti-PTB primary antibody SH54 [3] or anti-fibrillarin (Sigma Chemical Co., St. Louis, MO), a marker for the nucleolus, for 1 h at room temperature. Cells were rinsed in PBS and then incubated with Texas red–conjugated goat anti–human or FITC-conjugated goat anti–mouse antibody for 1 h at room temperature. The coverslips were mounted onto glass slides with mounting medium containing DAPI to visualize the nucleus. Cells were examined with a fluorescent microscope (FXA; Nikon Inc., Melville, NY). Images were captured by a SenSys cooled CCD camera (Photometrics, Tucson, AZ) using Oncor Image software. PNCs were counted based on an approximate 2-fold or more intense signaling of the PTB labeling than the nucleoplasm. Cells with PNC, as well as cells with multiple PNCs, were counted in four different fields of view. This experiment was performed in triplicate.

### Cell viability and invasion assays

SKOV3 and OVCAR3 cells were treated with vehicle or ML246 for 72 h at the indicated concentrations. Cell viability was measured using the WST-1 viability assay as per the manufacturer's instructions (Roche, Switzerland).

In vitro invasion assays were performed on SKOV3 and OVCAR3 using 24-well transwell units with polycarbonate filters (pore size: 8 µm) coated on the upper side with reconstituted basement membrane matrix, Matrigel (BD Biosciences, USA). $5 \times 10^5$ cells were added to the transwell in serum free media. Media with FBS was added to the outer compartment as the chemoattractant. Cells were treated with DMSO or ML246, and cultured for 72 h at 37 °C. Cells remaining on the upper side of the transwell were scraped off with a cotton swab. Cells remaining on the underside of the membrane were fixed and stained using the commercially available, Shandon Kwik-Diff stain kit (ThermoFisher Scientific). Cells were counted in four fields and the mean $\pm$ SEM was calculated. This experiment was performed in triplicate in three independent experiments.

## SKOV3 Xenografts

### Preparation of cell pellets

SKOV3 cells were prepared in collagen pellets for intrabursal xenoplantation. Cells were suspended in a rat-tail collagen (type I) solution (BD Bioscience, San Jose, CA) at $10^6$ cells per 10 µl as previously described [16]. The cell–collagen mixture was then dropped onto a 6-well plate and incubated at 37 °C in a humidified atmosphere of 95% air and 5% $CO_2$ for 30 min. The pellets were incubated overnight as floating cultures.

### Surgical procedure for implantation of xenografts in intraovarian bursa

The implantation of xenografts into the intraovarian bursa has been previously described [16]. Briefly, nude mice (Jackson Laboratories) at 8 weeks old were used for xenografting. All animal experiments were approved by the Institutional Animal Care and Use Committee of Northwestern University. Mice were anesthetized with ketamine/xylazine (90/8 mg/kg) by intraperitoneal (IP) injection. An incision was made in the skin just laterally to the midline of the lower back, and the left ovary was exteriorized. A tiny incision was made in the bursa of the ovary with the aid of a dissecting microscope and the cell pellet was grafted into the ovarian bursa. The pellet was fixed in place due to the tension of bursa. The ovary was placed back into the body cavity, and no bleeding was noted. The incision was surgically closed.

### Preparation of ML246 solution

ML246 solution was prepared by dissolving ML246 into 5% (v/v) N-methylpyrrolidine (NMP, Sigma), then adding 20% (v/v) Polyethylene glycol 400 (PEG-400, Sigma), followed by 75% (v/v) of 10% (2-Hydroxypropyl)-β-cyclodextrin (HP-β-CD, Sigma) dropwise into the tube. 200 µl of 1.5 mg/ml (for PDX) or 2.5 mg/ml (for SKOV3) of ML246 or vehicle (5% NMP, 20% PEG-400, and 75% of 10% HP-β-CD) were intraperitoneally injected into mice per 20 g body weight for the treatment dosage of 15 mg/kg or 25 mg/kg. Mice were treated once a day on the weekdays (Monday through Friday).

### ML246 treatment in mice

Treatment commenced 3 weeks after grafting of SKOV3 cell pellets. Twelve mice received ML246 by intraperitoneal injection at 25 mg/kg on a weekday schedule for a total of 7 weeks. Ten mice received cisplatin by intraperitoneal injection as a positive control and 12 mice received vehicle as the negative control. Mice were harvested 10 weeks post-xenografting. Organs and tumor deposits were weighed, processed and preserved. H&E analysis was performed by a pathologist to confirm the presence of tumor in the ovary and in suspected metastatic lesions.

Mice were monitored for behavior and activity on a daily basis, and weights obtained three times per week.

## Patient-derived xenografts

### Subcutaneous implantation of ovarian cancer PDX line

The OVCA4P PDX tumor line from the third passage (P3) [17] was used for subcutaneous xenografting into ten-week-old female adult non-obese diabetic (NOD)-scid IL2Rγ null (NSG) mice (The Jackson Laboratory). PDX tumor tissues were cut into small fragments, approximately $2 \times 2 \times 2$ mm. Two pieces were subcutaneously xenografted into two dorsal flanks of NSG mice, under anesthesia by intraperitoneal injection of ketamine/xylazine (90/8 mg/kg). The surgical site was shaved and disinfected with providone iodine prep pads and alcohol swab (70% isopropyl alcohol). A 1 cm incision was made in the skin at the midline of the mouse dorsum, and two separate tumor fragments were placed into the lower left and lower right of dorsal side. The skin was sutured, and mice were allowed to recover. Tumors were allowed to grow for 3 weeks. Five mice were treated with 15 mg/kg ML246 and 5 mice were treated with vehicle by intraperitoneal injection once a day on a 5-day schedule (Monday through Friday) for 5 weeks. Subcutaneous tumor size was monitored by palpation and measured with digital calipers weekly.

### Tissue processing

Tumors were fixed in modified Davidson's solution. All fixed tumor tissues were processed, embedded in paraffin, sectioned, and then stained with H&E. Tumor histology, differentiation, invasion and metastasis were examined by a gynecologic pathologist. Extra sections and slides were reviewed for areas in which extra-ovarian tumor deposits were suspected.

### Statistical analysis

Prism/GraphPad Software (LaJolla, California) was used for all statistical analysis. PNC prevalence and invasion assays were analyzed by a one-way ANOVA followed by Tukey's multiple comparisons test. The mean total tumor volumes of the subcutaneous xenografts were analyzed with the Mann-Whitney U test comparing vehicle and ML246 treated mice at each time point. $P < 0.05$ was considered significant.

## Results

### Effect of ML246 on PNCs in ovarian cancer cell lines

PNCs were detected in the ovarian cancer cell lines, SKOV3 and OVCAR3, using immunolabeling with SH54 antibody that specifically recognizes PTB, a key marker protein of PNCs. PNCs were present in both cell lines as seen by the bright green signal around the nucleolus, with a higher PNC prevalence in OVCAR3 cells than in SKOV3 cells (Fig. 1a). As ML246 was identified in a drug

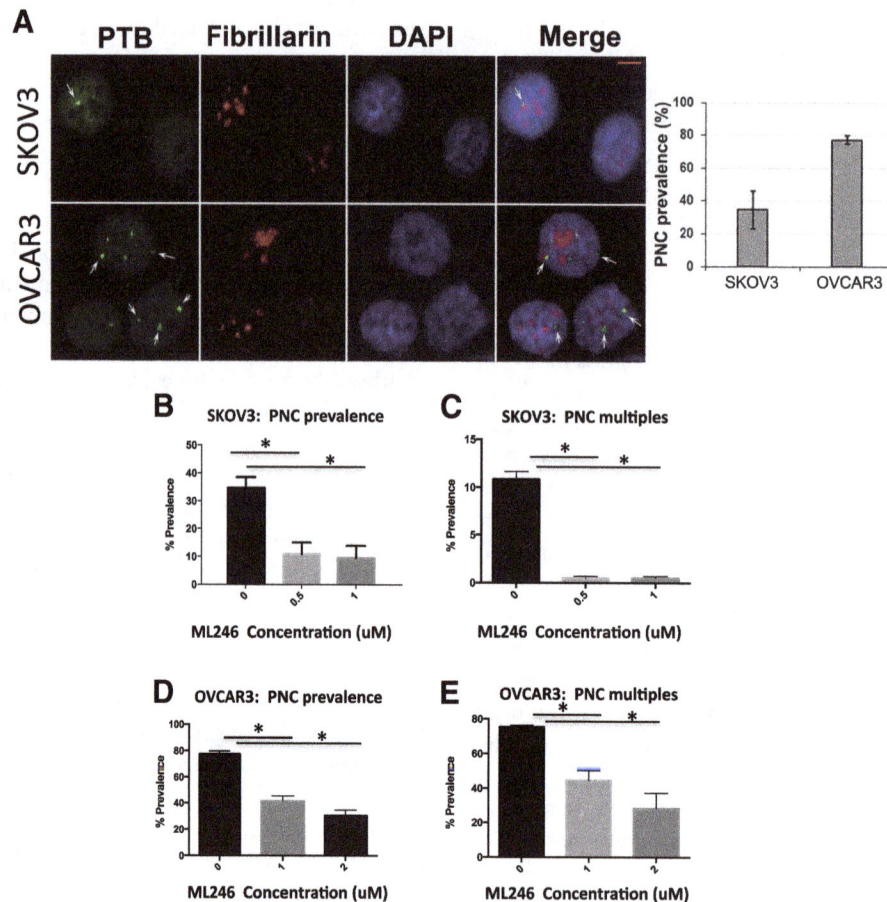

**Fig. 1** PNC prevalence in ovarian cancer cell lines. **a** Immunofluorescent staining was done in SKOV3 and OVCAR3 for PTB, a component of PNC (green, marked by arrows) that are located adjacent to nucleoli (fibrillarin staining in red) within the nucleus (DAPI staining in blue). Bar = 5 μm. **b** and **c** SKOV3 and **d** and **e** OVCAR3 cells were treated with ML246 at 0.05uM, 1uM or 2 uM or DMSO for 24 h and % PNC prevalence as well as cells carrying multiple PNCs was calculated. * $p < 0.05$

screen as a compound that effectively targeted PNCs in tumor cells [14, 18], the prevalence of PNCs was examined in SKOV3 and OVCAR3 cell lines before and after treatment with ML246. The PNC prevalence in both SKOV3 (Fig. 1b) and OVCAR3 (Fig. 1d) cells significantly decreased with ML246 treatment. The number of cells with multiple PNCs per nucleus also decreased in both SKOV3 and OVCAR3 cell lines with ML246 treatment (Fig. 1c, e). The increased incidence of multiple PNCs in the OVCAR3 cell line may reflect the aggressive nature of a serous ovarian cancer cell line, as opposed to SKOV3 which originated from an endometrioid ovarian tumor [19].

### Effect of ML246 on invasion of ovarian cancer cells in vitro
The effect of ML246 on the invasive properties of SKOV3 and OVCAR3 was assessed in vitro. SKOV3 and OVCAR3 cells were plated on Matrigel coated membranes of invasion chambers and subsequently treated with ML246 for 72 h. ML246 significantly attenuated invasion of both cell lines as there were less cells that

invaded through the membrane (Fig. 2a and b). The significant reduction in the number of cells on the underside of the membrane was not due to decreases in cell viability under these conditions (Fig. 2a and b).

### Effect of ML246 on ovarian cancer xenograft growth and spread
The SKOV3 cell line was xenografted under the ovarian bursa of mice and the effect of ML246 was assessed. Mice were treated with vehicle, cisplatin or ML246 and at the end of a 7-week treatment schedule, the primary tumor size was measured, then excised and analyzed by hematoxylin and eosin (H&E). Growth of SKOV3 tumors at the primary site was apparent (Fig. 3a; arrow). The tumor appeared as an endometrioid carcinoma given its cribriform and solid architecture, cytologic features including columnar cells, and mitotic index (Fig. 3b). There was high variability in tumor size at the ovary within each treatment group and thus no significant difference in tumor volume was noted between the treatments. Tumor

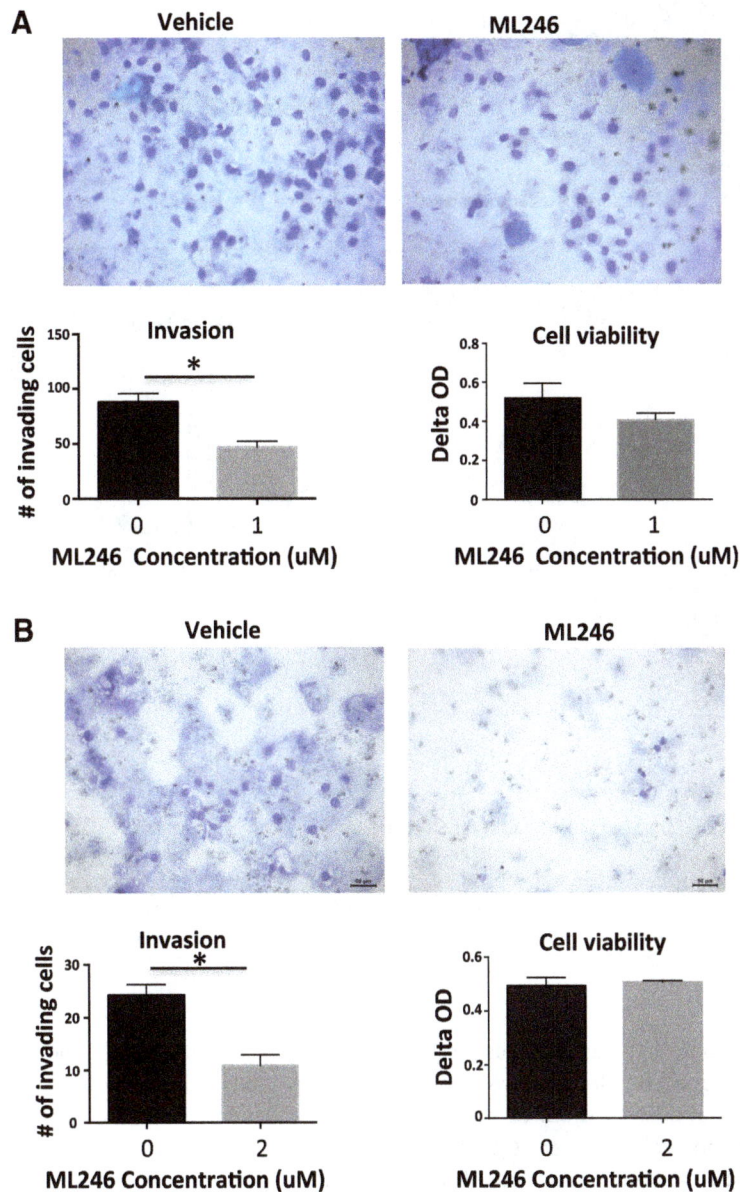

**Fig. 2** Effect of ML246 on invasive activity of ovarian cancer cells. **a** SKOV3 and **b** OVCAR3 cells were plated onto Matrigel coated invasion chambers and subsequently treated with 1uM or 2uM of ML246, respectively for 72 h. Cells that invaded and migrated through the Matrigel and porous membrane were stained and imaged at 40×. Cells were counted in four fields and the mean ± SEM was calculated. This experiment was performed in triplicate in three independent experiments. WST-1 viability assay was done on cells treated under the same conditions to assess viability after ML246 treatment. $p < 0.05$

lesions were also found in the abdominal cavity away from the primary site and confirmed by H&E staining in all treatment groups (Fig. 3c, Table 1). The number of extra-ovarian lesions differed between the treatment groups. Excluding mice that died, eight out of 11 (73%) mice had lesions outside of the primary site in the vehicle treated group (Table 1). In the cisplatin-treated group, one mouse did not have tumor on the primary site or anywhere else and overall, 3 out of 9 mice (33%) had lesions outside of the ovary. In the ML246 group, 4 out of 9 mice

did not have tumor at the primary site and among these 4, 2 mice did not have tumor anywhere in the abdominal cavity. Overall, 3 out of 9 mice (33%), had lesions outside of the ovary. The difference in the incidence of tumors outside of the primary site between the groups was statistically significant ($p = 0.012$). No obvious toxicities of ML246 and cisplatin were observed in the mice as total body weights and organ weights did not differ between treatment groups with the exception of a slight increase in liver weight with ML246 treatment (Fig. 3d).

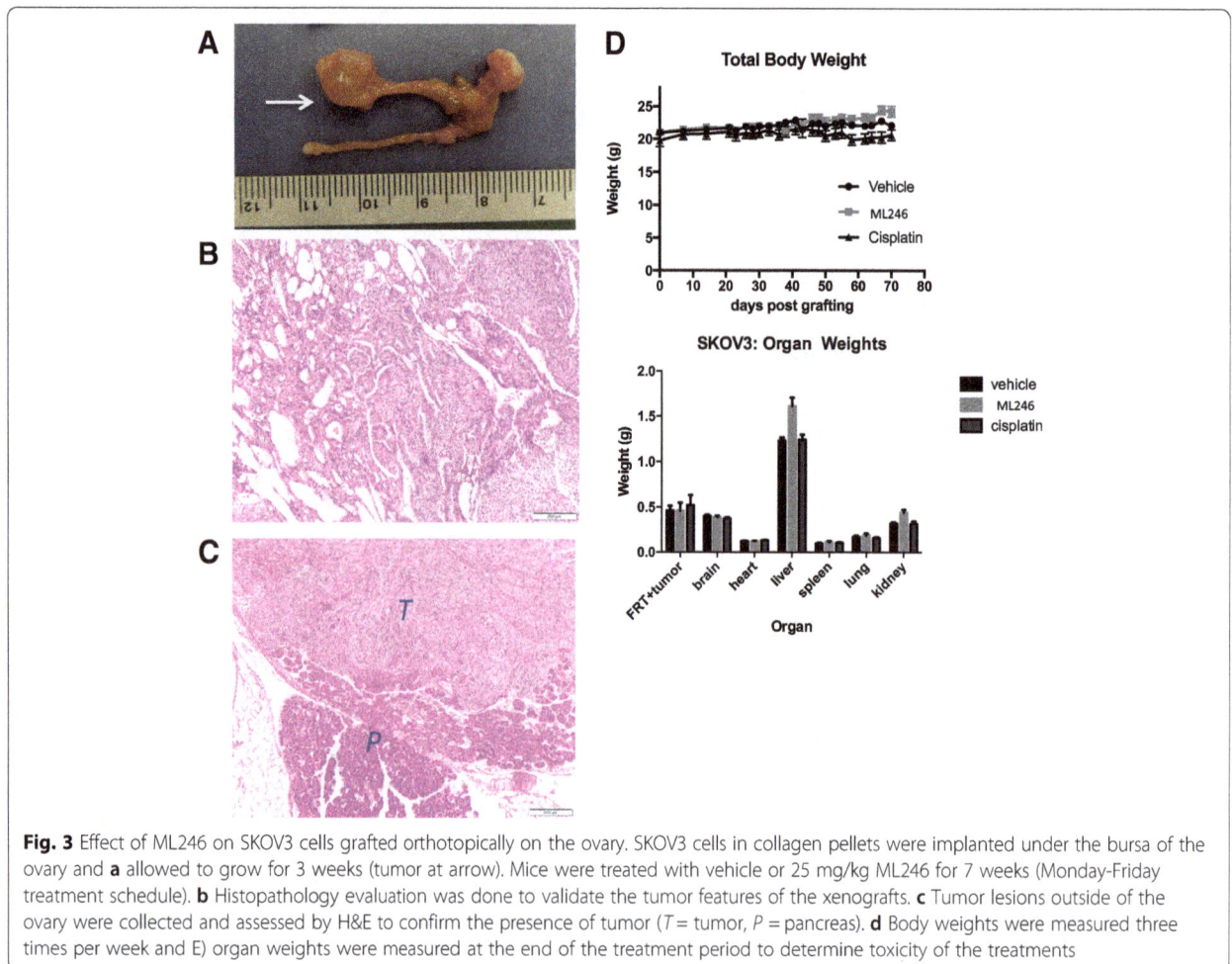

**Fig. 3** Effect of ML246 on SKOV3 cells grafted orthotopically on the ovary. SKOV3 cells in collagen pellets were implanted under the bursa of the ovary and **a** allowed to grow for 3 weeks (tumor at arrow). Mice were treated with vehicle or 25 mg/kg ML246 for 7 weeks (Monday-Friday treatment schedule). **b** Histopathology evaluation was done to validate the tumor features of the xenografts. **c** Tumor lesions outside of the ovary were collected and assessed by H&E to confirm the presence of tumor ($T$ = tumor, $P$ = pancreas). **d** Body weights were measured three times per week and E) organ weights were measured at the end of the treatment period to determine toxicity of the treatments

An ovarian cancer PDX line that was previously established in the lab [17] was grafted subcutaneously in the right and left flanks of the mouse to monitor growth of the tumors. The mean tumor volumes were significantly smaller at the end of the treatment period with ML246 compared to vehicle (Fig. 4a, b). Over a 5-week treatment period, ML246 attenuated growth of subcutaneous tumors (Fig. 4c). Body weight of the mice did not change indicating no apparent significant toxicity of ML246.

## Discussion

Platinum-based chemotherapy has been the mainstay of treatment paradigms for ovarian cancer, however, the disease remains highly lethal. Effective treatments, singular or in combination, that could significantly extend patient survival continues to be a key interest of research. Here we report that an anti-cancer small molecule, ML246, has the ability to attenuate growth and progression of ovarian cancer.

Cancer cells are highly heterogeneous among different individuals, among the affected organs of the same

patient, and even within the same primary tumor. Although many cellular pathways and mutations have been shown to contribute to tumorigenesis and progression, none have been found to be singularly necessary for metastatic transformation. Rather, a complex cellular structure may better reflect tumor behavior than a single gene or gene product. The PNC, a nuclear body, forms primarily in a subset of cancer cells and has been hypothesized to be a surrogate marker for metastatic behavior of cancer cells [6–9, 14]. In breast cancer, the prevalence of PNC was significantly correlated to stage and shows a stepwise increase from a median of 23% in primary tumors to approximately 100% in distant metastases [6, 9]. Similarly, PNC prevalence was associated with disease progression in colorectal carcinoma as high PNC prevalence was associated with poor patient outcome [8, 9]. This is the first report on PNC prevalence in ovarian carcinoma and interestingly, a higher PNC prevalence was observed in the OVCAR3 cell line derived from a high grade serous carcinoma, compared to the SKOV3 cell line which originated from an endometrioid ovarian carcinoma.

**Table 1** Effect of ML246 and cisplatin on SKOV3 xenograft growth and spread

| Mouse ID | Treatment | Primary tumor volume(mm$^3$) | Lesions outside of primary site (#) | Total # extraovarian lesions |
|---|---|---|---|---|
| 201 | cisplatin | 195.7 | | 0 |
| 203 | cisplatin | 738.2 | | 0 |
| 204 | cisplatin | 70.3 | | 0 |
| 205 | cisplatin | 287.3 | | 0 |
| 207 | cisplatin | 208.9 | back/subQ (1) | 1 |
| 211 | cisplatin | 25.9 | back/subQ (1) | 1 |
| 214 | cisplatin | 51.2 | | 0 |
| 217 | cisplatin | NR | mouse died | |
| 229 | cisplatin | NT | | 0 |
| 234 | cisplatin | 93.3 | back/subQ (1) | 1 |
| 206 | vehicle | small | back/subQ (1) | 1 |
| 208 | vehicle | NR | mouse died | |
| 209 | vehicle | 172.6 | back/subQ (1) | 1 |
| 210 | vehicle | 118.3 | | 0 |
| 212 | vehicle | 11.7 | pelvis (1); back/subQ (1) | 2 |
| 221 | vehicle | 3.4 | | 0 |
| 222 | vehicle | 35.9 | cecum (1); | 1 |
| 224 | vehicle | 323.8 | diaphram (2); pelvis (1); bowel (1); back/subQ (1); mesentery (1) | 6 |
| 225 | vehicle | 184.4 | back/subQ (1) | 1 |
| 223 | vehicle | 212.0 | | 0 |
| 230 | vehicle | 234.0 | bowel (2) | 2 |
| 233 | vehicle | small | pelvis (1) | 1 |
| 202 | ML246 | NR | mouse died | |
| 213 | ML246 | 14.3 | | 0 |
| 215 | ML246 | NT | | 0 |
| 216 | ML246 | 140.7 | back/subQ (1) | 1 |
| 218 | ML246 | NR | mouse died | |
| 219 | ML246 | 114.6 | back/subQ (1) | 1 |
| 220 | ML246 | 917.4 | | 0 |
| 226 | ML246 | NT | back/subQ (2) | 2 |
| 227 | ML246 | NR | mouse died | |
| 228 | ML246 | NT | | 0 |
| 231 | ML246 | NT | | 0 |
| 232 | ML246 | 213.3 | | 0 |

*NT* No tumor, *SubQ* Subcutaneous, *NR* Not recorded

ML246 was identified from a high throughput screen of compounds that reduced PNC prevalence [14, 18]. Here we tested the effects of ML246 on ovarian cancer growth, invasion and spread. Tumor growth was assessed in subcutaneous grafts of SKOV3 cells or PDX tissues. ML246 significantly attenuated growth of the PDX tumor while SKOV3 xenografts were unaffected. SKOV3 tumor sizes were highly variable and any affect of ML246 did not reach statistical significance. Grafting the human ovarian cancer cells under the bursa of the mouse ovary provided an orthotopic environment most similar to the primary disease site in humans. In addition, this site provided a niche to allow for peritoneal spread from the ovary to other intra-abdominal organs. The incidence of lesions outside of the grafting site in the ML246-treated mice carrying SKOV3 xenografts compared to the vehicle-treated mice was lower. In addition, a pilot study was done, grafting patient tumors (same PDX line used

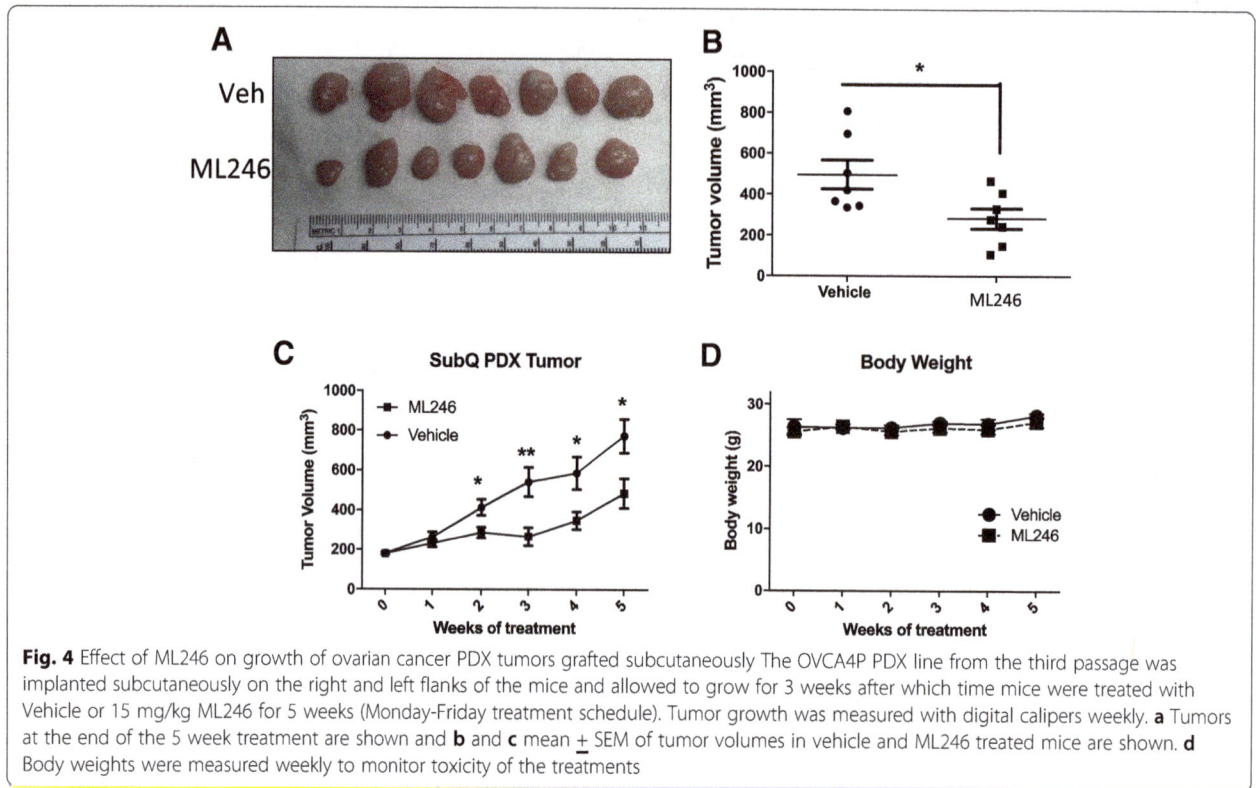

**Fig. 4** Effect of ML246 on growth of ovarian cancer PDX tumors grafted subcutaneously The OVCA4P PDX line from the third passage was implanted subcutaneously on the right and left flanks of the mice and allowed to grow for 3 weeks after which time mice were treated with Vehicle or 15 mg/kg ML246 for 5 weeks (Monday-Friday treatment schedule). Tumor growth was measured with digital calipers weekly. **a** Tumors at the end of the 5 week treatment are shown and **b** and **c** mean $\pm$ SEM of tumor volumes in vehicle and ML246 treated mice are shown. **d** Body weights were measured weekly to monitor toxicity of the treatments

in the subcutaneous model) under the ovarian bursa and similarly, ML246 treatment decreased the total number of lesions outside of the ovary (data not shown). The decrease in the number of lesions outside of the primary site could be due to the inability of tumor cells to metastasize, or the inability of tumor cells to adhere and propagate in a new microenviroment, distant from the primary tumor source. While the presence of tumor tissues outside of the ovarian bursa is suggestive of metastasis, it is noteworthy that an incision was made to place tumor cells under the bursa. It is possible that tumor cells escaped from the surgical site making it difficult to distinguish true metastasis (invasion and migration) from displacement, and thus a technical limitation of the intrabursal model.

As ML246 is an investigational agent, there was limited pharmacokinetic data, and the ideal dose for our studies was unknown. Although the therapeutic index still remains undefined, a higher dose of ML246 may have caused a more robust response in our systems. Furthermore, pathologic sectioning was done on visible tumor deposits and grossly abnormal organs with up to three sections analyzed. Additional metastatic lesions could have gone undetected. Ultrafine sectioning of the whole organ would have given a more thorough measurement of tumor cells outside the ovary.

ML246 has not been studied at the clinical level for any tumor type although there are plans to move ML246 into human trials. Given its ability to inhibit tumor growth and

metastases in preclinical models, one could foresee using this in first line, maintenance and recurrent settings, especially if it is well tolerated. Additional preclinical studies to evaluate the efficacy of ML246 in combination with platinum and/or taxane chemotherapy, would be warranted. Our data demonstrate that ML246 is as effective as cisplatin in inhibiting ovarian cancer growth and thus could be considered in platinum-resistant disease.

Our study reports for the first time, the effects of ML246, an inhibitor of PNC, in ovarian cancer. ML246 decreased invasive ability of ovarian cancer cell lines, attenuated tumor growth of human xenografts of ovarian cancer, and decreased abdominal spread of xenografts. These data warrant additional investigation into the therapeutic potential of ML246 for ovarian cancer as well as its mode of action. Given the significant heterogeneity and metastatic potential of ovarian cancer [20], the PNC structure may be a reliable target. ML246 is a promising compound that targets PNC and should be studied in greater detail in ovarian cancer.

## Conclusions

PNC's are present in ovarian cancer cells and treatment with ML246 decreases invasion in vitro and tumor growth and spread in vivo. Additional studies will determine the efficacy of ML246 as an inhibitor of metastatic disease in ovarian cancer and to determine its precise mechanism of action.

## Abbreviations

$CO_2$: Carbon dioxide; DAPI: 4',6-diamidino-2-phenylindole; DMEM: Dulbecco's modified Eagle's medium; DMSO: Dimethyl sulfoxide; DNA: Deoxyribonucleic acid; FBS: Fetal bovine serum; H&E: Hematoxylin and eosin; NSG: NOD-scid IL2Rγ null; PARP: Poly ADP ribose polymerase; PDX: Patient derived xenograft; PNC: Perinucleolar compartment; PTB: Polypyrimidine tract-binding protein; RNA: Ribonucleic acid

## Acknowledgements

We acknowledge Dr. Kevin Frankowski of the University of Kansas Specialized Chemistry Center for synthesizing the ML246 sample, which was supported through the Molecular Libraries Initiative (U54HG005031). We also acknowledge Dr. Sui Huang for providing the ML246 compound and for PNC staining of the cell lines.

## Funding

This work was funded by Institutional funds to the Division of Gynecologic Oncology by Northwestern University Feinberg School of Medicine. (MJK).

## Authors' contributions

Conceptualization: MK and JJK formulated overarching research goals and aims. Methodology: MK, WQ and JJK developed or designed methodology and created the models. Validation: Verification, whether as a part of the activity or separate, of the overall replication/reproducibility of results/experiments and other research outputs was done by MK, WQ, KM and JJK. Formal analysis: Application of statistical, mathematical, computational, or other formal techniques to analyze or synthesize study data was performed by MK, WQ, MP, KM and JJK. Investigation: Research and investigation process, specifically performing the experiments, or data/evidence collection were performed by MK WQ, MP and KM. Resources: WQ and JJK provided study materials, reagents, materials, patients, laboratory samples, animals, instrumentation, computing resources, or other analysis tools. Data curation: Management activities to annotate (produce metadata), scrub data and maintain research data (including software code, where it is necessary for interpreting the data itself) for initial use and later re-use was done by MK, WQ, JJK. Writing – original draft: Preparation, creation and/or presentation of the published work, specifically writing the initial draft (including substantive translation) were done by MK, WQ and JJK. Writing – review and editing: Preparation, creation and/or presentation of the published work by those from the original research group, specifically critical review, commentary or revision – including pre- or post-publication stages were done by MK, WQ, MP, KM and JJK. Visualization: Preparation, creation and/or presentation of the published work, specifically visualization/data presentation were done by MK, WQ, KM and JJK. Supervision: Oversight and leadership responsibility for the research activity planning and execution, including mentorship external to the core team were provided by MP and JJK. Project administration: Management and coordination responsibility for the research activity planning and execution was done by JJK. Funding acquisition: Acquisition of the financial support for the project leading to this publication was from MK and JJK. All authors read and approved the final manuscript.

## Consent for publication

Not applicable.

## Competing interests

The authors declare that they have no competing interests.

## Author details

[1]Division of Gynecology Oncology, Northwestern University Feinberg School of Medicine, Chicago, IL, USA. [2]Division of Reproductive Science in Medicine, Department of Obstetrics and Gynecology, Northwestern University Feinberg School of Medicine, Chicago, IL, USA. [3]Department of Pathology, Northwestern University Feinberg School of Medicine, Chicago, IL, USA. [4]Robert H. Lurie Comprehensive Cancer Center, Northwestern University, 303 E. Superior Street, 4-117, Chicago, IL 60611, USA.

## References

1. Siegel RL, Miller KD, Jemal A. Cancer statistics, 2017. CA Cancer J Clin. 2017; 67(1):7–30.
2. Coward JI, Middleton K, Murphy F. New perspectives on targeted therapy in ovarian cancer. Int J Womens Health. 2015;7:189–203.
3. Huang S, Deerinck TJ, Ellisman MH, Spector DL. The dynamic organization of the perinucleolar compartment in the cell nucleus. J Cell Biol. 1997; 137(5):965–74.
4. Huang S, Deerinck TJ, Ellisman MH, Spector DL. The perinucleolar compartment and transcription. J Cell Biol. 1998;143(1):35–47.
5. Matera AG, Frey MR, Margelot K, Wolin SL. A perinucleolar compartment contains several RNA polymerase III transcripts as well as the polypyrimidine tract-binding protein, hnRNP I. J Cell Biol. 1995;129(5):1181–93.
6. Kamath RV, Thor AD, Wang C, Edgerton SM, Slusarczyk A, Leary DJ, et al. Perinucleolar compartment prevalence has an independent prognostic value for breast cancer. Cancer Res. 2005;65(1):246–53.
7. Norton JT, Pollock CB, Wang C, Schink JC, Kim JJ, Huang S. Perinucleolar compartment prevalence is a phenotypic pancancer marker of malignancy. Cancer. 2008;113(4):861–9.
8. Slusarczyk A, Kamath R, Wang C, Anchel D, Pollock C, Lewandowska MA, et al. Structure and function of the perinucleolar compartment in cancer cells. Cold Spring Harb Symp Quant Biol. 2010;75:599–605.
9. Wen Y, Wang C, Huang S. The perinucleolar compartment associates with malignancy. Front Biol (Beijing). 2013;8(4). https://doi.org/10.1007/s11515-013-1265-z.
10. Even Y, Escande ML, Fayet C, Genevieve AM. CDK13, a kinase involved in pre-mRNA splicing, is a component of the Perinucleolar compartment. PLoS One. 2016;11(2):e0149184.
11. Norton JT, Huang S. The perinucleolar compartment: RNA metabolism and cancer. Cancer Treat Res. 2013;158:139–52.
12. Politz JC, Scalzo D, Groudine M. Something silent this way forms: the functional organization of the repressive nuclear compartment. Annu Rev Cell Dev Biol. 2013;29:241–70.
13. Pollock C, Daily K, Nguyen VT, Wang C, Lewandowska MA, Bensaude O, et al. Characterization of MRP RNA-protein interactions within the perinucleolar compartment. Mol Biol Cell. 2011;22(6):858–67.
14. Frankowski K, Patnaik S, Schoenen F, Huang S, Norton J, Wang C, et al. Discovery and development of small molecules that reduce PNC prevalence. Bethesda: Probe Reports from the NIH Molecular Libraries Program; 2010.
15. Frankowski KJ, Wang C, Patnaik S, Schoenen FJ, Southall N, Li D, et al. Metarrestin, a perinucleolar compartment inhibitor, effectively suppresses metastasis. Sci Transl Med. 2018;10(441). https://doi.org/10.1126/scitranslmed.aap8307.
16. Xu X, Ayub B, Liu Z, Serna VA, Qiang W, Liu Y, et al. Anti-miR182 reduces ovarian cancer burden, invasion, and metastasis: an in vivo study in orthotopic xenografts of nude mice. Mol Cancer Ther. 2014;13(7):1729–39.
17. Dong R, Qiang W, Guo H, Xu X, Kim JJ, Mazar A, et al. Histologic and molecular analysis of patient derived xenografts of high-grade serous ovarian carcinoma. J Hematol Oncol. 2016;9(1):92.
18. Frankowski KJ, Wang C, Patnaik S, Schoenen FJ, Southall N, Li D, et al. Metarrestin, a perinucleolar compartment inhibitor, effectively suppresses metastasis. Sci Transl Med. 2018; in press.
19. Domcke S, Sinha R, Levine DA, Sander C, Schultz N. Evaluating cell lines as tumour models by comparison of genomic profiles. Nat Commun. 2013;4:2126.
20. Cancer Genome Atlas Research N. Integrated genomic analyses of ovarian carcinoma. Nature. 2011;474(7353):609–15.

# 24

# Comprehensive knowledge and uptake of cervical cancer screening is low among women living with HIV/AIDS in Northwest Ethiopia

Daniel Asfaw Erku[1][*] ⓘ, Adeladlew Kassie Netere[1], Amanual Getnet Mersha[2], Sileshi Ayele Abebe[2], Abebe Basazn Mekuria[3] and Sewunet Admasu Belachew[1]

**Abstract**

**Background:** In Ethiopia, cervical cancer is ranked as the second most common type of cancer in women and it is about 8 times more common in HIV infected women. However, data on knowledge of HIV infected women regarding cervical cancer and acceptability of screening is scarce in Ethiopia. Hence, the present study was aimed at assessing the level of knowledge of about cervical cancer and uptake of screening among HIV infected women in Gondar, northwest Ethiopia.

**Methods:** A cross sectional, questionnaire based survey was conducted on 302 HIV infected women attending the outpatient clinic of University of Gondar referral and teaching hospital from March 1 to 30, 2017. Descriptive statistics, univariate and multivariate logistic regression analysis were also performed to examine factors associated with uptake of cervical cancer screening service.

**Results:** Overall, only 64 (21.2%) of respondent were knowledgeable about cervical cancer and screening and only 71 (23.5%) of respondents were ever screened in their life time. Age between 21 and 29 years old (AOR = 2.78, 95% CI = 1.71–7.29), perceived susceptibility to develop cervical cancer (AOR =2.85, 95% CI = 1.89–6.16) and comprehensive knowledge of cervical cancer (AOR = 3.02, 95% CI = 2.31–7.15) were found to be strong predictors of cervical cancer screening service uptake.

**Conclusion:** The knowledge and uptake of cervical cancer screening among HIV infected women was found to be very poor. Taking into consideration the heightened importance of comprehensive knowledge in boosting up the number of participants towards cervical cancer screening services, different stakeholders working on cancer and HIV/AIDS should provide a customized health promotion intervention and awareness creation to HIV-infected women, along with improving accessibility of cervical cancer screening services in rural areas.

**Keywords:** Cervical cancer, Ethiopia, HIV/AIDS, Screening, Knowledge, Women

* Correspondence: daniel.asfaw05@gmail.com
[1]Department of Clinical Pharmacy, School of Pharmacy, College of Medicine and Health Sciences, University of Gondar, Chechela Street, Lideta Sub city Kebele 16, P.O. Box: 196, Gondar, Ethiopia
Full list of author information is available at the end of the article

## Background

Cancer of the cervix, mainly attributed to persistent infection with a high risk oncogenic Human papillomavirus (HR-HPV), is one of the most common type of women's cancer globally, with more than 90% of new cases occurring in developing and resource-limited countries [1–3]. It is also associated with a higher rate of mortality with over 150,000 global mortality reported only in 2012, of which 87% of death occurred in developing countries [1, 2]. In Ethiopia, cervical cancer is ranked as the second most common type of cancer in women with crude incidence rate of 16.3 per 100,000 populations annually. In 2012 only, more than 27 million women of reproductive age in Ethiopia were at risk of developing cervical cancer and jeopardized the lives of more than 4500 women [4].

Evidences showed that, immunosuppression and low CD4 counts caused by HIV infection predisposes women living with HIV infection at an increased risk for cervical cancer and the development of squamous intraepithelial lesions [5–9]. Cervical cancer is about 8 times more common in HIV infected women than none infected ones [5]. From around 35 new cases diagnosed annually per 100, 000 population in sub-Saharan African countries, about 60% of the cases diagnosed among patients living with HIV infection [10, 11]. In a study done in southern Ethiopia, around 22% women infected with HIV were positive for precancerous cervical cancer [8].

Despite its preventable cause, global cervical cancer incidence rate is expected to be doubled by 2025 [12]. While performing regular screening is known to prevent the disease by a significant percentage [13, 14], the acceptability of regular screening in Ethiopia is limited and covers less than 1% of women [12, 15]. Moreover, comprehensive data on knowledge of women living with HIV/AIDS regarding cervical cancer and acceptability of screening is lacking in Ethiopia, which limits the development of cancer prevention efforts in these patient populations. Hence, the present study was aimed at assessing the level of knowledge about cervical cancer and uptake of screening among women living with HIV/AIDS in Gondar, northwest Ethiopia.

## Methods

### Study design and setting

A hospital-based cross-sectional survey was employed on 302 women attending ART clinic at University of Gondar Referral and Teaching Hospital (UoGRTH), northwest Ethiopia. UoGRTH is located in Gondar town, northwest Ethiopia, 738 km away from Addis Ababa (the capital city of Ethiopia).

### Sampling and recruitment strategies

All HIV infected women above age of 17 years who visited the outpatient clinic of UoGRTH for follow up and medication refill were taken as a study population. Single population proportion formula was used with the assumption of 95% confidence interval, 5% margin of error, the proportion (p) of cervical cancer screening in women living with HIV/AIDS (11%) [16] and 5% for possible non-response was taken to determine a final sample size of 317. A systematic random sampling technique was then applied to select participants until the final sample size was attained.

### Survey instrument

Data collection was performed by two of the principal investigators through interviewer-administered questionnaire. The investigators were properly trained on the instrument and ways of approaching the patients and securing potential participants permission for the interview prior to the commencement of the study. The data collection tool was developed after a thorough literature review of the published studies [17–20] and was primarily prepared in English. This was translated to local language (Amharic) and then back to English by an expert in the area in order to ensure that the translated version gives the proper meaning. The data collection instrument was also pretested on 20 women who were not included in the final analysis and relevant modifications were instituted before the commencement of actual data collection. The final questionnaire divided into three main parts. The first section was focusing on the socio-demographic and disease related information including age, marital status, educational level, CD4 count and WHO clinical stage. The second section, having 30 yes/no or true/false questions, assessed the knowledge about cervical cancer (CC) screening with five subcategories (risk factors for CC, prevention of CC, clinical symptoms of CC, benefits of screening, and meaning of positive results). The third section asked respondents regarding the uptake of cervical cancer screening services. Total scores for each category were then summed up to determine an overall score with a maximum score of 30. Using published literature as a reference [17], we classify respondents with a score of 60% or more as knowledgeable. The number of women who achieved this for any one score is defined as the knowledge rate. The third section included questions about the respondents' uptake of CC screening.

### Statistical analysis

All the statistical analyses were done using Statistical Package for the Social Sciences (SPSS) software version 21.0 for Windows (SPSS Inc., Chicago, IL). Frequencies and percentages were used to express different variables. Univariate and multivariate logistic regression analysis were used to determine predictors of knowledge about cervical cancer and acceptability of screening. The results were adjusted for patients' demographic and disease characteristics. Odds ratio (OR) with 95% CI were computed along with corresponding $p$-value ($p < 0.05$) as cut off points for determining statistical significance.

### Ethical considerations

This study was approved by the ethical review committee of University of Gondar with an approval number of UoG-SoP-92/2017. Written informed consent from the respondents was also obtained before conducting this study. Participants' information obtained was kept confidential.

### Operational definitions

CD4 Count: It is a laboratory value that measures the number of CD4 T lymphocytes (CD4 cells) in a sample of blood. In people with HIV, the CD4 count is the most important laboratory indicator of immune function and the predictor of HIV progression. Healthy individuals CD4 count ranges from 500 to 1700 cells/mm$^3$. However, in HIV positive individuals the CD4 count sharply drops down to less than 500 cells/mm$^3$, which shows immunodefiency.

WHO clinical Stage: WHO clinical staging is based on clinical findings that guide the diagnosis, evaluation, and management of HIV/AIDS, and it does not require a CD4 cell count. This staging system is used in many countries to determine eligibility for antiretroviral therapy, particularly in settings in which CD4 testing is not available like the case of Ethiopia. These stages are defined by specific clinical conditions or symptoms. With this, clinical stages are categorized as 1 through 4, progressing from primary HIV infection to advanced HIV/AIDS [21].

### Results

#### Characteristics of the study participants

Out of 317 patients approached, 302 of them were included in the study giving a response rate of 95.3%. The mean age of respondents was 33.72 years with a standard deviation of ±9.72. Majority of the respondents were urban residents (69.9%). A substantial proportion of respondents (36.7%) were at the stage of WHO clinical stage 2 and had a CD4 count of ≤500 cells/ul (66.9%). The sociodemographic and disease characteristics of study participants are depicted in Table 1.

#### Knowledge and uptake of cervical cancer screening

The majority of respondents in this study 265 (87.7%) had heard about cervical cancer and its screening. The average total knowledge score was found to be 10.8 ± 5.20 (a range possible from 0 to 30), with a mean score of 1.64 ± 1.27 for the risk factors of CC (a range possible from 0 to 7), 1.77 ± 1.81 for preventive measures of CC (a range possible from 0 to 7), 2.74 ± 1.67 for clinical symptoms of CC (a range possible from 0 to 9), 1.71 ± 1.23 for benefits of screening (a range possible from 0 to 3) and 2.72 ± 1.07

**Table 1** Sociodemographic characteristics and factors associated with uptake of cervical cancer screening, Gondar, 2017

| Variables | Total | Screening | | AOR (95% CI) |
|---|---|---|---|---|
| | | No ($n = 231$) | Yes ($n = 71$) | |
| Age group, in years | | | | |
| < 29 | 128 (42.4%) | 111 | 17 | 1 |
| 30–39 | 105 (34.8%) | 69 | 36 | 2.78 (1.71–7.29) |
| > 40 | 69 (22.8%) | 51 | 18 | 2.61 (1 .89–5.17) |
| Residence | | | | |
| Rural | 91 (30.1%) | 71 | 20 | – |
| Urban | 211 (69.9%) | 160 | 51 | – |
| Marital status | | | | |
| Unmarried | 123 (40.7%) | 112 | 11 | – |
| Ever married | 179 (59.3%) | 119 | 60 | – |
| Educational status | | | | |
| Illiterate | 33 (10.9%) | 28 | 5 | 1 |
| Primary | 145 (48%) | 133 | 12 | 0.87 (0.33–1.79) |
| Secondary | 80 (26.5%) | 66 | 14 | 1.08 (0.54–1.91) |
| Tertiary | 44 (14.6%) | 4 | 40 | 0.41 (0.21–1.29) |
| Average monthly income | | | | |
| < 100 | 148 (49%) | 119 | 29 | – |
| 100–150 | 85 (28.2%) | 59 | 16 | – |
| > 150 | 69 (22.8%) | 43 | 26 | – |
| Age at first sex | | | | |
| ≤ 16 | 63 (20.9%) | 46 | 17 | – |
| > 16 | 239 (79.1%) | 185 | 54 | – |
| Had multiple sexual partner | | | | |
| No | 123 (40.7%) | 89 | 34 | 1 |
| Yes | 179 (59.3%) | 142 | 37 | 1.01 (0.43–1.72) |
| Comprehensive knowledge about CC | | | | |
| Not knowledgeable | 238 (78.8%) | 129 | 9 | 1 |
| Knowledgeable | 64 (21.2%) | 2 | 62 | 3.02 (2.31–7.15) |
| CD4 count | | | | |
| < 500 cells/ul | 202 (66.9%) | 170 | 32 | – |
| > 500 cells/ul | 100 (33.1%) | 61 | 39 | – |
| WHO clinical stage | | | | |
| One | 91 (30.1%) | 80 | 11 | 1 |
| Two | 111 (36.7%) | 90 | 21 | 0.62(0.39–1.72) |
| Three | 67 (22.2%) | 52 | 15 | 1.01(0.41–1.52) |
| Four | 33 (11%) | 9 | 24 | 0.91(0.40–1.69) |
| Perceived susceptibility | | | | |
| None receptive | 118 (39.1%) | 105 | 13 | 1 |
| Receptive | 184 (60.9%) | 126 | 58 | 2.85 (1.89–6.16) |

for understanding about the positive results of CC (a range possible from 0 to 4). Overall, only 64 (21.2%) of respondent were knowledgeable about CC and screening as per the definition set in our study.

The majority of respondents correctly answered that CC is both preventable 238 (78.8%) and curable 223 (73.8%) disease. However, a significant proportion of respondents 103 (34.1%) didn't know the risk factors of CC or identified only one 57 (18.9%) or two 45 (14.9%) risk factors. While a highest proportion of patients correctly identified "early onset of sexual activity" 112 (37.1%) as a risk factor for CC, hormonal contraceptive use and HPV infection were identified as risk factors for CC only by 57 (18.9%) and 53 (17.5%) of respondents respectively. Similarly, over half of the respondents 172 (56.9%) knew that CC screening could prevent CC occurrence. Yet, only 88 (29.1%) respondents believed that CC screening could enable early diagnosis of the disease. Even though majority of respondents knew at least one of the clinical symptoms of CC 274 (90.7%), a substantial proportion of respondents 63 (20.8%) incorrectly stated "vulvar itching or burning sensation" as one of the clinical symptoms of CC. The detailed frequency of correct answer for each knowledge items are presented in Table 2. According to the findings our study, only 71 (23.5%) of respondents were ever tested for CC in their life time, of which 29 (40.8%) of them screened after 1 year of HIV/AIDS diagnosis. Among the 231 (76.5%) of respondents who were not screened for CC, absence of symptoms 205 (88.7%) and emotional barriers like fear of test result 164 (71%) and embarrassment 159 (68.8%) were the main reasons for not undergoing CC screening (Table 3).

### Predictors of CC screening service uptake

Logistic regression analysis was employed to assess possible associations between different sociodemographic variables and women's CC screening service uptake. According to the results from bivariate logistic regression, there were statistically significant differences in age, history of multiple sexual partners, educational status, WHO clinical stage, comprehensive knowledge of CC and screening and perceived susceptibility to develop CC between women who underwent CC screening and those who didn't. Variables that were significantly associated with CC screening service uptake in the bivariate analysis (those with $p$-value < 0.20) were further examined in multivariate logistic regression. Accordingly, age, perceived susceptibility to develop CC and comprehensive knowledge of CC and screening remained to be significant in the multivariate logistic model. The odds of CC screening service uptake among women in the age range of 30–39 years were 1.78 times higher than women aged less than 29 years old (AOR = 2.78, 95% CI = 1.71–7.29). The odds of CC screening uptake among

**Table 2** Frequency of correct answer for knowledge items about CC among participants, Gondar, Ethiopia, 2017

| Knowledge items | Correct answers (%) |
|---|---|
| Risk factor for CC | |
| Prolonged use of oral contraceptive | 57 (18.9%) |
| Sexually transmitted infection | 77 (25.5%) |
| Early onset of sexual activity | 112 (37.1%) |
| Smoking | 54 (17.9%) |
| Multiple sexual partner | 49 (16.2%) |
| History of HPV infection | 53 (17.5%) |
| Aged 30–65 | 65 (21.5%) |
| Symptoms of cervical cancer | |
| Bleeding and pain after sexual intercourse | 60 (19.9%) |
| Vulvar itching or burning sensation | 63 (20.8%) |
| Post-menopausal bleeding | 54 (17.9%) |
| Excessive vaginal discharge | 71 (23.5%) |
| Abnormal vaginal discharge | 68 (22.5%) |
| Inter-menstrual bleeding | 67 (22.2%) |
| Longer or heavier menstrual periods | 55 (18.2%) |
| Pelvic pain | 48 (15.9%) |
| Urinary frequency, urgency | 38 (12.6%) |
| Preventive measures for CC | |
| CC screening | 172 (56.9%) |
| Reduce numbers of sexual partners | 61 (20.2%) |
| Vaccine for HPV | 27 (8.9%) |
| Late marriage and late childbirth | 21 (6.9%) |
| No smoking | 57 (18.9%) |
| Consistent condom use | 29 (9.6%) |
| Prompt treatment of STIs | 71 (23.5%) |
| Benefits of screening for CC | |
| Early detection | 71 (23.5%) |
| Early diagnosis | 88 (29.1%) |
| Early treatment | 101 (33.4%) |
| Understanding of the positive results | |
| Negative screening result means cervix without any lesion, needing no more screening | 142 (47%) |
| Positive screening result means suffering from CC | 224 (74.2%) |
| Positive screening result means there is cervical lesion, it needs further diagnosis | 76 (25.2%) |
| CC is a curable disease | 223 (73.8%) |

women who had positive perception on their susceptibility to develop CC were 1.85 times higher than those who had negative perception (AOR =2.85, 95% CI = 1.89–6.16). Similarly, the odds of undergoing CC screening among women who had a comprehensive knowledge on CC and screening were 2.02 times higher than those

**Table 3** Acceptance of CC screening service among study participants, Gondar, Ethiopia, 2017

| Variables | Frequency (%) |
|---|---|
| Have you ever had CC screening in your life time? | |
| No | 231 (76.5%) |
| Yes | 71 (23.5%) |
| If yes, when was the last time you screened for cervical cancer? (N = 71) | |
| Before HIV/AIDS diagnosis | 19 (26.8%) |
| Within 1 year of HIV/AIDS diagnosis | 23 (32.4%) |
| After 1 year of HIV/AIDS diagnosis | 29 (40.8%) |
| If no, what are the reasons for not being screened? (N = 231) | |
| Absence of symptoms | 205 (88.7%) |
| High cost of the test | 64 (27.7%) |
| Not prescribed by the doctor | 76 (32.9%) |
| Embarrassment | 159 (68.8%) |
| Time consuming | 44 (19%) |
| Fear of test result | 164 (71%) |
| Screening center too far | 87 (37.7%) |
| No reason | 46 (19.9%) |
| Others[a] | 19 98.2%) |
| Are you willing to be screened in the near future? (N = 302) | |
| No | 88 (29%) |
| Yes | 214 (71%) |

[a]Others include Religious denial, partner acceptance, no symptom

who didn't have comprehensive knowledge on CC and screening (AOR = 3.02, 95% CI = 2.31–7.15).

## Discussion

Exploring the comprehensive knowledge towards the causative/risk factors, benefits of screening, pertinent manifestations and prevention of cervical cancer is so indispensable in women care. According to the finding of this study, majority of (87.7%) respondents heard about cervical cancer and its screening. The overall knowledge rate of CC was 21.2%, which is higher compared to the study done in Nigeria where 11.8% of the rural and 17.6% of urban women had knowledge of CC [19]. In line with this, the average total knowledge score women had was found to be merely $10.8 \pm 5$, which is higher than the study conducted in china, which is $6.91 \pm 3.42$ [18]. The difference in knowledge score could be attributed to the difference in time period and the characteristics of the study population as both of the studies were conducted among the general population in Nigeria and China and did not account whether the respondents had HIV/AIDS or not. This could potentially account for the variation in the level of knowledge as patients living with HIV/AIDS expected to have a higher level of awareness about CC due to their frequent contact with healthcare providers compared to the general population. In our study, only

33.8% of the study respondents were capable of identifying one or two risk factors for CC, which is lower than the study conducted among rural communities of South Africa in which about 64% of the respondents gave one or more risk factors [22]. This might be due to the absence of a comprehensive cancer prevention and treatment center in Ethiopia unlike countries like South Africa..Majority of respondents in this study (73.8%) believed that CC is curable, which is lower than the study conducted in China (80.8%) [18]. This might be due to the difference in the background of study population as the study conducted in China included respondents from Wufeng, a high-incidence region of cervical cancer in China.

According to the findings of our study, only 23.5% of respondents were ever tested for CC in their life time, which is significantly higher compared with the study done in among patients living with HIV/AIDS in Addis Ababa, Ethiopia, where only 11.5% of women screened for CC [16]. The uptake of screening in our study is also higher compared with the study conducted in Nigeria (9.4%) [23]. The enhanced uptake of screening service in our study could be partially explained by the increased nation-wide advocacy, community sensitization and awareness creation about the CC screening that has been put into effect in recent years. It might also be due to the improved expansion and access of screening centers across the country and integration of CC screening into the standard care for women who are living with HIV/AIDS. Yet, the proportion of women screened for CC in our study is still low compared to developed countries such as Ottawa (58%) [24], despite the recent effort to screen all HIV positive women who are on antiretroviral therapy (ART) who were not screened before. Among 76.5% of patients who were not screened in our study, absence of symptoms (88.7%) and emotional barriers like fear of test result (71%) and embarrassment (68.8%) were the main reasons for not undergoing screening, which was consistent with the study conducted in China [18]. According to the results from multivariate logistic regression analysis, age, perceived susceptibility to develop CC and comprehensive knowledge of CC and screening remained to be strong predictors of CC screening service uptake. The odds of CC screening service uptake among women in the age range of 30–39 years were 2.78 times higher than women aged 21–29 years old. Similar findings were also reported both in developing and developed countries [25, 26]. This is not surprising as women at the age of 30s and 60s are more likely to be symptomatic due to the bimodal distribution nature of the CC, which may enhance their probability of screening for CC. Similarly, the odds of CC screening uptake among women who had positive perception on their susceptibility to develop CC were 2.85 times higher than those who had negative perception, which could be explained by the assumption of behavioral model, which assumes that belief and attitudes, including self-vulnerability to illness, are important predictors of their health-related activities [27]. Furthermore, the odds of undergoing CC screening among women who had a comprehensive knowledge on CC and screening were 3.02 times higher than those who didn't have comprehensive knowledge on CC and screening, which corroborates the findings of studies conducted among patients living with HIV/AIDS in Addis Ababa, Ethiopia and Botswana [16, 28].

## Limitation of the study

Even though this survey highlights an area of research where there is lack of literature in Ethiopia, caution should be exercised when generalizing to other regions in Ethiopia as the study was a cross-sectional and conducted only in Gondar, northwest Ethiopia. Nevertheless, this survey has significant implications for improving uptake of CC screening services and provide a foundation for planning future in-depth research prior to developing educational materials. A larger-scale and multi centered survey that includes more diverse participants is warranted to validate our findings and to provide more accurate findings. Furthermore, our study could be used as an input for future studies aiming at exploring the difference in knowledge about cervical cancer and cervical cancer screening uptake experience between HIV positive and negative women.

## Conclusion and recommendation

The results of the present study revealed that the knowledge and uptake of cervical cancer screening among HIV infected women was very poor. Our findings emphasize the need to reform the existing national strategies of cervical cancer screening so as to strengthen the health education and promotion, beyond providing screening services. Taking into consideration the heightened importance of comprehensive knowledge in participating in cervical cancer screening services, different stakeholders working on cancer and HIV/AIDS should provide a customized health promotion intervention and awareness creation among HIV-infected women. Furthermore, interventions should focus on overcoming the identified barriers for not being screened including improving accessibility of cervical cancer screening services in rural areas.

## Abbreviations

CC: Cervical cancer; CI: Confidence interval; HIV/AIDS: Human immunodeficiency virus/Acquired immune deficiency syndrome; HPV: Human papillomavirus; HR-HPV: High risk oncogenic Human papillomavirus; OR: Odds ratio; SPSS: Statistical package for the social sciences; UoGRTH: University of Gondar Referral and Teaching Hospital; WHO: World health organization

## Acknowledgements

The authors acknowledge the Support of School of pharmacy, University of Gondar and UOGRTH in facilitating the data collection process.

## Funding

No financial support was gained to conduct this study.

## Authors' contributions

DAE, SAB involved in conceptualization, project administration, formal analysis, investigation, methodology and supervision; ABM, SAA and AKN involved in data curation, resources, writing and original draft of the manuscript; AGM and DAE involved in methodology, investigation and writing, review & editing of the final manuscript. All authors read and approved the final manuscript.

## Consent for publication

Not applicable.

## Competing interests

The authors declare that they have no competing interests.

## Author details

[1]Department of Clinical Pharmacy, School of Pharmacy, College of Medicine and Health Sciences, University of Gondar, Chechela Street, Lideta Sub city Kebele 16, P.O. Box: 196, Gondar, Ethiopia. [2]Department of Gynecology and obstetrics, College of Medicine and Health Sciences, University of Gondar, Chechela Street, Lideta Sub city Kebele 16, Gondar, Ethiopia. [3]Department of Pharmacology, School of Pharmacy, University of Gondar, Chechela Street, Lideta Sub city Kebele 16, Gondar, Ethiopia.

## References

1. Integrated Africa Cancer Factsheet. Focusing on cervical cancer, Girls & Women Health, Sexual & Reproductive Health, HIV & Maternal Health. 2014.
2. WHO. International agency for research on cancer: Latest world cancer statistics; 2013.
3. Zur Hausen H. Papillomaviruses in the causation of human cancers – a brief historical account. Virology. 2009;384:260–5.
4. Bruni L, Barrionuevo-Rosas L, Albero G, Aldea M, Serrano B, Valencia S, et al. ICO information Centre on HPV and cancer (HPV information Centre). Human Papillomavirus and Related Diseases in Ethiopia. 2014;12:18. Summary Report http://www.hpvcentre.net/.
5. Tanon A, Jaquet A, Ekouevi DK, Akakpo J, Adoubi I, et al. The pectrum of cancers in West Africa: associations with human immunodeficiency virus. PLoS One. 2012;7(10):e48108.
6. Moscicki AB, Ellenberg JH, Vermund SH, Holland CA, Darragh T, Crowley-Nowick PA, et al. Prevalence of and risks for cervical human papillomavirus infection and squamous intraepithelial lesions in adolescent girls: impact of infection with human immunodeficiency virus. Arch Pediatr Adolesc Med. 2000;154(2):127–34.
7. Meijer CJ, Rozendaal L, Voorhorst FJ, Verheijen R, Helmerhorst TJ, Walboomers JM. Human papillomavirus and screening for cervical cancer: state of art and prospects. Ned Tijdschr Geneeskd. 2000;144(35):1675–9.
8. Gedefaw A, Astatkie A, Tessema GA. The prevalence of precancerous cervical cancer lesion among HIV-infected women in southern Ethiopia: a cross-sectional study. PLoS One. 2013;8(12):e84519.
9. Sun X-W, Kuhn L, Ellerbrock TV, Chiasson MA, Bush TJ, Wright TC Jr. Human Papillomavirus infection in women infected with the human immunodeficiency virus. N Engl J Med. 1997;337:1343–9.
10. Sam MM, Kishor B, Clement A, Annie JS. HIV and cancer in Africa: mutual collaboration between HIV and cancer programs may provide timely research and public health data. Infect Agents Cancer. 2011;6:16. https://doi.org/10.1186/1750-9378-6-16.
11. UNAIDS. AIDS epidemic update Geneva, Switzerland. November 2009. http://www.unaids.org/. Global report UNAIDS report on the global aids epidemic. 2010. http://www.unaids.org/en.
12. WHO/ICO Information Centre on HPV and Cervical Cancer (HPV Information Centre). Human Papillomavirus and Related Cancers in World. Summary Report 2010. http://www.hpvcentre.net.
13. Cancer Research UK Registered charity in England and Wales (1089464), Scotland (SC041666) and the Isle of Man (1103). 2014. cruk.org/cancerstats.
14. Minjee L, Eun-Cheol P, Hoo-Sun C, Jeoung AK, Ki Bong Y, et al. Socioeconomic disparity in cervical cancer screening among Korean women: 1998–2010. MC Public Health. 2013;13:553.

15. Joint United Nations Program on HIV/AIDS. (UNAIDS) report on the global AIDS epidemic. 2010.

16. Belete N, Tsige Y, Mellie H. Willingness and acceptability of cervical cancer screening among women living with HIV/AIDS in Addis Ababa, Ethiopia: a cross sectional study. Gynecologic Oncology Research and Practice. 2015;2: 6. https://doi.org/10.1186/s40661-015-0012-3.

17. Di J, Rutherford S, Wu J, Song B, Ma L, Chen J, et al. Knowledge of cervical cancer screening among women across different socio- economic regions of China. PLoS One. 2015;10(12):e0144819. https://doi.org/10.1371/journal.pone.0144819.

18. Jia Y, Li S, Yang R, Zhou H, Xiang QY, Hu T, et al. Knowledge about cervical cancer and barriers of screening program among women in Wufeng County, a high-incidence region of cervical cancer in China. PLoS One. 2013;8(7):e67005. https://doi.org/10.1371/journal.pone.0067005.

19. Nwankwo K, Aniebue U, Aguwa E, Anarado A, Agunwah E. Knowledge attitudes and practices of cervical cancer screening among urban and rural Nigerian women: a call for education and mass screening. European journal of cancer care. 2011;20(3):362–7. https://doi.org/10.1111/j.1365-2354.2009. 01175.x.

20. Getahun F, et al. Comprehensive knowledge about cervical cancer is low among women in Northwest Ethiopia. BMC Cancer. 2013;13:2.

21. HIV Classification: CDC and WHO Staging Systems https://www.aidsetc.org/guide/hiv-classification-cdc-and-who-staging-systems.

22. Hoque M, Hoque E, Kader SB. Evaluation of cervical cancer screening program at a rural community of South Africa. East Afr J Publ Health. 2008;5(2):111.

23. Oliver CE, Chidinma VGO, Per OO, Karen OP. Willingness and acceptability of cervical cancer screening among HIV positive Nigerian women. BMC Public Health. 2013;13:46.

24. Pamela L, Claire K, Claire T, Kevin P, Jonathan BA, James J. Cervical cancer screening among HIV-positive women retrospective cohort study from a tertiary care HIV clinic. Can Fam Physician. 2010;56:e425–31.

25. Sawaya GF, Sung H-Y, Kathleen A, Marie M, Walter K, Robert A, et al. Advancing age and cervical cancer screening and prognosis. J Am Geriatr Soc. 2001;49:1499–504.

26. Smith AM, Heywood W, Ryall R, Shelley JM, Pitts MK, Richters J, et al. Association between sexual behavior and cervical cancer screening. J Women's Health. 2011;20:1091–6.

27. Ndikom CM, Ofi BA. Awareness, perception and factors affecting utilization of cervical cancer screening services among women in Ibadan, Nigeria: a qualitative study. Reprod Health. 2012;9:11.

28. Mingo AM, Panozzo CA, Taylor DiAngi Y, Smith J, Steenhoff AP, et al. Cervical cancer awareness and screening in Botswana. International journal of gynecological cancer: official journal of the International Gynecological Cancer Society. 2012;22:638–51.

# 25

# Safety and feasibility of contained uterine morcellation in women undergoing laparoscopic hysterectomy

Sarah Dotson[1]* (ID), Alejandro Landa[2], Jessie Ehrisman[3] and Angeles Alvarez Secord[3]

## Abstract

**Background:** Widespread concerns have been raised regarding the safety of power morcellation of uterine specimens because of the potential to disseminate occult malignancy. We sought to assess the safety and feasibility of contained manual uterine morcellation within a plastic specimen bag among women with uterine neoplasms.

**Methods:** A retrospective single-institution descriptive cohort study was conducted from 2003 to 2014. Patients with leiomyoma and/or uterine malignancy who underwent minimally invasive surgery with contained uterine manual morcellation were identified from surgical logs. Demographic data, pathology results, operative details and adjuvant treatments were abstracted.

**Results:** Eighty-eight patients were identified; 35 with leiomyoma and 53 with endometrial cancer. The mean age was 48 and 60, respectively. Uterine size/weight was greater in women with leiomyoma compared to those with cancer (15.1 weeks/448 g vs. 10.7 weeks/322 g). Mean operative time was 206 min (range 115–391) for leiomyoma cases and 238 min (range 131–399) for cancer cases. Median length of stay was 1 day (range 0–3 days). There were no cases of occult leiomyosarcoma and all specimens were successfully manually morcellated within a bag. There were no intraoperative complications. Thirty-day postoperative complications occurred in 7 patients, including one readmission for grade (G) 1 vaginal cuff separation after intercourse, G1 port-site hematoma (1), G2 port-site cellulitis (1), G2 vaginal cuff cellulitis (2), G2 bladder infection (2), G2 pulmonary edema (1), and G1 musculoskeletal injury (1).

**Conclusions:** Contained uterine hand morcellation is a feasible procedure with low peri-operative complication rates that allows for minimally invasive surgical procedures for women with large uterine neoplasms. Further evaluation is needed to assess survival outcomes for uterine malignancies.

**Keywords:** Leiomyoma, Malignancy, Morcellation, Total laparoscopic hysterectomy

## Background

Minimally invasive surgery (MIS) for hysterectomy provides patients with an alternative to laparotomy, particularly for uteri enlarged by leiomyomas or malignancy that are not amenable to vaginal hysterectomy. MIS can be performed either through conventional laparoscopic approaches or by utilizing the robotic platform. Advantages of MIS include faster return to normal activities, better cosmesis, decreased length of hospital stay, less blood loss, lower rates of infection and wound complications, less pain, and lower incidence of venous thromboembolism compared to laparotomy [1]. These benefits have been reported in women undergoing hysterectomy for both benign [1] and malignant conditions [2]. MIS for enlarged uteri presents gynecologic surgeons with the challenge of removing the uterus from the abdomen. Options for removal of the uterus traditionally include the following: laparotomy or "mini-laparotomy," removal through the vagina with or without morcellation of the specimen, and removal via 10–15 mm laparoscopic port sites with intracorporeal morcellation, including the use of a power morcellator.

Concerns about the dissemination of undiagnosed uterine cancer using power morcellation have been raised.

---

* Correspondence: sarah.dotson1@hsc.wvu.edu
[1]Department of Obstetrics and Gynecology, West Virginia University, 1 Medical Center Dr. PO Box 9186, HSC 4th floor, Morgantown, WV 26501-9186, USA
Full list of author information is available at the end of the article

The FDA cautioned use of power morcellators in April 2014 after a patient undergoing hysterectomy for presumed leiomyoma was found to have leiomyosarcoma, disseminated throughout the abdomen by use of a power morcellator [3]. In November 2014, the FDA released a safety communication defining contraindications to power uterine morcellation: 1) removal of suspected fibroid tissue in peri- and postmenopausal women who are candidates for en-bloc resection (vaginal or via mini-laparotomy), and 2) removal of tissue known or suspected to contain malignancy [4]. The prevalence of occult uterine malignancy in patients with suspected leiomyoma is not known exactly, but multiple retrospective studies have estimated rates of malignancy at 0.2–1% in women undergoing uterine morcellation [5] compared to 0.23–0.49% in non-morcellated specimens [6]. Despite the low probability of malignancy, the risk of tumor dissemination has caused significant concerns regarding power morcellation, a moratorium of the procedure at select centers, and removal of some morcellation devices from the market.

In response to concerns over dissemination of uterine pathology, contained uterine morcellation within a specimen bag has been suggested as an approach to maintain a minimally invasive approach to hysterectomy [5–7]. However, the FDA warns that there are no studies examining the efficacy of contained "bag" morcellation. At our institution, we have used the technique of contained uterine manual (hand) morcellation within a specimen bag for more than a decade. The purpose of the study was to investigate the feasibility and safety of contained uterine morcellation. Our primary objectives were to describe intraoperative and postoperative complications, to determine the frequency of occult uterine leiomyosarcoma among patients with suspected leiomyoma, and to assess cancer outcomes among patients with known uterine malignancy following laparoscopic hysterectomy with contained "bag" morcellation.

## Methods

A retrospective single-institution descriptive cohort study was performed using chart review of cases from January 1, 2003 to December 31, 2014. The study was approved by the Duke University Institutional Review Board. Patients who underwent laparoscopic hysterectomy with contained uterine manual morcellation within a specimen bag were identified using chart review. Eligible study subjects were identified through a large institutional database of patients with endometrial cancer, as well as through review of surgical case logs maintained by the Division of Gynecologic Oncology for quality assurance purposes. Not all case logs were available for review and therefore this cohort may not include every eligible case during the study period. Two authors (SD and AL) reviewed available

charts of patients who underwent laparoscopic hysterectomy to identify cases which included specimen morcellation within a bag. Patients with a post-operative diagnosis of endometrial cancer or uterine fibroids were included. All cases were performed by one of five Gynecologic Oncologists at our institution. While the study was not restricted to a particular type of specimen bag, the most commonly used technique at our institution is to place a 15 mm Endo Catch™ specimen retrieval bag through the vagina with a vaginal occlusion balloon, place the specimen in the bag under direct visualization and pull the opening of the bag through the vagina to expose the specimen. Morcellation was performed by hand using scissors or a scalpel to remove the specimen in small pieces that fit through the vagina. A similar technique is used via extended laparoscopic port sites. The decision to morcellate the uterus within a specimen bag was made intraoperatively when the uterus was too large to fit through the vagina intact, but the surgeon felt it could be safely removed using contained morcellation.

The two groups are described as separate cohorts, given two distinct patient populations for which uterine morcellation may be needed during minimally invasive hysterectomy. Data was abstracted by one of the authors (SD). Demographic data, pathology results, operative details, adjuvant treatments, disease recurrence and most recent disease status were abstracted. All data is descriptive for the two cohorts.

## Results

### Patient characteristics and operative findings

Eighty-eight patients were identified from retrospective chart review: 35 with leiomyoma and 53 with endometrial cancer. Baseline characteristics for the two groups are shown in Table 1. The mean age for patients with leiomyoma and uterine cancer was 48 and 60, respectively. The mean uterine size estimate on pre-operative exam was 15.1 and 10.7 weeks for women with leiomyoma and uterine cancer, respectively. Additional pre-operative diagnoses are outlined in Table 1.

Intraoperative and postoperative findings are shown in Table 2. The majority of cases were performed using a robotic platform. Mean operative time was 206 min (range 115–391) for leiomyoma cases and 238 min (range 131–399) for cancer cases. The mean uterine weight was 448 g (140 g - 1076 g) in women with leiomyoma and 322 g (135 g - 611 g) in those with malignancy. Length of inpatient hospital stay was 1 day, range 0–3 days) in both groups. The most frequent method for uterine specimen morcellation was contained manual morcellation within a specimen bag inside the vagina (82.9% for leiomyoma and 98.1% for uterine cancer). Alternative methods used included contained manual

**Table 1** Baseline characteristics

| Characteristic | Leiomyoma (N = 35) | Uterine Cancer (N = 53) |
|---|---|---|
| Age | 48 ± 6.5 [range 36–60] | 60.1 ± 9.9 [range 38–81] |
| Race/ethnicity | | |
|   Caucasian | 27 (77.1) | 29 (54.7) |
|   African American | 5 (14.3) | 23 (43.4) |
|   Asian | 0 (0) | 1 (1.9) |
|   Hispanic | 2 (5.7) | 0 (0) |
|   Other | 1 (2.9) | 0 (0) |
| BMI | 32.8 ± 9.2 [range 19.7–56.3] | 37.5 ± 11.0 [range 19.2–64.5] |
| Parity[a] | 1.5 ± 1.0 [range 0–3] | 1.9 ± 1.8 [range 0–7] |
| Pre-op uterine size estimate (weeks)[b] | 15.1 ± 2.7 [range 10–20] | 10.7 ± 2.7 [range 6–14] |
| Menopausal | 7 (20) | 40 (75.5) |
| Prior Abdominal Surgery | 23 (65.7) | 27 (50.9) |
| Pre-op Diagnosis | | |
|   Leiomyoma | 33 (94.3) | 6 (11.3) |
|   Endometrial cancer | 0 | 50 (94.3) |
|   Ovarian cyst/mass | 10 (30.3) | 2 (3.8) |
|   Other[c] | 10 (30.3) | 7 (13.2) |

Data are n(%) or mean ± SD unless otherwise specified. Data are presented as two separate cohorts given different disease states
[a]Missing data: n = 34 for leiomyoma group
[b]Missing data: n = 21 for leiomyoma group, n = 17 for uterine cancer group
[c]Includes endometrial intraepithelial neoplasia (3), abnormal uterine bleeding (4), family history of cancer (1), terminal ileum cancer (1), anemia (1), breast cancer (1), pelvic pain (1) and history of rectovaginal fistula repair (1) in the leiomyoma group and postmenopausal bleeding (2), atypical glandular cells (2), cirrhosis (1), cervical stenosis (2), chronic kidney disease (1), ventral hernia (1), atypical spindle cells (1) and pelvic organ prolapse (1) for the endometrial cancer group

morcellation through an extended laparoscopic port site and contained vaginal morcellation of a fibroid separate from the uterus. In one case, the cervix and lower portion of the uterus were morcellated within a bag in the vagina, but the remainder of the specimen was removed via mini-laparotomy, still contained within the specimen bag. No cases of occult leiomyosarcoma were identified. There were no intraoperative complications in either group. One patient received planned transfusion of fresh frozen plasma to correct INR secondary to known coagulopathy from cirrhosis (estimated blood loss 100 mL). Thirty-day postoperative complications occurred in 7 patients, including one readmission for grade (G) 1 vaginal cuff separation after intercourse, as well as G1 port-site hematoma (1), G2 port-site cellulitis (1), G2 vaginal cuff cellulitis (2), G2 bladder infection (2), G2 pulmonary edema (1), and G1 musculoskeletal injury (1). Two patients were suspected of having small vaginal cuff hematomas, but no imaging was obtained for confirmation, and symptoms resolved without intervention. Mean length of follow-up was 24 (range 1–85) months for patients with uterine cancer and 31 (range 3–89) months for patients with leiomyoma.

**Uterine malignancies**

Fifty-three patients underwent hysterectomy for uterine cancer and the histologic subtypes were as follows: 75.5% endometrioid, 9.4% serous and 1.9% clear cell adenocarcinomas, and 13.2% carcinosarcoma (Table 3). One case of grade 1 endometrioid adenocarcinoma contained sections with grade 3 signet ring cell differentiation. Among the 40 cases of endometrioid adenocarcinoma, 55% were grade 1, 42.5% grade 2 and 7.5% grade 3. Cytologic washings were positive in 5 cases (9.4%), suspicious or indeterminate in 6 cases (11.3%), and not collected in one case. Spillage of tumor was described in 2 cases, which occurred during hysterectomy and prior to placing the specimen in the plastic bag. One of these patients died of recurrent IB carcinosarcoma within 1 year, and the second patient (IB, grade 2 endometrioid adenocarcinoma) was offered and declined radiation therapy, and was alive at 2.5 months following surgery with no evidence of disease. Distribution of cancer stage is shown in Table 3.

Fifteen patients with uterine cancer received adjuvant treatment with chemotherapy or radiation, and four patients received hormonal therapy (Table 3). Median length of follow up was 546 days (range 34–2535 days). There were 7 deaths in the uterine cancer group (13.2%), and 5 were attributable to the patient's cancer (9.4%) (Table 4). Patients who died of their cancer had the following disease stages, histologic subtypes and adjuvant therapies: 1B serous adenocarcinoma who received adjuvant pelvic radiation and died with disseminated disease

**Table 2** Operative and postoperative characteristics

| Perioperative characteristics | Leiomyoma (N = 35) | Uterine cancer (N = 53) |
|---|---|---|
| Robotic platform | 26 (74.3) | 34 (64.2) |
| Uterine weight (grams)[a] | 448.35 ± 194.9 [range 140–1076] | 321.77 ± 102.1 [range 135–611] |
| Intra-op size estimate (weeks)[b] | 14.8 ± 2.6 [range 10–20] | 12.5 ± 2.2 [range 6–16] |
| Operative time (minutes)[c] | 206.0 ± 76.3 [range 115–391] | 237.5 ± 67.0 [range 131–399] |
| Abdominal/pelvic Adhesions | 13 (37.1) | 35 (34.0) |
| Length of stay[d] | 0.97 ± 0.5 [range 0–3] | 1.12 ± 0.4 [range 0–3] |
| Mode of morcellation | | |
|   Port site | 3 (8.6) | 0 (0) |
|   Vaginal | 29 (82.9) | 52 (98.1) |
|   Other | 3 (8.6) | 1 (1.9) |
| Post-op Diagnosis | | |
|   Leiomyoma | 35 (100) | 40 (75.5) |
|   Endometrial cancer[e] | 1 (2.9) | 53 (100) |
|   Benign ovarian neoplasm | 9 (25.7) | 6 (11.3) |
|   Adenomyosis | 13 (37.1) | 18 (33.9) |
|   Pelvic adhesive disease | 8 (22.9) | 9 (17.0) |
|   Other[f] | 18 (51.4) | 12 (22.6) |
| Post-op complications[g] | 3 (8.6) | 4 (7.5) |
| Length of follow-up (months) | 31 ± 21 [range 3–89] | 24 ± 21 [range 1–85] |

Data are n (%) or mean ± SD unless otherwise specified
[a]Missing data: n = 34 for leiomyoma group, n = 52 for uterine cancer group
[b]Missing data: n = 30 for leiomyoma group, n = 24 for uterine cancer group
[c]Missing data: n = 33 for leiomyoma group, n = 52 for uterine cancer group
[d]Missing data: n = 52 for uterine cancer group
[e]Incidental finding of Stage IA, grade 1 endometrioid adenocarcinoma, no adjuvant therapy
[f]Includes endometrial intraepithelial neoplasia (3), abnormal uterine bleeding (4), family history of cancer (1), terminal ileum cancer (1), anemia (1), breast cancer (1), pelvic pain (1), abdominal wall mesothelioma (1), retroperitoneal fibrosis (2), urethral diverticulum (1) ovarian cancer (1), endometrial polyp (3), endometriosis (3)and history of rectovaginal fistula repair (1) in the leiomyoma group and hydrosalpinx (1), endometriosis (1), ventral hernia (1) and appendicitis (1) for the endometrial cancer group
[g]Includes readmission for grade (G) 1 vaginal cuff separation after intercourse, as well as G1 port-site hematoma (1), G2 port-site cellulitis (1), G2 vaginal cuff cellulitis (2), G2 bladder infection (2), G2 pulmonary edema (1), and G1 musculoskeletal injury (1)

in the setting of end-stage renal disease; recurrent IA, grade 2 endometrioid who received no adjuvant therapy; IVB carcinosarcoma who declined adjuvant therapy; IIIC-2 and IIIA serous adenocarcinoma who each received adjuvant chemotherapy and pelvic radiation. One patient with Stage IA, grade 1 endometrioid adenocarcinoma died of severe pulmonary disease unrelated to malignancy 10 months after surgery. One patient with Stage IIIC-1 endometrioid adenocarcinoma died of unknown cause, but in the setting of recurrent, progressive disease for 1 year. Mean survival time among patients whose death was attributed to their uterine malignancy was 342 days (range 84–549 days).

## Discussion

Determining alternative and safe procedural techniques for uterine morcellation and specimen extraction are necessary to permit MIS for women with large uteri, not amenable to vaginal hysterectomy. MIS has several advantages over laparotomy, including better surgical

outcomes and quality of life in the majority of patients [1, 8]. Siedoff et al. published a decision analysis comparing surgical risks of laparotomy with risks of disseminated occult malignancy during laparoscopy for women with large leiomyoma, and predicted that laparoscopic hysterectomy was associated with slightly better 5-year overall survival and improved quality-adjusted life years [9]. Thus, on a population level, the benefits of MIS for the large majority of patients may outweigh the very small risk of disseminating occult malignancy in very few patients. This brings into consideration the key medical principle of "primum non nocere" or non-maleficence. The conflict regarding power morcellation highlights the juxtaposition of utilitarianism and non-maleficence, emphasizing the need to develop procedural techniques to provide safe MIS options for women with enlarged uteri.

Our cohort of patients with leiomyoma and uterine malignancy represents the largest published series of patients undergoing contained uterine morcellation to date. Contained uterine hand morcellation within a

**Table 3** Uterine cancer characteristics, adjuvant therapy and disease status

| Characteristic | Uterine cancer (N = 53) |
|---|---|
| Pre-op Histology (n = 49) | |
| Endometrioid | 34 (69.4) |
| Serous | 6 (12.2) |
| Clear cell | 3 (6.1) |
| Carcinosarcoma | 3 (6.1) |
| Other/unspecified | 7 (14.3) |
| Post-op Histology | |
| Endometrioid | 40 (75.5) |
| Serous | 5 (9.4) |
| Clear cell | 1 (1.9) |
| Carcinosarcoma | 7 (13.2) |
| Grade | |
| 1 | 21 (39.6) |
| 2 | 15 (28.3) |
| 3 | 17 (32.1) |
| Stage | |
| IA | 28 (52.8) |
| IB[a] | 15 (28.3) |
| II | 1 (1.9) |
| IIIA | 2 (3.8) |
| IIIC1 | 3 (5.7) |
| IIIC2 | 2 (3.8) |
| IVB | 2 (3.8) |
| Lymph nodes | |
| Positive | 6 (11.32) |
| Negative | 29 (54.7) |
| Not collected | 18 (34.0) |
| Pelvic Washings | |
| Positive | 5 (9.4) |
| Negative | 41 (77.4) |
| Indeterminate/suspicious | 6 (11.3) |
| Not collected | 1 (1.9) |
| Adjuvant Therapy[b] | |
| Radiation | 13 (24.5) |
| Chemotherapy | 10 (18.9) |
| Hormonal | 4 (7.6) |
| Recurrence rate | 7 (13.2) |
| Median time to recurrence (days) | 395 [range 128–539] |

**Table 3** Uterine cancer characteristics, adjuvant therapy and disease status (Continued)

| Characteristic | Uterine cancer (N = 53) |
|---|---|
| Status of disease | |
| No evidence of disease | 43 (81.1) |
| Alive with disease[c] | 3 (5.7) |
| Died of disease | 5 (9.4) |
| Died of intercurrent disease | 1 (1.9) |
| Died of unknown cause[d] | 1 (1.9) |

Data are n(%) unless otherwise specified
[a]Depth of invasion could not be determined in one case and is included in the Stage 1B group
[b]Chemotherapy: Carboplatin/Taxol (6), Carboplatin/Taxol + Cisplatin (with radiation) (1), Carboplatin/Taxol + Doxil (1); Ifosfamide/Taxol (2). Radiation: vaginal brachytherapy (5), external beam radiation (4), IMRT (2), vaginal brachytherapy + external beam radiation (1). Hormonal: Megace (2), Megace + Tamoxifen (1), Megace + Anastrozole (1)
[c](1) IIIC-2, grade 2 endometrioid, disease-free survival 7.8 months (2) IA, grade 2 endometrioid, disease-free survival 13.2 months (3) IB, grade 3 endometrioid, disease-free survival 4.3 months
[d]Most likely this patient died of disease given her disease distribution with distant metastases

specimen bag appears to be a feasible technique based on our experience with a large group of patients undergoing minimally invasive hysterectomy for both benign and malignant uterine neoplasms. Our patient population was diverse with respect to uterine size, body mass index, previous abdominal surgeries and pelvic adhesions, and safe removal of the uterus was achieved with no intraoperative complications. The technique uses relatively low cost specimen bags and does not require additional advanced surgical skills. Furthermore, for patients with uterine cancer who require adjuvant therapy, minimally invasive surgery allows for more rapid recovery with fewer wound complications leading to fewer delays in starting subsequent therapy. Further evaluation is needed to support our findings, particularly with respect to uterine cancer outcomes.

Multiple other studies have used similar techniques for contained uterine morcellation for both benign [10, 11] and malignant uterine neoplasms [12, 13]. Cohen et al. described power morcellation through a laparoscopic port site within a specimen bag for patients with leiomyoma (n = 73), demonstrating efficiency in operative time and no complications with a wide range of uterine sizes [10]. Favero et al. and Montella et al. have published small prospective case series (n = 30, 12 respectively) of patients with uterine cancer who underwent contained uterine hand morcellation through the vagina, both demonstrating the feasibility of the technique [12, 13]. Serur et al. described contained hand morcellation via an extended laparoscopic port site for patients with benign pathology [11]. Together, these studies and our findings indicate that contained uterine morcellation is

**Table 4** Clinicopathologic characteristics, adjuvant therapy, and survival outcomes of the deceased

| Stage, grade, histology | Uterine size (weeks) | Adjuvant therapy | Site of recurrence | Progression free survival (months) | Overall survival (months) | Death status |
|---|---|---|---|---|---|---|
| IA, 1 endometrioid | 14 | none | N/A | N/A | 51.2 | DICD (pulmonary disease) |
| IA, 2 endometrioid | 14 | none | carcinomatosis | 16.1 | 18.3 | DOD |
| IB carcinosarcoma | 12 | WPRT | RLQ mass | 8.3 | 10.7 | DOD |
| IIIA serous | Not recorded | Carboplatin/ Taxol IMRT | carcinomatosis | 14.1 | 17.4 | DOD |
| IIIC-1, 3 endometrioid | 13 | Carboplatin/ Taxol | Pulmonary, mediastinal | 18.0 | 30.6 | Unknown cause[a] |
| IIIC-2 serous | 15 | Carboplatin/ Taxol External beam pelvic radiation | N/A | N/A | 7.7 | DOD |
| IVB carcinosarcoma | 10 | none | carcinomatosis | 1.6 | 2.8 | DOD |

*WPRT* whole pelvic radiation therapy, *IMRT* intensity-modulate radiation therapy, *DOD* died of disease, *DICD* died of intercurrent disease
[a]Most likely this patient died of disease given her disease distribution with distant metastases

feasible with low rates of complications and conversion to laparotomy.

Different types of specimen bags were used in each study, demonstrating that specific specialty equipment is not required for this technique. Currently there are three FDA approved tissue retrieval devices (Applied Medical Specimen Retrieval System and Tissue Containment System (Rancho Santa Margarita, CA) and Cook LapSac Tissue Entrapment Pouch (Mudellein, IL)) [14]. These devices are approved to contain and isolate tissue during, or prior to, surgical removal and/or extracorporeal manual morcellation, but are contraindicated for use with powered cutting devices (power morcellators, electrosurgical and laser instruments). Solima et al. performed a prospective evaluation of the Endo Catch™ bag in 12 patients and revealed no gross rupture during morcellation, but identified four minimal ruptures using diluted methylene blue. These findings demonstrate concern over bag integrity and a potential route for tumor dissemination. Our study was retrospective and no specific integrity testing was performed on the bags before or after morcellation so unnoticed small spillage of tissue could have occurred.

In our series, none of the women who underwent laparoscopic hysterectomy and contained manual uterine morcellation for leiomyoma had an occult malignancy. In addition, we had no reports of postoperative intra-abdominal dissemination of benign uterine pathology including leiomyomatosis and endometriosis which have been described with an estimated prevalence of 0.5–1.2% following mechanical morcellation [5, 15–17]. During the time period of the study we did not routinely conduct preoperative testing such as endometrial biopsies or MRIs to assess for malignancy. Recent research efforts have focused on preoperative risk stratification of patients with

large leiomyoma considering minimally invasive surgery in order to correctly select appropriate candidates for laparoscopic hysterectomy. Known risk factors for uterine malignancy include older age, menopausal status, exposure to tamoxifen or radiation therapy and a history of certain hereditary cancer syndromes [18]. Past studies have shown that large uterine size [19, 20] and rapidly increasing uterine size [21] are not associated with an increased risk of uterine sarcoma. The International Society for Gynecologic Endoscopy (ISGE) identified black race, increasing age, ≥ 5 years tamoxifen use, hereditary leiomyomatosis and renal cell carcinoma (HLRCC), prior pelvic radiation, and personal history of childhood retinoblastoma as risk factors for sarcoma. The ISGE has published clear guidelines for preoperative evaluation and consent prior to hysterectomy for uterine leiomyoma. Using a retrospective cohort design, Ricci et al. demonstrated that young age is associated with very low risk of occult malignancy and no cases of leiomyosarcoma were identified among a cohort of reproductive age women [22]. A combined approach of preoperative risk stratification and contained uterine morcellation may allow gynecologic surgeons to offer a minimally-invasive approach to hysterectomy for the majority women with large uteri, while quelling fears of intra-abdominal dissemination of malignant tissue.

With regard to endometrial cancer, MIS became the standard surgical approach based on the initial experience reported by Walker et al. [2], which showed short-term advantages of laparoscopy compared to laparotomy, including shorter hospital stays, fewer perioperative complications, reduced blood loss, similar incidence of metastatic disease (17% of patients in both groups) and similar recurrence rates (11.4% in the laparoscopy group and 10.2% in the laparotomy group; hazard ratio for laparoscopy 1.14; 95% CI, 0.92 to 1.46) [23]. However, the study results were inconclusive because laparoscopy could not be demonstrated with 95% confidence to have a hazard ratio below the predetermined threshold of 1.4 for noninferiority [24]. While the study may have been underpowered to detect differences in survival between groups, particularly certain high-risk histologic subtypes, laparoscopy has become the dominant surgical approach for women with earlier stage endometrial cancer [23, 24]. Significant uterine enlargement that precluded a vaginal hysterectomy was an exclusion criterion for the LAP2 study. Therefore, the findings from LAP2 may not be generalizable to women with larger uteri or to the patients in our study who had enlarged uteri requiring morcellation. However, recent SEER data indicated that MIS hysterectomy was not associated with worse overall (HR, 0.89; 95% CI, 0.75–1.04) or cancer-specific (HR, 0.83; 95% CI, 0.59–1.16) mortality compared to abdominal hysterectomy [25].

Evaluation of survival outcomes in our study is difficult given that our sample size is small and heterogeneous, and follow-up time is limited. Overall five-year survival rates for women with endometrial cancer range widely based on stage of disease: stage IA, 88%; stage IB, 75%; stage II, 69%; stage IIIA, 58%; stage IIIB, 50%; stage IIIC, 47%; stage IVA, 17%; and stage IVB, 15% [26]. Many women with endometrial cancer who died in our study had advanced disease or aggressive histologic subtypes associated with worse survival (serous adenocarcinoma, carcinosarcoma, and grade 3 endometrioid adenocarcinoma). One patient with stage IA, grade 2 endometrioid carcinoma was diagnosed with carcinomatosis at the time of recurrence. Carcinomatosis is a pattern of recurrence that is concerning in the setting of morcellation. Intraperitoneal spillage was not reported during her initial surgery, but in general we suspect that gross spillage of tumor in the peritoneal cavity may worsen prognosis. While tumor spillage may occur during laparotomy, it may be more frequent during MIS where manipulation of the uterus through the vagina or into a bag for extraction is required. Montella et al. have reported short-term cancer outcomes for 12 endometrial cancer patients who underwent contained uterine morcellation [13]. All patients had grade 1 or 2 endometrioid adenocarcinoma. Nine patients had Stage IA, two had Stage 1B, and one had Stage IIIA disease. All were alive without evidence of recurrence at a median of 18 months of follow-up. Favero et al. had a median follow up of 20 months and reported 24-month survival of 74%. Four patients with metastatic nodal disease had died with distant metastasis [12]. In addition to concern of spreading malignant cells, morcellation raises new challenges in pathology interpretation of disrupted tissue specimens. [27] Pathologic evaluation of morcellated uteri is more challenging and there is a possibility that smaller uterine tumors were missed.

Strengths of this study include the relatively large sample size for describing a single surgical technique and the diversity of patients with respect to age, BMI, uterine size and pathology. Limitations include retrospective design, inability to identify all cases performed at the institution, lack of comparison group for outcomes, heterogeneity of tumor specimen retrieval bags and methodology for extraction, and short length of follow-up with respect to cancer-related outcomes. Additionally, hand morcellation can be a time-consuming process, particularly for large uteri. More research is needed to compare different techniques for specimen morcellation and extraction with respect to operative time and complications. The safety of power morcellation within a specimen bag should be further investigated as this particular technique has the potential to maximize efficiency while protecting against dissemination of tissue. Furthermore, the complexity of this technique may require more advanced training to ensure safety in the hands of novice users.

## Conclusions

Our initial results indicate that contained manual morcellation of uterine specimens is both feasible and safe from an intra-operative and immediate postoperative perspective for women with leiomyoma. Our study, however does not address the safety of the technique among the small number of women who are found to have leiomyosarcoma at the time of surgery. Further prospective research is needed to confirm the safety of FDA-approved specimen retrieval devices, to develop a systematic approach to preoperative risk stratification for patients considering MIS for large uterine neoplasms, and to assess this technique further in women with uterine malignancies to determine safety with respect to long-term oncologic outcomes.

**Abbreviations**
FDA: Food and Drug Administration; MIS: Minimally invasive surgery

**Acknowledgements**
None

**Funding**
This study was funded by the Duke University Department of Obstetrics & Gynecology.

**Authors' contributions**
SD designed the research study with guidance from AS. SD performed relevant literature review, chart review, data abstraction and analysis and the majority of the manuscript preparation. AL assisted with chart review to identify eligible subjects, as well as with literature review and manuscript editing. JE made significant contributions to manuscript preparation and editing include reference management. AS provided general mentorship to SD on all components of the project, with significant contributions to manuscript preparation and editing. All authors read and approved the final manuscript.

**Consent for publication**

Not applicable.

**Competing interests**

The authors declare that they have no competing interests.

**Author details**

[1]Department of Obstetrics and Gynecology, West Virginia University, 1 Medical Center Dr. PO Box 9186, HSC 4th floor, Morgantown, WV 26501-9186, USA. [2]Department of Obstetrics and Gynecology, Duke University Medical Center, Durham, NC 27710, USA. [3]Division of Gynecology Oncology, Department of Obstetrics and Gynecology, Duke Cancer Institute, Duke University Medical Center, Durham, NC 27710, USA.

**References**

1. Nieboer TE, Johnson N, Lethaby A, Tavender E, Curr E, Garry R, van Voorst S, Mol BW, Kluivers KB. Surgical approach to hysterectomy for benign gynaecological disease. Cochrane Database Syst Rev. 2009;(3):CD003677.
2. Walker JL, Piedmonte MR, Spirtos NM, Eisenkop SM, Schlaerth JB, Mannel RS, Spiegel G, Barakat R, Pearl ML, Sharma SK. Laparoscopy compared with laparotomy for comprehensive surgical staging of uterine cancer: gynecologic oncology group study LAP2. J Clin Oncol. 2009;27:5331–6.
3. Food and Drug Administration. Laparoscopic Uterine Power Morcellation in Hysterectomy and Myomectomy: FDA Safety Communication. 2014. Available at: http://wayback.archive-it.org/7993/20170722215731/https://www.fda.gov/MedicalDevices/Safety/AlertsandNotices/ucm393576.htm. Retrieved Mar 10, 2015.
4. Food and Drug Administration. UPDATED Laparoscopic uterine power Morcellation in hysterectomy and myomectomy: FDA safety communication. Silver Spring (MD):FDA; 2014. Available at: http://wayback.archive-it.org/7993/20170722215727/https://www.fda.gov/MedicalDevices/Safety/AlertsandNotices/ucm424443.htm. Retrieved Mar 10, 2015
5. Senapati S, Tu FF, Magrina JF. Power morcellators: a review of current practice and assessment of risk. Am J Obstet Gynecol. 2015;212:18–23.
6. Seidman MA, Oduyebo T, Muto MG, Crum CP, Nucci MR, Quade BJ. Peritoneal dissemination complicating morcellation of uterine mesenchymal neoplasms. PLoS One. 2012;7:e50058.
7. Kho KA, Nezhat CH. Evaluating the risks of electric uterine morcellation. JAMA. 2014;311:905–6.
8. Kornblith AB, Huang HQ, Walker JL, Spirtos NM, Rotmensch J, Cella D. Quality of life of patients with endometrial cancer undergoing laparoscopic international federation of gynecology and obstetrics staging compared with laparotomy: a gynecologic oncology group study. J Clin Oncol. 2009; 27:5337–42.
9. Siedhoff MT, Wheeler SB, Rutstein SE, Geller EJ, Doll KM, Wu JM, Clarke-Pearson DL. Laparoscopic hysterectomy with morcellation vs abdominal hysterectomy for presumed fibroid tumors in premenopausal women: a decision analysis. Am J Obstet Gynecol. 2015;212:e591–8.
10. Cohen SL, Einarsson JI, Wang KC, Brown D, Boruta D, Scheib SA, Fader AN, Shibley T. Contained power Morcellation within an insufflated isolation bag. Obstet Gynecol. 2014;124:491–7.
11. Serur E, Lakhi N. Laparoscopic hysterectomy with manual morcellation of the uterus An original technique that permits the safe and quick removal of a large uterus. Am J Obstet Gynecol. 2011;204:566–e562.
12. Favero G, Anton C, Silva e Silva A, Ribeiro A, Araujo MP, Miglino G, Baracat EC, Carvalho JP. Vaginal morcellation: a new strategy for large gynecological malignant tumor extraction: a pilot study. Gynecol Oncol. 2012;126:443–7.
13. Montella F, Riboni F, Cosma S, Dealberti D, Prigione S, Pisani C, Rovetta E. A safe method of vaginal longitudinal morcellation of bulky uterus with endometrial cancer in a bag at laparoscopy. Surg Endoscopy Other Interventional Techniques. 2014;28:1949–53.
14. Department of Health and Human Services, Food and Drug Administration. Section 510(k) premarket notification. 2014;K142427 (Applied Medical Tissue Containment System).
15. Bisceglia M, Galliani CA, Pizzolitto S, Ben-Dor D, Giannatempo G, Bergoli AL, Aieta M. Selected case from the Arkadi M. Rywlin international pathology slide series: Leiomyomatosis peritonealis disseminata: report of 3 cases with extensive review of the literature. Adv Anat Pathol. 2014;21:201–15.
16. Park BJ, Kim YW, Maeng LS, Kim TE. Disseminated peritoneal leiomyomatosis after hysterectomy: a case report. J Reprod Med. 2011;56: 456–60.
17. Ramos A, Fader AN, Roche KL. Surgical cytoreduction for disseminated benign disease after open power uterine morcellation. Obstet Gynecol. 2015;125:99–102.
18. Power morcellation and occult malignancy in gynecologic surgery. A special report. Washington, DC: American College of Obstetricians and Gynecologists; 2014.
19. Giuntoli RL, Metzinger DS, DiMarco CS, Cha SS, Sloan JA, Keeney GL, Gostout BS. Retrospective review of 208 patients with leiomyosarcoma of the uterus: prognostic indicators, surgical management, and adjuvant therapy. Gynecol Oncol. 2003;89:460–9.
20. West S, Ruiz R, Parker WH. Abdominal myomectomy in women with very large uterine size. Fertil Steril. 2006;85:36–9.
21. Parker WH, Fu YS, Berek JS. Uterine sarcoma in patients operated on for presumed leiomyoma and rapidly growing leiomyoma. Obstet Gynecol. 1994;83:414–8.
22. Ricci S, Angarita A, Cholakian D, Ramos A, Sinno AK, Long KC, Tanner EJ, Stone RL, Levinson K, Fader AN. Preoperative patient stratification results in low rates of occult uterine malignancy in women undergoing uterine surgery and morcellation. Gynecol Oncol. 2015;137:11–2.
23. Walker JL, Piedmonte MR, Spirtos NM, Eisenkop SM, Schlaerth JB, Mannel RS, Barakat R, Pearl ML, Sharma SK. Recurrence and survival after random assignment to laparoscopy versus laparotomy for comprehensive surgical staging of uterine cancer: gynecologic oncology group LAP2 study. J Clin Oncol. 2012;30:695–700.
24. Berchuck A, Alvarez Secord A, Havrilesky LJ. Minimally invasive surgery for endometrial cancer: the horse is already out of the barn. Proc Am Soc Clin Oncol. 2012;30(7):681–2.
25. Wright JD, Herzog TJ, Neugut AI, Burke WM, Lu YS, Lewin SN, Hershman DL. Comparative effectiveness of minimally invasive and abdominal radical hysterectomy for cervical cancer. Gynecol Oncol. 2012;127:11–7.
26. AJCC Cancer Staging Manual (8th edition). Springer International Publishing: American Joint Commission on Cancer; 2017.
27. Rivard C, Salhadar A, Kenton K. New challenges in detecting, grading, and staging endometrial cancer after uterine morcellation. J Minim Invasive Gynecol. 2012;19:313–6.

# 26

# EZH2 inhibition in *ARID1A* mutated clear cell and endometrioid ovarian and endometrioid endometrial cancers

Jill K. Alldredge[1] and Ramez N. Eskander[2*]

## Abstract

Clear cell carcinoma and endometrioid adenocarcinoma are histologic subtypes of ovarian and uterine cancer that demonstrate unique clinical behavior but share common underlying genomic aberrations and oncogenic pathways. *ARID1A* mutations are more frequently identified in these tumors, in comparison to other gynecologic histologies, and loss of *ARID1A* tumor suppressor function is thought to be an essential component of carcinogenic transformation. Several therapeutic targets in *ARID1A* mutated cancers are in development, including EZH2 inhibitors. EZH2 facilitates epigenetic methylation to modulate gene expression, and both uterine and ovarian cancers show evidence of EZH2 over expression. EZH2 inhibition in *ARID1A* mutated tumors acts in a synthetically lethal manner to suppress cell growth and promote apoptosis, revealing a unique new therapeutic opportunity. Several phase 1 and 2 clinical trials of EZH2 inhibitors are ongoing currently and there is considerable promise in translational trials for utilization of this new targeted therapy, both to capitalize on *ARID1A* loss of function and to increase sensitivity to platinum-based adjuvant chemotherapies. This review will synthesize the molecular carcinogenesis of these malignancies and their unique clinical behavior, as a foundation for an emerging frontier of targeted therapeutics – the synergistic inhibition of EZH2 in *ARID1A* mutated cancers.

**Keywords:** ARID1A, EZH2, Targeted therapy, Molecular carcinogenesis, Synthetic lethality

## Introduction

Ovarian and uterine cancer represent gynecologic malignancies with significant morbidity and mortality in the advanced and recurrent settings. Clear cell carcinoma (CCC) and endometrioid adenocarcinoma are histologic subtypes of both ovarian and uterine cancer that demonstrate unique clinical behavior, although emerging literature suggests that they may share underlying genomic aberrations and oncogenic pathways. This review explores the evolving paradigm of targeted therapeutics, as the understanding of the pathogenesis of these cancers becomes paramount to exploring new therapeutic frontiers and achieving improved oncologic outcomes.

## Low grade endometrioid and clear cell uterine carcinoma

Endometrial cancer is the most common gynecologic malignancy, with 61,380 estimated new cases and 10,920 estimated deaths in 2017 [1]. Approximately 75% of women are diagnosed with stage I disease, confined to the uterus, and have excellent 5-year survival [2]. While the majority of patients are diagnosed with well differentiated, International Federation of Gynecology and Obstetrics (FIGO) grade 1 and 2 endometrioid adenocarcinoma, a subset of patients have estrogen-independent histologies, including grade 3 endometrioid adenocarcinoma, serous carcinoma, clear cell carcinoma, carcinosarcoma, uterine sarcomas and undifferentiated cell types.

Clear cell endometrial carcinoma is rare, accounting for 1–6% of all endometrial cancers. Endometrial CCC is more likely to present with extra-uterine spread compared to low grade endometrioid histologies and is an independent predictor of poor prognosis. The proportion of patients with FIGO stage III-IV disease at the time of diagnosis is 36% with a 5-year disease specific

* Correspondence: reskander@ucsd.edu
[2]University of California, San Diego Moores Cancer Center, 3855 Health Sciences Drive, La Jolla, CA 92029-S0987, USA
Full list of author information is available at the end of the article

survival of 68% [2]. Given its rarity, optimal management strategies are not well defined and treatment is extrapolated from large studies primarily comprised of the more common endometrioid histology. Management of endometrial CCC includes comprehensive surgical staging and typically adjuvant platinum-based chemotherapy and/or radiotherapy.

## Endometrioid and clear cell ovarian carcinoma

Ovarian cancer, while less common than uterine cancer, is generally diagnosed at a more advanced stage, resulting in compromised long term outcomes, with an estimated 5-year survival of 46%. In 2017 there were an estimated 22, 440 new cases and 14, 080 deaths [1]. Ovarian cancers are broadly categorized by origin, into epithelial and non-epithelial neoplasms. The most common epithelial histology, high grade serous carcinoma, accounts for nearly 70% of ovarian cancers, and is disproportionately represented in clinical trials exploring novel therapeutic paradigms. In addition to high grade serous histology, epithelial ovarian cancers include endometrioid, clear cell, mucinous, carcinosarcoma, mixed epithelial and undifferentiated.

Ovarian endometrioid carcinoma accounts for approximately 10% of epithelial ovarian cancers. Clinically, these often present with disease confined to the pelvis, may be bilateral in up to 28% of cases, and are generally low grade and early stage, portending a more favorable prognosis when compared to high grade serous carcinoma [3]. Approximately 20% of patients with ovarian endometrioid carcinomas will also have simultaneous endometrial adenocarcinomas, and both histologies are thought to share molecular aberrations [4, 5]. Furthermore, endometriosis is highly prevalent in patients with endometrioid ovarian cancer, reported in up to 35.9% of cases [6]. Management paradigms are analogous to the more common high grade serous histology, and include surgical cytoreduction followed by adjuvant platinum based combination chemotherapy [7].

Ovarian CCC constitutes approximately 5–10% of all ovarian malignancies. Although commonly identified at an early stage, with ovarian confined disease, patients may be diagnosed with advanced stage disease, or suffer recurrence, both of which are difficult to treat given the relative resistance of this histology to standard chemotherapy [8]. When compared to high grade serous carcinoma, stage-for-stage survival is lower in patients with ovarian CCC [8]. As discussed above, treatment is dependent on surgical cytoreduction followed by combination platinum-based cytotoxic chemotherapy for patients with stage 1C or greater disease.

Given the rarity of these histologies as well as their unique characteristics, additional therapeutic strategies are urgently needed to improve survival in patients suffering from advanced stage or recurrent endometrioid and clear cell ovarian cancer.

## Review
### What is ARID1A?

Gene expression relies on the complex interplay of transcription factors, cofactors and chromatin regulators. The role of transcription dysregulation as a mechanism for cancer is well established. With the emergence of genome-wide analyses, the significant role of chromatin remodeling complexes on gene expression levels through modified transcription, replication, repair, recombination and methylation of DNA has been identified [9]. One such complex is the Switch/Sucrose Non-Fermentable (SWI/SNF) complex which is involved in activation and inhibition of transcription. The SWI/SNF complex plays a unique role in carcinogenesis and may be mutated in over 20% of human cancers [10]. *ARID1A*, an acronym for the gene AT-rich interacting domain-containing protein 1A, encodes a component of the SWI/SNF complex and has high mutation rates across multiple malignancies [11]. Mutations are typically frameshift or nonsense mutations, often occurring at either the nuclear-export signal sequence or at the *ARID1A* interaction site with the SWI/SNF complex resulting in protein complex instability [12]. This complex modifies expression of multiple genes, including p53, through direct interaction, SMAD3, CDKN1A (p21), MLH1 and PIK3IP1 through transcription regulation of downstream effectors, and transformation of cells through the PI3K/AKT pathway [13].

### ARID1A as a tumor suppressor gene

*ARID1A* mutations typically results in loss of protein function with implications for cell proliferation, differentiation and apoptosis – essential roles of a tumor suppressor gene. Initial efforts into understanding its role in tumorigenesis began approximately a decade ago. The knockout of *ARID1A* in embryonic stem cells resulted in loss of self-renewal properties and substantially modified cellular differentiation [14]. In *ARID1A* knockout leukemia cell populations, Fas-mediated cell death is inhibited, supporting altered apoptosis [11, 15]. In 2011, Guan et al. restored wild-type *ARID1A* expression in ovarian cancer cells harboring deleterious mutations and noted reactivation of protein function. Additional work by Guan et al. in 2014 utilizing xenograft models confirmed that silencing *ARID1A* expression in nontransformed cells promoted cellular proliferation [13, 16]. These cumulative efforts were essential in establishing the role of *ARID1A* as a tumor suppressor gene.

### ARID1A in ovarian cancers

As the molecular characterization of solid malignancies expanded, it became evident that *ARID1A* mutations were most pronounced in gynecologic cancers. Within ovarian cancer cohorts, mutation rates of 46–57% were identified in clear cell adenocarcinoma and 30% in endometrioid adenocarcinoma [17, 18]. This is contrasted with the absence of identifiable *ARID1A* mutations in high-grade serous carcinomas.

Endometrioid and clear cell ovarian carcinomas are uniquely associated with endometriosis, and have been recently referred to as endometriosis-associated ovarian cancer (EAOC). Between 14 and 42% of endometrioid and 20–36% of clear cell carcinomas are associated with endometriotic lesions or patient reported symptoms of endometriosis [6, 19]. Common genetic alterations, particularly in *ARID1A*, have been recognized within atypical endometriosis and adenocarcinoma, suggesting a significant carcinogenic role [20, 21]. Loss of *ARID1A* is more frequent in endometriosis associated neoplasms, with loss of *ARID1A* immunohistochemical expression in 61% of endometriosis associated clear cell carcinomas [22]. While it is unclear if *ARID1A* mutations alone are sufficient to induce cancer progression, concurrent mutations in alternate pathways, including the PI3K/AKT pathway are frequent and appear to occur simultaneously to facilitate tumorigenesis [22, 23].

### ARID1A in endometrial cancers

*ARID1A* mutations are also found frequently among women with endometrial cancers, with mutation frequency of 40% in uterine endometrioid adenocarcinoma [24]. Low grade endometrioid carcinoma is the most predominant histology, with 29% of grade 1 and 2 tumors showing loss of expression, in contrast to 39% with grade 3 tumors, 26% of uterine clear cell carcinomas, and 18% of uterine serous carcinomas [25]. The Cancer Genome Atlas further confirmed that *ARID1A* is mutated in a high proportion of type I uterine cancers, particularly in the POLE hypermutated, microsatellite unstable (MSI) hypermutated, and copy-number low subgroups. These often occurred concurrently with inactivating PTEN mutations [26].

### ARID1A as a biomarker

Given the heterogeneity of gynecologic cancers, a consistent relationship between the presence of an *ARID1A* mutation and prognosis has been elusive. In a 2015 meta-analysis of 5651 patients with a variety of tumor types, *ARID1A* was evaluated via genetic analysis and immunohistochemistry with findings that *ARID1A* deficient tumors had significantly increased cancer-specific mortality (HR = 2.55) and cancer recurrence (HR = 1.93) when compared to a matched *ARID1A* positive population [27]. Conversely, in patient cohorts with high grade endometrioid and clear cell endometrial cancer, *ARID1A* mutations were not associated with clinical stage, depth

of myometrial invasion, lymph node metastasis, or overall survival [28–30]. In a separate study, Yokoyama et al. found that *ARID1A* expression levels using immunohistochemistry correlated with prognosis and chemoresistance in stage III and IV epithelial ovarian cancers. Women with low *ARID1A* expression more frequently had incomplete response to chemotherapy ($p = 0.026$) and were more likely to experience relapse after achieving a complete response ($p = 0.07$). *ARID1A*-negative tumors had significantly worse progression free survival than *ARID1A*-positive tumors [31]. Additionally, Itamochi et al. confirmed an association between *ARID1A* immunohistochemical expression and FIGO stage as well as prognosis, with stage I and II patients having 91% 5-year survival with normal *ARID1A* expression and 74% 5-year survival with negative *ARID1A* expression [32] (Fig. 1).

### Potential molecular therapeutic targets in *ARID1A* mutated cancers

Loss of *ARID1A* function facilitates tumorigenesis through its chromatin-mediated dysregulation of gene expression and loss of tumor suppressor gene function. As *ARID1A* plays an integral role in cell-cycle control and DNA damage repair pathways, the loss of *ARID1A* function with concurrent dysfunction in p53, p21, MLH1, or the PI3K/AKT/mTOR pathway allow malignant progression, and have revealed several potential therapeutic targets in *ARID1A* mutated cancers. These are detailed in Table 1 and Fig. 2 and several are being actively investigated for the treatment of epithelial ovarian cancer.

### The role of EZH2 in cancer

Functional studies of ovarian cancer cell lines reveal numerous gene targets of the SWI/SNF complex which may be impacted by *ARID1A* mutation, including cyclins, c-myc, and the Polycomb complexes [33, 34]. The enhancer of zeste homolog 2 (EZH2) protein is the enzymatically active core of the polycomb repressive complex 2/3 (PRC2), responsible for trimethylation of lysine 27 of histone H3 (H3K27) and can induce gene suppression through promoter binding [35, 36]. EZH2 plays a role in cancer progression through several mechanisms, including gain-of-function and loss-of-function mutations, overexpression of EZH2, mutations in the H3K27 demethylase gene, and through antagonistic mutations in the SWI/SNF chromatin remodeling complex. Within the gynecologic cancer arena, the predominant mechanisms are EZH2 overexpression and SWI/SNF antagonism of the Polycomb complex. EZH2 overexpression manifests through histone hypermethylation, resulting in tumor proliferation, cell cycle dysregulation, metastatic spread, and angiogenesis [37–39].

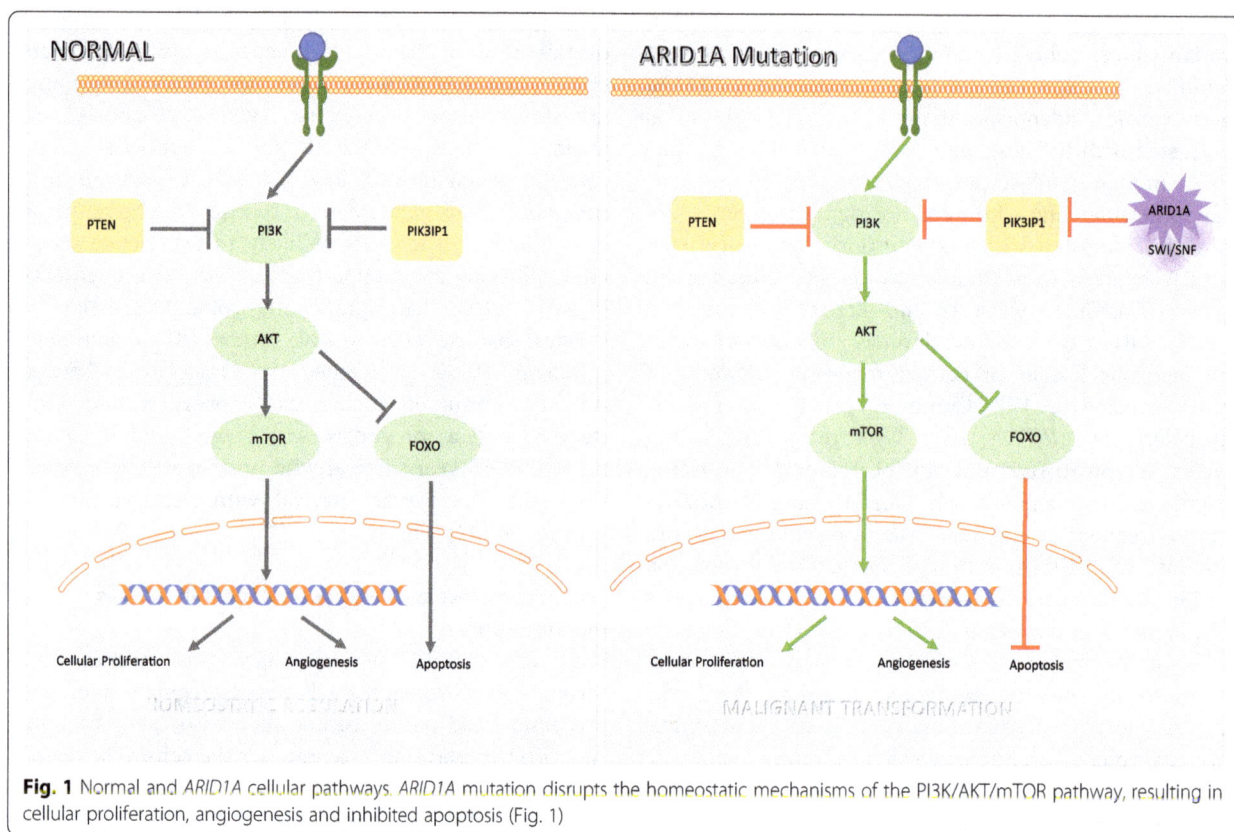

**Fig. 1** Normal and *ARID1A* cellular pathways. *ARID1A* mutation disrupts the homeostatic mechanisms of the PI3K/AKT/mTOR pathway, resulting in cellular proliferation, angiogenesis and inhibited apoptosis (Fig. 1)

**Table 1** Therapeutic targets being explored in *ARID1A* mutated cancers

| | | | |
|---|---|---|---|
| EZH-2 | Epigenetic synthetic lethality, promotion of apoptosis | GSK126 | [33, 34] |
| | PIK3IP1 mediated inhibition of PI3K/AKT pathway | | |
| mTOR | Inhibition of downstream regulator of PI3K/AKT pathway | Temsirolimus | [35, 36] |
| | | Ridaforolimuus | |
| | | Everolimus | |
| | | AP23573 | |
| TP53 | Stabilization of wild-type p53 to overcome ARID1A loss, resume tumor suppressor function | Nutlin 3 | [13, 37] |
| PI3K/AKT | Inhibit upregulated AKT phosphorylation caused by concurrent mutations | Sorafenib | [38, 39] |
| | | Copanlisib | [36] |
| | | BKM120 | |
| | | XL147 | |
| BRCA | Enhance DNA-damaging effects of platinum chemotherapies EZH2 modulated function of BRCA1 | | [40, 41] |
| ARID1B | Inhibition of residual AWI/SNF complex to suppress cell growth | | [42, 43] |
| Anti-IL6 | Inhibit inflammatory microenvironment and escape from anti-tumor immune response | | [44] |

## EZH2 in ovarian cancers

EZH2 overexpression is found in 50–85% of ovarian carcinomas, with high expression correlating with high grade, more advanced stage disease and poor survival [40, 41]. EZH2 plays an integral role in cellular proliferation, apoptosis and invasion in human epithelial ovarian cancer cell lines ([39, 42]. EZH2 is often overexpressed in ovarian clear cell carcinomas [42]. Additionally, these tumors are characterized by genomic instability and thus, epigenetic modification of gene expression may play a critical role in tumorigenesis.

## EZH2 in uterine cancers

EZH2 targets genes which may exhibit modified function in endometrial cancer including: p16, E-cadherin, SFRP1, DKK3, and β-catenin [43–45]. EZH2 overexpression was identified in complex hyperplasia, atypical hyperplasia, and endometrial carcinoma but not in simple hyperplasia or normal endometrial tissue [45]. Overexpression has been associated with high proliferation rates and aggressive tumor subgroups of endometrial cancers ([43, 44]). EZH2 expression correlated with high tumor grade, deep myometrial invasion, lymphovascular space invasion and enhanced cellular proliferation, as well as decreased overall survival, suggesting a role as both a prognostic and therapeutic marker in endometrial cancer [44–46].

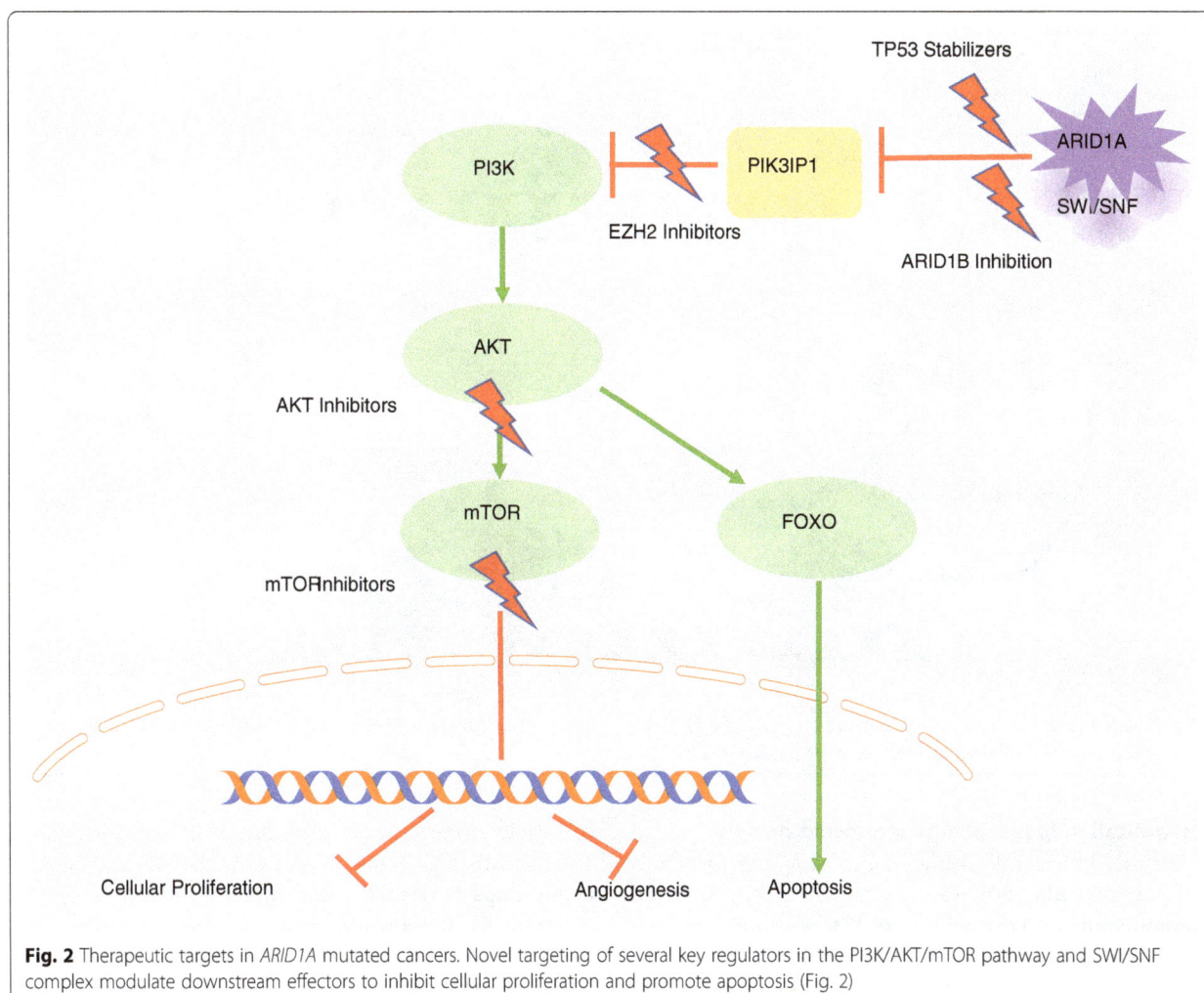

**Fig. 2** Therapeutic targets in *ARID1A* mutated cancers. Novel targeting of several key regulators in the PI3K/AKT/mTOR pathway and SWI/SNF complex modulate downstream effectors to inhibit cellular proliferation and promote apoptosis (Fig. 2)

## Synthetic lethality

Given the reversible epigenetic modifications which drive tumorigenesis, EZH2 methyltransferase activity is an ideal target for cancer therapeutics. Several new selective small molecules targeting EZH2 have been developed, including GSK126 [47], EPZ005687 [48] and EI1 [49], all of which inhibit EZH2 without otherwise effecting the PCR2 complex.

Homeostasis requires balanced action of *ARID1A* and EZH2 through chromatin-mediated gene expression. Loss of *ARID1A* expression results in imbalanced EZH2 activity, and is hypothesized to drive tumorigenesis (Figs. 3 and 4). Mechanistically, both *ARID1A* and EZH2 target PI3K-interacting protein 1 gene (PIK3IP1), with resultant silencing causing cell proliferation and promotion of anti-apoptotic effects through the PI3K-AKT pathway. In a pivotal study by Bitler et al., it was demonstrated that targeted EZH2 inhibition triggers apoptosis in *ARID1A* mutated cells and upregulates PIK3IP1 expression, thereby suppressing cell growth [50]. This cooperation of *ARID1A* mutation and EZH2 targeted

inhibition represents a synthetically lethal interaction. This is particularly exciting in that drug-gene synthetic lethality often allows utilization of low concentrations of drugs, minimal toxicity, and limited treatment resistance (Table 2).

## EZH2 targeted therapeutics

GSK126 was shown to be well tolerated in mouse xenograft models of ovarian CCC [47]. Of numerous available targeted small molecules, GSK126 exhibited the highest sensitivity against *ARID1A* deficient ovarian CCC cells [50]. Bitler et al. showed that GSK126 significantly decreased tumor burden and reduced the number of metastatic peritoneal tumor implants in a mouse clear cell ovarian xenograft model when compared to controls. On a mechanistic level, immunohistochemical analysis showed decreased H3K27Me3 levels, increased PIK3IP1 activity, as well as cleaved caspase 3 in the GSK126 treated mice. This further confirmed the PIK3PI1 shared gene target, allowing synthetic lethality in *ARID1A*-deficient tumors via EZH2 inhibition [50].

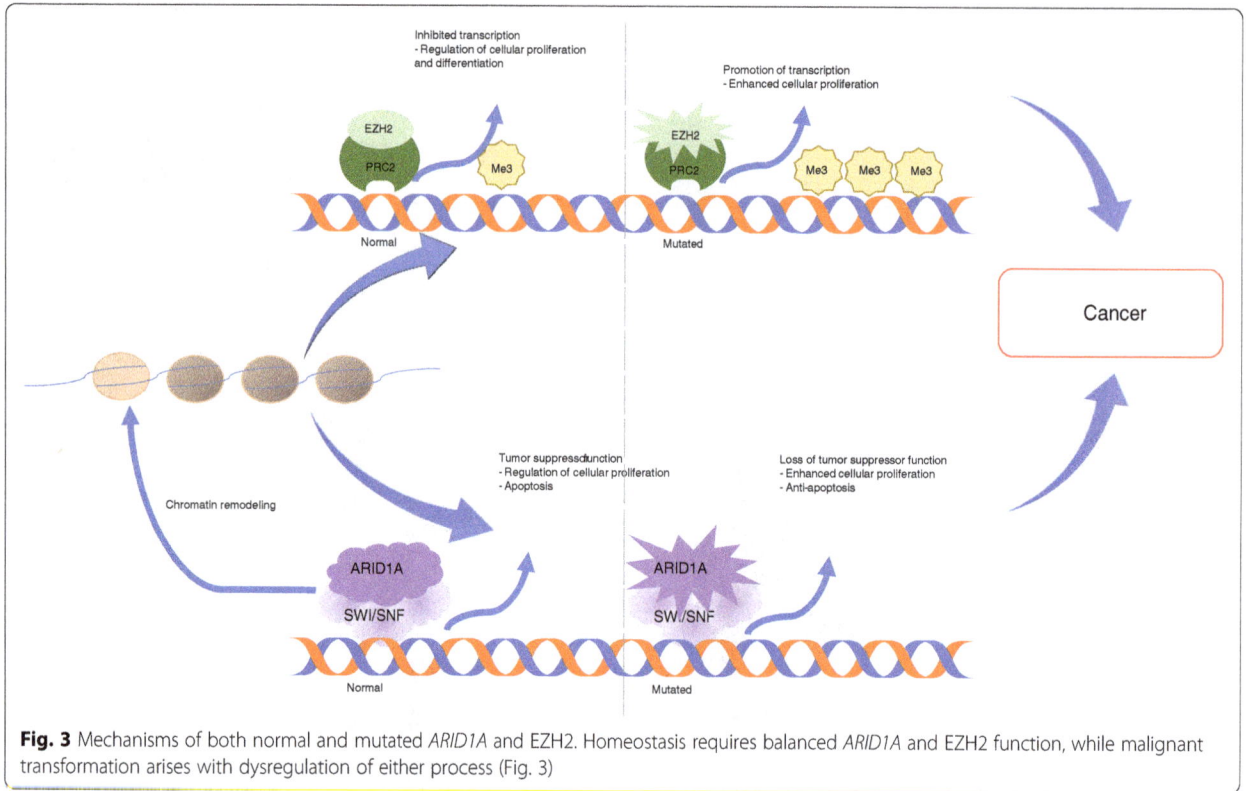

**Fig. 3** Mechanisms of both normal and mutated *ARID1A* and EZH2. Homeostasis requires balanced *ARID1A* and EZH2 function, while malignant transformation arises with dysregulation of either process (Fig. 3)

## Resensitization to platinum based chemotherapies

In advanced clear cell ovarian carcinoma, approximately half of patients progress while on platinum-based chemotherapy, in comparison to 29% of those with high grade serous histology. Additionally, patients with advanced stage clear cell carcinoma have compromised survival outcomes, with a median overall survival overall of approximately 12 months, significantly less than those with high grade serous histology [51]. This compromised outcome in patients with clear cell carcinoma is thought

to result from relative platinum resistance, and thus mechanisms to increase platinum sensitivity may significantly impact morbidity and mortality in this subset of patients. EZH2 downregulation in ovarian cancer has been shown to sensitize tumor cells to cisplatin and EZH2 overexpression is associated with resistance to cisplatin through H3K27 tri-methylation of drug-resistance genes [52, 53].

Translational research suggests that combination therapies utilizing platinum-based cytotoxic chemotherapy

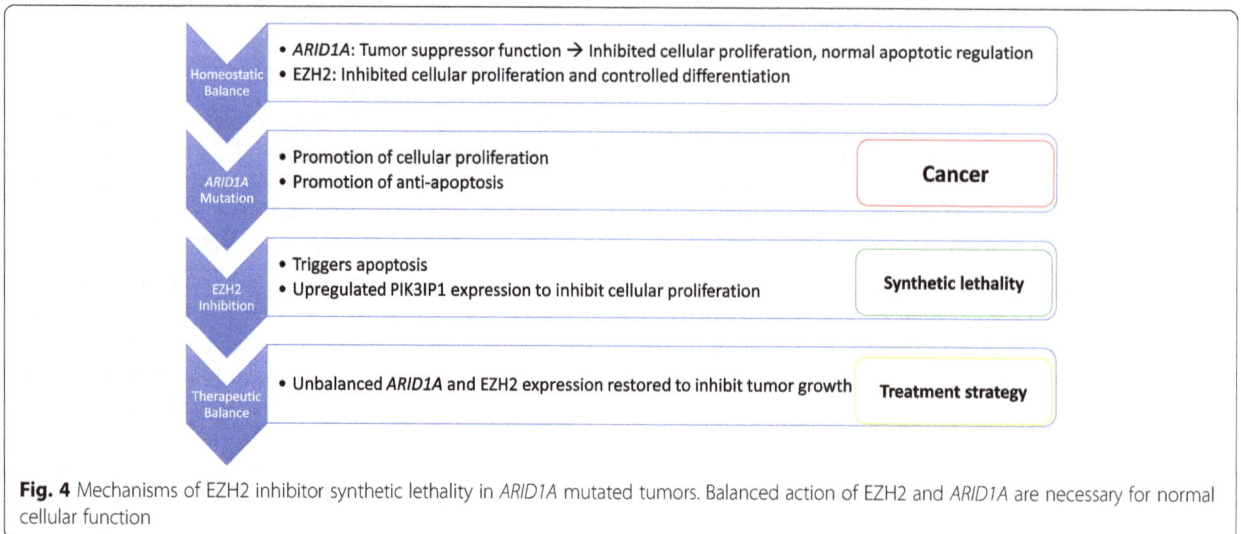

**Fig. 4** Mechanisms of EZH2 inhibitor synthetic lethality in *ARID1A* mutated tumors. Balanced action of EZH2 and *ARID1A* are necessary for normal cellular function

**Table 2** Ongoing EZH2 targeted clinical trials

| Targeted Agent | Trade Name | Route | Trial | Tumor | Status/Adverse Events (Grade 3–4) | References |
|---|---|---|---|---|---|---|
| EPZ-6438 | Tazemetostat | PO | Phase 1 | NHL | Thrombocytopenia Neutropenia Hypertension Anorexia Transaminitis | [58] |
| | | PO | Phase 1/2 | B-cell lymphoma or advanced solid tumor | Recruiting actively NCT01897571 Nausea Asthenia Thrombocytopenia Neutropenia Fatigue | (Clinicaltrials.Gov. (2.13.2017)), (Epizyme pharmaceuticals website. (2.13.2017)) |
| | | PO | Phase 1 | Pediatric INI1 negative tumors or synovial sarcoma | Recruiting actively NCT02601937 | (Clinicaltrials.Gov. (2.13.2017)), (Epizyme pharmaceuticals website. (2.13.2017)) |
| | | PO | Phase 2 | Adult INI1 negative tumors or synovial sarcoma | Recruiting actively NCT02601950 | (Clinicaltrials.Gov. (2.13.2017)), (Epizyme pharmaceuticals website. (2.13.2017)) |
| | | PO | Phase 2 | Malignant mesothelioma | Recruiting actively NCT02860286 | (Clinicaltrials.Gov. (2.13.2017)), (Epizyme pharmaceuticals website. (2.13.2017)) |
| GSK 2,816,126 | GSK126 | IV | Phase 1/2 | Diffuse large B-cell lymphoma | Fatigue Nausea Vomiting Anemia | [59] |
| EPZ-5676 | Pinometostat | IV | Phase 1 | Leukemia | Hypophosphatemia Neutropenia Reduced ejection fraction Transaminitis | [60] |
| CPI-1205 | | IV | Phase 1 | B cell lymphoma | Recruiting actively NCT02395601 | (Clinicaltrials.Gov. (2.13.2017)), |

and EZH2 inhibitors, may be particularly potent and synergistic in ARID1A mutated tumors [54]. Within non-Hodgkin's lymphoma tumors with EZH2 mutations, a combination of EPZ-6438 and traditional targeted chemotherapy prevented tumor growth [55]. Prostate cancer cell lines had increased tumor death when treated with combined etoposide and GSK126, again suggesting synergistic therapeutic effect [56]. Interestingly, EZH2 inhibition had varying effects in a preclinical study of non-small cell lung cancers, with increased sensitization to topoisomerase II inhibitors in the tumor subset demonstrating BRG1/SMARCA4 loss-of-function mutations or EGFR gain-of-function mutations [57]. These findings in non-gynecologic tumors provide a foundation for exploring the cooperative effects of chemotherapy and EZH2 inhibition within ovarian and uterine malignancies.

**Future directions**

The potential therapeutic role of EZH2 inhibition in *ARID1A* mutated gynecologic cancers may represent a novel and exciting treatment paradigm in a subset of patients with limited treatment options. Capitalizing on the concept of synthetic lethality induced in this population using EZH2 inhibitors, as well as the potential synergistic effects with platinum-based chemotherapies, may help translate into improved oncologic outcomes.

Given the frequency of *ARID1A* mutations in patients with clear cell and endometrioid ovarian and uterine cancer, and the prognostic implications of loss of *ARID1A* expression, it is natural to explore the impact of EZH2 inhibition in these patient subsets. Given the above, clinical trialists are currently designing a basket trial concept of the EZH2 inhibitor, Tazemetostat, in patients with recurrent, measurable, clear cell and endometrioid ovarian cancer, as well as recurrent endometrioid endometrial cancer. In this study, subjects with recurrent, measurable disease, will be enrolled and treated with single agent Tazemetostat at the recommended phase 2 dose of 800 mg orally twice daily until disease progression or unacceptable toxicity. *ARID1A* mutation status will be an integrated biomarker, and will be assessed via BAF250a IHC, as well as next generation sequencing, allowing investigators to determine the correlation between *ARID1A* mutation status and IHC expression. Furthermore, sequencing studies will facilitate assessment of the mutation status of all other SWI/SNF members.

Ultimately, if single agent regimens using EZH2 inhibitors are shown to be effective in this subset of patients, then novel combinatorial approaches utilizing platinum-based chemotherapy, TP53 stabilizers, PI3K/AKT inhibitors, or mTOR inhibitors may be warranted.

## Conclusions

In an effort to expand the therapeutic portfolio for patients with advanced stage and recurrent ovarian and endometrial cancer, molecular characterization of theses lesions has emerged as a clinical priority. Using both institutional genomic data, and data from the NCI sponsored cancer genome atlas, *ARID1A* mutations were frequently identified as mutated tumor suppressor genes, in clear cell and endometrioid ovarian cancer as well as low grade endometrioid endometrial cancer. Ultimately, clinicians will look to capitalize on this molecular aberration via novel targeted therapies, such as tazemetostat, as single agents or in combination regimens. As our understanding of the molecular mechanisms underlying malignant transformation evolves, the discovery of novel targeted therapies that lead to meaningful survival gains may become a reality.

### Abbreviations
ARID1A: AT-rich interacting domain-containing protein 1A; CCC: Clear cell carcinoma; EZH2: Enhancer of zeste homolog 2; FIGO: International Federation of Gynecology and Obstetrics; PRC2: Polycomb repressive complex 2/3; SWI/SNF: Switch/Sucrose Non-Fermentable

### Acknowledgements
Not applicable.

### Funding
This manuscript was supported by the Ruth L Kirschstein NRSA Institutional Training Research Grant, T32 CA06039611.

### Authors' contributions
Both JA and RE contributed to the literature review and manuscript preparation and editing. Both contributed to creation of novel figures and tables. Both authors read and approved the final manuscript.

### Consent for publication
Not applicable.

### Competing interests
The authors declare that they have no competing interests. RNE has served as a speaker and received honoraria from Genetech Roche, Clovis Oncology and AZ Oncology.

### Author details
[1]University of California, 101 The City Drive South Orange, Irvine, CA 92868, USA. [2]University of California, San Diego Moores Cancer Center, 3855 Health Sciences Drive, La Jolla, CA 92029-S0987, USA.

### References
1.  Siegel RL, Miller KD, Jemal A. Cancer statistics, 2017. CA Cancer J Clin. 2017;67:7–30.
2.  Institute, N.C. Surveillance, epidemiology and end results program. https://seer.cancer.gov/statfacts/
3.  Bouchard-Fortier G, Panzarella T, Rosen B, Chapman W, Gien LT. Endometrioid carcinoma of the ovary: outcomes compared to serous carcinoma after 10 years of follow-up. J Obstet Gynaecol Can. 2017;39:34–41.
4.  Zaino R, Whitney C, Brady MF, DeGeest K, Burger RA, Buller RE. Simultaneously detected endometrial and ovarian carcinomas–a prospective clinicopathologic study of 74 cases: a gynecologic oncology group study. Gynecol Oncol. 2001;83:355–62.
5.  Eifel P, Hendrickson M, Ross J, Ballon S, Martinez A, Kempson R. Simultaneous presentation of carcinoma involving the ovary and the uterine corpus. Cancer. 1982;50:163–70.
6.  Van Gorp T, Amant F, Neven P, Vergote I, Moerman P. Endometriosis and the development of malignant tumours of the pelvis. A review of literature. Best Pract Res Clin Obstet Gynaecol. 2004;18:349–71.
7.  Chen S, Leitao MM, Tornos C, Soslow RA. Invasion patterns in stage i endometrioid and mucinous ovarian carcinomas: a clinicopathologic analysis emphasizing favorable outcomes in carcinomas without destructive stromal invasion and the occasional malignant course of carcinomas with limited destructive stromal invasion. Mod Pathol. 2005;18:903–11.
8.  Sugiyama T, Kamura T, Kigawa J, Terakawa N, Kikuchi Y, Kita T, Suzuki M, Sato I, Taguchi K. Clinical characteristics of clear cell carcinoma of the ovary: a distinct histologic type with poor prognosis and resistance to platinum-based chemotherapy. Cancer. 2000;88:2584–9.
9.  Clapier CR, Cairns BR. The biology of chromatin remodeling complexes. Annu Rev Biochem. 2009;78:273–304.
10. Kadoch C, Hargreaves DC, Hodges C, Elias L, Ho L, Ranish J, Crabtree GR. Proteomic and bioinformatic analysis of mammalian swi/snf complexes identifies extensive roles in human malignancy. Nat Genet. 2013;45:592–601.
11. Lawrence MS, Stojanov P, Mermel CH, Robinson JT, Garraway LA, Golub TR, Meyerson M, Gabriel SB, Lander ES, Getz G. Discovery and saturation analysis of cancer genes across 21 tumour types. Nature. 2014;505:495–501.
12. Guan B, Gao M, Wu C-H, Wang T-L, Shih I-M. Functional analysis of in-frame indel arid1a mutations reveals new regulatory mechanisms of its tumor suppressor functions. Neoplasia. 2012;14:986–93.
13. Guan B, Wang TL, Shih Ie M. Arid1a, a factor that promotes formation of swi/snf-mediated chromatin remodeling, is a tumor suppressor in gynecologic cancers. Cancer Res. 2011;71:6718–27.
14. Gao X, Tate P, Hu P et al. Es cell pluripotency and germ-layer formation require the swi/snf chromatin remodeling componenet baf250a. Proc Natl Acad Sci U S A. 2008;105(18):6656-61.
15. Luo B, W.C. Cheung, Subramanian A et al. Highly parallel identification of essential genes in cancer cells. Proc Natl Acad Sci USA. 2008;105(51):20380-5.
16. Guan, B.; Rahmanto, Y.S.; Wu, R.C.; Wang, Y.; Wang, Z.; Wang, T.L.; Shih Ie, M. Roles of deletion of arid1a, a tumor suppressor, in mouse ovarian tumorigenesis. J Natl Cancer Inst. 2014;106(7).

17. Wiegand KC, Shah SP, Al-Agha OM, Zhao Y, Tse K, Zeng T, Senz J, McConechy MK, Anglesio MS, Kalloger SE, et al. Arid1a mutations in endometriosis-associated ovarian carcinomas. N Engl J Med. 2010;363:1532–43.

18. Jones S, Wang TL, Shih Ie M, Mao TL, Nakayama K, Roden R, Glas R, Slamon D, Diaz LA Jr, Vogelstein B, et al. Frequent mutations of chromatin remodeling gene arid1a in ovarian clear cell carcinoma. Science. 2010;330:228–31.

19. Pearce CL, Templeman C, Rossing MA, Lee A, Near AM, Webb PM, Nagle CM, Doherty JA, Cushing-Haugen KL, Wicklund KG, et al. Association between endometriosis and risk of histological subtypes of ovarian cancer: a pooled analysis of case–control studies. Lancet Oncol. 2012;13:385–94.

20. Chene G, Ouellet V, Rahimi K, Barres V, Provencher D, Mes-Masson AM. The arid1a pathway in ovarian clear cell and endometrioid carcinoma, contiguous endometriosis, and benign endometriosis. Int J Gynaecol Obstet. 2015;130:27–30.

21. Kobayrashi H. Molecular pathogenesis of endometriosis-associated clear cell carcinoma of the ovary (review). Oncol Rep. 2009;22(2):233-40.

22. Yamamoto S, Tsuda H, Takano M, Tamai S, Matsubara O. Loss of arid1a protein expression occurs as an early event in ovarian clear-cell carcinoma development and frequently coexists with pik3ca mutations. Mod Pathol. 2012;25:615–24.

23. Yamamoto S, Tsuda H, Takano M, Tamai S, Matsubara O. Pik3ca mutations and loss of arid1a protein expression are early events in the development of cystic ovarian clear cell adenocarcinoma. Virchows Arch. 2012;460:77–87.

24. Guan B, Mao TL, Panuganti PK, Kuhn E, Kurman RJ, Maeda D, Chen E, Jeng YM, Wang TL, Shih Ie M. Mutation and loss of expression of arid1a in uterine low-grade endometrioid carcinoma. Am J Surg Pathol. 2011;35:625–32.

25. Wiegand KC, Lee AF, Al-Agha OM, Chow C, Kalloger SE, Scott DW, Steidl C, Wiseman SM, Gascoyne RD, Gilks B, et al. Loss of baf250a (arid1a) is frequent in high-grade endometrial carcinomas. J Pathol. 2011;224:328–33.

26. Kandoth C, Schultz N, Cherniack AD, Akbani R, Liu Y, Shen H, Robertson AG, Pashtan I, Shen R, Benz CC, et al. Integrated genomic characterization of endometrial carcinoma. Nature. 2013;497:67–73.

27. Luchini C, Veronese N, Solmi M, Cho H, Kim JH, Chou A, Gill AJ, Faraj SF, Chaux A, Netto GJ, et al. Prognostic role and implications of mutation status of tumor suppressor gene arid1a in cancer: a systematic review and meta-analysis. Oncotarget. 2015;6:39088–97.

28. Zhang ZM, Xiao S, Sun GY, Liu YP, Zhang FH, Yang HF, Li J, Qiu HB, Liu Y, Zhang C, et al. The clinicopathologic significance of the loss of baf250a (arid1a) expression in endometrial carcinoma. Int J Gynecol Cancer. 2014;24:534–40.

29. Fadare O, Gwin K, Desouki MM, Crispens MA, Jones HW 3rd, Khabele D, Liang SX, Zheng W, Mohammed K, Hecht JL, et al. The clinicopathologic significance of p53 and baf-250a (arid1a) expression in clear cell carcinoma of the endometrium. Mod Pathol. 2013;26:1101–10.

30. Fadare O, Renshaw IL, Liang SX. Does the loss of arid1a (baf-250a) expression in endometrial clear cell carcinomas have any clinicopathologic significance? A pilot assessment. J Cancer. 2012;3:129–36.

31. Yokoyama Y, Matsushita Y, Shigeto T, Futagami M, Mizunuma H. Decreased arid1a expression is correlated with chemoresistance in epithelial ovarian cancer. J Gynecol Oncol. 2014;25:58–63.

32. Itamochi H, Oumi N, Oishi T, Shoji T, Fujiwara H, Sugiyama T, Suzuki M, Kigawa J, Harada T. Loss of arid1a expression is associated with poor prognosis in patients with stage i/ii clear cell carcinoma of the ovary. Int J Clin Oncol. 2015; 20:967–73.

33. Nagl NG Jr, Patsialou A, Haines DS, Dallas PB, Beck GR Jr, Moran E. The p270 (arid1a/smarcf1) subunit of mammalian swi/snf-related complexes is essential for normal cell cycle arrest. Cancer Res. 2005;65:9236–44.

34. Nagl NG Jr, Zweitzig DR, Thimmapaya B, Beck GR Jr, Moran E. The c-myc gene is a direct target of mammalian swi/snf-related complexes during differentiation-associated cell cycle arrest. Cancer Res. 2006;66:1289–93.

35. Yoo KH, Hennighausen L. Ezh2 methyltransferase and h3k27 methylation in breast cancer. Int J Biol Sci. 2012;8:59–65.

36. Cao R, Wang L, Wang H, Xia L, Erdjument-Bromage H, Tempst P, Jones RS, Zhang Y. Role of histone h3 lysine 27 methylation in polycomb-group silencing. Science. 2002;298:1039–43.

37. Choi JH, Song YS, Yoon JS, Song KW, Lee YY. Enhancer of zeste homolog 2 expression is associated with tumor cell proliferation and metastasis in gastric cancer. APMIS. 2010;118:196–202.

38. Fan T, Jiang S, Chung N, Alikhan A, Ni C, Lee CC, Hornyak TJ. Ezh2-dependent suppression of a cellular senescence phenotype in melanoma cells by inhibition of p21/cdkn1a expression. Mol Cancer Res. 2011;9:418–29.

39. Lu C, Han HD, Mangala LS, Ali-Fehmi R, Newton CS, Ozbun L, Armaiz-Pena GN, Hu W, Stone RL, Munkarah A, et al. Regulation of tumor angiogenesis by ezh2. Cancer Cell. 2010;18:185–97.

40. Rao ZY, Cai MY, Yang GF, He LR, Mai SJ, Hua WF, Liao YJ, Deng HX, Chen YC, Guan XY, et al. Ezh2 supports ovarian carcinoma cell invasion and/or metastasis via regulation of tgf-beta1 and is a predictor of outcome in ovarian carcinoma patients. Carcinogenesis. 2010;31:1576–83.

41. Guo J, Cai J, Yu L, Tang H, Chen C, Wang Z. Ezh2 regulates expression of p57 and contributes to progression of ovarian cancer in vitro and in vivo. Cancer Sci. 2011;102:530–9.

42. Li H, Cai Q, Godwin AK, Zhang R. Enhancer of zeste homolog 2 promotes the proliferation and invasion of epithelial ovarian cancer cells. Mol Cancer Res. 2010;8:1610–8.

43. Bachmann IM, Halvorsen OJ, Collett K, Stefansson IM, Straume O, Haukaas SA, Salvesen HB, Otte AP, Akslen LA. Ezh2 expression is associated with high proliferation rate and aggressive tumor subgroups in cutaneous melanoma and cancers of the endometrium, prostate, and breast. J Clin Oncol. 2006;24:268–73.

44. Eskander RN, Ji T, Huynh B, Wardeh R, Randall LM, Hoang B. Inhibition of enhancer of zeste homolog 2 (ezh2) expression is associated with decreased tumor cell proliferation, migration, and invasion in endometrial cancer cell lines. Int J Gynecol Cancer. 2013;23:997–1005.

45. Jia N, Li Q, Tao X, Wang J, Hua K, Feng W. Enhancer of zeste homolog 2 is involved in the proliferation of endometrial carcinoma. Oncol Lett. 2014;8:2049–54.

46. Zhou J, Roh JW, Bandyopadhyay S, Chen Z, Munkarah AR, Hussein Y, Alosh B, Jazaerly T, Hayek K, Semaan A, et al. Overexpression of enhancer of zeste homolog 2 (ezh2) and focal adhesion kinase (fak) in high grade endometrial carcinoma. Gynecol Oncol. 2013;128:344–8.

47. McCabe MT, Ott HM, Ganji G, Korenchuk S, Thompson C, Van Aller GS, Liu Y, Graves AP, Della Pietra A 3rd, Diaz E, et al. Ezh2 inhibition as a therapeutic strategy for lymphoma with ezh2-activating mutations. Nature. 2012;492:108–12.

48. Knutson SK, Wigle TJ, Warholic NM, Sneeringer CJ, Allain CJ, Klaus CR, Sacks JD, Raimondi A, Majer CR, Song J, et al. A selective inhibitor of ezh2 blocks h3k27 methylation and kills mutant lymphoma cells. Nat Chem Biol. 2012;8:890–6.

49. Qi W, Chan H, Teng L, Li L, Chuai S, Zhang R, Zeng J, Li M, Fan H, Lin Y, et al. Selective inhibition of ezh2 by a small molecule inhibitor blocks tumor cells proliferation. Proc Natl Acad Sci U S A. 2012;109:21360–5.

50. Bitler BG, Aird KM, Garipov A, Li H, Amatangelo M, Kossenkov AV, Schultz DC, Liu Q, Shih Ie M, Conejo-Garcia JR, et al. Synthetic lethality by targeting ezh2 methyltransferase activity in arid1a-mutated cancers. Nat Med. 2015;21:231–8.

51. Goff BA, Sainz de la Cuesta R, Muntz HG, Fleischhacker D, Ek M, Rice LW, Nikrui N, Tamimi HK, Cain JM, Greer BE, et al. Clear cell carcinoma of the ovary: a distinct histologic type with poor prognosis and resistance to platinum-based chemotherapy in stage iii disease. Gynecol Oncol. 1996;60:412–7.

52. Hu S, Yu L, Li Z, Shen Y, Wang J, Cai J, Xiao L, Wang Z. Overexpression of ezh2 contributes to acquired cisplatin resistance in ovarian cancer cells in vitro and in vivo. Cancer Biol Ther. 2010;10:788–95.

53. Li T, Cai J, Ding H, Xu L, Yang Q, Wang Z. Ezh2 participates in malignant biological behavior of epithelial ovarian cancer through regulating the expression of brca1. Cancer Biol Ther. 2014;15:271–8.

54. Kim KH, Roberts CW. Targeting ezh2 in cancer. Nat Med. 2016;22:128–34.

55. Knutson SK, Warholic NM, Johnston LD, Klaus CR, Wigle TJ, Iwanowicz D, Littlefield BA, Porter-Scott M, Smith JJ, Moyer MP, et al. Synergistic anti-tumor activity of ezh2 inhibitors and glucocorticoid receptor agonists in models of germinal center non-hodgkin lymphomas. PLoS One. 2014;9:e111840.

56. Kirk JS, Schaarschuch K, Dalimov Z, Lasorsa E, Ku S, Ramakrishnan S, Hu Q, Azabdaftari G, Wang J, Pili R, et al. Top2a identifies and provides epigenetic rationale for novel combination therapeutic strategies for aggressive prostate cancer. Oncotarget. 2015;6:3136–46.

57. Fillmore CM, Xu C, Desai PT, Berry JM, Rowbotham SP, Lin YJ, Zhang H, Marquez VE, Hammerman PS, Wong KK, et al. Ezh2 inhibition sensitizes brg1 and egfr mutant lung tumours to topoii inhibitors. Nature. 2015;520:239–42.

58. Vincent Ribrag, J.-C.S, Jean-Marie Michot, et al. Phase 1 study of tazemetostat (epz-6438), an inhibitor of enhancer of zeste-homolog 2 (ezh2): Preliminary safety and activity in relapsed or refractory nonhodgkin lymphoma (nhl) patients. Blood. 2015;126:473.

59. Timothy A Yap, J.N.W, John P. Leonard, et al. A phase i study of gsk2816126, an enhancer of zeste homolog 2(ezh2) inhibitor, in patients (pts) with relapsed/refractory diffuse large b-cell lymphoma (dlbcl), other non-hodgkin lymphomas (nhl), transformed follicular lymphoma (tfl), solid tumors and multiple myeloma (mm). Blood. 2016;128:4203.

60. Eytan M Stein, G.G.-M, David A Rizzieri et al. A phase 1 study of the dot1l inhibitor, pinometostat (epz-5676), in adults with relapsed or refractory leukemia: Safety, clinical activity, exposure and target inhibition. Blood.2015:126:2547.

# 27

# Multidisciplinary approach to manage antenatally suspected placenta percreta: updated algorithm and patient outcomes

Paula S. Lee[1,2,6*] [iD], Samantha Kempner[1], Michael Miller[4], Jennifer Dominguez[7], Chad Grotegut[1,3], Jessie Ehrisman[2], Rebecca Previs[1,2,6], Laura J. Havrilesky[1,2,6], Gloria Broadwater[5], Sarah C. Ellestad[1,3] and Angeles Alvarez Secord[1,2,6]

## Abstract

**Background:** Due to the significant morbidity and mortality associated with placenta percreta, alternative management options are needed. Beginning in 2005, our institution implemented a multidisciplinary strategy to patients with suspected placenta percreta. The purpose of this study is to present our current strategy, maternal morbidity and outcomes of patients treated by our approach.

**Methods:** From 2005 to 2014, a retrospective cohort study of patients with suspected placenta percreta at an academic tertiary care institution was performed. Treatment modalities included immediate hysterectomy at the time of cesarean section (CHYS), planned delayed hysterectomy (interval hysterectomy 6 weeks after delivery) (DH), and fertility sparing (uterine conservation) (FS). Prognostic factors of maternal morbidity were identified from medical records. Complications directly related to interventional procedures and DH was recorded. Descriptive statistics were utilized.

**Results:** Of the 21 patients with suspected placenta percreta, 7 underwent CHYS, 13 underwent DH, and 1 had FS with uterine preservation. Of the 20 cases that underwent hysterectomy, final pathology showed 11 increta, 7 percreta, and 2 inconclusive. 19/20 cases underwent interventional radiology (IR) procedures. Selective embolization was utilized in 14 cases (2/7 CHYS; 12/13 DH). The median time from cesarean section (CS) to DH was 41 [26–68] days. There were no cases of emergent hysterectomy, delayed hemorrhage, or sepsis in the DH group. Both estimated blood loss and number of packed red blood cell transfusions were significantly higher in the CHYS group. 3/21 cases required massive transfusion (2 CHYS, 1 FS) with median total blood product transfusion of 13 units [12–15]. The four IR-related complications occurred in the DH group. Incidence of postoperative complications was similar between both groups. Median hospital length of stay (LOS) after CHYS was 4 days [3–8] compared to DH cohort: 7 days [3–33] after CS and 4 days [1–10] after DH. The DH cohort had a higher rate of hospital readmission of 54% (7/13) compared to 14% (1/7) CHYS, most commonly due to pain. There were no maternal deaths.

**Conclusion:** This multidisciplinary strategy may appear feasible; however, further investigation is warranted to evaluate the effectiveness of alternative approaches to cesarean hysterectomy in cases of morbidly adherent placenta.

**Keywords:** Conservative management of placenta percreta, Delayed hysterectomy, Postpartum hemorrhage, Uterine artery embolization

* Correspondence: paula.s.lee@duke.edu
[1]Department of Obstetrics and Gynecology, Duke University Hospital, Durham, North Carolina 27710, USA
[2]Division of Gynecologic Oncology, Department of Obstetrics and Gynecology, Duke University Hospital, Durham, USA
Full list of author information is available at the end of the article

## Background

Placenta accreta includes various degrees of placental penetration into the myometrium that defines accreta, increta, and percreta. Placenta percreta is the most severe and least common form of placenta accreta (5–7% of cases) in which villi penetrate the entire myometrial thickness and reach or penetrate the serosa to involve adjacent organs. Although the specific incidence of placenta percreta is not known, the incidence of placenta accreta has risen over the past several decades likely due to the increasing cesarean delivery rate in this country, with a 10-fold increase in placenta accreta over the past 50 years [1]. By the year 2020, there are projected to be nearly nine-thousand cases of placenta accreta in the United States annually [2].

Abnormal placental attachment disorders are associated with a high rate of hemorrhage, coagulopathy, infection, urologic injury, and maternal death. The Society for Maternal-Fetal Medicine (SMFM) recognizes these risks and advocates that when clinical suspicion for placenta accreta exists, arrangements be made for delivery at an institution with appropriate expertise and facilities. Specifically, resources must be available for anticipated massive transfusion [3]. Despite advances in medical and surgical management of these patients, there continues to be an unacceptably high risk of maternal mortality, which is as high as 5.6% in women with placenta percreta [4].

There is no randomized study that evaluates cesarean hysterectomy compared to delayed hysterectomy (DH) in the setting of placenta accreta. Experience of delayed hysterectomy is obtained from case series of conservative approach to placenta accreta for women who desire fertility, whereby the placenta is left within the uterus, and *unplanned* hysterectomy is performed after cesarean delivery due to clinical deterioration [5, 6]. In the largest multicenter retrospective study of this conservative approach, 36/167 women required unplanned hysterectomy [7] 18/36 hysterectomies occurred within 24 h of delivery and all were the result of postpartum hemorrhage. The remaining 18 hysterectomies occurred after 24 h, with a median duration of 39 days (range 9–105 days). Reasons for delayed hysterectomy included hemorrhage, sepsis, uterine necrosis, vesicouterine fistula, arteriovenous malformation, and maternal request. Six percent (10/167 cases) had severe maternal morbidity with the most common causes due to sepsis and hemorrhage. There was one maternal death. Of these 10 severe morbidity cases, 8/10 underwent delayed hysterectomy and interestingly, the majority did not have severe placentation abnormality (only 2 percreta, 8 accretas). Of the 18/167 cases of percreta, severe maternal morbidity occurred in two. In these series, delayed hysterectomy was not planned since the primary intent was uterine conservation. Thus there is limited data on morbidity and outcomes related to *planned* delayed

hysterectomy after delivery. Given the potential morbidity associated with delayed hysterectomy, only the morbidly adherent cases with potential extrauterine organ involvement should be considered as candidates.

Beginning in 2005, our institution has developed an algorithm for patients with suspected placenta percreta that involves integral communication and planning between multiple specialties. Our management algorithm has evolved since our initial reported cases [8] based on patient outcomes and ongoing experience. The objective of this study is to present our current strategy, maternal morbidity and outcomes of patients treated by our multidisciplinary approach, with careful attention to morbidity associated with planned delayed hysterectomy.

## Methods

After the Duke University Health System Institutional Review Board granted approval, retrospective identification for women with placenta percreta was conducted through SNOMED (Systematized Nomenclature of Medicine) diagnostic retrieval of the Duke pathology database. The search terms "Accreta," "Increta," and "Percreta" were utilized. The ICD-9 codes for these diagnoses were also used as search terms within the D.E.D.U.C.E. (Duke Enterprise Data Unified Content Explorer), an on-line research tool (http://deduce.duhs.duke.edu). All patients scheduled for elective DH from 2005 to 2011 were identified from the Gynecologic Oncology and Maternal-Fetal Medicine (MFM) operative scheduling logs. From August 2011 to 2014, patients with antenatally suspected placenta percreta were consented to participate in a prospective abnormal placentation database at Duke University Medical Center. Patients were identified during initial consultation with the gynecologic oncologist. For this study, only patients with a suspected diagnosis of placenta percreta since 2005 were included for analysis, given our contemporary approach began at this time.

Medical records were extracted for type of surgery performed, anesthetic technique, interventional radiology procedures utilized, suspected preoperative diagnosis by imaging, and final diagnosis based on pathology. Demographic data including age, race, gravidity, parity, body mass index, and number of prior cesarean deliveries were recorded. Prognostic factors of maternal morbidity such as duration of hospital stay, hospital readmission, administration of anti-fibrinolytic agents, use of cell salvage, blood transfusion, coagulopathy, activation of massive obstetric hemorrhage protocol, thrombosis, urologic injury, infection, unplanned intensive care unit (ICU) admission, sepsis, pulmonary edema, heart failure, bowel injury, and fistula formation were identified from medical records. We recorded complications related to specific treatment strategies including interventional procedures, methotrexate use, and DH. In addition, complications related to each treatment phase, including at time of cesarean section (CS), interval between CS and DH, and at time of DH, were recorded.

Descriptive statistics were used to analyze demographic and clinical characteristics. Statistical analysis was performed using SAS 9.3 (SAS Institute, Cary, NC). Wilcoxon rank sum tests were used to compare the number of blood transfusion units and estimated blood loss. Fisher's Exact test (2-sided) was used to compare the total infection rates.

### Overview of multidisciplinary approach

Once antenatal diagnosis of placenta percreta is suspected on ultrasound, the MFM team coordinates communication and consultations with the Gynecologic Oncology, Interventional Radiology (IR), and Women's Anesthesia divisions. Additional imaging with pelvic MRI is recommended to assist with surgical planning especially in cases with posterior or lateral placental involvement. The decision to proceed with immediate cesarean hysterectomy (CHYS) versus DH is an informed one between the patient and the multidisciplinary team. Criteria to offer the DH approach include: 1) prenatal imaging with ultrasound and/or MRI showing suspicion for placenta percreta with concern for extra-uterine placental invasion or loss of planes between placenta and surrounding tissues; 2) no desire for future fertility; 3) clinical stability; 4) access to tertiary care center; and 5) patient willingness to comply with close follow up between delivery and interval hysterectomy. In the rare instance that patients desire future fertility, close expectant management occurs until placental resorption. Given the many steps and consulting services involved, a treatment algorithm has been developed at our institution (Fig. 1). This algorithm reflects our current practice at our institution and is updated from our initial approach in 2005.

### Delivery management

Delivery between 34 and 36 weeks gestation is performed in the hybrid operating room that has angiography capability. The recommendation for delivery during this gestational period is supported by a decision tree model that compared 11 strategies for optimal delivery timing in patients with vasa previa [9]. Our initial cases were performed in the main operating room (OR) and patients were transferred to and from the IR suite from the main OR for catheter placement and embolization after CS. Initially the patient came to the IR suite where bilateral femoral access was obtained and 7 French Flexor® Check-Flo® ANL2 sheaths (Cook® Medical, Bloomington In.) were placed and 8.5 mm occlusion balloons left in the internal iliac artery. Due to lack of use of the balloons and some CHYS not having

embolization or balloon use, we converted to a single femoral artery 6 French vascular sheath to allow for selective embolization post-delivery by the IR team since 2011. Prophylactic balloon catheters are no longer utilized.

Neuraxial anesthesia remains the anesthetic of choice for cesarean delivery. Currently, neuraxial anesthesia is considered for delivery in both groups [10]. In these cases, it provides anesthesia for the placement of the femoral arterial sheath and the operative procedure, as well as post-operative analgesia. The interventional radiologist places the arterial sheath following placement of central venous access, arterial catheter and combined spinal epidural (CSE), if indicated. This order is necessary because the patient cannot be positioned for the neuraxial block placement after the sheath is in place. General anesthesia is performed in some cases based on patient preference and/or surgical indications, and should be considered for anticipated difficult airways.

The obstetrical team performs a modified midline periumbilical vertical incision that is *not* extended to the symphysis pubis and is made just large enough for delivery of the infant. For those cases in which the patient was deemed eligible for and desire DH, the final decision about whether to proceed with DH versus CHYS is made upon entry into the abdomen based on the intraoperative findings. A classical cesarean delivery is then performed in the awake parturient by a fundal incision under ultrasound guidance to avoid the placenta. The umbilical cord is ligated and transected at its placental insertion and the placenta is left undisturbed. Retraction on the cord is avoided. The uterine and abdominal incisions are closed in the usual fashion.

Intraoperative transfusion is at the discretion of the anesthesiologist, but we have had an institutional massive obstetric hemorrhage protocol in place since 2010 that can be activated to mobilize resources in these cases. We also have cell salvage available in the room for all cases. Recently, a tranexamic acid (TXA) 1000 mg slow intravenous bolus has been administered immediately after cord clamping.

Initially, bilateral uterine artery embolization was only performed for subjects who were having a DH. We now perform bilateral uterine artery embolization following delivery for both patients having an immediate CHYS and those having a DH. Bilateral uterine arteries and any branches recruited from other arterial distributions supplying the placental bed are embolized prior to removal of the groin catheter. Particle embolization ranging from 710 to 1000 μm up to 1000–1180 μm Contour™ polyvinyl alcohol (PVA) embolization particles (Boston Scientific Inc. Natick MA) are used until there is no visible supply to the placenta from the internal iliac artery. For subjects having an immediate hysterectomy, the

**MFM coordinates multidisciplinary care:**
1. Schedule delivery date 34-36weeks
2. Schedule consultation with:
✓ IR (or vascular surgery if no IR available)
✓ GynOnc (and/or other surgical specialties) to determine if candidate for DH and assist with surgical planning
✓ Anesthesia
  ○ CSE for delivery; General if needed
  ○ Cell saver
  ○ Consider tranexamic acid 1g
  ○ Activate Transfusion Protocol for massive hemorrhage
**Consents:**
✓ Surgical, IR, anesthesia
  ○ If DH is considered, document discussion with patient regarding possible risks (delayed hemorrhage, sepsis, coagulopathy) that may occur during interval period and need for close follow up

**ANTENATAL DIAGNOSIS**

**MULTIDISCIPLINARY COMMUNICATION**

**CRITERIA MET FOR DELAYED HYSTERECTOMY?**
✓ Suspicion or evidence of extrauterine placental invasion
✓ Hemodynamically stable
✓ Access to tertiary care
✓ Excellent patient compliance
✓ No desire for future fertility

**Ultrasound suspicious for percreta:**
✓ Obtain pelvic MRI at 25-28 wks, request "placenta accreta protocol"
✓ Review MRI images with radiologist and examine for:
  ○ Loss of fat planes between placenta and surrounding tissues
  ○ Suspicion or evidence of extrauterine placental invasion

Yes ← / → No

**DELAYED HYSTERECTOMY**

**DELIVERY IN HYBRID OR or MAIN OR**

**IR**
Single femoral access 6fr sheath under CSE

**OR**
1. All surgical specialties available
2. Patient preparation
  a. Supine
  b. Consider 3-way foley
3. Delivery
  a. Modified vertical skin incision: periumbilical, do not extend to symphysis
  b. Classical c-section
  c. Ultrasound to aid fundal uterine incision
  d. Clamp and tie cord at placental insertion
  e. DO NOT ATTEMPT to remove placenta, NO TRACTION
  f. Repair hysterotomy
  g. Abdominal and skin closure

**IR**
Uterine artery and selective embolization PVA particles ≥710microns

**IMMEDIATE HYSTERECTOMY**

**DELIVERY IN HYBRID OR or MAIN OR**

**IR**
Single femoral access 6fr sheath under CSE

**OR**
1. Available blood products
2. Cell saver available
3. All surgical specialties available
4. Patient preparation
  a. Supine
  b. Consider 3-way foley if concern for bladder involvement
5. Delivery
  a. Vertical skin incision
  b. Classical c-section
  c. Ultrasound to aid fundal uterine incision
  d. Clamp and tie cord at placental insertion
  e. DO NOT ATTEMPT to remove placenta
  f. Repair hysterotomy
  g. Abdominal packing, skin closure or sterile covering in preparation for embolization

**IR**
1. Selective artery embolization with PVA particles ≥710microns to target placental blood supply and reduce blood loss
2. Wait ~30 minutes prior to hysterectomy

**HYSTERECTOMY**
1. Avoid midline dissection of bladder in cases of bladder invasion
2. Anticipate resection of involved bladder and use of intentional cystotomy
3. Cell saver
4. Use vessel sealing devices
5. Activate transfusion protocol in cases of severe hemorrhage
6. Early intraoperative involvement of gyn onc or other surgical specialties

**IMMEDIATE POSTOP CARE**
1. Monitor for vaginal bleeding as partial placental separation may occur. Continue conservative approach only if patient is clinically stable
2. Designate primary provider/team for outpatient follow up care prior to discharge from hospital

**IMMEDIATE POSTOP CARE**
1. Consider planned admission to ICU
2. Monitor for bleeding, coagulopathy

**OUTPATIENT MANAGEMENT**
1. Weekly to every other week evaluation until hysterectomy
2. Obtain imaging and/or labs only if clinically indicated
3. Pain management
4. Monitor for infection, pain, bleeding, coagulopathy; avoid routine pelvic exams, if needed perform sterile speculum exam
5. Schedule delayed hysterectomy ~6 weeks postpartum
6. Patient and team prepared to proceed to emergent hysterectomy-communicate with on call teams
7. Do NOT attempt transcervical placental removal-can lead to catastrophic hemorrhage

**DELAYED HYSTERECTOMY**
1. Schedule ~6weeks after csection
2. Avoid midline dissection of bladder in cases of bladder invasion
3. Anticipate resection of involved bladder and use of intentional cystotomy
4. Use vessel sealing devices
5. Consider minimally invasive approach in appropriate candidates with removal of uterus transvaginally within endocatch bag

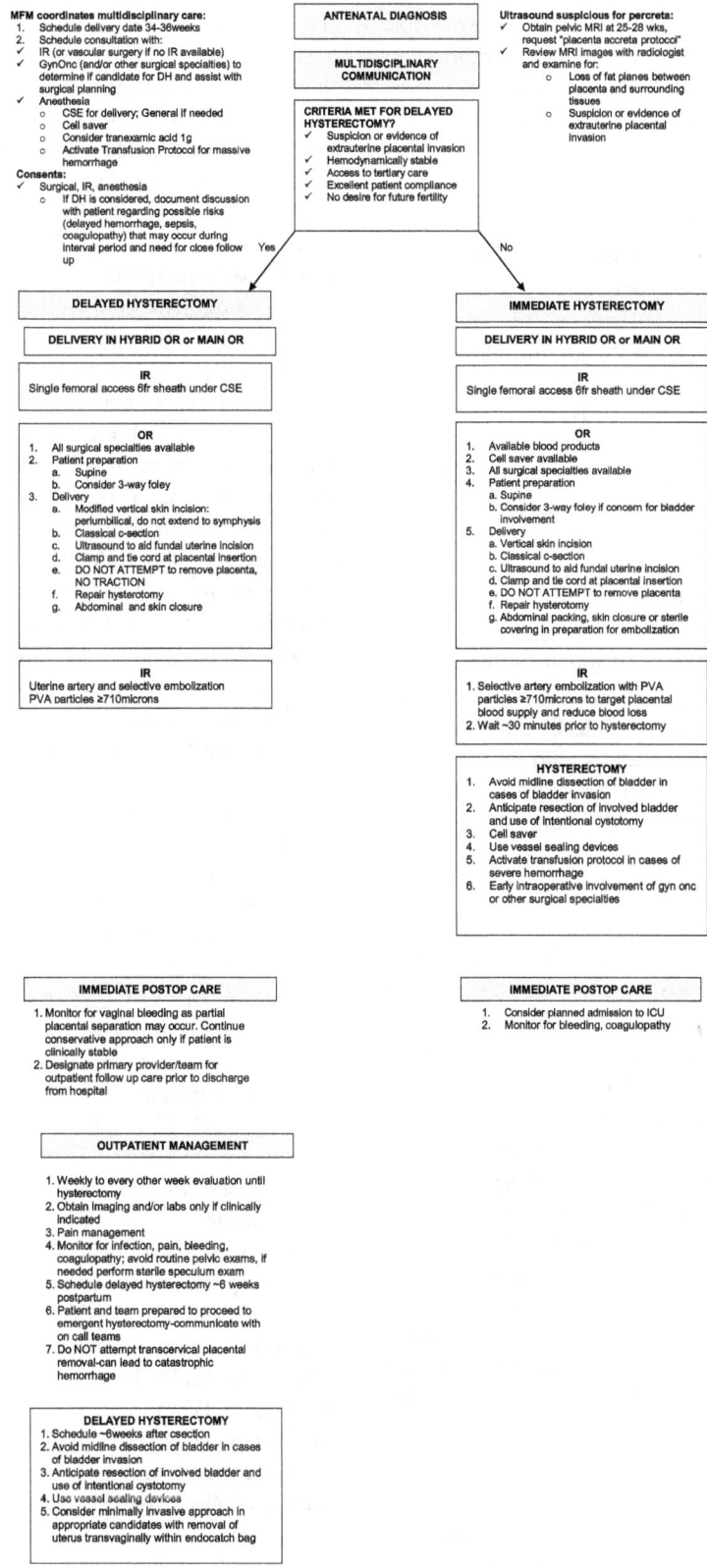

**Fig. 1** Algorithm for Placenta Percreta Management. Summary of considerations for each stage of treatment

embolization is performed following delivery while the abdomen is still open and just prior to hysterectomy. For women having a DH, the uterus and abdomen are first closed and then the patient undergoes embolization. The catheter is then removed from the femoral access site and the patient is transferred to recovery.

## Post-cesarean management

Prophylactic antibiotics for the retained placenta have not been administered routinely as our experience has not indicated benefit. Postpartum antibiotics are given when clinically indicated. Although used in our initial cases, methotrexate is no longer utilized. Patients are followed weekly to biweekly after cesarean delivery by the gynecologic oncologist until DH. Routine pelvic exams are avoided and are performed only when clinically indicated. For example, if patients present with increased vaginal bleeding and/or pain with the concern for partial expulsion of the placenta or infection. Transcervical removal of the placenta is avoided as this could lead to catastrophic hemorrhage. Pain management is emphasized and includes oral narcotics and anti-inflammatory medications until delayed hysterectomy. Laboratory and radiologic testing are performed only when clinically indicated. Routine imaging with either pelvic ultrasound or MRI is not performed prior to DH. Women desiring to breast feed are allowed and encouraged to do so during the period between delivery and DH.

## Delayed hysterectomy

The rationale for the six week interval between cesarean section and delayed hysterectomy is to allow time for return to normal maternal blood volume physiology, placental resorption, and uterine involution which would accommodate for transvaginal uterine removal for those cases having a laparoscopic approach to hysterectomy. The surgical technique to control the uterine arteries in the presence of an expanded lower uterine segment from the retained placenta has moved away from a modified radical hysterectomy approach with the use of vessel sealing instruments. However, caution should be used with these devices on thin walled placental vessels as shearing of the vessels can occur during attempted sealing or during release of the instrument. Laparoscopic approach has been performed in select cases with removal of the uterus transvaginally within a large endocatch bag.

## Results

Among 21 consecutive cases of antenatally suspected placenta percreta occurring between November 2005 and September 2014, seven underwent CHYS, 13 underwent DH, and one patient strongly desired future fertility and had successful uterine preservation. Given only the one case of uterine preservation, data is presented only for patients who underwent hysterectomy.

Nineteen of the 20 patients were diagnosed antenatally with imaging suspicious of placenta percreta and majority underwent both antenatal ultrasound and MRI (7/7 CHYS; 11/13 DH). There was one diagnosis of antenatal increta "cannot rule out percreta" on ultrasound and outside MRI did not confirm percreta. In this case, percreta was diagnosed at time of CHYS with visible placental involvement of the lower uterine segment. The median outpatient follow-up was 17 [0–108] days after CHYS and 55 [13–184] days after DH. Demographic and clinical characteristics are shown in Table 1. There were no differences between maternal age, gravidity, parity, gestational age, body mass index, or number of prior cesarean deliveries. In both groups, most had ≥2 prior cesarean deliveries (3/7 CHYS; 7/13 DH). The majority of patients had an additional prenatal placental diagnosis of placenta previa and/or vasa previa (6/7 CHYS, 13/13 DH). Forty-five percent (9/20) of cases were delivered on their scheduled date and the median gestational age at delivery was 35 weeks [18–37]. Reasons to deliver earlier included contractions, bleeding, fetal growth restriction, and premature rupture of membranes. There were no emergent cesarean deliveries performed. The final pathology revealed 11/20 increta and 7/20 percreta cases, while in 2 cases the diagnosis was indeterminate.

Table 2 summarizes surgical approaches, anesthetic, interventional radiologic and postoperative management. The decision to proceed to CHYS included no extrauterine involvement (3/7), patient preference (2/7), second trimester (1/7), and placental separation at time of CS (1/7). Initially general anesthesia was used for cesarean delivery in both groups. More recently, the majority of CS are now performed under neuraxial blockade with or without conversion to general anesthesia when indicated after delivery of the fetus (4/7 CHYS; 8/13 DH). Three patients received intraoperative TXA (2 CHYS, 1 DH). Intentional cystotomy to assess the necessary degree of bladder resection was performed in 3/20 cases (1/7 CHYS; 2/7 DH). All but one patient underwent an IR procedure. In both groups where prophylactic occlusion balloons were placed, none required inflation of the balloons to control hemorrhage. Prophylactic embolization occurred in 14 cases (2/7 CHYS and 12/13 DH). Only 2/13 DH cases received prophylactic IV antibiotics of 1–2 doses immediately after CS. Two patients were treated with extended antibiotics for endometritis and pyelonephritis, respectively. Three patients received weekly methotrexate with a median of 4 cycles given. There were no grade 3 or 4 toxicities related to methotrexate therapy. Methotrexate was last utilized in 2010. In the delayed cohort, the median time from cesarean delivery to delayed hysterectomy was 41 days [26–68]. Ten hysterectomies were performed via an open

**Table 1** Demographic and Clinical Characteristics

| | Cesarean Hysterectomy<br>N = 7<br>n (%) | Delayed Hysterectomy<br>N = 13<br>n (%) |
|---|---|---|
| Maternal Age at Delivery, years | 37 ± 3.7 | 31 ± 1.3 |
| Maternal Race | | |
| African-American | 2 (29) | 2 (15) |
| Hispanic | 0 | 3 (23) |
| White | 5 (71) | 6 (46) |
| Other/Not Specified | 0 | 2 (15) |
| Gravidity | 4 [2–6] | 3[2–8] |
| Parity | 2 [1–3] | 2 [1–4] |
| Gestational Age, weeks | 35 [18–37] | 34 [28–37] |
| BMI | 28 [20–54] | 30 [22–53] |
| Prior Cesarean Delivery | | |
| 1 | 4 (57) | 6 (46) |
| 2 | 2 (29) | 6 (46) |
| 3 | 1 (14) | 1 (8) |
| Other Prior Uterine Surgery | | |
| Uterine curettage | 1 (14) | 3 (23) |
| Hysteroscopic myomectomy | 0 | 1 (8) |
| Concurrent Placental Diagnosis | | |
| Partial previa | 2 (29) | 3 (23) |
| Complete previa | 3 (43) | 9 (69) |
| Vasa previa | 1 (14) | 1 (18) |
| Indication for Delivery | | |
| Scheduled | 3 (43) | 6 (46) |
| Contractions | 1 (14) | 3 (23) |
| Vaginal bleeding | 1(14) | 1 (8) |
| Hematuria | 1 (14) | 1 (8) |
| Fetal growth restriction | 1 (14) | 1 (8) |
| Premature rupture of membranes | 0 | 1 (8) |
| Final Pathology | | |
| Accreta | 0 | 0 |
| Increta | 4 (57) | 7 (54) |
| Percreta | 3 (43) | 4 (31) |
| Inconclusive[a] | 0 | 2 (15) |

Data are n (%), mean ± mean standard error, or median with [range]
[a]Inconclusive pathology in two cases: 1) extensive degree of post-embolization myometrial infarction significantly hampered ability to recognize infiltrating chorionic villi and 2) changes in anterior myometrium may be consistent with prior placental involvement; however no retained placental identified

approach and three were performed laparoscopically, with two using the robotic platform.

Table 3 summarizes maternal morbidity at time of CHYS and for the DH cohort, at time of CS and at DH. 71% (5/7) of patients in the CHYS group required blood transfusion compared to 46% (6/13) in the total DH cohort. The median estimated blood loss was significantly higher in the CHYS cohort compared to both treatment phases of DH group, including at time of CS and at time of DH (2800 ml [400–4500] CHYS vs. 900 ml [400–1500] CS vs. 750 ml [50–2000] DH, $p$ = 0.01). The median packed red blood cells (PRBC) transfusion was higher in the CHYS group compared to both phases in the DH group (2 [0–10] CHYS vs. 0 [0–3] CS vs. 0 [0–4] DH, $p$ = 0.006). Massive transfusion (defined as greater than 4 units PRBCs) occurred in 2 cases (2 CHYS cases

**Table 2** Management Strategies for Patients with Placenta Percreta

|  | Cesarean Hysterectomy N = 7 n (%) | Delayed Hysterectomy N = 13 n (%) |
|---|---|---|
| Reason to proceed to Cesarean Hysterectomy |  |  |
| Placental separation occurred at time of delivery | 1 (14) | N/A |
| No extra-uterine involvement | 3 (43) | N/A |
| Patient preference | 2 (29) | N/A |
| Second trimester | 1 (14) | N/A |
| Anesthetic Technique at time of delivery |  |  |
| General | 3 (43) | 5 (38) |
| Neuraxial | 1 (14) | 7 (54) |
| Neuraxial followed by general | 3 (43) | 1 (8) |
| Non-operative blood loss strategies |  |  |
| Tranexamic acid (1 g) | 2 (29) | 1 (8) |
| Cell saver | 2 (29) | 0 |
| Urologic Procedures |  |  |
| Cystoscopy only | 0 | 1 (8) |
| Ureteral stents | 1 (14) | 5 (38) |
| Intentional cystotomy | 1 (14) | 2 (15) |
| Interventional radiology procedures |  |  |
| Prophylactic occlusion balloons only | 3 (43) | 0 |
| Prophylactic occlusion balloon +embolization | 1 (14) | 7 (54) |
| Prophylactic embolization | 2 (29) | 5 (38) |
| Femoral access only | 1 (14) | 0 |
| Prophylactic antibiotic after delivery for placenta left in situ | N/A | 2 (15) |
| Methotrexate administration | N/A | 3 (23) |
| Median number of cycles [range] |  | 4 [4–5] |
| Interval of time (days) between delivery to hysterectomy | N/A | 41 [26–68] |
| Surgical approach | N/A |  |
| Modified radical |  | 6 (46) |
| Total abdominal |  | 4 (31) |
| Laparoscopic |  | 3 (23) |

required 7 and 10 units, respectively) with a median total blood transfusion (including fresh frozen plasma, platelets, and cryoprecipitate) of 13 units [11–14]. Massive transfusion was not required in any of the DH cases. Although the infection rate was higher in the DH cohort (69% DH vs. 43% CHYS, $p = 0.4$), this was not significant and majority was due to urinary tract infections. The rate of coagulopathy, venous thromboembolism, and urologic injury were similar between all groups. Urologic injury included four cases of unintentional cystotomy (2 CHYS, 2 DH) and one ureteral injury in the DH group. There were no cases of unplanned ICU admission, fistula, bowel injury, pulmonary edema, or heart failure. In the DH cohort, there were no cases of delayed hemorrhage, sepsis, or emergent hysterectomy. There were no maternal deaths.

Of the 19/20 hysterectomy patients who underwent interventional radiology procedures, there were no catheter-related injuries to the common femoral artery accessed for the procedure. Of the 14 total embolization procedures performed, none required re-embolization. The four possible IR-related complications occurred in the DH cohort where embolization was performed. One patient had transient paresthesia of the thigh, which may have been related to her embolization procedure or local anesthesia of the femoral nerve during access into the femoral artery. A second patient was found to have transient hypoxia during embolization. During the procedure, embolization with 700 to 900 µm Embospheres® (Merit Medical™, South Jordan, UT) was initially used. Following development of hypoxia, the decision was made to change to 710–1000 µm

**Table 3** Maternal Morbidity

| | Cesarean Hysterectomy N = 7 n (%) | Cesarean section prior to Delayed Hysterectomy N = 13 n (%) | Delayed Hysterectomy N = 13 n(%) |
|---|---|---|---|
| Estimated blood loss | 2800 [400–4500] | 900 [400–1500] | 750 [50–2000] |
| Total number of PRBC units transfused | 2[0–10] | 0[0–3] | 0[0–4] |
| Total number of *patients* requiring PRBC | 5 (71) | 1 (8) | 5 (38) |
| ≤ 4 units | 3 (43) | 1 (8) | 5 (38) |
| 4 units | 2 (29) | 0 | 0 |
| Infection | | | |
| Total | 3 (43) | 4 (31) | 5 (38) |
| Endometritis | N/A | 2 (15) | N/A |
| Wound Infection | 3 (43) | 0 | 2 (15) |
| Urinary Tract | 0 | 2 (15) | 2 (15) |
| Vaginal cuff Cellulitis | 0 | N/A | 1 (8) |
| Coagulopathy[a] | 2 (29) | 0 | 2 (15) |
| Unplanned admission to the ICU | 0 | 0 | 0 |
| Venous thromboembolism | 1 (14) | 1 (8) | 0 |
| Urologic injury | | | |
| Total | 2 (29) | 0 | 3 (23) |
| Ureteral | 0 | 0 | 1 (8) |
| Unintentional cystotomy | 2 (29) | 0 | 2 (15) |
| Interventional radiology complications | 0 | 4 (31) | N/A |
| Paresthesia | 0 | 1 (8) | |
| Transient hypoxia | 0 | 1 (8) | |
| Ischemia (uterus) | 0 | 1 (8) | |
| Gluteal ulcer | 0 | 1 (8) | |
| Methotrexate toxicity | N/A | 0 | N/A |
| Spontaneous delivery of placenta prior to DH | N/A | 1 (8) | N/A |
| Length of hospital stay (days) | 3 [3–4] | 4 [3–30] | 4[1–10] |
| Hospital readmission | 1 (14) | 5 (38) | 2 (15) |
| Wound infection | 1 (14) | 0 | 0 |
| Pain | 0 | 4 (31) | 0 |
| Bleeding | 0 | 1 (8) | 0 |
| Ileus | 0 | 0 | 1 (8) |
| Drainage of Uroma | 0 | 0 | 1 (8) |
| Emergency department visit | 1 (14) | 2 (15) | 0 |

Data are n (%) or median [range]
[a]Coagulopathy that required correction

Contour™ PVA particles (Boston Scientific, Natick, MA) to reduce the potential for presumed shunting. It was difficult to determine if this was due to shunting or a pulmonary embolus. The patient subsequently was diagnosed with a pulmonary embolism. It is not clear if uterine artery embolization caused the pulmonary embolism. Following this case no additional hypoxic events occurred during embolization. This may have been due to converting to the use of 710–1000 μm Contour™ PVA particles (Boston Scientific, Natick, MA) or larger with the patients that followed this event. The last two possible IR related injuries include: 1) anterior uterine wall necrosis found on subsequent final pathology from hysterectomy and 2) an ulcer at the superior gluteal fold found approximately one month after delivery which may have been related to a radiation burn from fluoroscopy at time of procedure and/or nondirected embolization to this area.

The length of hospital stay (LOS) was similar between groups. However, there was one case in the DH cohort with an extended LOS of 33 days. This patient was not discharged after CS due to significant anemia and blood refusal status, as well as her long-distance residence. She remained inpatient receiving erythropoietin and IV iron per recommendations from our hospital's Center for Blood Conservation until her hematocrit increased safely to proceed with delayed hysterectomy. The DH cohort had a higher rate of hospital readmission (including after CS and DH) as compared to the CHYS cohort (54% (7/13) vs. 14% (1/7)). In the DH cohort, pain was the most common reason for hospital readmission between delivery and delayed hysterectomy. One patient was readmitted during this interval period for observation secondary to bleeding but did not require transfusion.

## Discussion

With the rising incidence of abnormal placentation, it is important to define management strategies with a focus on reducing maternal morbidity and mortality. In the current study, we have shown that delayed hysterectomy may provide a feasible alternative to cesarean hysterectomy in patients with placenta percreta. Women with placenta percreta are known to have a high rate of hemorrhage, infection, urologic injury, and ICU admission despite treatment at a tertiary center [4]. Significant maternal bleeding is the most common complication, with an average reported estimated blood loss ranging between 3000 ml and 5000 ml [15]. Blood transfusion is required in 80–90% of cases, with large volume transfusion in 42% of cases [11–13]. Our delayed hysterectomy approach was associated with a significantly lower blood loss and transfusion rates. Furthermore, none of these patients required a massive transfusion. In our series, we demonstrate that planned DH occurring between four and six weeks following delivery is feasible. This duration of time allows for normalization of the hypervascular changes of the puerperal pelvis and therefore decrease the potential risk of massive hemorrhage and coagulopathy associated with cesarean hysterectomy [14, 16].

Methotrexate chemotherapy may increase the placental resorption rate, though not all investigators advocate for its use given that trophoblasts are not dividing in this setting [17–19]. Though rare, there can be severe adverse events such as immunosuppression and hepatotoxicity in patients who receive this medication. In our limited experience, we did not appreciate a significant clinical impact of methotrexate on the resorption of the placenta and therefore discontinued using this agent in 2010. Given the lack of data supporting the use of methotrexate we feel that further study is warranted

prior to routine use, especially since it is contraindicated with breast feeding.

Our approach utilizes prophylactic uterine artery embolization (UAE) to reduce the risk of post-delivery hemorrhage while the placenta remains in situ. Initially, the rationale for *prophylactic* UAE was supported by higher success rates of UAE when used in a non-emergent setting [20]. This has been again demonstrated in a recent series that showed embolization failure was associated with disseminated intravascular coagulation and transfusions of more than ten units [21]. Furthermore, Angstmann et al. demonstrated a statistically significant reduction in blood loss in patients who underwent embolization prior to hysterectomy when compared to those who underwent immediate cesarean hysterectomy without embolization [11]. Thus, we have recently incorporated this into our algorithm when CHYS is planned for placenta percreta cases. The decreased transfusion requirements in our DH cohort may be related to prophylactic UAE, which was performed in 12/13 DH cases compared to only 2/7 CHYS cases. Prophylactic UAE may be helpful in decreasing potential delayed hemorrhage and may contribute to placental resorption in the period between delivery and delayed hysterectomy. However, there is no evidence to support or refute the use of prophylactic UAE when the placenta is left in situ and further investigation is required.

Prophylactic placement of arterial balloon-occlusion catheters in the anterior divisions of the internal iliac arteries can provide temporary hemostasis if severe hemorrhage is encountered during cesarean hysterectomy [22, 23]. However, previous studies have shown no impact of balloons on risk of transfusion [24]. Other investigators have found an unacceptably high rate of complications related to catheter placement (including artery thrombosis and dissection) and recommended against the use of prophylactic intravascular balloon catheters [25, 26]. In our series, occlusion-catheters that were placed in 12 women prior to delivery were only inflated in the fertility-sparing case. Thus, our current algorithm has moved away from routine placement of balloon occlusion catheters.

Patients have a consultation with an obstetric anesthesiologist prior to surgery to discuss anesthetic options, and are routinely offered neuraxial anesthesia for the cesarean delivery in both CHYS and DH approaches. Neuraxial anesthesia is the preferred mode of anesthesia for obstetric patients, as it is associated with fewer airway complications and less bleeding than general anesthesia [27, 28]. Many patients wish to remain awake to experience the birth of their child, and we do allow a support person to remain in the room with the patient until the birth of the baby. Light sedation is often employed for placement of lines and interventional radiology groin access prior to delivery. In some cases that required massive transfusion, general anesthesia was induced after the birth of the infant.

Non-operative blood conserving strategies such as pre-operative treatment of anemia and the use of cell saver, should be considered at time of delivery and hysterectomy [29, 30]. Acute normovolemic hemodilution was utilized for both delivery and hysterectomy in our one case of blood refusal and is described elsewhere in detail [31].

The antifibrinolytic agent, tranexamic acid (TXA), has been shown to decrease the need for blood transfusion in a wide range of planned surgeries, without an increased risk of thrombotic events, [32] and to decrease mortality in bleeding trauma patients [33]. More recently it has been described for the management of obstetric hemorrhage [34] and is currently under investigation in a randomized clinical trial [33]. Although further study is needed to confirm the use and safety of TXA in this population, we have incorporated low-dose TXA (1 g) as a standard part of the protocol for these cases. This dose has been used in a number of trials for the prevention of postpartum hemorrhage, and few adverse events have been reported [32]. However, none of the randomized-controlled trials that have been conducted to date have reported neonatal outcomes, and TXA does cross the placenta. Therefore, until more robust, larger trials confirm neonatal safety, we have chosen to administer TXA after cord clamping.

Our study is limited by its retrospective nature, duration of the study, and its small sample size. Although the numbers of placenta percreta cases are likely increasing, the low incidence is a barrier to conduct prospective randomized controlled studies. An important limitation is our inability to assess the relative value of each component of our algorithm for women with placenta percreta. For example, "What is the benefit of prophylactic UAE relative to awaiting placental resorption and delaying hysterectomy?" However, our algorithm is undergoing real-time assessment and continues to mature based on our clinical experience and hopefully will help us address these important questions. Other considerations that were not measured in this study are the potential psychosocial impact of undergoing a second surgery in the postpartum period and cost effectiveness of treatment. Discussion of accurate antenatal diagnosis of placenta percreta is beyond the scope of this study; however, given our experience we have recommended pelvic MRI to be performed at our institution and reviewed by our interventional radiology team. Finally, all of our patients were treated at the same tertiary care center with strict criteria to offer the delayed hysterectomy approach and thus our results may have limited generalizability.

It is important to emphasize that multidisciplinary care for a rare condition requires appropriate coordination. Identifying an interested faculty attending, rather than a trainee, from each specialty to be the point person to contact for each case is imperative. As these cases will likely be treated in larger academic centers where trainees are involved, we have learned that because of trainee turnover and infrequency of cases, primary coordination by a designated MFM attending, involvement of consistent faculty from each specialty, and having a written protocol are critical to avoid inconsistencies and maximize patient outcomes.

## Conclusion

We present our current multidisciplinary management strategy for those select patients with the most severe forms of abnormal placentation. The maternal morbidity and outcomes of these patients reflect that uterine artery embolization with delayed hysterectomy appears to be feasible. Given the significant morbidity and mortality of placenta percreta cases, further study is warranted to investigate potential alternatives to cesarean hysterectomy for those women who are at highest risk of maternal morbidity.

**Abbreviations**
CHYS: Immediate hysterectomy after cesarean section; CS: Cesarean section; CSE: Combined spinal epidural; DH: Delayed hysterectomy; FS: Fertility sparing; IR: Interventional radiology; LOS: Length of stay; MFM: Maternal fetal medicine; OR: Operating room; PRBC: Packed red blood cells; PVA: Polyvinyl alcohol; TXA: Tranexamic acid; UAE: Uterine artery embolization

**Acknowledgements**
Dr. Ashraf Habib (Duke Women's Anesthesia) and Dr. David Sopko (Duke Interventional Radiology) for their support of this study.

**Funding**
Not applicable.

**Authors' contributions**
PL, SK, MM, JD, JE, RP, LH, SE, and AS contributed to the acquisition of data, analysis, coordination, drafting and revising the manuscript. CG contributed to coordination and manuscript revision. PL and AS also contributed to conception and design of the study. GB performed statistical analysis and manuscript review. All authors read and approved the final manuscript.

**Consent for publication**
Not applicable.

**Competing interests**
The authors declare that they have no competing interests.

**Author details**
[1]Department of Obstetrics and Gynecology, Duke University Hospital, Durham, North Carolina 27710, USA. [2]Division of Gynecologic Oncology, Department of Obstetrics and Gynecology, Duke University Hospital,

Durham, USA. [3]Division of Maternal Fetal Medicine, Department of Obstetrics and Gynecology, Duke University Hospital, Durham, USA. [4]Department of Interventional Radiology, Duke University Hospital, Durham, USA. [5]Cancer Statistical Center, Duke Cancer Institute, Durham, USA. [6]Duke Cancer Institute, Durham, USA. [7]Department of Anesthesiology, Duke University Hospital, Durham, USA.

## References

1.  Miller DA, Chollet JA, Goodwin TM. Clinical risk factors for placenta previa-placenta accreta. Am J Obstet Gynecol. 1997;177:210–4.

2.  Solheim KN, Esakoff TF, Little SE, Cheng YW, Sparks TN, Caughey AB. The effect of cesarean delivery rates on the future incidence of placenta previa, placenta accreta, and maternal mortality. J Matern Fetal Neonatal Med. 2011;24:1341–6.

3.  Publications Committee SfM-FM, Belfort MA. Placenta accreta. Am J Obstet Gynecol. 2010;203:430–9.

4.  Washecka R, Behling A. Urologic complications of placenta percreta invading the urinary bladder: a case report and review of the literature. Hawaii Med J. 2002;61:66–9.

5.  Clausen C, Lonn L, Langhoff-Roos J. Management of placenta percreta: a review of published cases. Acta Obstet Gynecol Scand. 2014;93:138–43.

6.  Pather S, Strockyj S, Richards A, Campbell N, de Vries B, Ogle R. Maternal outcome after conservative management of placenta percreta at caesarean section: a report of three cases and a review of the literature. Aust N Z J Obstet Gynaecol. 2014;54:84–7.

7.  Sentilhes L, Ambroselli C, Kayem G, Provansal M, Fernandez H, Perrotin F, Winer N, Pierre F, Benachi A, Dreyfus M, et al. Maternal outcome after conservative treatment of placenta accreta. Obstet Gynecol. 2010;115:526–34.

8.  Lee PS, Bakelaar R, Fitpatrick CB, Ellestad SC, Havrilesky LJ, Alvarez Secord A. Medical and surgical treatment of placenta percreta to optimize bladder preservation. Obstet Gynecol. 2008;112:421–4.

9.  Robinson BK, Grobman WA. Effectiveness of timing strategies for delivery of individuals with vasa previa. Obstet Gynecol. 2011;117:542–9.

10. Lilker SJ, Meyer RA, Downey KN, Macarthur AJ. Anesthetic considerations for placenta accreta. Int J Obstet Anesth. 2011;20:288–92.

11. Angstmann T, Gard G, Harrington T, Ward E, Thomson A, Giles W. Surgical management of placenta accreta: a cohort series and suggested approach. Am J Obstet Gynecol. 2010;202:38. e31-39

12. Eller AG, Porter TF, Soisson P, Silver RM. Optimal management strategies for placenta accreta. BJOG. 2009;116:648–54.

13. Stotler B, Padmanabhan A, Devine P, Wright J, Spitalnik SL, Schwartz J. Transfusion requirements in obstetric patients with placenta accreta. Transfusion. 2011;51:2627–33.

14. Edman CD, Toofanian A, MacDonald PC, Gant NF. Placental clearance rate of maternal plasma androstenedione through placental estradiol formation: an indirect method of assessing uteroplacental blood flow. Am J Obstet Gynecol. 1981;141:1029–37.

15. Hudon L, Belfort MA, Broome DR. Diagnosis and management of placenta percreta: a review. Obstet Gynecol Surv. 1998;53:509–17.

16. Shellhaas CS, Gilbert S, Landon MB, Varner MW, Leveno KJ, Hauth JC, Spong CY, Caritis SN, Wapner RJ, Sorokin Y, et al. The frequency and complication rates of hysterectomy accompanying cesarean delivery. Obstet Gynecol. 2009;114:224–9.

17. Ramoni A, Strobl EM, Tiechl J, Ritter M, Marth C. Conservative management of abnormally invasive placenta: four case reports. Acta Obstet Gynecol Scand. 2013;92:468–71.

18. Steins Bisschop CN, Schaap TP, Vogelvang TE, Scholten PC. Invasive placentation and uterus preserving treatment modalities: a systematic review. Arch Gynecol Obstet. 2011;284:491–502.

19. Tam Tam KB, Dozier J, Martin JN Jr. Approaches to reduce urinary tract injury during management of placenta accreta, increta, and percreta: a systematic review. J Matern Fetal Neonatal Med. 2012;25:329–34.

20. Badawy SZ, Etman A, Singh M, Murphy K, Mayelli T, Philadelphia M. Uterine artery embolization: the role in obstetrics and gynecology. Clin Imaging. 2001;25:288–95.

21. Cheong JY, Kong TW, Son JH, Won JH, Yang JI, Kim HS. Outcome of pelvic arterial embolization for postpartum hemorrhage: a retrospective review of 117 cases. Obstet Gynecol Sci. 2014;57:17–27.

22. Salazar GM, Petrozza JC, Walker TG. Transcatheter endovascular techniques for management of obstetrical and gynecologic emergencies. Tech Vasc Interv Radiol. 2009;12:139–47.

23. Teixidor Vinas M, Chandraharan E, Moneta MV, Belli AM. The role of interventional radiology in reducing haemorrhage and hysterectomy following caesarean section for morbidly adherent placenta. Clin Radiol. 2014;69:e345–51.

24. Bodner LJ, Nosher JL, Gribbin C, Siegel RL, Beale S, Scorza W. Balloon-assisted occlusion of the internal iliac arteries in patients with placenta accreta/percreta. Cardiovasc Intervent Radiol. 2006;29:354–61.

25. Bishop S, Butler K, Monaghan S, Chan K, Murphy G, Edozien L. Multiple complications following the use of prophylactic internal iliac artery balloon catheterisation in a patient with placenta percreta. Int J Obstet Anesth. 2011;20:70–3.

26. Shrivastava V, Nageotte M, Major C, Haydon M, Wing D. Case-control comparison of cesarean hysterectomy with and without prophylactic placement of intravascular balloon catheters for placenta accreta. Am J Obstet Gynecol. 2007;197:402. e401-405

27. Endler GC, Mariona FG, Sokol RJ, Stevenson LB. Anesthesia-related maternal mortality in Michigan, 1972 to 1984. Am J Obstet Gynecol. 1988;159:187–93.

28. Heesen M, Hofmann T, Klohr S, Rossaint R, van de Velde M, Deprest J, Straube S. Is general anaesthesia for caesarean section associated with postpartum haemorrhage? Systematic review and meta-analysis. Acta Anaesthesiol Scand. 2013;57:1092–102.

29. Goucher H, Wong CA, Patel SK, Toledo P. Cell salvage in obstetrics. Anesth Analg. 2015;121:465–8.

30. Liumbruno GM, Meschini A, Liumbruno C, Rafanelli D. The introduction of intra-operative cell salvage in obstetric clinical practice: a review of the available evidence. Eur J Obstet Gynecol Reprod Biol. 2011;159:19–25.

31. Mauritz AA, Dominguez JE, Guinn NR, Gilner J, Habib AS. Blood-Conservation Strategies in a Blood-Refusal Parturient with Placenta Previa and Placenta Percreta. A A Case Rep. 2016;6(5):111–3.

32. Henry DA, Carless PA, Moxey AJ, O'Connell D, Stokes BJ, Fergusson DA, Ker K. Anti-fibrinolytic use for minimising perioperative allogeneic blood transfusion. Cochrane Database Syst Rev. 2011;3:CD001886.

33. CRASH-2 collaborators, Shakur H, Roberts I, Bautista R, Caballero J, Coats T, Dewan Y, El-Sayed H, Gogichaishvili T, Gupta S, et al. Effects of tranexamic acid on death, vascular occlusive events, and blood transfusion in trauma patients with significant haemorrhage (CRASH-2): a randomised, placebo-controlled trial. Lancet. 2010;376:23–32.

34. Sentilhes L, Lasocki S, Ducloy-Bouthors AS, Deruelle P, Dreyfus M, Perrotin F, Goffinet F, Deneux-Tharaux C. Tranexamic acid for the prevention and treatment of postpartum haemorrhage. Br J Anaesth. 2015;114:576–87.

# Permissions

All chapters in this book were first published in GORP, by BioMed Central; hereby published with permission under the Creative Commons Attribution License or equivalent. Every chapter published in this book has been scrutinized by our experts. Their significance has been extensively debated. The topics covered herein carry significant findings which will fuel the growth of the discipline. They may even be implemented as practical applications or may be referred to as a beginning point for another development.

The contributors of this book come from diverse backgrounds, making this book a truly international effort. This book will bring forth new frontiers with its revolutionizing research information and detailed analysis of the nascent developments around the world.

We would like to thank all the contributing authors for lending their expertise to make the book truly unique. They have played a crucial role in the development of this book. Without their invaluable contributions this book wouldn't have been possible. They have made vital efforts to compile up to date information on the varied aspects of this subject to make this book a valuable addition to the collection of many professionals and students.

This book was conceptualized with the vision of imparting up-to-date information and advanced data in this field. To ensure the same, a matchless editorial board was set up. Every individual on the board went through rigorous rounds of assessment to prove their worth. After which they invested a large part of their time researching and compiling the most relevant data for our readers.

The editorial board has been involved in producing this book since its inception. They have spent rigorous hours researching and exploring the diverse topics which have resulted in the successful publishing of this book. They have passed on their knowledge of decades through this book. To expedite this challenging task, the publisher supported the team at every step. A small team of assistant editors was also appointed to further simplify the editing procedure and attain best results for the readers.

Apart from the editorial board, the designing team has also invested a significant amount of their time in understanding the subject and creating the most relevant covers. They scrutinized every image to scout for the most suitable representation of the subject and create an appropriate cover for the book.

The publishing team has been an ardent support to the editorial, designing and production team. Their endless efforts to recruit the best for this project, has resulted in the accomplishment of this book. They are a veteran in the field of academics and their pool of knowledge is as vast as their experience in printing. Their expertise and guidance has proved useful at every step. Their uncompromising quality standards have made this book an exceptional effort. Their encouragement from time to time has been an inspiration for everyone.

The publisher and the editorial board hope that this book will prove to be a valuable piece of knowledge for researchers, students, practitioners and scholars across the globe.

# List of Contributors

**Alex Laios, Iryna Terekh, Hooman Soleymani Majd, Pubudu Pathiraja and Krishnayan Haldar**
Gynaecologic Oncology Unit, Churchill Hospital, Oxford University Hospitals, NHS Trust, Oxford, UK

**Sanjiv Manek**
Department of Cellular Pathology, Oxford University Hospitals, Oxford, UK

**Hanoon P Pokharel**
Department of Obstetrics and Gynaecology, B P Koirala Institute of Health Sciences, Dharan, Nepal

**Neville F Hacker**
Royal Hospital for Women, Randwick, Australia
School of Women's and Children's Health, University of New South Wales, Sydney, Australia

**Lesley Andrews**
School of Women's and Children's Health, University of New South Wales, Sydney, Australia
Prince of Wales Hospital, Randwick, Australia

**Teresa C. Longorla and Ramez N. Eskander**
University of California, Irvine Medical Center, 101 The City Drive South, Bldg 56, Ste 800, Orange, CA 92868, USA

**Michelle Glasgow and Peter Argenta**
Department of Obstetrics, Gynecology and Women's Health, Division of Gynecologic Oncology, University of Minnesota, Minneapolis, MN, USA

**Rachel Isaksson Vogel**
Department of Obstetrics, Gynecology and Women's Health, Division of Gynecologic Oncology, University of Minnesota, Minneapolis, MN, USA
Biostatistics and Bioinformatics Core, Masonic Cancer Center, University of Minnesota, Minneapolis, MN, USA

**Melissa A. Geller**
Department of Obstetrics, Gynecology and Women's Health, Division of Gynecologic Oncology, University of Minnesota, Minneapolis, MN, USA.
University of Minnesota, MMC 395, 420 Delaware St. SE, Minneapolis, MN 55445, USA

**Jennifer Burgart**
Eastern Virginia Medical School, Norfolk, VA, USA

**Kathryn Dusenbery**
Radiation Oncology, University of Minnesota, Minneapolis, MN, USA

**Brittany A. Davidson, Jonathan Foote, Laura J. Havrilesky and Angeles Alvarez Secord**
Division of Gynecologic Oncology, Duke University Medical Center, Duke University, DUMC Box 3079, Durham, NC 27710, USA

**Stacey L. Brower and Chunqiao Tian**
Product Development, Helomics Corporation, Pittsburgh, PA, USA

**Mohammed Elmarjany, Khalid Andaloussi, Amine Bazine, Issam Lalya, Noha Zaghba, Khalid Hadadi, Hassan Sifat and Hamid Mansouri**
Department of Radiotherapy, Mohamed V Military Hospital, Rabat, Morocco

**Abdelhak Maghous and Elamin Marnouche**
National Institute of Oncology, Rabat, Morocco

**Rachid Razine**
Department of Public Health, Laboratory of Biostatics, Clinical Research and Epidemiology, School of Medicine and Pharmacy of Rabat, Rabat, Morocco

**Baba Habib and Jaouad Kouach**
Department of Gynecology, Mohamed V Military Hospital, Rabat, Morocco

**A. Talhouk**
Department of Pathology and Laboratory Medicine, University of British Columbia and BC Cancer Agency, Vancouver, BC, Canada

**J. N. McAlpine**
Department of Gynecology and Obstetrics, Division of Gynecologic Oncology, University of British Columbia, 2775 Laurel St. 6th Floor, Vancouver, BC, CanadaV5Z 1M9

**Michael Feichtinger**
Department of Obstetrics and Gynecology, Division of Gynecological Endocrinology and Reproductive Medicine, Medical University of Vienna, Vienna, Austria
Wunschbaby Institut Feichtinger, Vienna, Austria
Department of Obstetrics and Gynecology, Section of Reproductive Medicine, Karolinska University Hospital, Novumhuset Plan 4, SE-141 86 Stockholm, Sweden

**Kenny A. Rodriguez-Wallberg**
Department of Oncology – Pathology, Karolinska Institutet, Stockholm, Sweden

Department of Obstetrics and Gynecology, Section of Reproductive Medicine, Karolinska University Hospital, Novumhuset Plan 4, SE-141 86 Stockholm, Sweden

**Austin Huy Nguyen, Ahmed I. Tahseen and Adam M. Vaudreuil**
Creighton University School of Medicine, 2500 California Plaza, Omaha, NE 68102, USA

**Gabriel C. Caponetti**
Department of Pathology and Laboratory Medicine, Perelman School of Medicine, University of Pennsylvania, 3400 Spruce Street, Philadelphia, PA, USA

**Christopher J. Huerter**
Division of Dermatology, Creighton University School of Medicine, 2500 California Plaza, Omaha, NE 68102, USA

**Lindsey E. Minion**
Dignity Health St. Joseph's Hospital and Medical Center, 500 West Thomas Road, Suite 660, Phoenix, AZ 85013, USA

**Dana M. Chase, John H. Farley, Lyndsay J. Willmott and Bradley J. Monk**
Division of Gynecologic Oncology, Department of Obstetrics and Gynecology, University of Arizona Cancer
Center at Dignity Health St. Joseph's Hospital and Medical Center, 500 West Thomas Road, Suite 660, Phoenix, AZ 85013, USA

**Lauren Patterson Cobb and Angeles Alvarez Secord**
Division of Gynecologic Oncology, Department of Obstetrics and Gynecology, Duke Cancer Institute, Duke University Medical Center, Durham, NC 27710, USA

**Stephanie Gaillard**
Division of Medical Oncology, Department of Internal Medicine, Duke University Medical Center, Durham, NC 27710, USA

**Yihong Wang and Ie-Ming Shih**
Department of Gynecology and Obstetrics, Johns Hopkins University School of Medicine, Baltimore, MD 21205, USA

**Bradley J. Monk**
Arizona Oncology (US Oncology Network), University of Arizona College of Medicine, Creighton University School of Medicine at St. Joseph's Hospital, Phoenix, AZ, USA

**Warner K. Huh**
University of Alabama at Birmingham, Birmingham, AL, USA

**Julie Ann Rosenberg**
Pfizer, Groton, CT, USA

**Ira Jacobs**
Early Oncology Development and Clinical Research, Pfizer, 219 East 42nd Street, New York, NY 10017-5755, USA.

**Munetaka Takekuma**
The Division of Gynecology, Shizuoka Cancer Center, Shizuoka 411-8777, Japan

**Kwong K. Wong and Robert L. Coleman**
Department of Gynecologic Oncology and Reproductive Medicine, University of Texas, M.D. Anderson Cancer Center, 1155 Herman Pressler Dr., CPB6.3590, Houston, TX 77030, USA.

**Victor Rodriguez-Freixinos and Helen J. Mackay**
Division of Medical Oncology and Hematology, Princess Margaret Hospital, University of Toronto, 610 University Avenue, Toronto, Ontario M5G 2 M9, Canada

**Stéphanie L. Gaillard**
Department of Medicine, Division of Medical Oncology, Duke Cancer Institute, 200 Trent Drive, Durham, NC 27710, USA

**Angeles A. Secord**
Department of Obstetrics and Gynecology, Division of Gynecologic Oncology, Duke Cancer Institute, 200 Trent Drive, Durham, NC 27710, USA

**Bradley Monk**
Department of Obstetrics and Gynecology, Division of Gynecologic Oncology, University of Arizona College of Medicine, 2222 E. Highland Ave., Suite 400, Phoenix, AZ 85016, USA.

**Siqing Fu, Naiyi Shi, Jennifer Wheler, Aung Naing, Filip Janku, Sarina Piha-Paul, Jing Gong, David Hong, Apostolia Tsimberidou, Ralph Zinner, Vivek Subbiah, Ming-Mo Hou and Funda Meric-Bernstam**
Department of Investigational Cancer Therapeutics, Unit 0455, The University of Texas MD Anderson Cancer Center, 1515 Holcombe Boulevard, Houston, TX 77030, USA.

**Pedro Ramirez, Lois Ramondetta and Karen Lu**
Department of Gynecologic Oncology, The University of Texas MD Anderson Cancer Center, Houston, TX, USA

**Brandon-Luke L. Seagle, Emily S. Miller, Anna E. Strohl and Shohreh Shahabi**
Department of Obstetrics and Gynecology, Prentice Women's Hospital, Northwestern University, Feinberg School of Medicine, 250 E Superior Street, Suite 05-2168, Chicago, IL 60611, USA

**Anna Hoekstra**
West Michigan Cancer Center and Western Michigan University, Homer Stryker School of Medicine, Kalamazoo, MI, USA

**Graziela Zibetti Dal Molin**
Department of Gynecologic Oncology and Reproductive Medicine, The University of Texas MD Anderson Cancer Center, Houston, TX, USA

**Carina Meira Abrahão**
Hospital BP Mirante, São Paulo, Brazil

**Robert L. Coleman**
Department of Gynecologic Oncology and Reproductive Medicine, The University of Texas MD Anderson Cancer Center, Houston, TX, USA

**Fernando Cotait Maluf**
Hospital BP Mirante, Martiniano de Carvalho Street, 965, São Paulo 01323-90, Brazil

**Matthew Schlumbrecht, Guillermo Morales, Marilyn Huang and Brian Slomovitz**
Division of Gynecologic Oncology, Sylvester Comprehensive Cancer Center, University of Miami, 1121 NW 14th St, Suite 345C, Miami, FL 33136, USA

**John Siemon**
Department of Obstetrics and Gynecology, University of Miami, Miami, USA

**Mekonnen Sisay**
Department of Pharmacology and Toxicology, School of Pharmacy, College of Health and Medical Sciences, Haramaya University, Harar, Ethiopia

**Dumessa Edessa**
Department of Clinical Pharmacy, School of Pharmacy, College of Health and Medical Sciences, Haramaya University, Harar, Ethiopia.

**Rachel Grisham**
Memorial Sloan Kettering Cancer Center and Weil Cornell Medical College, New York, NY, USA

**Bonnie Ky**
Perelman School of Medicine, University of Pennsylvania, Philadelphia, PA, USA

**Krishnansu S. Tewari**
Division of Gynecologic Oncology, University of California Irvine, Orange, CA, USA

**David J. Chaplin**
Mateon Therapeutics, South San Francisco, CA, USA

**Joan Walker**
The Stephenson Cancer Center, University of Oklahoma, Oklahoma City, OK, USA

**Thomas J. Herzog**
University of Cincinnati Cancer Institute, University of Cincinnati, Medical Sciences Bldg, Suite 2005H, ML0662, 231 Albert Sabin Way, Cincinnati, OH 45267-0662, USA

**Bradley J. Monk**
Arizona Oncology (US Oncology Network), University of Arizona College of Medicine and Creighton University School of Medicine at Dignity Health St. Joseph's Hospital and Medical Center, Phoenix, AZ 85013, USA

**Margaux J. Kanis and Mario Pineda**
Division of Gynecology Oncology, Northwestern University Feinberg School of Medicine, Chicago, IL, USA

**Wenan Qiang**
Division of Reproductive Science in Medicine, Department of Obstetrics and Gynecology, Northwestern University Feinberg School of Medicine, Chicago, IL, USA
Department of Pathology, Northwestern University Feinberg School of Medicine, Chicago, IL, USA

**J. Julie Kim**
Division of Reproductive Science in Medicine, Department of Obstetrics and Gynecology, Northwestern University Feinberg School of Medicine, Chicago, IL, USA
Robert H. Lurie Comprehensive Cancer Center, Northwestern University, 303 E. Superior Street, 4-117, Chicago, IL 60611, USA

**Kruti P. Maniar**
Department of Pathology, Northwestern University Feinberg School of Medicine, Chicago, IL, USA

**Daniel Asfaw Erku, Adeladlew Kassie Netere and Sewunet Admasu Belachew**
Department of Clinical Pharmacy, School of Pharmacy, College of Medicine and Health Sciences, University of Gondar, Chechela Street, Lideta Sub city Kebele 16, Gondar, Ethiopia

**Amanual Getnet Mersha and Sileshi Ayele Abebe**
Department of Gynecology and obstetrics, College of Medicine and Health Sciences, University of Gondar, Chechela Street, Lideta Sub city Kebele 16, Gondar, Ethiopia

**Abebe Basazn Mekuria**
Department of Pharmacology, School of Pharmacy, University of Gondar, Chechela Street, Lideta Sub city Kebele 16, Gondar, Ethiopia

**Sarah Dotson**
Department of Obstetrics and Gynecology, West Virginia University, 1 Medical Center Dr. PO Box 9186, HSC 4th floor, Morgantown, WV 26501-9186, USA

**Alejandro Landa**
Department of Obstetrics and Gynecology, Duke University Medical Center, Durham, NC 27710, USA

**Jessie Ehrisman and Angeles Alvarez Secord**
Division of Gynecology Oncology, Department of Obstetrics and Gynecology, Duke Cancer Institute, Duke University Medical Center, Durham, NC 27710, USA

**Jill K. Alldredge**
University of California, 101 The City Drive South Orange, Irvine, CA 92868, USA

**Ramez N. Eskander**
University of California, San Diego Moores Cancer Center, 3855 Health Sciences Drive, La Jolla, CA 92029-S0987, USA

**Samantha Kempner**
Department of Obstetrics and Gynecology, Duke University Hospital, Durham, North Carolina 27710, USA

**Paula S. Lee, Rebecca Previs, Laura J. Havrilesky and Angeles Alvarez Secord**
Department of Obstetrics and Gynecology, Duke University Hospital, Durham, North Carolina 27710, USA
Division of Gynecologic Oncology, Department of Obstetrics and Gynecology, Duke University Hospital, Durham, USA
Duke Cancer Institute, Durham, USA

**Chad Grotegut and Sarah C. Ellestad**
Department of Obstetrics and Gynecology, Duke University Hospital, Durham, North Carolina 27710, USA
Division of Maternal Fetal Medicine, Department of Obstetrics and Gynecology, Duke University Hospital, Durham, USA

**Jessie Ehrisman**
Division of Gynecologic Oncology, Department of Obstetrics and Gynecology, Duke University Hospital, Durham, USA

**Michael Miller**
Department of Interventional Radiology, Duke University Hospital, Durham, USA

**Gloria Broadwater**
Cancer Statistical Center, Duke Cancer Institute, Durham, USA

**Jennifer Dominguez**
Department of Anesthesiology, Duke University Hospital, Durham, USA

# Index

www.ingramcontent.com/pod-product-compliance
Lightning Source LLC
Chambersburg PA
CBHW080508200326
41458CB00012B/4127